89.50 2vol. 1995

# THE CIBA COLLECTION OF MEDICAL ILLUSTRATIONS

Volume 1

# Nervous System

Part I

Anatomy and Physiology

A compilation of paintings depicting
anatomy and embryology,
physiology and functional neuroanatomy

Prepared by

Frank H. Netter, M.D.

Edited by

Alister Brass, M.D.

Regina V. Dingle
Managing Editor

Commissioned and published by

CIBA

Other published volumes of
THE CIBA COLLECTION OF MEDICAL ILLUSTRATIONS
prepared by
Frank H. Netter, M.D.

**Nervous System, Part II: Neurologic and Neuromuscular Disorders**

**Reproductive System**

**Digestive System, Part I: Upper Digestive Tract**

**Digestive System, Part II: Lower Digestive Tract**

**Digestive System, Part III: Liver, Biliary Tract and Pancreas**

**Endocrine System and Selected Metabolic Diseases**

**Heart**

**Kidneys, Ureters, and Urinary Bladder**

**Respiratory System**

**Musculoskeletal System, Part I: Anatomy, Physiology, and Metabolic Disorders**

**Musculoskeletal System, Part II: Developmental Disorders, Tumors,**
    **Rheumatic Diseases, and Joint Replacement**

*See page 239 for additional information*

First Printing, 1983
Second Printing, 1986
Third Printing, 1991

ISBN 0-914168-10-X
Library of Congress Catalog No: 53-2151

Printed in U.S.A.

Book printed offset by The Hennegan Co.
Offset color photoengraving by R.R. Donnelley & Sons Company
Layout and typographic design by Pierre J. Lair
Text photocomposed in Mergenthaler Garamond No. 3 by Arrow Typographers, Inc.
Contents printed on Cameo dull text, basis 80, by S.D. Warren Company
Smyth-sewn case binding by The Riverside Group
Endpapers: White Flannel text, basis 80, by Curtis Paper Division, James River Corporation
Cover material: Buckram linen cloth by Industrial Coatings Group Inc.
Front and spine cover design by Philip Grushkin
Index by Steele/Katigbak Indexers

# Foreword

When the late John F. Fulton, M.D., then Sterling Professor of Physiology, Yale University, wrote the foreword to the original Volume 1, of THE CIBA COLLECTION OF MEDICAL ILLUSTRATIONS in March 1953, it is doubtful he had any idea it would still be appropriate 30 years later. We include it here for the sake of continuity and because there is no better way to introduce the first of what is intended to be a series of new editions of THE CIBA COLLECTION OF MEDICAL ILLUSTRATIONS.

In the early texts of anatomy the central nervous system of human beings was seldom adequately depicted because, although the art of embalming was known, this procedure was rarely used for the preservation of the brain and spinal cord. The result was that by the time the anatomist or the pathologist came to expose the brain, it was generally soft and disintegrated and not well suited for anatomical study. The first adequate illustrations of cerebral structure are those found in the *Fabrica* of Andreas Vesalius, published in 1543. His plates representing the nervous system show many more of the major structures, but the sulci are flattened and the hemispheres themselves have the appearance of being more or less collapsed. However, Vesalius had depicted the major gross structures of the human brain, including the cerebellum, the cerebral ventricles, and the majority of the cranial nerves.

It was discovered later that the cerebral ventricles had been much more clearly portrayed some years earlier in the manuscript notebooks of Leonardo. He injected the ventricular system with wax and, on macerating the surrounding cortical tissue, he emerged with an accurate cast of the ventricles which he had drawn in his notebook; but unfortunately these excellent drawings did not become public property for nearly four centuries.

There were many other anatomists in the sixteenth century who made anatomical illustrations of various parts of the central nervous system — Eustachio, whose plates of the cranial nerves, including the vagus, represent a conspicuous advance over the vesalian portrayal of corresponding structures. And then the Florentine Guidi, better known as Vidius (the Latin form of his name), grandson of Ghirlandajo, made good use of the artistic talent which he inherited and published an illustrated anatomical and also a surgical text. Vidius' contemporary, Costanzo Varolio, in 1573, issued a monograph on the optic nerves which contains a plate illustrating the base of the brain that was more accurate than anything before him and was only matched by the celebrated plate which Thomas Willis issued in 1674 in his *Cerebri anatome*. The latter plate, showing the vascular circle which still bears Willis' name, was designed by the young Christopher Wren, who had learned the art of injection of blood vessels in London while working as an assistant in the anatomical theatre of Sir Charles Scarborough. Wren introduced the new technique at Oxford, and I have always suspected that it was Wren rather than Willis who discovered the arterial circle.

In the seventeenth and eighteenth centuries there were a number of other notable illustrations of the brain and spinal cord in monographs such as those of Vieussens (1685) and Ridley (1695). In the eighteenth century the most remarkable plates of the nervous system were the colored portrayals of Jan Ladmiral and Jacques Fabian Gautier d'Agoty. The color process employed by these artists, although they claimed it as their own invention, was probably that of the German LeBlon, since they had both worked with him as assistants.

There was little progress in anatomical illustration of the nervous system during the nineteenth century, although note should be made of the plates published by Charles Bell who was as much artist as he was anatomist and of

# Foreword

whom it is generally said that he colored his anatomical plates by hand. Those of Cruveilhier should also be mentioned. His plates depicting tumors of the central nervous system are as fine as anything that had appeared before or has been published since.

With the advent of the modern period, hand coloring has largely disappeared and in its place we have the three-color process employed by the German anatomists such as Spalteholtz. The present volume, composed of the beautiful plates of Dr. Frank H. Netter, makes use of every modern device to present the structural relations of the nervous system with care and precision. At a time when a high value is placed on visual aids as an accompaniment to the written word in the educational process, these exquisite and highly accurate illustrations commend themselves to all who are either teaching or learning the functions of the nervous system. Although there have been a number of artists throughout medical history who have achieved lasting acclaim for the excellence of their work even though they were not themselves physicians, this collection of drawings well illustrates the happy result of artist and physician being combined in one person. Dr. Netter's knowledge of function cannot but lend clarity to his plates.

The legends and descriptions to the illustrations as provided by Doctors Kaplan, Kuntz and von Bonin (in the new edition by Doctors Angevine, Crelin, Mauro, Mitchell, Peterson, Sheldon and Wood) of course do not substitute for a textbook but are comprehensive and yet masterpieces of conciseness. Both illustrations and text together are quite obviously the result of a most cheerful and successful cooperation. The consultant experts have left their imprint also on the pictures and in the method of demonstrating a variety of details, since one may readily recognize traces of their own scientific contributions in their respective fields.

One common source of confusion to students—the position of the Island of Reil—is beautifully resolved in one of Dr. Netter's diagrams to be found in Plate 17 (now Section II, Plate 1). His portrayal of the Circle of Willis in Plate 16 (now Section III, Plate 4) is probably the clearest that one will find in any modern anatomical text. His diagram of the relations of the cerebellum in Plate 44 (now Section VIII, Plate 38) is also highly illuminating and the diagram in Plate 72 (now Section IV, Plate 21) of the innervation of the female genital system is excellent.

These are but a few selections from a work of consistently high quality. CIBA Pharmaceutical Company, in offering this new volume in their series of anatomical illustrations, adds another to their enviable list of contributions to the progress and the history of medicine.

JOHN F. FULTON, M.D.
NEW HAVEN, MARCH, 1953

# Introduction

THE CIBA COLLECTION OF MEDICAL ILLUSTRATIONS was originally conceived as a series of atlases picturing the anatomy, embryology, physiology, pathology and diseases of mankind, system by system. The creation of these atlases has been for me a labor of love to which I have devoted most of my working career. The first volume of this series was *Nervous System*. That volume was very well received and acclaimed by students, physicians and members of allied professions throughout the world. It has been reprinted many times and published in a number of languages. The multitude of letters of appreciation I have received in the more than thirty years since its first publication have been a great source of satisfaction to me, even as I progressed with other volumes in the series.

From the beginning, however, certain deficiencies in the *Nervous System* volume became evident. It contained, for example, practically no coverage of the peripheral nervous system, of embryology, of basic neurophysiology, ie, nerve impulse transmissions and synapse; and the presentation of the neurologic and neuromuscular diseases was far too skimpy and incomplete. Furthermore, as time progressed and our knowledge advanced, the deficiencies became more significant. Advances in neuroradiology and neurosurgery made it important to update the illustrations of the blood vessels of the brain and spinal cord. The advent of the CT scan as a valuable diagnostic tool necessitated its inclusion as a specific procedure. Our improved understanding of the neuromuscular diseases and increased application of electromyography, electroencephalography and nerve conduction studies called for a better presentation of basic neurophysiology and nerve-muscle relationships. The great progress in the study of neurologic disorders such as poliomyelitis, Parkinsonism, myasthenia gravis, stroke, trauma, Alzheimer's disease, and many others demanded amplification of the section on specific diseases of the nervous system. Finally, the better definition of congenital and developmental disorders not only prompted presentation of those disorders but emphasized the importance of including a section on neuroembryology.

Accordingly, it has for many years been my desire to revise and expand this atlas in a new edition. I was, however, so busy with preparing other volumes of the CIBA COLLECTION that it took me a long time to accomplish it. This was, to a certain extent, fortuitous, for it allowed me to include newer material which would not have been available for an earlier revision. But the volume of illustrations and accompanying texts grew to such an extent that they could not all be included in a single book. It was therefore decided to issue the atlas in two parts; part one to include anatomy, embryology, physiology, and functional neuroanatomy; and part two, shortly forthcoming, to include all the neurologic and neuromuscular diseases.

At the same time that I was working on this revision I was also occupied with preparing an atlas on the musculoskeletal system, and the great overlap between the fields of orthopedics, ie, musculoskeletal disorders and neurologic or neurosurgical disorders became apparent. Indeed, many of the disorders to be covered lay in the realm of both specialities. Thus, the two-part presentation of this atlas is advantageous, since Part II bridges the gap between the two fields, and I believe will be pertinent to both neurology-neurosurgery and orthopedics, as well as to the fields of general practice and internal medicine. Part I, on the other hand, will serve as a reference for basic understanding of much of the material in Part II, and will be very useful for the student and for

# Introduction

those in allied professions such as physical therapy, speech therapy and psychology. All in all, I believe that in this revised edition of *Nervous System* I have corrected the deficiencies referred to above, as well as many others, and I hope it will prove as useful and helpful to all those who refer to it as the original edition apparently was in its day.

I take this opportunity to express my appreciation to all the collaborators and consultants who helped me with preparing this volume. They are all credited separately herein. I admire their erudition and I thank them for the time they gave me and the knowledge they imparted to me. It was a great pleasure for me to learn from them, and I cherish the friendships we established during our collaboration. The creation of this volume would have been impossible without their help. I also thank the CIBA-GEIGY Corporation and its executives for the free hand they have given me in this project, and the members of the editorial staff for their very helpful and dedicated cooperation.

Since the foundation for this volume was laid in its earlier edition, I reiterate here, with much nostalgia, my appreciation for the great men who guided me through that original endeavor. They were: Dr. Abraham Kaplan, neurosurgeon and gifted student of Dr. Harvey Cushing; Dr. Albert Kuntz, pioneer in unraveling the mysteries of the autonomic nervous system, Dr. Gerhardt von Bonin, brilliant neurophysiologist; and Dr. W.R. Ingram, professor of anatomy at the University of Iowa, who devoted much of his career to the study of hypothalamus. In regard to the editor of that original edition, I quote herewith the last paragraph from my introduction to that volume. "Every artist thrives on appreciation, understanding, and encouragement. In this respect I have been doubly fortunate. First, the warm reception which the medical profession has accorded my pictures has been a wonderful source of satisfaction to me. Second, more personal and close at hand, has been the inspiring personality of Dr. Ernst Oppenheimer. His understanding of the things I was trying to do, his appreciation of what I had done, and his encouragement to do more were a constant assurance that I was not alone. In addition, his vision of the scope and value of this atlas and his many co-ordinating activities in its behalf have been vital factors in the project."

Frank H. Netter, M.D.

# Preface

Mention the name Netter to a physician or a medical student anywhere in the world and you evoke instant recognition. For in its 30-year history, THE CIBA COLLECTION OF MEDICAL ILLUSTRATIONS—of which the present volume is both the latest addition and the first of the Netter atlases to be completely updated and rewritten—has successfully conveyed the essentials of human anatomy, physiology and pathology to generations of medical professionals. Dr. Frank Netter's extraordinary paintings are to the learning and practice of contemporary medicine what Andreas Vesalius' revolutionary anatomical drawings were to renaissance medical thought; they intrigue, they delight, they clarify, and they subtly highlight key information. Through their vivid coloring and startlingly fresh viewpoint, they make ideas that have lost their edge through overfamiliarity newly memorable. A Netter painting of, say, the bones of the skull or—one of the most famous illustrations from the first *Nervous System* (and reproduced in the present volume with scant alteration)— the components of the rage reaction, automatically becomes for the reader the definitive visual metaphor for the subject from the moment of first viewing.

The burden of responsibility such compelling illustrations carry is, therefore, considerable. It is for this reason, as he has explained in the introductory essays to other books in the series, that Dr. Netter, at all stages in the development of a plate, checks closely with the expert collaborator for that particular subject, and also consults the published and unpublished reference materials on the topic. In the event there remains a lingering question or a conflict of authority, he goes directly to the cadaver to resolve the issue.

For this new atlas, Dr. Netter has created 119 new plates and reworked 69 from the original book. The accompanying texts have been prepared afresh by a new board of distinguished collaborators from both sides of the Atlantic. As regards the ongoing debate among the experts about the exact mechanism of this or that event in the nervous system, and all the unanswered questions about neurophysiology at the molecular level, Dr. Netter summed up his attitude in his preface to the original volume, and his views have not changed. He wrote: "The complexity of the central nervous system is such that one must be guided by the fundamental requirements of simplicity if effectiveness in presentation is to be achieved... The backbone of this collection is, of course, generally accepted information. While minute details and controversial theories have been avoided, this was not done at the expense of accuracy or completeness. Clinical significance has been the guiding principle." As readers will discover, these intentions have been amply fulfilled.

Only over the matter of terminology has there been some difference of opinion among the experts, primarily in this first, basic science part of the new *Nervous System*. As is customary in preparing a volume for the CIBA COLLECTION, whenever possible we have used the particular vocabulary chosen by the collaborator concerned as being the most appropriate and up-to-date, using as our backup resource Gould's Medical Dictionary, fourth edition. Yet to maintain a consistent style of terminology for the text and plates throughout the book, we have arrived at what we believe is a satisfactory compromise.

For the anatomical plates, Dr. Mitchell expressed a preference for using the internationally agreed-on language of anatomy as codified in the fourth edition of Nomina Anatomica. However, an editor seeking to reconcile the strict logic of this reference source with the less precise language of practising physicians encounters problems, particularly with some of the more recently identified sub-regions of the brain. In those cases in which the N.A. system seems too academic for contemporary concepts in neuroarchitecture, we have opted for the vernacular of American clinical practice. Also, where it seemed wise to retain both the formal and the informal terminology, especially for those items

# Preface

with long-familiar eponyms, we have inserted the alternative title in parentheses. Dr. Mitchell graciously acceded to our request to retain several clinical conventions in the interest of unity throughout the book; in particular, we chose to bypass "cranial", "caudal", "dorsal" and "ventral" as synonyms for the less scientific but more familiar "superior", "inferior", "posterior" and "anterior" modifiers in almost every situation where they appear.

In the section on functional neuroanatomy, we have again attempted to follow the terminology preferred by our American collaborators. As before, we have given the alternatives in parentheses – for instance, "amygdaloid body" and "amygdala," and have only occasionally exercised editorial fiat, as in the case of our using "pineal gland" instead of "pineal body." The naming of the ascending and descending tracts of the spinal cord is another area in which anatomists and neurophysiologists have their own firm opinions. We hope that the reader will benefit from our attempt to choose clarity and clinical usefulness above all else.

This new Volume 1 of the CIBA COLLECTION, after all the years of preparatory work, far surpasses the scope of the original *Nervous System*. We trust that it and its subsequent companion, which will include the diseases of the nervous and neuromuscular systems, will prove of lasting benefit to future generations of medical and health science students, physicians, nurses, teachers, and all those interested in learning about the wonders of the human nervous system.

ALISTER BRASS, M.D.

# Acknowledgements

One of the real pleasures of working with a publishing project like THE CIBA COLLECTION OF MEDICAL ILLUSTRATIONS is the virtually unanimous and continuing shower of praise which greets those of us connected with it. This praise, of course, is not for us but for the man who created the project and the many talents he has brought to it. There is between the users of the books and the man who created them a very personal association which is evoked each time a perusal of the pages brings back a memory of a moment in medical school or in practice which was somehow illuminated by his work. There is a desire to know the man, to understand his inner workings, and to somehow touch him personally.

Thus, all of us who work with the CIBA COLLECTION are continually called upon to talk about our perceptions of the man and his talent and to listen to stories of those moments when a Netter illustration suddenly unlocked for a previously uncomprehending viewer a door of understanding for him. In all these stories, the phrase most often repeated is "Without the *Nervous System* book, I never would have passed neuroanatomy." Clearly the ultimate tribute!

With the original book continuing to earn this kind of praise, some would ask "why prepare a new edition?" Dr. Netter has clearly answered this question in his introduction and we have long been in agreement with his view. In fact, this project has been in preparation for more than a dozen years and in that time has been picked up, worked on and put aside no less than four times – not because it was not desirable to complete, but because Dr. Netter's prolific output continually moved other volumes of the CIBA COLLECTION into first place in terms of priority. Thus, it has been a monumental task to once again pick up the pieces, meld them into a useful whole, and move on to completion with efficiency.

Imagine, for instance, the differences in terminology which have developed since 1969 or the growth in understanding of mechanisms of neuroscience which has come about in the same time. Even the changes which have taken place in the technology of color separation and printing have had a profound effect on the development of this book. Like building a new house versus trying to renovate an old home, it is often easier to start with a clean slate. On the other hand, there is nothing like the patina of old wood to enhance a contemporary renovation, even though it means much agony and hard work. And so it is with this first volume in a continuing series of new editions. With it we introduce a new cover design, slightly modified page graphics and a variety of technical improvements. These changes are intended to signal the new beginning but to in no way alter the patina of the original.

It is a pleasure to salute all those who worked on this project. In particular, we appreciate the understanding and patience of our authors who reworked their manuscripts several times during the revision process. We thank the craftsmen at the Crawfordsville, Indiana plant of R. R. Donnelley & Sons, where the color separation of the artwork and the printing was done. Their special skills have made it possible to convey on paper the unique delicacy of color, of shading and of shape that is the essence of Dr. Netter's painting. We also thank Cesareo Studio, our long-time collaborator on the Netter volumes, for the preparation of caption and line overlays.

Within the CIBA organization, our sincere appreciation is tendered to Ms. Anne Trench and Ms. Barbara Bekiesz for their assistance in the early stages of preparation; to Mr. Pierre Lair, Art Director and Production Manager, who designed the layout and supervised the production of the book, and to Ms. Gina Dingle, Managing Editor, who coordinated the project from start to finish.

In all, we are proud to have been a part of a unique project and hope the end result brings much pleasure and enlightenment to all who use it.

PHILIP B. FLAGLER
DIRECTOR
MEDICAL EDUCATION

# Contributors
# and Consultants

*The artist, editors and publishers express
their appreciation for the dedicated
collaboration of these contributing
authors:*

## Jay B. Angevine Jr., Ph.D.

Professor and Associate Head, Anatomy;
Lecturer, Neurology, College of Medicine, The University of Arizona,
Arizona Health Sciences Center,
Tucson, Arizona

## Edmund S. Crelin, Ph.D., D.Sc.

Professor and Chief, Section of Anatomy, Department of Surgery;
Chairman, Human Growth and Development Study Unit,
Yale University School of Medicine,
New Haven, Connecticut

## Alexander Mauro, Ph.D.

Professor of Biophysics,
The Rockefeller University,
New York, New York

## G.A.G. Mitchell, O.B.E., T.D., Ch.M., D.Sc., F.R.C.S.*

Hon. Alumnus, The University of Louvain, Belgium;
Chevalier (1st Cl.) Order of the Dannebrog;
Emeritus Professor of Anatomy and Director of the Anatomical Laboratories,
University of Manchester,
Manchester, England

## Barry W. Peterson, Ph.D.

Professor of Physiology and Rehabilitation Medicine,
Northwestern University Medical School,
Chicago, Illinois

## Jerome J. Sheldon, M.D., F.A.C.R.

Chief, Section of Neuroradiology and Computed Tomography, Department of Radiology,
Mount Sinai Medical Center, Miami Beach;
Associate Professor of Radiology,
University of Miami School of Medicine,
Miami, Florida

## Joe G. Wood, Ph.D.

Professor and Chairman, Department of Neurobiology and Anatomy,
The University of Texas Health Science Center at Houston,
Houston, Texas

*Deceased

# Contents

Section I

# Bony Coverings of Brain and Spinal Cord

Frank H. Netter, M.D.

*in collaboration with*

**G.A.G. Mitchell, Ch.M., D.Sc., F.R.C.S.**  *Plates 1–18*

# Anterior and Lateral Aspects of Skull

## Anterior Aspect

The anterior, or facial, aspect of the skull is composed of the frontal part of the calvaria (skull-cap) above and the facial bones below. The facial contours and proportions are largely determined by the underlying bones, and it is a commonplace observation that they show considerable variations associated with age, sex and race. The outer surface of the frontal bone underlies the brow. The facial skeleton is irregular, a feature accentuated by the presence of the orbital openings, the piriform aperture, and the superior and inferior dental arches of the oral cavity.

The convex anterior surface of the frontal bone is relatively smooth, but there are frontal tuberosities, or elevations, on each side. In early life, a median suture separates the two halves of the developing bone (Plate 8). This suture normally fuses between ages 6 and 10, but occasionally persists as the metopic suture.

*The two orbital openings* are roughly quadrangular and have supraorbital, infraorbital, medial and lateral borders. The supraorbital notch, or fissure, carries the corresponding nerve and vessels. The infraorbital foramen, located about 1 cm below the infraorbital margin, transmits the nerve and vessels of the same name. The orbits are somewhat pyramidal in shape, with the quadrangular openings, or bases, directed forward and slightly outward, while the apexes correspond to the medial ends of the superior orbital fissures.

The *superior wall (roof)* separates the orbital contents from the brain and meninges in the anterior cranial fossa. Anteromedially, it is hollowed out by a variably sized frontal sinus, and anterolaterally, there is a shallow lacrimal fossa for the orbital part of the lacrimal gland. Posteriorly, the optic canal (foramen) lies between the two roots of the lesser wing of the sphenoid bone, just above the medial end of the superior orbital fissure; it transmits the optic (II) nerve and ophthalmic artery.

The *inferior wall (floor)* is formed mainly by the orbital surface of the maxilla, which separates the orbit from the maxillary sinus (antrum). A groove for the infraorbital nerve and vessels ends in the infraorbital foramen.

The thin *medial wall* separates the orbit from the ethmoidal air cells, the anterior part of the sphenoidal sinus and the nasal cavity. At its anterior end, the lacrimal fossa is continuous below with the short nasolacrimal canal that opens into the inferior nasal meatus.

The thicker *lateral wall* separates the orbit from the temporal fossa anteriorly and from the middle cranial fossa posteriorly. The orbital surface of the zygomatic bone shows a foramen for the zygomatic nerve, which bifurcates within the bone to emerge on the cheek and temporal fossa as the

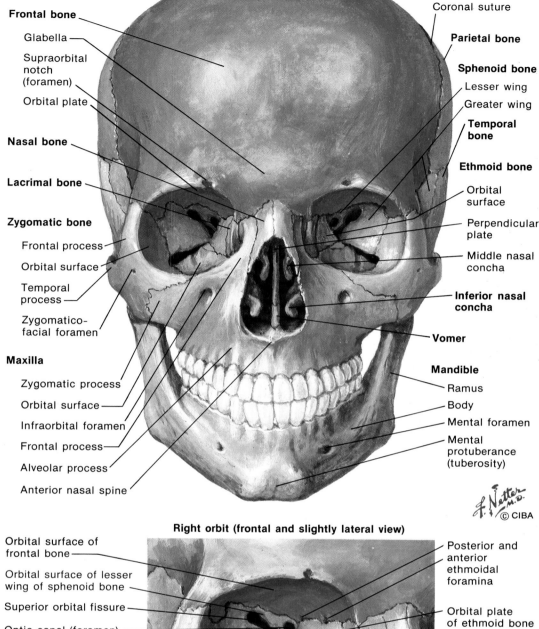

**Anterior Aspect of Skull**

Frontal bone
Glabella
Supraorbital notch (foramen)
Orbital plate
Nasal bone
Lacrimal bone
Zygomatic bone
Frontal process
Orbital surface
Temporal process
Zygomatico-facial foramen
Maxilla
Zygomatic process
Orbital surface
Infraorbital foramen
Frontal process
Alveolar process
Anterior nasal spine

Coronal suture
Parietal bone
Sphenoid bone
Lesser wing
Greater wing
Temporal bone
Ethmoid bone
Orbital surface
Perpendicular plate
Middle nasal concha
Inferior nasal concha
Vomer
Mandible
Ramus
Body
Mental foramen
Mental protuberance (tuberosity)

**Right orbit (frontal and slightly lateral view)**

Orbital surface of frontal bone
Orbital surface of lesser wing of sphenoid bone
Superior orbital fissure
Optic canal (foramen)
Orbital surface of greater wing of sphenoid bone
Orbital surface of zygomatic bone
Inferior orbital fissure
Infraorbital sulcus

Posterior and anterior ethmoidal foramina
Orbital plate of ethmoid bone
Lacrimal bone
Fossa of lacrimal sac
Orbital process of palatine bone
Orbital surface of maxilla

zygomaticofacial and zygomaticotemporal nerves, respectively.

The lateral wall and roof are continuous anteriorly, but diverge posteriorly to bound the *superior orbital fissure*, which lies between the greater and lesser wings of the sphenoid bone and opens into the middle cranial fossa. The fissure transmits the oculomotor (III) and trochlear (IV) nerves, the lacrimal, frontal and nasociliary branches of the ophthalmic nerve, the abducens (VI) nerve, the ophthalmic veins and small meningeal vessels.

The lateral wall and floor of the orbit are also continuous anteriorly, but are separated posteriorly by the *inferior orbital fissure*, most of which is

located between the greater wing of the sphenoid bone and the orbital surface of the maxilla. The inferior orbital fissure connects the orbit with the pterygopalatine and infratemporal fossae. The maxillary nerve passes from the pterygopalatine fossa into the orbit through the inferior orbital fissure and continues forward as the infraorbital nerve. Anastomotic channels between the orbital and pterygoid venous plexuses, and orbital fascicles from the pterygopalatine ganglion also traverse this fissure.

*The anterior nasal (piriform) aperture* is bounded by the nasal and maxillary bones. The nasal bones articulate with each other in the

## Anterior and Lateral Aspects of Skull
(*Continued*)

midline, with the frontal bone above, and with the frontal processes of the maxillae behind. The irregular lower borders of the nasal bones give attachment to the lateral nasal cartilages.

*The lower face* is supported by both the maxillary alveolar processes and the mandible. The inferior margin of each *maxilla* projects downward as the curved alveolar process, which unites in front with its fellow to form the U-shaped alveolar arch containing the sockets for the upper teeth. The roots of the teeth produce slight surface elevations, the most obvious of which are produced by the canine teeth. The upper border of the body of the *mandible* is called the alveolar part and contains sockets for the lower teeth, whose roots also produce slight surface elevations between faint grooves. The mental protuberance is at the lower end of a slight ridge representing the symphysis menti, the line of fusion of the two halves of the fetal bone. The mental foramen lies below the interval between the premolar teeth and transmits the mental nerves and vessels. In the adult, this foramen lies about halfway between the upper and lower borders of the body of the mandible. At birth, the opening is near the lower border, because most of the body of the mandible is still occupied by unerupted teeth.

### Lateral Aspect

Viewed from the side, the skull is divided into the larger ovoid braincase and the smaller facial skeleton. The two are connected by the zygomatic bone, which acts as a yoke (zygon) between the temporal, sphenoid (greater wing) and frontal bones and the maxilla. Other features on the lateral aspect of the skull include parts of the sutures between the frontal, parietal, sphenoid and temporal bones (which form most of the braincase), and the sutures between such facial bones as the nasal, lacrimal, ethmoid and maxilla. Clearly seen are the parts of the mandible and the temporomandibular joint, the external acoustic meatus and the various foramina that transmit nerves and vessels of the same name. Not readily visible are the foramen ovale and the foramen spinosum (Plates 5 and 7).

Certain features deserve particular mention. The curved *superior* and *inferior temporal lines* arch upward and backward over the frontal bone from the vicinity of the frontozygomatic suture, pass over the coronal suture and the parietal bone, and then turn downward and forward across the temporal squama to end above the mastoid process. The superior and inferior temporal lines provide attachments, respectively, for the temporal fascia and the upper margin of the temporal muscle, which occupies most of the *temporal fossa*. This fossa is bounded above by the superior temporal line, and below it is bounded by the infratemporal crest separating the greater wing of the sphenoid bone from the pterygoid processes. The anteroinferior corner of the parietal bone usually fills the angle between the greater wing of the sphenoid and the frontal bone, although sometimes the squamous part of the temporal bone may extend forward to articulate directly with the frontal bone, thus excluding the sphenoid. This area is the *pterion*, and its internal surface is deeply grooved by the anterior branches of the middle meningeal vessels. It is situated about 3.5 cm behind the frontozygomatic suture (usually palpable as a slight ridge) and 4 cm above the zygomatic arch. As the most common site of damage to these vessels from a skull fracture, it is a surgical landmark.

The *infratemporal fossa* is an irregular space lying below the infratemporal crest. It is continuous above with the temporal fossa through the gap between the crest and the zygomatic arch. It is bounded medially by the lateral plate of the pterygoid process and the infratemporal surface of the maxilla, and laterally, by the ramus of the mandible. It communicates through the pterygomaxillary fissure with the pterygopalatine fossa. □

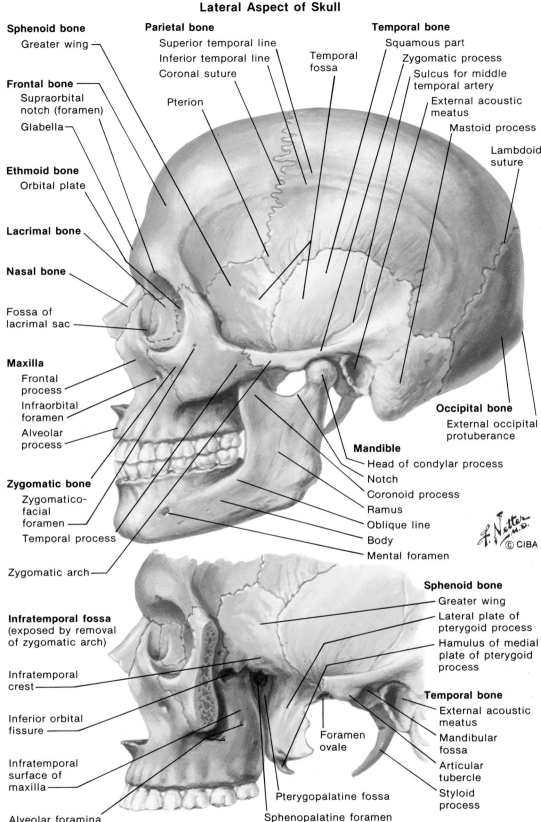

**Lateral Aspect of Skull**

Sphenoid bone
  Greater wing
Frontal bone
  Supraorbital notch (foramen)
  Glabella
Ethmoid bone
  Orbital plate
Lacrimal bone
Nasal bone
Fossa of lacrimal sac
Maxilla
  Frontal process
  Infraorbital foramen
  Alveolar process
Zygomatic bone
  Zygomaticofacial foramen
  Temporal process
Zygomatic arch

Parietal bone
  Superior temporal line
  Inferior temporal line
  Coronal suture
Pterion

Temporal fossa

Temporal bone
  Squamous part
  Zygomatic process
  Sulcus for middle temporal artery
  External acoustic meatus
  Mastoid process
Lambdoid suture

Occipital bone
  External occipital protuberance
Mandible
  Head of condylar process
  Notch
  Coronoid process
  Ramus
  Oblique line
  Body
  Mental foramen

Infratemporal fossa (exposed by removal of zygomatic arch)
Infratemporal crest
Inferior orbital fissure
Infratemporal surface of maxilla
Alveolar foramina
Pterygopalatine fossa
Sphenopalatine foramen
Foramen ovale

Sphenoid bone
  Greater wing
  Lateral plate of pterygoid process
  Hamulus of medial plate of pterygoid process
Temporal bone
  External acoustic meatus
  Mandibular fossa
  Articular tubercle
  Styloid process

## Midsagittal Section of Skull

The rigid braincase is formed by the bones of the calvaria (Plate 4) and the base of the skull (Plate 5), which is divided into anterior, middle and posterior cranial fossae (Plates 6 and 7). These divisions are less visible on a sagittal section of the skull.

The *occipital bone* bounds most of the posterior cranial fossa. It is pierced by the foramen magnum, through which the medulla oblongata and spinal cord, surrounded by their meninges, become continuous; it also transmits the vertebral arteries, a few small veins, the spinal roots of the accessory (XI) nerves and the recurrent meningeal branches from the upper spinal nerves. The occipital condyle articulates with the homolateral superior atlantoarticular process. The hypoglossal (XII) nerve passes through the corresponding canal. The jugular foramen lodges the superior bulb of the internal jugular vein (in which the sigmoid and inferior petrosal sinuses end); the glossopharyngeal (IX), vagus (X) and accessory nerves pass through it anteromedial to the bulb, and it provides an entry for the recurrent meningeal branches of the vagus and small meningeal branches of the ascending pharyngeal and occipital arteries. The basilar part of the occipital bone unites with the body of the sphenoid to form a sloping platform anterior to the pons and medulla oblongata.

The squamous part of the *temporal bone* is grooved by the posterior branches of the middle meningeal vessels, and the sulcus along the superior border of its petrous part is for the superior petrosal sinus. The inferior petrosal sinus lies in the sulcus between the petrous temporal and occipital bones. The internal acoustic meatus is a canal about 1 cm long, ending in a cribriform septum that separates it from the internal ear. It transmits the facial (VII) nerve and its nervus intermedius, the vestibulocochlear (VIII) nerve and the internal auditory (labyrinthine) artery.

The *sphenoid bone* has a central body from which two greater and two lesser wings and two pterygoid processes arise. The body contains two air sinuses separated by a septum that is often incomplete. Its concave upper surface, the sella turcica, houses the pituitary gland. The optic canal transmits the optic (II) nerve and the ophthalmic artery. (For a full description of the blood vessels of the skull and the cranial nerves, see Sections III and V.)

*The nasal cavity* is roofed over mainly by the cribriform plate of the ethmoid bone, augmented anteriorly by small parts of the frontal and nasal bones, and posteriorly, by the anteroinferior surface of the sphenoidal body. Its floor is formed by the palatine processes of the maxillae and by the horizontal plates of the palatine bones. The *incisive canal* transmits the nasopalatine nerves and branches of the greater palatine arteries. Each lateral wall is formed above by the nasal surface of

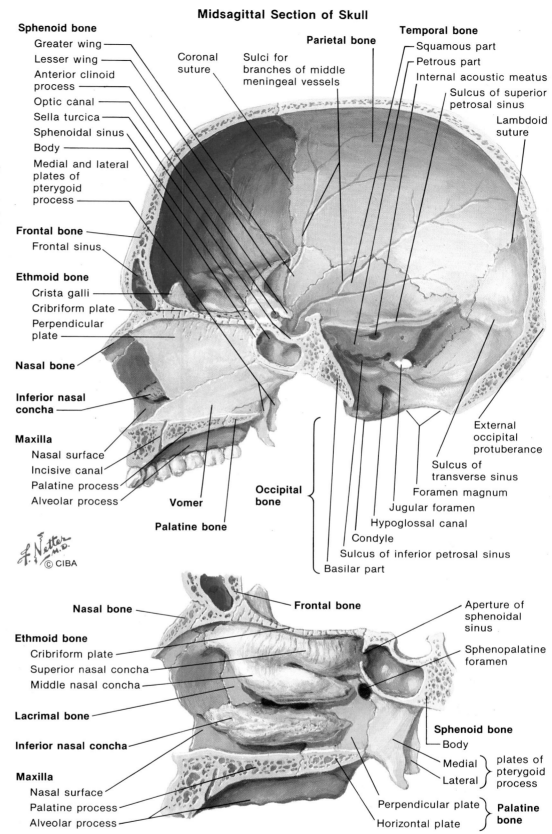

**Midsagittal Section of Skull**

Sphenoid bone
— Greater wing
— Lesser wing
— Anterior clinoid process
— Optic canal
— Sella turcica
— Sphenoidal sinus
— Body
— Medial and lateral plates of pterygoid process

**Frontal bone**
— Frontal sinus

**Ethmoid bone**
— Crista galli
— Cribriform plate
— Perpendicular plate

**Nasal bone**

**Inferior nasal concha**

**Maxilla**
— Nasal surface
— Incisive canal
— Palatine process
— Alveolar process

**Vomer**

**Palatine bone**

Coronal suture
Sulci for branches of middle meningeal vessels

**Parietal bone**

**Temporal bone**
— Squamous part
— Petrous part
— Internal acoustic meatus
— Sulcus of superior petrosal sinus
— Lambdoid suture

External occipital protuberance
Sulcus of transverse sinus
Foramen magnum
Jugular foramen
Hypoglossal canal
Condyle
Sulcus of inferior petrosal sinus
Basilar part

**Occipital bone**

*F. Netter M.D.*
© CIBA

Nasal bone

**Ethmoid bone**
— Cribriform plate
— Superior nasal concha
— Middle nasal concha

**Lacrimal bone**

**Inferior nasal concha**

**Maxilla**
— Nasal surface
— Palatine process
— Alveolar process

Frontal bone

Aperture of sphenoidal sinus

Sphenopalatine foramen

**Sphenoid bone**
— Body
— Medial / Lateral } plates of pterygoid process

Perpendicular plate / Horizontal plate } **Palatine bone**

the ethmoid bone that covers the ethmoidal labyrinth and supports thin, shell-like projections, the *superior* and *middle nasal conchae*. These overhang the corresponding nasal meatuses. Below, each lateral wall is formed by the nasal surface of the maxilla, the perpendicular plate of the palatine bone and the medial pterygoid plate. The maxillary and palatine bones articulate with a separate bone, the *inferior nasal concha*, overhanging the inferior nasal meatus. The sphenoidal air sinuses open into the nose through the *sphenoidal aperture* in the sphenoethmoidal recess posterosuperior to the superior concha. The frontal

and maxillary air sinuses open into the middle meatus through a *semilunar hiatus*, and the multiple air cells forming the ethmoidal labyrinth open into the superior and middle meatuses. The lower opening of the *nasolacrimal duct* is near the anterior end of the inferior meatus. The *sphenopalatine foramen* behind the middle concha transmits the nasopalatine nerve.

The nasal cavity is subdivided by a more-or-less vertical *septum* formed by the perpendicular ethmoidal plate and the vomer. The triangular gap between them anteriorly is filled in by the nasal *septal cartilage* (not shown in the illustration). □

# The Calvaria

**The Calvaria**

**Viewed from above**

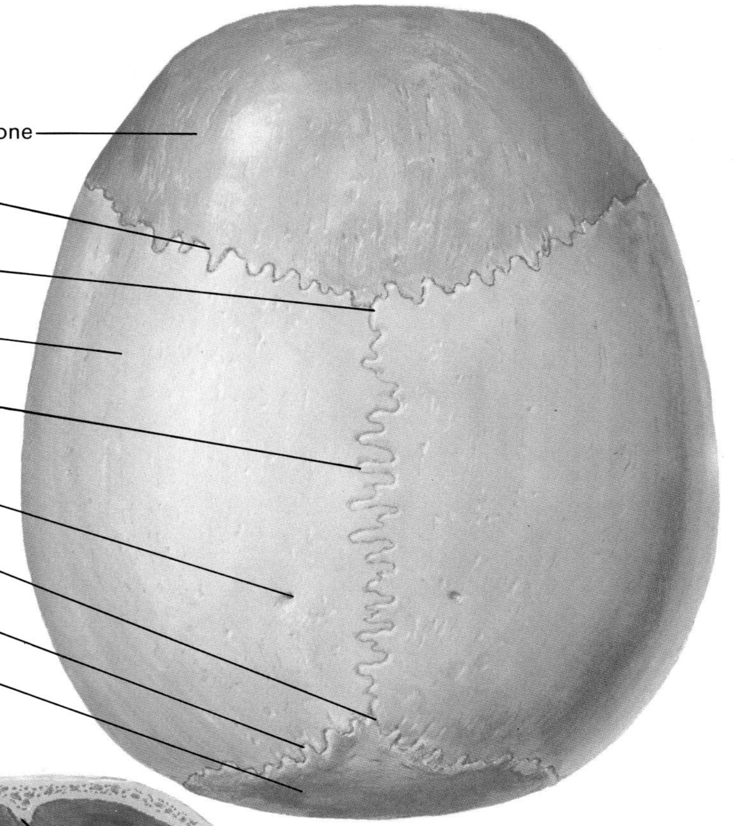

Frontal bone

Coronal suture

Bregma

Parietal bone

Sagittal suture

Parietal foramen
(for emissary vein)

Lambda

Lambdoid suture

Occipital bone

**Viewed from within**

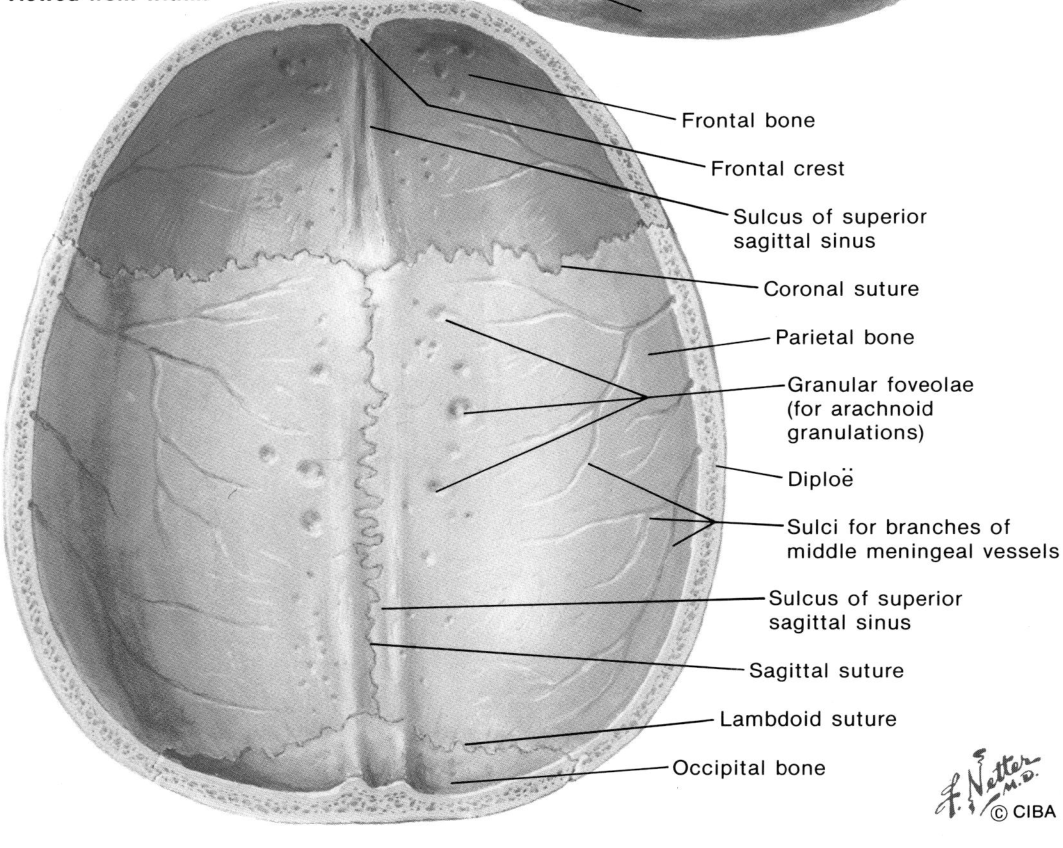

Frontal bone

Frontal crest

Sulcus of superior
sagittal sinus

Coronal suture

Parietal bone

Granular foveolae
(for arachnoid
granulations)

Diploë

Sulci for branches of
middle meningeal vessels

Sulcus of superior
sagittal sinus

Sagittal suture

Lambdoid suture

Occipital bone

The *calvaria*, or skullcap, is the roof of the cranium and is formed by the frontal, parietal and occipital bones. It is ovoid in shape and widest toward the posterior parts of the parietal bones, but there are individual variations in size and shape associated with age, race and sex; thus, minor degrees of asymmetry are common.

The anterior part, or brow, is formed by the frontal bone, which extends backward to the *coronal suture* between the frontal bone and the parietal bones. The latter curve upward and inward to meet at the midline *sagittal suture*. Posteriorly, the parietal bones articulate with the triangular upper part of the occipital squama along the *lambdoid suture*. The meeting points of the sagittal suture with the coronal and lambdoid sutures are termed, respectively, *bregma* and *lambda*. In the fetal skull, they are the sites of the anterior and posterior fontanelles (Plate 8). The *vertex*, or highest point, of the skull lies near the middle of the sagittal suture. Parietal foramina are usually present; they transmit emissary veins passing between the superior sagittal sinus and the veins of the scalp.

The deeply concave internal, or endocranial, surface of the calvaria is made up of the inner aspects of the bones, sutures and foramina mentioned above. The bones show indistinct impressions produced by related cerebral gyri, more evident grooves for dural venous sinuses and meningeal vessels, and small pits, or *foveolae*, for arachnoid granulations. Thus, there is a median groove in the frontal, parietal and occipital bones extending backward from the frontal crest to the internal occipital protuberance; it increases in

width from before backward and lodges the *superior sagittal sinus*. The frontal crest seen in the midline is produced by the coalescence of the anterior ends of the lips of the groove for the superior sagittal sinus. There are other, narrower grooves for meningeal vessels. The largest of these, the *middle meningeal arteries and veins*, leave their imprints in particular on the parietal bones, and the channels containing them may become tunnels where the anteroinferior angles of the parietal bones meet the greater wings of the sphenoid bone (the *pterion* of surface anatomy, Plate 2). The skull varies in thickness, and the area around the pterion is thin. It is relatively easily fractured

by a blow to the side of the head, with possible tearing of the middle meningeal vessels. The resulting hemorrhage can be serious if it is not recognized and treated promptly.

The cut edge of the skullcap reveals that the constituent bones possess outer and inner laminae of compact bone separated by the *diploë*, a layer of cancellous bone. The outer lamina is thicker and tougher than the more brittle inner lamina. (See Section III, Plates 11 and 12 for more information on blood vessels of the diploë and emissary veins and on arachnoid granulations, Plate 7 on meningeal arteries, and Plate 13 on dural venous sinuses.) ☐

# External Aspect of Base of Skull

The inferior surface of the base of the skull, the *norma basilaris*, is formed anteriorly by the arched hard palate, fringed by the maxillary alveolar processes and teeth; posteriorly, by the wider occipital squama, pierced by the foramen magnum; and in between, by an irregular area comprising several bony processes for muscular and tendinous attachments, articular and other fossae and many foramina. The bones and fissures shown in the illustration need no added description, but the nerves and vessels traversing the foramina will be listed (Plates 6 and 7; see also Sections III and V).

The *incisive foramen* transmits the terminal branches of the nasopalatine nerves and greater palatine vessels. The *major* and *minor palatine foramina* are traversed by the corresponding arteries and nerves. The *choanae* are the posterior nasal apertures.

The *foramen ovale* pierces the greater sphenoidal wing near the lateral pterygoid plate and the sulcus for the auditory tube; the mandibular nerve, the accessory meningeal artery and communications between the cavernous sinuses and pterygoid venous plexus pass through it. The *foramen spinosum*, anteromedial to the sphenoidal spine, transmits the middle meningeal artery and the meningeal branch of the mandibular nerve.

The *foramen lacerum* is an irregular canal between the sphenoidal body, the apex of the petrous part of the temporal bone and the basilar part of the occipital bone. The upper end of the carotid canal opens into it, and the internal carotid artery with its nerves and veins, on emerging from the canal, turn upward to enter the cavernous sinus. Meningeal branches of the ascending pharyngeal artery and emissary veins from the cavernous sinus pass through the foramen lacerum, and the deep and greater petrosal nerves unite within it to form the nerve of the pterygoid canal.

The anterior part of the *mandibular fossa* articulates with the mandibular head and belongs to the temporal squama, but the posterior nonarticular part is derived from the tympanic plate. The *tympanosquamous fissure* between them is continued medially as the *petrotympanic fissure*, through which the chorda tympani nerve emerges. The *stylomastoid foramen* behind the root of the styloid process transmits the facial (VII) nerve and the stylomastoid branch of the posterior auricular artery.

The lower opening of the *carotid canal* is anterior to the *jugular fossa*, which lodges the superior bulb of the internal jugular vein. The canal bends at right angles within the petrous part of the temporal bone, and its upper end opens into the foramen lacerum. The *tympanic canaliculus* pierces the ridge between the carotid canal and the jugular fossa and conveys the tympanic branch of the glossopharyngeal (IX) nerve to the tympanic plexus. The *mastoid canaliculus* opens on the lateral wall of the fossa and transmits the auricular branch of the vagus (X) nerve. The *jugular foramen* in the depth of the fossa may be partly or completely divided into three parts by bony spicules. The anteromedial compartment transmits the inferior petrosal sinus and a meningeal branch of

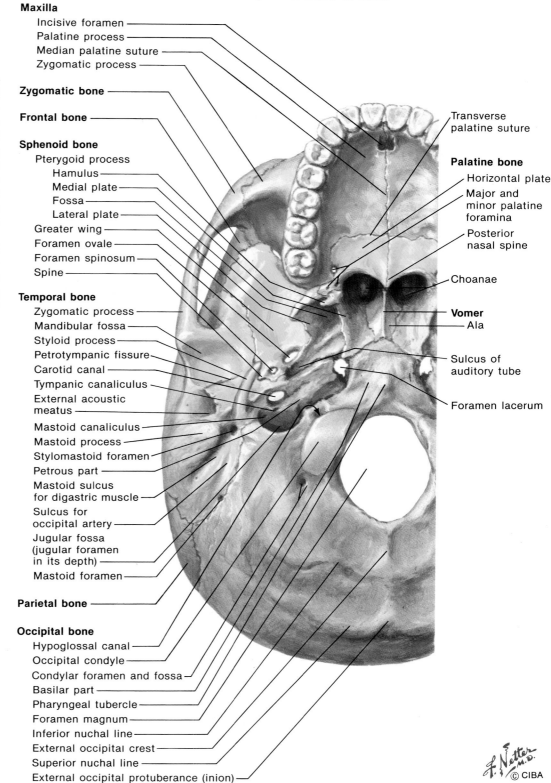

**Maxilla**
Incisive foramen
Palatine process
Median palatine suture
Zygomatic process

**Zygomatic bone**

**Frontal bone**

**Sphenoid bone**
Pterygoid process
Hamulus
Medial plate
Fossa
Lateral plate
Greater wing
Foramen ovale
Foramen spinosum
Spine

**Temporal bone**
Zygomatic process
Mandibular fossa
Styloid process
Petrotympanic fissure
Carotid canal
Tympanic canaliculus
External acoustic meatus
Mastoid canaliculus
Mastoid process
Stylomastoid foramen
Petrous part
Mastoid sulcus for digastric muscle
Sulcus for occipital artery
Jugular fossa (jugular foramen in its depth)
Mastoid foramen

**Parietal bone**

**Occipital bone**
Hypoglossal canal
Occipital condyle
Condylar foramen and fossa
Basilar part
Pharyngeal tubercle
Foramen magnum
Inferior nuchal line
External occipital crest
Superior nuchal line
External occipital protuberance (inion)

Transverse palatine suture

**Palatine bone**
Horizontal plate
Major and minor palatine foramina
Posterior nasal spine

Choanae

**Vomer**
Ala

Sulcus of auditory tube

Foramen lacerum

the ascending pharyngeal artery; the intermediate part transmits the glossopharyngeal, vagus and accessory (XI) nerves; and the posterolateral part conveys the sigmoid sinus to the superior bulb of the internal jugular vein. Often seen near the posterior border of the mastoid process is a *mastoid foramen*, which is traversed by an emissary vein from the sigmoid sinus and a meningeal twig from the occipital artery. The anterior end of the *hypoglossal canal* (for the hypoglossal (XII) nerve and some small meningeal vessels) is above the anterior end of the occipital condyle. Behind the condyle is a shallow condylar fossa, usually pierced by a *condylar foramen* conveying

an emissary vein between the sigmoid sinus and cervical veins.

The posterior part of the base of the skull is formed predominantly by the occipital squama; these are marked by nuchal lines, occipital crest, etc, which serve mainly for muscular and ligamentous attachments. However, the most notable feature is the *foramen magnum*, through which the medulla oblongata and spinal cord become continuous. The vertebral arteries, spinal roots of the accessory nerves and recurrent meningeal branches from the upper cervical nerves ascend through the foramen magnum, while down through it pass the anterior and posterior spinal arteries. □

# Bones, Markings and Orifices in Base of Skull

The internal surface of the base of the skull has adapted its shape to the configuration of the adjacent parts of the brain. It consists of three cranial fossae, the anterior, middle and posterior, which are separated by conspicuous ridges and increase in size and depth from before backward.

*The anterior cranial fossa* is the shallowest of the three fossae and lodges the lower parts of the frontal lobes of the brain. The sulci and gyri of the lobes are mirrored in the irregularities of the bony surfaces. It is limited anteriorly and laterally by the frontal bone. On each side, the floor is formed by the slightly domed and ridged *orbital plate of the frontal bone*, which supports the orbital surface of the homolateral frontal lobe of the brain and its meninges and separates them from the orbit. Posterior extensions from the frontal air sinuses may expand the orbital plates for variable distances, and the medial parts of these plates overlie the ethmoidal labyrinths.

On each side of the midline *crista galli* are the grooved *ethmoidal cribriform plates* that help to form the roof of the nasal cavity, lodge the olfactory bulbs, and provide numerous orifices for the delicate olfactory nerves. A small pit exists between the frontal crest and the crista galli, the *foramen cecum*, which occasionally transmits a tiny vein from the nose to the superior sagittal sinus. The crista galli and frontal crest give attachment to the anterior end of the falx cerebri.

Posterior to the ethmoid and frontal bones, the floor of the anterior cranial fossa is formed by the anterior part of the body of the sphenoid bone, the *jugum sphenoidale*, and on each side, by the *lesser wings* of this bone. These lesser wings slightly overlap the anterior part of the middle cranial fossa and project into the stems of the lateral cerebral sulci, thus forming the upper boundaries of the superior orbital fissures.

The medial ends of the posterior borders of the lesser wings end in small, rounded projections, the *anterior clinoid processes*, which provide attachments for the anterior ends of the free border of the tentorium cerebelli. Each anterior process is grooved on its medial side by the internal carotid artery, and each may be joined to the inconstant middle clinoid process by a thin osseous bar, thus forming a narrow bony ring around the artery as it emerges from the cavernous sinus.

*The middle cranial fossa* is intermediate in depth between the anterior and posterior fossae. It is narrow and elevated medially, but expands and becomes deeper at each side to lodge and protect the temporal lobes of the brain. It is bounded anteriorly by the posterior borders of the lesser wings of the sphenoid bone and the anterior

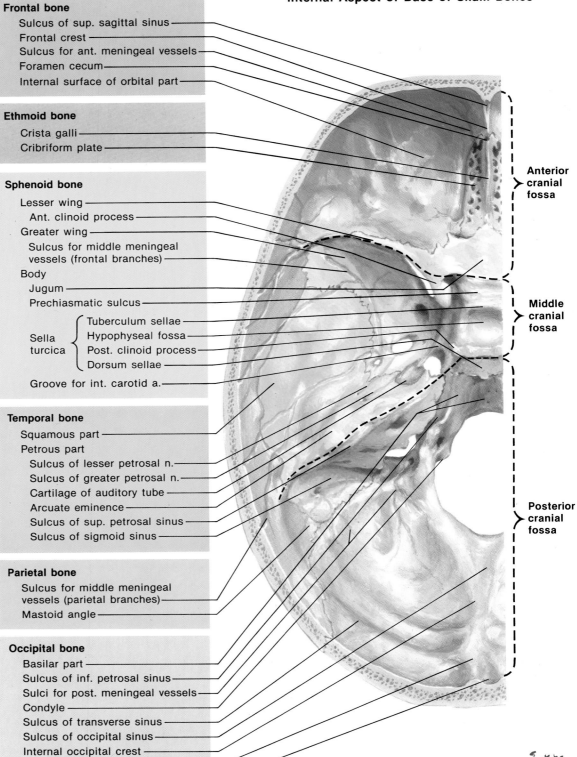

**Frontal bone**
Sulcus of sup. sagittal sinus
Frontal crest
Sulcus for ant. meningeal vessels
Foramen cecum
Internal surface of orbital part

**Ethmoid bone**
Crista galli
Cribriform plate

**Sphenoid bone**
Lesser wing
Ant. clinoid process
Greater wing
Sulcus for middle meningeal vessels (frontal branches)
Body
Jugum
Prechiasmatic sulcus
Sella turcica {
Tuberculum sellae
Hypophyseal fossa
Post. clinoid process
Dorsum sellae }
Groove for int. carotid a.

**Temporal bone**
Squamous part
Petrous part
Sulcus of lesser petrosal n.
Sulcus of greater petrosal n.
Cartilage of auditory tube
Arcuate eminence
Sulcus of sup. petrosal sinus
Sulcus of sigmoid sinus

**Parietal bone**
Sulcus for middle meningeal vessels (parietal branches)
Mastoid angle

**Occipital bone**
Basilar part
Sulcus of inf. petrosal sinus
Sulci for post. meningeal vessels
Condyle
Sulcus of transverse sinus
Sulcus of occipital sinus
Internal occipital crest
Internal occipital protuberance
Sulcus of sup. sagittal sinus

Anterior cranial fossa

Middle cranial fossa

Posterior cranial fossa

margin of the prechiasmatic sulcus; posteriorly, by the superior borders of the petrous parts of the temporal bones, which are grooved by the superior petrosal sinuses and by the dorsum sellae of the sphenoid; and laterally, by the greater wings of the sphenoid, the frontal angles of the parietal bones and the temporal squamae.

The floor in the median area is formed by the *body of the sphenoid bone*, containing the sphenoidal air sinuses. The lesser wings of the sphenoid are attached to its body by two roots, separated from each other by the *optic canals* that transmit the optic (II) nerves and ophthalmic arteries. Behind the prechiasmatic sulcus is a median elevation,

the *tuberculum sellae*, and the *hypophyseal fossa* housing the pituitary gland. The fossa is limited behind by the *dorsum sellae*, an upward-projecting bony plate with a concave upper border expanding laterally into the *posterior clinoid processes*. Lateral to the sellae is a shallow, sinuous *groove for the internal carotid artery*; at its anterior end on the medial side may be a small tubercle, the *middle clinoid process* (see CIBA COLLECTION, Volume 4, page 8).

The lateral parts of the middle fossa are related in front to the orbits; on each side, to the temporal fossae; and below, to the infratemporal fossae. The middle fossa communicates with the orbits through the *superior orbital fissures* (Plate 1).

**Internal Aspect of Base of Skull: Orifices**

## Bones, Markings and Orifices in Base of Skull

*(Continued)*

Various other, more-or-less symmetrical openings exist on each side. The *foramen rotundum* pierces the greater wing of the sphenoid bone just below and behind the inner end of the superior orbital fissure, and then it opens anteriorly into the pterygopalatine fossa. The *foramen ovale* also penetrates the greater sphenoidal wing posterolateral to the foramen rotundum and leads downward into the infratemporal fossa. The smaller *foramen spinosum* lies posterolateral to the foramen ovale and opens below into the infratemporal fossa close to the sphenoidal spine; the sulcus for the middle meningeal vessels starts at this foramen. The *foramen lacerum* is an irregular aperture between the body and greater wing of the sphenoid bone and the apex of the petrous part of the temporal bone; it marks the point of entry of the internal carotid artery into the cavernous sinus. Behind the foramen lacerum is the shallow *depression for the trigeminal (semilunar) ganglion* on the anterior surface of the petrous temporal bone, and lateral to this are two narrow grooves leading to the hiatuses for the lesser (minor) and greater (major) petrosal nerves.

The *arcuate eminence* is produced by the superior semicircular canal of the internal ear. Anterolateral to this eminence is a thin plate of bone, the *tegmen tympani*, forming the roof of the tympanic cavity and mastoid antrum and extending forward and medially to cover the bony part of the auditory (pharyngotympanic) tube.

*The posterior cranial fossa* is the largest and deepest of the cranial fossae and lodges the cerebellum, pons and medulla oblongata. It is bounded anteriorly by the dorsum sellae, the back of the body of the sphenoid bone and the basilar part of the occipital bones; posteriorly, by the squama of the occipital bone below the sulci for the transverse sinuses and the internal occipital protuberance; and laterally, by the petrous and mastoid parts of the temporal bones, the mastoid angles of the parietal bones, and the lateral parts of the occipital bone.

The posterior fossa is pierced by a number of foramina and is grooved by various dural venous sinuses. A large median opening in the floor of the fossa, the *foramen magnum*, penetrates the occipital bone. The medulla oblongata and spinal cord and their surrounding meninges become directly continuous immediately below the foramen. The petrous part of the temporal bone and the occipital bone are separated by the *petrooccipital fissure* and the *sulcus for the inferior petrosal sinus*; the fissure ends behind, in the *jugular foramen*. The inferior petrosal and sigmoid sinuses pass through

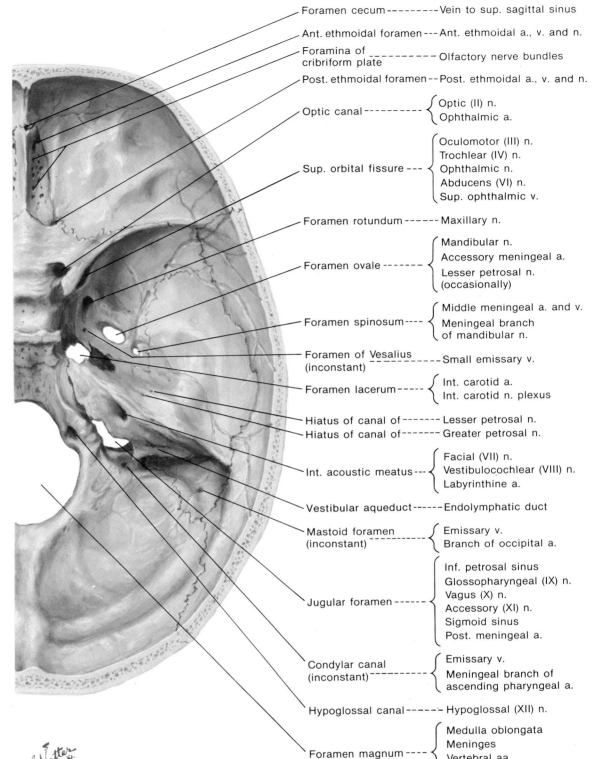

Foramen cecum -------- Vein to sup. sagittal sinus

Ant. ethmoidal foramen --- Ant. ethmoidal a., v. and n.

Foramina of cribriform plate --------- Olfactory nerve bundles

Post. ethmoidal foramen -- Post. ethmoidal a., v. and n.

Optic canal ---------
- Optic (II) n.
- Ophthalmic a.

Sup. orbital fissure ---
- Oculomotor (III) n.
- Trochlear (IV) n.
- Ophthalmic n.
- Abducens (VI) n.
- Sup. ophthalmic v.

Foramen rotundum ------ Maxillary n.

Foramen ovale -------
- Mandibular n.
- Accessory meningeal a.
- Lesser petrosal n. (occasionally)

Foramen spinosum ----
- Middle meningeal a. and v.
- Meningeal branch of mandibular n.

Foramen of Vesalius (inconstant) ----------- Small emissary v.

Foramen lacerum -----
- Int. carotid a.
- Int. carotid n. plexus

Hiatus of canal of ------- Lesser petrosal n.

Hiatus of canal of ------- Greater petrosal n.

Int. acoustic meatus ---
- Facial (VII) n.
- Vestibulocochlear (VIII) n.
- Labyrinthine a.

Vestibular aqueduct ------ Endolymphatic duct

Mastoid foramen (inconstant)
- Emissary v.
- Branch of occipital a.

Jugular foramen ------
- Inf. petrosal sinus
- Glossopharyngeal (IX) n.
- Vagus (X) n.
- Accessory (XI) n.
- Sigmoid sinus
- Post. meningeal a.

Condylar canal (inconstant)
- Emissary v.
- Meningeal branch of ascending pharyngeal a.

Hypoglossal canal ------ Hypoglossal (XII) n.

Foramen magnum ----
- Medulla oblongata
- Meninges
- Vertebral aa.
- Spinal roots of accessory nn.

*F. Netter M.D.* © CIBA

the anterior and posterior parts of this foramen, respectively, while the glossopharyngeal (IX), vagus (X) and accessory (XI) nerves occupy an intermediate position as they leave the skull.

Two canals are associated with the occipital condyles: the *hypoglossal canal*, for the twelfth cranial nerve, and the *condylar canal*.

Above the jugular foramen, the *internal acoustic meatus* tunnels into the petrous part of the temporal bone. It is about 1 cm long and is separated laterally from the internal ear by a thin bony plate pierced by many apertures for fascicles of the facial (VII) and vestibulocochlear (VIII) nerves. Behind the orifice of this meatus is the slitlike opening of

the *vestibular aqueduct*, which lodges the blind end of the endolymphatic duct.

The internal opening of the inconstant *mastoid foramen* is close to the *sulcus for the sigmoid sinus*, which winds downward from the transverse sinus to the jugular foramen, where it ends in the superior bulb of the internal jugular vein. The *internal occipital protuberance* is related to the confluence of the superior sagittal, straight, occipital and transverse sinuses. The margins of the sulci for the transverse sinuses give attachment to the tentorium cerebelli. (For a detailed account of the blood vessels of the brain and skull and of the cranial nerves, see Sections III and V.) ☐

# Skull of the Newborn

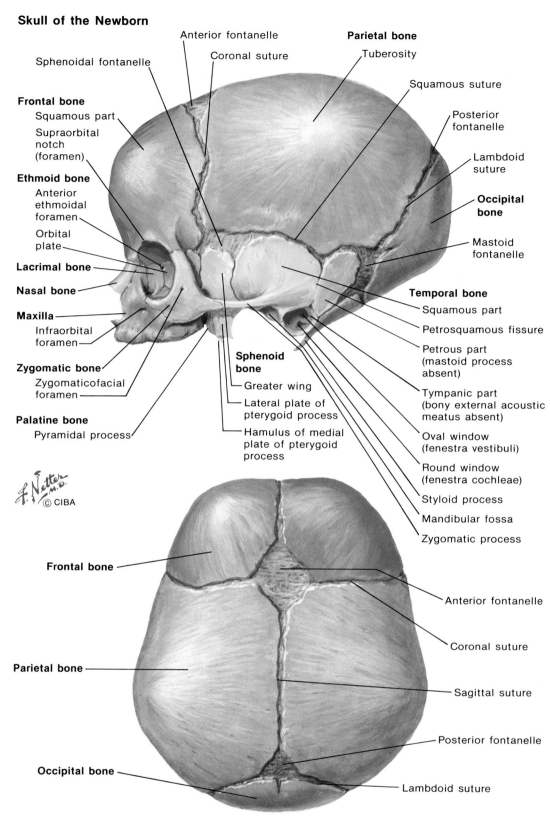

**Skull of the Newborn**

Anterior fontanelle
Coronal suture
**Parietal bone**
Tuberosity
Sphenoidal fontanelle
Squamous suture
**Frontal bone**
Squamous part
Supraorbital notch (foramen)
Posterior fontanelle
Lambdoid suture
**Ethmoid bone**
Anterior ethmoidal foramen
Orbital plate
**Occipital bone**
**Lacrimal bone**
Mastoid fontanelle
**Nasal bone**
**Maxilla**
Infraorbital foramen
**Temporal bone**
Squamous part
Petrosquamous fissure
**Zygomatic bone**
Zygomaticofacial foramen
**Sphenoid bone**
Greater wing
Petrous part (mastoid process absent)
**Palatine bone**
Pyramidal process
Lateral plate of pterygoid process
Hamulus of medial plate of pterygoid process
Tympanic part (bony external acoustic meatus absent)
Oval window (fenestra vestibuli)
Round window (fenestra cochleae)
Styloid process
Mandibular fossa
Zygomatic process

*f. Netter M.D.*
© CIBA

**Frontal bone**
Anterior fontanelle
**Parietal bone**
Coronal suture
Sagittal suture
Posterior fontanelle
**Occipital bone**
Lambdoid suture

At birth, the cranial part of the skull is comparatively large, but the facial part is small due to the relative underdevelopment of the maxilla and mandible, the absence of erupted teeth, the small size of the nasal cavity, and the rudimentary state of the paranasal sinuses. The squamous part of the frontal bone bulges forward, slightly overhanging the nasal bones and orbits, although the superciliary arches and glabella are not yet evident. At this stage, the nasal cavity lies almost entirely between the orbits. Individual bones are easily identifiable because ossification is still incomplete, especially along their margins.

The comparatively large cranial part of the skull accommodates the relatively large brain. In the newborn, it is about 25% of its adult size, and it reaches about 75% of its adult size by the end of the first year after birth.

The newborn calvaria is ovoid in shape and, as is the case in the adult, its widest part usually lies between the parietal tuberosities. At this stage, the component bones are thin, consisting of a single, pliable layer without diploë. They ossify in fibrous membranes, whereas most of the bones in the base of the skull develop in cartilage. The frontal bone develops in two halves; its midline suture is normally obliterated by the eighth year, but it may persist (in some races more often than in others), and is then known as the *metopic suture.*

At birth, the edges of the calvarial bones are not serrated, as they are in later years. They are separated by fibrous or membranous tissue, continuous externally with the bony periosteum, and internally, with the endosteal layer of the dura mater. These membranous gaps are larger at the corners of the parietal bones, where they form the anterior, posterior, sphenoidal and mastoid fontanelles (literally, small springs, or fountains, which fluctuate with changes in intracranial pressure). The largest, the diamond-shaped *anterior fontanelle,* is the most important clinically. It does not

become fully ossified until 18 to 24 months after birth, whereas the other fontanelles are usually closed within 2 to 3 months. A minor posterior extension from the mastoid fontanelle indicates the original subdivision between the upper interparietal and lower supraoccipital parts of the occipital bone.

The tympanic part of the temporal bone is an incomplete, slender ring, and the bony part of the adult external acoustic meatus is absent. The tympanic membrane is thus relatively superficial and is inclined more downward rather than laterally, as is the case in adults. If it is removed (as in the illustration), the round and oval windows and

other features on the medial wall of the narrow tympanic cavity are visible. The mastoid process is still undeveloped, so that the styloid process and stylomastoid foramen are exposed. The mandibular fossa is shallow, and the articular tubercle is lacking.

Parts of other neonatal skull bones are also relatively undeveloped—for example, the sphenoidal wings and pterygoid processes and the pyramidal processes of the palatine bones—but parts of a few bones are relatively large. Thus, although the maxillae are comparatively small, their alveolar arches, which contain the unerupted upper teeth, are disproportionately conspicuous. □

## Spinal Column

The spinal column is built up from alternating bony vertebrae and fibrocartilaginous discs, which are intimately connected by strong ligaments and supported by powerful musculotendinous masses. The individual bony elements and ligaments are described in Plates 10 to 18.

There are 33 vertebrae (7 cervical, 12 thoracic, 5 lumbar, 5 sacral and 4 coccygeal), although the sacral and coccygeal vertebrae are usually fused to form the sacrum and coccyx. All vertebrae conform to a basic plan, but individual variations occur in the different regions. A typical vertebra consists of an anterior, more-or-less cylindrical *body* and a posterior *arch* composed of two *pedicles* and two *laminae*, the latter united posteriorly to form a *spinous process*. These processes vary in shape, size and direction in the various regions of the spine. On each side, the arch also supports a *transverse process* and *superior* and *inferior articular processes*; the latter form synovial joints with corresponding processes on adjacent vertebrae, and the spinous and transverse processes provide levers for the many muscles attached to them. The increasing size of the vertebral bodies from above downward is related to the increasing weights and stresses borne by successive segments, and the sacral vertebrae are fused to form a solid wedge-shaped base—the keystone in a bridge whose arches curve down toward the hip joints. The *intervertebral discs* act as elastic buffers to absorb the numerous mechanical shocks sustained by the spinal column.

Only limited movements are possible between adjacent vertebrae, but the sum of these movements confers a considerable range of mobility on the vertebral column as a whole. Flexion, extension, lateral bending, rotation and circumduction are all possible, and these actions are freer in the cervical and lumbar regions than in the thoracic. Such differences exist because the discs are thicker in the cervical and lumbar areas, the splinting effect produced by the thoracic cage is lacking, the cervical and lumbar spinous processes are shorter and less closely apposed, and the articular processes are shaped and arranged differently.

At birth, the spinal column presents a general dorsal convexity, but later, the cervical and lumbar regions become curved in the opposite directions—when the infant reaches the stages of holding up its head (3 to 4 months) and sitting upright (6 to 9 months). The dorsal convexities are *primary curves* associated with the fetal uterine position, whereas the cervical and lumbar ventral *secondary curves* are compensatory to permit the assumption of the upright position. There may

be additional slight lateral deviations due to unequal muscular traction in right-handed and left-handed persons.

Man's evolution from a quadrupedal to a bipedal posture was mainly effected by the tilting of the sacrum between the hip bones, by an increase in lumbosacral angulation, and by minor adjustments of the anterior and posterior depths of various vertebrae and discs. An erect posture greatly increases the load borne by the lower spinal joints, and, good as these ancestral adaptations were, some static and dynamic imperfections remain and predispose to strain and backache. The length of the vertebral column averages 72 cm in the

adult male and 7 to 10 cm less in the female. The *vertebral canal* extends through the entire length of the column and provides an excellent protection for the spinal cord, the cauda equina and their coverings. The spinal vessels and nerves pass through *intervertebral foramina* formed by notches on the superior and inferior borders of the pedicles of adjacent vertebrae, bounded anteriorly by the corresponding intervertebral discs, and posteriorly, by the joints between the articular processes of adjoining vertebrae. Pathological or traumatic conditions affecting any of these structures may produce pressure on the nerves or vessels they transmit (see Section II, Plates 14 to 16). □

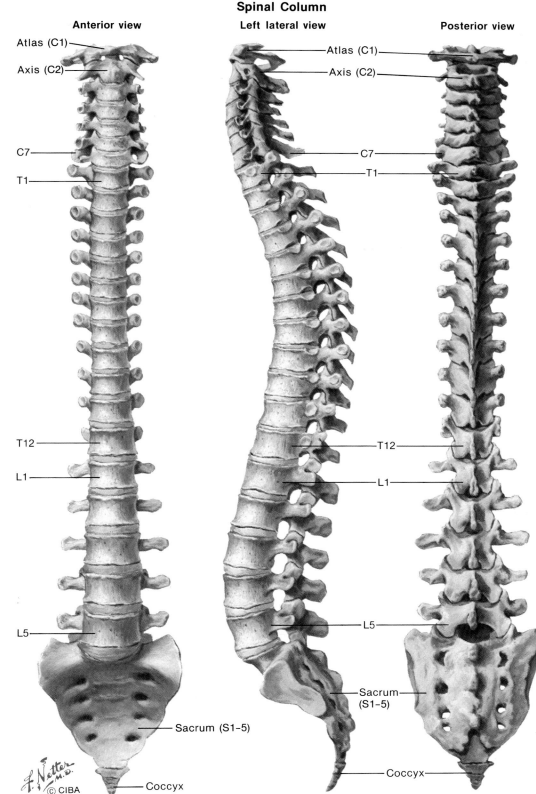

**Spinal Column**

**Anterior view**

Atlas (C1)
Axis (C2)
C7
T1
T12
L1
L5
Sacrum (S1–5)
Coccyx

**Left lateral view**

Atlas (C1)
Axis (C2)
C7
T1
T12
L1
L5
Sacrum (S1–5)
Coccyx

**Posterior view**

Atlas (C1)
Axis (C2)
C7
T1
T12
L1
L5

# Atlas and Axis

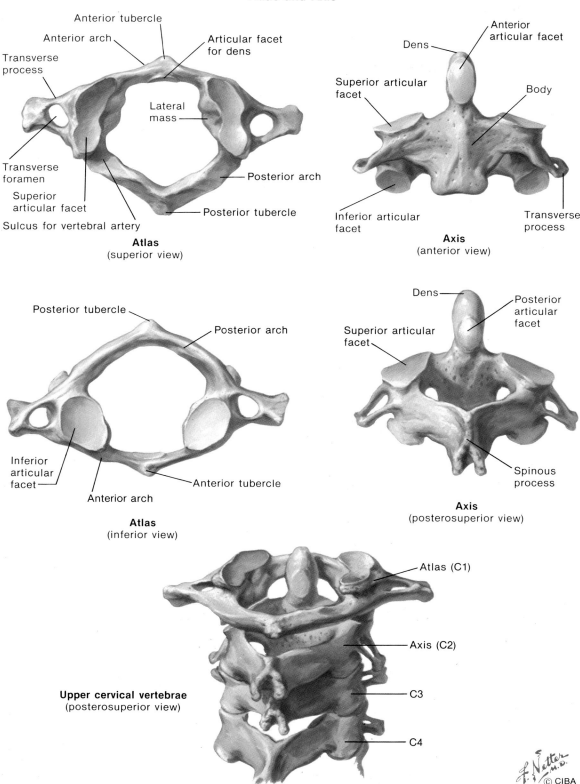

**Atlas**
(superior view)

Anterior tubercle
Anterior arch
Transverse process
Articular facet for dens
Lateral mass
Transverse foramen
Superior articular facet
Sulcus for vertebral artery
Posterior arch
Posterior tubercle

**Axis**
(anterior view)

Dens
Anterior articular facet
Superior articular facet
Body
Inferior articular facet
Transverse process

**Atlas**
(inferior view)

Posterior tubercle
Posterior arch
Inferior articular facet
Anterior tubercle
Anterior arch

**Axis**
(posterosuperior view)

Dens
Posterior articular facet
Superior articular facet
Spinous process

**Upper cervical vertebrae**
(posterosuperior view)

Atlas (C1)
Axis (C2)
C3
C4

The atlas and axis are the first and second cervical vertebrae, and both are atypical. They are linked together and to the skull and other cervical vertebrae by a layered pattern of craniocervical ligaments (Plates 12 and 13).

*The atlas* (named after the mythical giant who carried the earth on his shoulders) supports the globe of the skull. It lacks a body and forms a ring consisting of shorter anterior and longer posterior arches, with two lateral masses. The enclosed *vertebral foramen* is relatively large.

The *anterior arch* is slightly curved, with an anterior midline tubercle and a posterior midline facet for articulation with the dens of the axis.

The *lateral masses* bear superior and inferior articular facets and transverse processes. The *superior articular facets* are concave and ovoid (often waisted, or reniform) and are directed upward and inward as shallow cups, or foveae, for the reception of the occipital condyles. Nodding movements of the head mainly occur at these atlantooccipital joints. The *inferior articular facets* are almost circular, gently concave, and face downward and slightly medially and backward; they articulate with the superior articular facets on the axis. The *transverse processes* are each pierced by a foramen for the vertebral artery, and project so far laterally that they can be easily palpated by pressing inward between the mandibular angles and the mastoid processes. They provide attachments and levers for some of the muscles involved in head rotation. On the anteromedial aspect of each lateral mass is a small tubercle for the attachment of the transverse ligament of the atlas.

The *posterior arch* is more curved than the anterior and has a small *posterior tubercle*, which is a rudimentary spinous process. Just behind each superior articular facet is a shallow *groove for the vertebral artery* and first cervical spinal nerve, the nerve lying between the artery and the bone.

*The axis*, or second cervical vertebra, has a toothlike process, or dens, projecting upward from its body. The *dens* is really the divorced body of the atlas that has united with the axis to form a pivot around which the atlas and the superjacent skull can rotate. Its anterior surface has an oval *anterior facet* for articulation with the facet on the

back of the anterior arch of the atlas, and a smaller *posterior facet* lower down on its posterior surface, which is separated from the transverse ligament of the atlas by a small bursa. The apex of the dens is attached to the lower end of the apical ligament, and the alar ligaments are attached to its sides.

The *body* of the axis has a lower liplike projection that overlaps the anterosuperior border of the third cervical vertebra. Its anterior surface shows a median ridge separating slight depressions for slips of the longus colli muscles. The posteroinferior border of the body is less prominent, and attached to it are the tectorial membrane and the posterior longitudinal spinal ligament.

The *pedicles* and *laminae* are stout, and the latter end in a strong, bifid *spinous process*. The *vertebral foramen* of the axis is somewhat smaller than that of the atlas. On each side of the body are superior and inferior articular and transverse processes. The *articular processes* are offset, since the superior pair is anterior in position to the inferior pair. They articulate with the adjoining processes of the atlas and third cervical vertebra. The *transverse processes* are smaller and shorter than those of the atlas, and their foramina are inclined superolaterally to allow the contained vertebral arteries and nerves to pass easily into the more widely spaced transverse foramina of the atlas. □

## Cervical Vertebrae

# Cervical Vertebrae

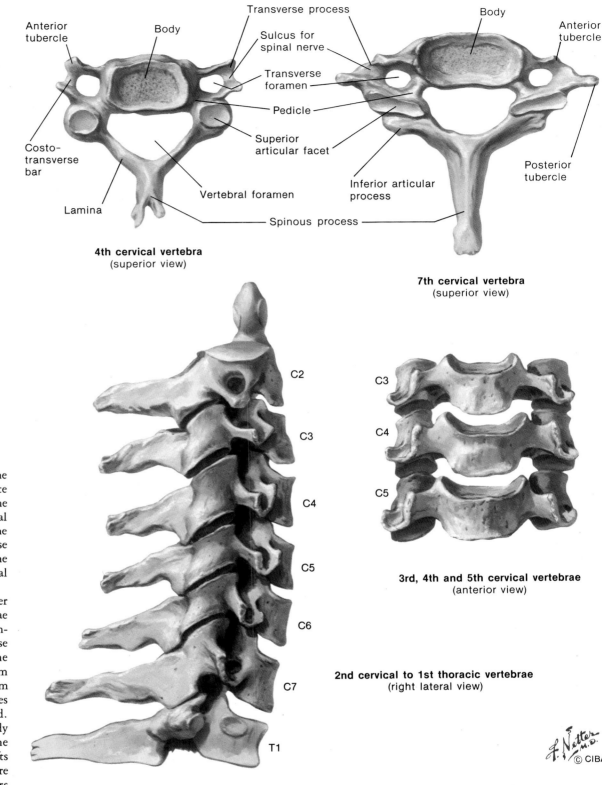

**4th cervical vertebra**
(superior view)

Labels on 4th cervical vertebra: Anterior tubercle, Body, Transverse process, Sulcus for spinal nerve, Transverse foramen, Pedicle, Superior articular facet, Costo-transverse bar, Vertebral foramen, Lamina, Spinous process

**7th cervical vertebra**
(superior view)

Labels on 7th cervical vertebra: Body, Anterior tubercle, Posterior tubercle, Inferior articular process

**3rd, 4th and 5th cervical vertebrae**
(anterior view)

**2nd cervical to 1st thoracic vertebrae**
(right lateral view)

Labels: C2, C3, C4, C5, C6, C7, T1

The first two cervical vertebrae, the atlas and the axis, are illustrated in Plate 10. The other five (C3 to C7) show the general vertebral features, but cervical vertebrae are easily distinguishable by the presence of foramina in their transverse processes, which (except in the case of the seventh vertebra) transmit the vertebral vessels and nerves (Plate 12).

The cervical *vertebral bodies* are smaller than those of the other movable vertebrae and increase in size from above downward; they are broader in the transverse diameter than anteroposteriorly. The superior body surfaces are concave from side to side and slightly convex from front to back, while the inferior surfaces are reciprocally curved or saddle-shaped. The lateral edges of the superior body surface are raised, while those of the lower surface are beveled and small clefts exist between them. Some claim these are miniature synovial joints, but others believe they are merely spaces in the lateral parts of the corresponding intervertebral discs.

The *vertebral foramina* are comparatively large in order to accommodate the cervical enlargement of the spinal cord; they are bounded by the bodies, pedicles and laminae of the vertebrae. The *pedicles* project posterolaterally from the bodies and are grooved by superior and inferior vertebral notches, almost equal in depth, which form the intervertebral foramina by connecting with similar notches on adjacent vertebrae. The medially directed *laminae* are thin and relatively long, and fuse posteriorly to form short, bifid *spinous processes*. Projecting laterally from the junction of the

pedicles and laminae are articular pillars supporting *superior* and *inferior articular facets*.

Each *transverse process* is pierced by a foramen, bounded by narrow bony bars ending in anterior and posterior tubercles; these are interconnected lateral to the foramen by the so-called *costotransverse bar*. Only the medial part of the posterior bar represents the true transverse process; the anterior and costotransverse bars and the lateral portion of the posterior bar constitute the costal element. Abnormally, these elements, especially in the seventh and/or sixth cervical vertebrae, develop to form cervical ribs. The upper surfaces of the costotransverse bars are grooved and lodge the anterior

primary rami of the spinal nerves. The anterior tubercles of the sixth cervical vertebra are large and are termed the *carotid tubercles*, because the common carotid arteries lie just anteriorly and can be compressed against them.

The seventh cervical vertebra is called the *vertebra prominens*, because its spinous process is long and ends in a tubercle that is easily palpable at the lower end of the nuchal furrow; the spinous process of the first thoracic vertebra is just as prominent. The seventh cervical vertebra sometimes lacks a transverse foramen on one or both sides; when present, the foramina transmit only small accessory vertebral veins. □

## External Craniocervical Ligaments

# External Craniocervical Ligaments

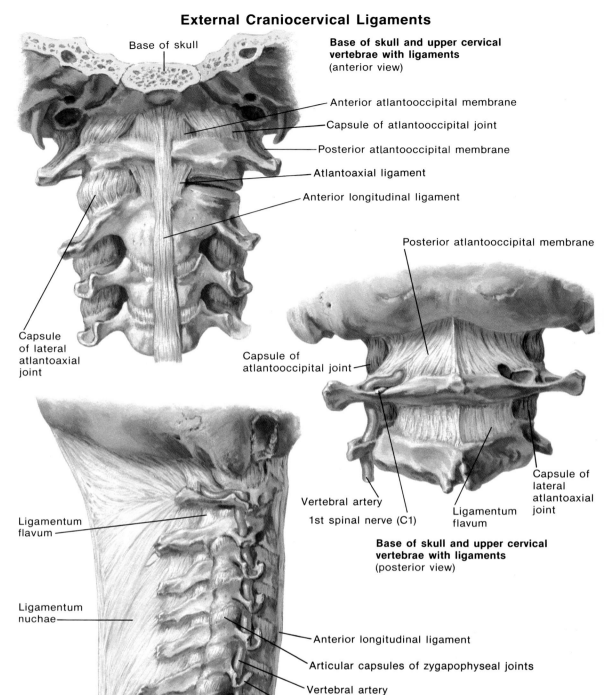

**Base of skull and upper cervical vertebrae with ligaments**
(anterior view)

Base of skull

Anterior atlantooccipital membrane

Capsule of atlantooccipital joint

Posterior atlantooccipital membrane

Atlantoaxial ligament

Anterior longitudinal ligament

Posterior atlantooccipital membrane

Capsule of atlantooccipital joint

Capsule of lateral atlantoaxial joint

Capsule of lateral atlantoaxial joint

Vertebral artery

1st spinal nerve (C1)

Ligamentum flavum

**Base of skull and upper cervical vertebrae with ligaments**
(posterior view)

Ligamentum flavum

Ligamentum nuchae

Spinous process (C7)

Interspinal ligament

Supraspinal ligament

Anterior longitudinal ligament

Articular capsules of zygapophyseal joints

Vertebral artery

Carotid tubercle

Intervertebral disc

**Base of skull and cervical vertebrae with ligaments**
(right lateral view)

The ligaments uniting the cranium, atlas and axis allow free yet safe movement of the head, and extra security is provided by the ligamentous action of the surrounding muscles. Ligaments best seen from the external aspect are shown in the illustration.

The *anterior atlantooccipital membrane* is a wide, dense, fibroelastic band extending between the anterior margin of the foramen magnum and the upper border of the anterior arch of the atlas. Laterally, it is continuous with the articular capsules of the atlantooccipital joints. In the midline, it is reinforced by the upward continuation of the anterior longitudinal ligament.

The *posterior atlantooccipital membrane* is broader and thinner than the anterior, and connects the posterior margin of the foramen magnum with the upper border of the posterior arch of the atlas. On each side, it arches over the groove for the vertebral artery, leaving an opening for the upward passage of the artery and the outward passage of the first cervical spinal nerve.

*Articular capsules* surround the joints between the occipital condyles and the superior atlantal

facets. The capsules are rather loose, allowing nodding movements of the head, and are thin medially; laterally, they are thickened and form the *lateral atlantooccipital ligaments*, which limit lateral tilting of the head.

The *anterior longitudinal ligament* extends from the base of the skull to the sacrum. Its uppermost part reinforces the anterior atlantooccipital membrane in the midline. The part between the anterior tubercle of the atlas and the anterior median ridge on the axis may have lateral extensions—the *atlantoaxial (epistrophic) ligaments*.

The *ligamentum nuchae* is a dense fibroelastic membrane stretching from the external occipital

protuberance and crest to the posterior tubercle of the atlas and the spinous processes of all the other cervical vertebrae. It provides areas for muscular attachments and forms a midline septum between the posterior cervical muscles. The ligamentum nuchae is better developed in quadrupeds than in humans.

The *ligamenta flava* contain a high proportion of yellow elastic fibers and connect the laminae of adjacent vertebrae. They are present between the posterior arch of the atlas and the laminae of the axis, but absent between the atlas and skull.

Intervertebral discs are lacking between the occiput and atlas, and between the atlas and axis. □

# Internal Craniocervical Ligaments

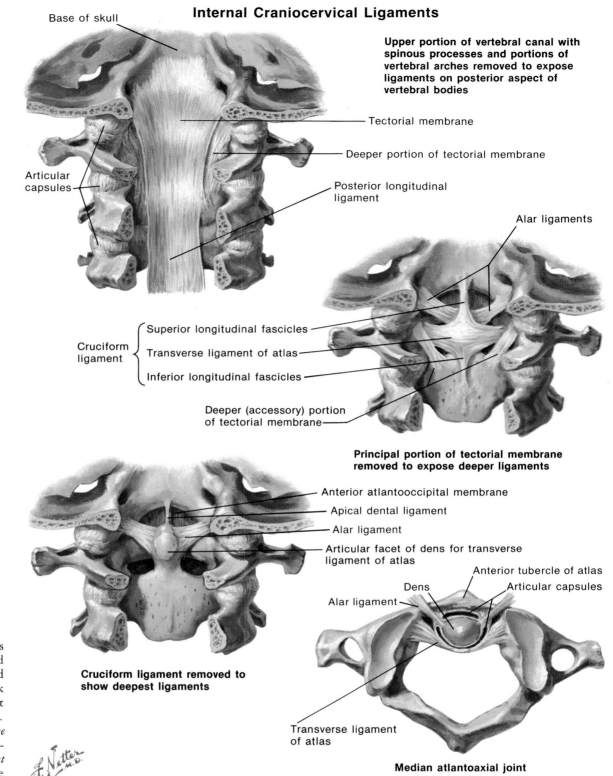

Base of skull

**Upper portion of vertebral canal with spinous processes and portions of vertebral arches removed to expose ligaments on posterior aspect of vertebral bodies**

Tectorial membrane

Deeper portion of tectorial membrane

Articular capsules

Posterior longitudinal ligament

Alar ligaments

Cruciform ligament {
Superior longitudinal fascicles

Transverse ligament of atlas

Inferior longitudinal fascicles
}

Deeper (accessory) portion of tectorial membrane

**Principal portion of tectorial membrane removed to expose deeper ligaments**

Anterior atlantooccipital membrane

Apical dental ligament

Alar ligament

Articular facet of dens for transverse ligament of atlas

Anterior tubercle of atlas

Dens

Articular capsules

Alar ligament

**Cruciform ligament removed to show deepest ligaments**

Transverse ligament of atlas

**Median atlantoaxial joint**
(superior view)

The ligaments on the posterior aspects of the vertebral bodies contribute added strength to the craniocervical region, and some are specifically arranged to check excessive movements, such as rotation at the median and lateral atlantoaxial joints.

The broad, strong *tectorial membrane* lies within the vertebral canal. It prolongs the *posterior longitudinal ligament* upward from the posterior surface of the body of the axis to the anterior and anterolateral margins of the foramen magnum, where it blends with the dura mater. It covers the dens and its ligaments and gives added protection to the junctional area between the medulla oblongata and spinal cord.

The *median atlantoaxial pivot joint* lies between the dens of the axis and the ring formed by the anterior arch and transverse ligament of the atlas (Plate 10). Two small synovial cavities surrounded by thin articular capsules are present between the dens and the anterior arch in front, and the transverse ligament of the atlas behind.

The *transverse ligament of the atlas* is a strong band passing horizontally behind the dens and attached on each side to a tubercle on the medial side of the lateral mass of the atlas. From its midpoint, bands pass vertically upward and downward to become fixed, respectively, to the basilar part of the occipital bone between the tectorial membrane and the apical ligament of the dens and to the posterior surface of the body of the axis—the *superior* and *inferior longitudinal fascicles*. These transverse and vertical bands together form the *cruciform ligament*.

The *apical ligament* is a slender cord connecting the apex of the dens to the anterior midpoint of the foramen magnum, lying between the anterior atlantooccipital membrane and the upper limb of the cruciform ligament.

The *alar ligaments* are two fibrous bands stretching upward and outward from the superolateral aspects of the dens to the medial sides of the occipital condyles. They check excessive rotation at the median atlantooccipital joint.

*Lateral atlantoaxial joints* are formed between the almost-flat inferior articular facets on the lateral masses of the atlas and the superior articular facets of the axis. They are synovial joints with thin, loose articular capsules. An *accessory ligament* extends from near the base of the dens to the lateral mass of the atlas, close to the attachment of the transverse ligament. It assists the alar ligaments in restricting atlantoaxial rotation. □

**Thoracic Vertebrae**

# Thoracic Vertebrae

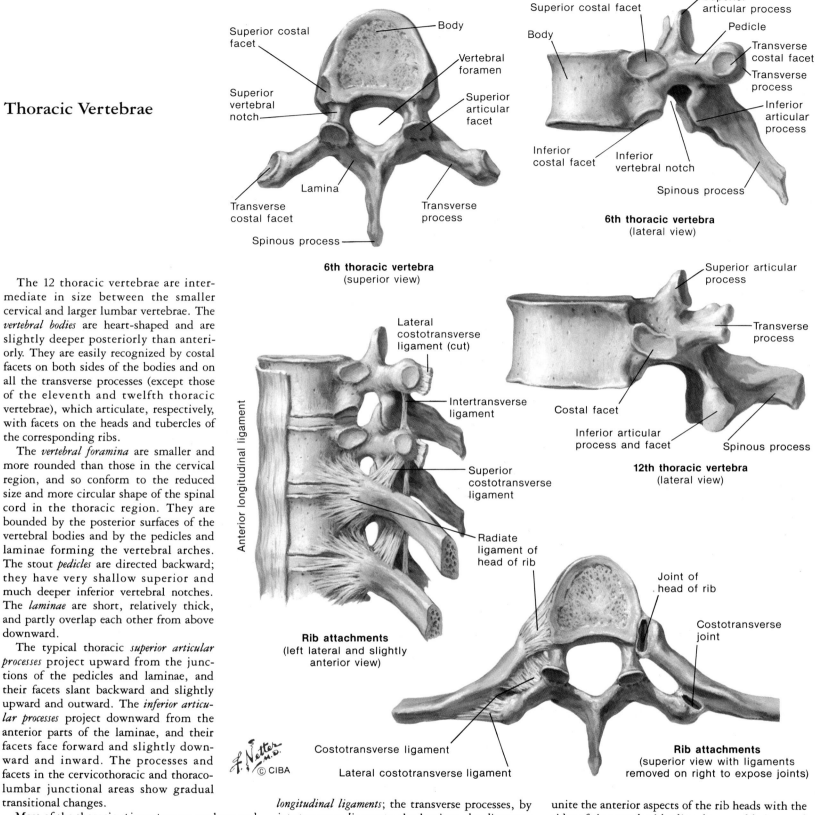

Superior costal facet

Body

Vertebral foramen

Superior vertebral notch

Superior articular facet

Lamina

Transverse costal facet

Transverse process

Spinous process

**6th thoracic vertebra**
(superior view)

Superior costal facet

Body

Superior articular process

Pedicle

Transverse costal facet

Transverse process

Inferior articular process

Inferior costal facet

Inferior vertebral notch

Spinous process

**6th thoracic vertebra**
(lateral view)

Lateral costotransverse ligament (cut)

Anterior longitudinal ligament

Intertransverse ligament

Superior costotransverse ligament

Radiate ligament of head of rib

**Rib attachments**
(left lateral and slightly anterior view)

Costotransverse ligament

Lateral costotransverse ligament

Superior articular process

Transverse process

Costal facet

Inferior articular process and facet

Spinous process

**12th thoracic vertebra**
(lateral view)

Joint of head of rib

Costotransverse joint

**Rib attachments**
(superior view with ligaments removed on right to expose joints)

The 12 thoracic vertebrae are intermediate in size between the smaller cervical and larger lumbar vertebrae. The *vertebral bodies* are heart-shaped and are slightly deeper posteriorly than anteriorly. They are easily recognized by costal facets on both sides of the bodies and on all the transverse processes (except those of the eleventh and twelfth thoracic vertebrae), which articulate, respectively, with facets on the heads and tubercles of the corresponding ribs.

The *vertebral foramina* are smaller and more rounded than those in the cervical region, and so conform to the reduced size and more circular shape of the spinal cord in the thoracic region. They are bounded by the posterior surfaces of the vertebral bodies and by the pedicles and laminae forming the vertebral arches. The stout *pedicles* are directed backward; they have very shallow superior and much deeper inferior vertebral notches. The *laminae* are short, relatively thick, and partly overlap each other from above downward.

The typical thoracic *superior articular processes* project upward from the junctions of the pedicles and laminae, and their facets slant backward and slightly upward and outward. The *inferior articular processes* project downward from the anterior parts of the laminae, and their facets face forward and slightly downward and inward. The processes and facets in the cervicothoracic and thoracolumbar junctional areas show gradual transitional changes.

Most of the thoracic *spinous processes* are long and are inclined downward and backward. Those of the upper and lower thoracic vertebrae are more horizontal. The *transverse processes* are also relatively long and extend posterolaterally from the junctions of the pedicles and laminae. Except for those of the lowest two or, occasionally, three thoracic vertebrae, the transverse processes have small oval facets near their tips, which articulate with similar facets on the corresponding rib tubercles.

Adjacent vertebral bodies are connected by *intervertebral discs* and by *anterior* and *posterior*

*longitudinal ligaments*; the transverse processes, by *intertransverse ligaments*; the laminae, by *ligamenta flava*; and the spinous processes, by *supraspinal* and *interspinal ligaments*. The joints between the articular processes are surrounded by fibrous *articular capsules*.

**Costovertebral Joints.** The ribs are connected to the vertebral bodies and transverse processes by various ligaments. The *costocentral joints* between the bodies and rib heads have *articular capsules*, and the second to tenth costal heads, each of which articulates with two vertebrae, are connected to the corresponding intervertebral discs by *intraarticular ligaments*. *Radiate (stellate) ligaments*

unite the anterior aspects of the rib heads with the sides of the vertebral bodies above and below, and with the intervening discs.

The *costotransverse joints* between the facets on the transverse processes and on the tubercles of the ribs are also surrounded by *articular capsules*. They are reinforced by a (middle) *costotransverse ligament* between the rib neck and the adjoining transverse process, a *superior costotransverse ligament* between the rib neck and the transverse process of the vertebra above, and a *lateral costotransverse ligament* interconnecting the end of a transverse process to the nonarticular part of the related costal tubercle.  □

**Lumbar Vertebrae and Intervertebral Disc**

## Lumbar Vertebrae and Intervertebral Disc

*The five lumbar vertebrae* are the largest separate vertebrae and are distinguished by the absence of transverse foramina and costal facets. The *vertebral bodies* are wider from side to side than from front to back, and the upper and lower surfaces are kidney-shaped and almost parallel, except in the case of the fifth vertebral body, which is slightly wedge-shaped. The triangular *vertebral foramina* are larger in the thoracic vertebrae and smaller in the cervical vertebrae.

The *pedicles* are short and strong and arise from the upper and posterolateral aspects of the bodies; the superior vertebral notches are therefore less deep than the inferior notches. The *laminae* are short, broad plates that meet in the midline to form the quadrangular and almost horizontal *spinous processes*. The intervals between adjacent laminae and spinous processes are relatively wide.

The *articular processes* project vertically upward and downward from the junctional areas between the pedicles and the laminae. The superior facets are gently concave and face posteromedially to embrace the inferior facets of the vertebra above, which are curved and disposed in a reciprocal fashion. This arrangement permits some flexion and extension, but very little rotation. The *transverse processes* of the upper three lumbar vertebrae are long and slender, while those of the fourth, and especially of the fifth, are more pyramidal.

Near the roots of each transverse process are small *accessory processes*; other small, rounded *mamillary processes* protrude from the posterior margins of the superior articular processes. The former may represent the true transverse processes (or their tips), since many of the so-called transverse processes are really costal elements. In the first lumbar vertebra, these elements occasionally develop into lumbar ribs.

The *fifth lumbar vertebra* is atypical. It is the largest, its body is deeper anteriorly, its inferior articular facets face almost forward and are set more widely apart, and the roots of its stumpy transverse processes are continuous with the posterolateral parts of the body and with the entire lateral surfaces of the pedicles.

*The intervertebral discs* are interposed between the adjacent vertebral bodies from the axis to the sacrum, and are immensely strong fibrocartilaginous structures that provide powerful bonds and elastic buffers. They consist of outer concentric layers of fibrous tissue—the *anulus fibrosus* (the fibers in adjacent layers are arranged

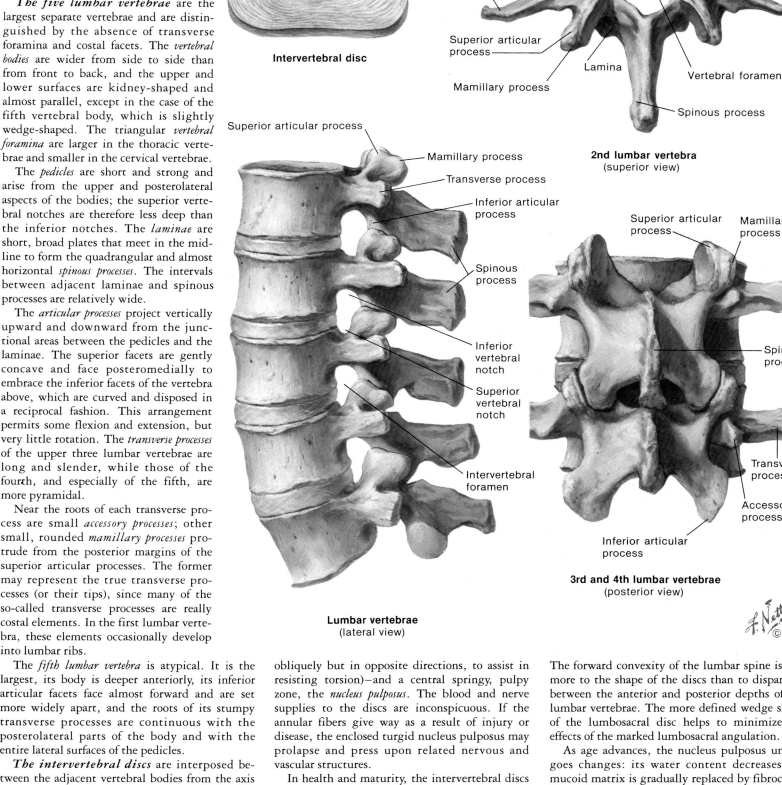

**Intervertebral disc**

Anulus fibrosus   Nucleus pulposus

**Lumbar vertebrae**
(lateral view)

Superior articular process

Mamillary process

Transverse process

Inferior articular process

Spinous process

Inferior vertebral notch

Superior vertebral notch

Intervertebral foramen

Body

Pedicle

Transverse process

Superior articular process

Lamina

Mamillary process

Vertebral foramen

Spinous process

**2nd lumbar vertebra**
(superior view)

Superior articular process   Mamillary process

Spinous process

Transverse process

Accessory process

Inferior articular process

**3rd and 4th lumbar vertebrae**
(posterior view)

*F. Netter*
© CIBA

obliquely but in opposite directions, to assist in resisting torsion)—and a central springy, pulpy zone, the *nucleus pulposus*. The blood and nerve supplies to the discs are inconspicuous. If the annular fibers give way as a result of injury or disease, the enclosed turgid nucleus pulposus may prolapse and press upon related nervous and vascular structures.

In health and maturity, the intervertebral discs account for almost 25% of the length of the vertebral column; they are thinnest in the upper thoracic region and thickest in the lumbar region. In vertical section, the lumbar discs are rather wedge-shaped, with the thicker edge anteriorly.

The forward convexity of the lumbar spine is due more to the shape of the discs than to disparities between the anterior and posterior depths of the lumbar vertebrae. The more defined wedge shape of the lumbosacral disc helps to minimize the effects of the marked lumbosacral angulation.

As age advances, the nucleus pulposus undergoes changes: its water content decreases, its mucoid matrix is gradually replaced by fibrocartilage, and it ultimately comes to resemble the anulus fibrosus. The resultant loss of depth in each disc is small, but overall it may amount to a decrease of 2 to 3 cm in the height of the spinal column. □

# Ligaments of Spinal Column

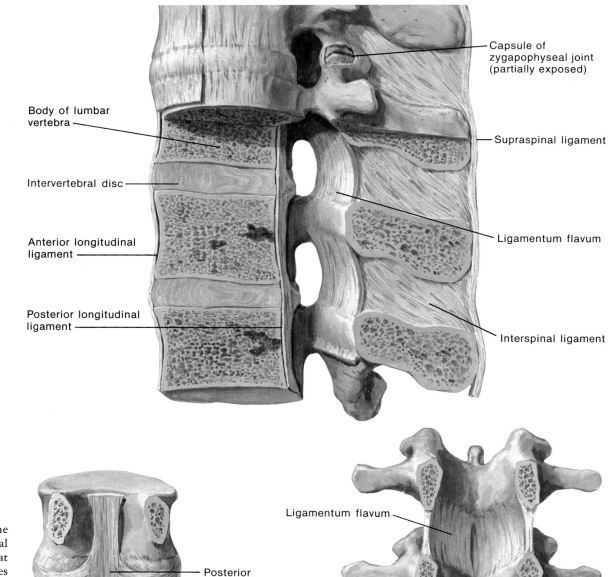

Capsule of zygapophyseal joint (partially exposed)

Body of lumbar vertebra

Intervertebral disc

Anterior longitudinal ligament

Posterior longitudinal ligament

Supraspinal ligament

Ligamentum flavum

Interspinal ligament

Posterior longitudinal ligament

Ligamentum flavum

The vertebrae from the axis to the upper sacrum are united by intervertebral discs and by various other ligaments that interconnect the vertebral bodies, arches and processes. Additional ligaments link the skull, atlas and axis (Plates 12 and 13), the ribs and the thoracic vertebrae (Plate 14), and the lower lumbar, sacral and coccygeal vertebrae and the hip bones (Plate 18).

The *anterior longitudinal ligament* is a straplike band that increases in width from above downward and extends from the anterior tubercle of the atlas to the sacrum. It is firmly attached to the anterior margins of the vertebral bodies and the intervertebral discs. The superficial fibers cross over several vertebrae, and the shorter, deeper fibers interconnect adjacent bodies and discs. The anterior longitudinal ligament is thicker in the thoracic region than in the other regions of the spinal column.

The *posterior longitudinal ligament* is broader above than below and lies within the vertebral canal behind the vertebral bodies. Its upper end is continuous with the tectorial membrane, and it extends from the axis to the sacrum. The edges of the ligament are serrated, especially in the lower thoracic and lumbar regions, because it spreads outward between its attachments to the borders of the vertebral bodies to blend with the annular fibers of the discs. It is separated from the posterior surfaces of the vertebral bodies by the

basivertebral veins that join the anterior internal vertebral venous plexus (see Section III, Plate 21).

The *ligamenta flava*, largely composed of yellow elastic tissue, join adjacent laminae. They extend from the anteroinferior aspect of the lamina above to the posterosuperior surface of the lamina below, and from the midline to the articular capsules laterally. Small gaps for the passage of veins from the internal to the external vertebral venous plexuses exist between them in the midline. The ligaments increase in thickness from the cervical to the lumbar region.

The *supraspinal ligaments* interconnect the tips of the spinous processes from the seventh cervical

vertebra to the sacrum. They are continuous with the ligamentum nuchae above and with the interspinal ligaments in front, and increase in thickness from above down. The *interspinal ligaments* are thin, membranous structures extending between the roots and apexes of the spines; they are best developed in the lumbar region.

*Articular capsules* surround the joints between adjacent articular processes. They are relatively lax in the cervical region.

The *intertransverse ligaments* connect adjoining transverse processes. They are often filamentous in the cervical and lumbar regions, but form distinct cords in the thoracic region. □

# Sacrum and Coccyx

**The sacrum** consists of five fused vertebrae and is wedge-shaped from above down and from before back. It forms most of the posterior pelvic wall and is fixed between the hip bones at an angle, so that its curved pelvic surface is inclined downward and forward.

The broader *base* of the sacrum faces anterosuperiorly toward the abdomen; its elevated central third is the upper part of the first sacral vertebral body and bears a smooth oval area for the attachment of the lumbosacral intervertebral disc. Its projecting anterior border is the sacral *promontory*. On each side, the costotransverse elements of the first vertebra are fused to form a wing-shaped lateral mass (sacral *ala*), separated from the pelvic surface by a curved line, which is the sacral portion of the arcuate pelvic brim. The articular processes are fused, like most of the other components of the sacral vertebrae, but the *superior articular processes* of the first vertebra remain and project upward for articulation with the inferior articular processes of the fifth lumbar vertebra. They are flattened and face almost directly backward to assist in preventing subluxation (spondylolisthesis) of the last lumbar vertebra at the angulated lumbosacral junction.

The narrow *apex* is the lower end of the sacrum and articulates with the coccyx.

The pelvic surface is concave both vertically and horizontally and shows four *transverse ridges* indicating the lines of fusion between the bodies of the original five vertebrae. On either side of the ridges, four *pelvic sacral foramina* permit the passage of the ventral rami of the first four sacral nerves and their associated vessels.

The convex dorsal surface shows irregular *median, intermediate* and *lateral sacral crests* representing, respectively, the fused spinous, articular and transverse processes. The areas between the median and intermediate crests are the fused laminae, and there are four pairs of *dorsal sacral foramina* for the passage of the dorsal rami of the upper four sacral nerves. The laminae of the fifth and, occasionally, the fourth vertebra fail to unite and thus leave a *hiatus*, which is exploited for the injection of epidural anesthetics. The hiatus is bounded on each side by a *cornu*, a relic of the inferior articular process, and transmits the small fifth sacral and coccygeal nerves.

The parts of the sacrum lateral to the sacral foramina are produced by the fusion of the costal, transverse and pedicular elements of the five vertebrae. The upper, broader parts of their lateral surfaces bear uneven *auricular*, or ear-shaped, surfaces for articulation with similar surfaces on the iliac parts of the hip bones.

Transverse sections of the sacrum reveal the triangular sacral end of the *vertebral canal*. This canal surrounds and protects the terminations of the dural and arachnoid sheaths and the subarachnoid space, which end at about the level of the second sacral vertebra and enclose the sacral and coccygeal roots of the cauda equina and the lower intrathecal portion of the filum terminale (see Section II, Plate 14). The dura mater is separated from the walls of the canal by fibrofatty tissue, fine arteries and nerves and sacral internal vertebral venous plexuses.

*Coccyx.* The small, triangular coccyx is formed by the fusion of four (occasionally, three or five) rudimentary tail vertebrae. Its base articulates with the sacral apex, and its apex is a mere button of bone. Most of the features of a typical vertebra are lacking, but the first coccygeal vertebra has small *transverse processes* and a *cornu* on each side, which is sometimes large enough to articulate with the corresponding sacral cornu. (For a detailed description of the nerves of the sacral and coccygeal plexuses, see Section VI, Plate 10.) □

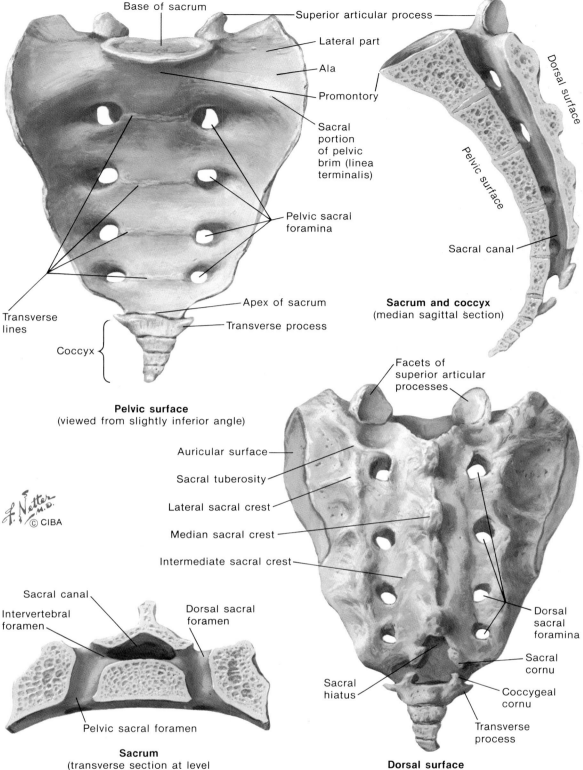

**Sacrum and Coccyx**

- Base of sacrum
- Superior articular process
- Lateral part
- Ala
- Promontory
- Sacral portion of pelvic brim (linea terminalis)
- Pelvic sacral foramina
- Apex of sacrum
- Transverse process
- Transverse lines
- Coccyx

**Pelvic surface**
(viewed from slightly inferior angle)

- Dorsal surface
- Pelvic surface
- Sacral canal

**Sacrum and coccyx**
(median sagittal section)

- Sacral canal
- Intervertebral foramen
- Dorsal sacral foramen
- Pelvic sacral foramen

**Sacrum**
(transverse section at level of superior sacral foramina)

- Facets of superior articular processes
- Auricular surface
- Sacral tuberosity
- Lateral sacral crest
- Median sacral crest
- Intermediate sacral crest
- Sacral hiatus
- Dorsal sacral foramina
- Sacral cornu
- Coccygeal cornu
- Transverse process

**Dorsal surface**
(viewed from slightly superior angle)

**Ligaments of Sacrum and Coccyx**

# Ligaments of Sacrum and Coccyx

Because the lumbosacral and sacroiliac joints transmit the entire weight of the body to the hip bones and thence to the lower limbs, their ligaments are most important.

*The lumbosacral junction* is mechanically imperfect because of its angulation and the consequent sloping platform provided for the fifth lumbar vertebra by the first sacral vertebra (Plate 17). The tendency to subluxation (spondylolisthesis) is resisted by the impingement of the almost sagittally arranged lumbosacral articular processes, and this bony check is strongly augmented by the last *intervertebral disc*, the *anterior* and *posterior longitudinal ligaments*, the *ligamenta flava* and the *supraspinal* and *interspinal ligaments*. These ligaments are further reinforced by the erector spinae and other muscles and by the *iliolumbar ligaments*—strong bands uniting the transverse processes of the fourth and fifth lumbar vertebrae and the posterior parts of the iliac crests and sacral alae. The iliolumbar ligaments are really the expanded lower margins of the anterior and middle layers of the thoracolumbar fascia that encloses the quadratus lumborum muscles. They blend below with the ventral (anterior) sacroiliac ligaments.

*The sacroiliac joints* between the auricular surfaces of the sacrum and ilia are synovial in type. Movements are limited, however, because of the interlocking elevations and depressions on the opposed articular surfaces, the way the sacrum is wedged between the hip bones, and the restraining influence of the ventral, dorsal and interosseous sacroiliac ligaments and the accessory sacrotuberal and sacrospinal ligaments.

The *ventral (anterior) sacroiliac ligament* is a thin, wide, fibrous layer reinforcing the anterior part of the articular capsule and stretching from the ala and pelvic surface of the sacrum to the adjoining parts of the iliac bone.

The *dorsal (posterior) sacroiliac ligament* consists of more superficial, longer bundles and deeper, shorter bundles. The fibers of the long dorsal sacroiliac ligament interconnect the posterior superior iliac spine and the lateral parts of the third and fourth sacral segments; its outer fibers interdigitate with those of the sacrotuberal ligament. The short dorsal sacroiliac ligament interconnects the medial surface of the iliac bone to the lateral parts of the first and second sacral segments, and is often considered to be a part of the interosseous ligament.

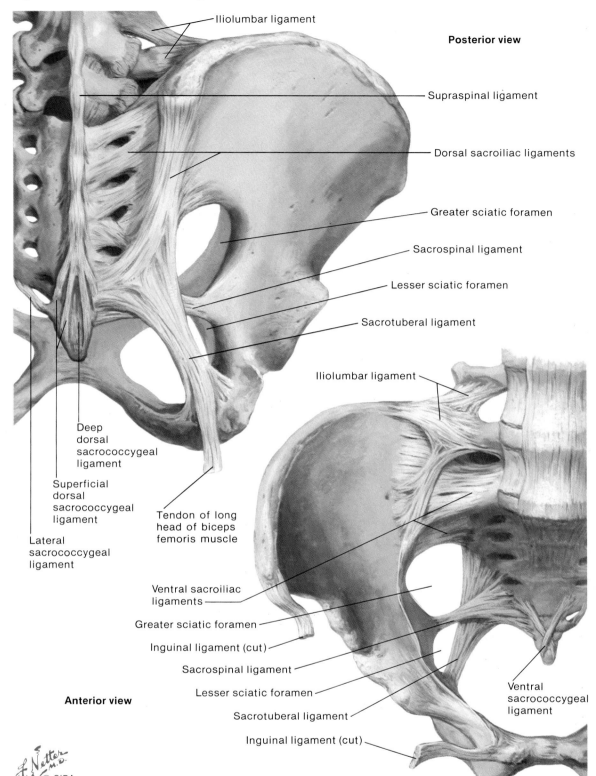

The *interosseous sacroiliac ligament* is formed by short, thick bundles of fibers interconnecting the sacral and iliac tuberosities—the rough areas behind and above the auricular surfaces of both bones. It is the most powerful bond between the bones and, indeed, is one of the strongest ligaments in the body. It lies deep to the dorsal sacroiliac ligament and is not shown in the illustration.

The *sacrotuberal* and *sacrospinal ligaments* act as accessory ligaments of the sacroiliac joints because they assist in regulating joint movements. The downward thrust at the lumbosacral junction tends to push the upper part of the sacrum down, with coincident upward tilting of its lower part as the sacrum seesaws on a transverse axis through the middle of the sacroiliac joints. The illustration shows how these accessory ligaments anchor the lower sacrum and coccyx to the ischial tuberosity and spine, thus limiting the seesaw movement.

*The sacrum and coccyx* are connected by a small, fibrocartilaginous *intervertebral disc* and by thin bands on the anterior, posterior and lateral sides of the junction—the *ventral, dorsal* and *lateral sacrococcygeal ligaments*. The dorsal ligament has a superficial part, which partly fills in the sacral hiatus, and a deep part, which represents the posterior spinal longitudinal ligament. □

Section II

# Gross Anatomy of Brain and Spinal Cord

Frank H. Netter, M.D.

*in collaboration with*

**G.A.G. Mitchell, Ch.M., D.Sc., F.R.C.S.**  *Plates 1–16*

**Barry W. Peterson, Ph.D.**  *Plate 17*

**Superolateral Surface of Brain**

## Surfaces of Cerebrum

The cerebrum is divided into *right* and *left hemispheres* by a longitudinal fissure. Each hemisphere has three surfaces—superolateral, medial and inferior—all of which have irregular fissures, or sulci, demarcating convolutions, or gyri (see Section III, Plates 4 to 6 and Section VII, Plates 4 and 5). Although there are variations in arrangement between the two hemispheres in the same brain and in those from different persons, a basic similarity in the pattern allows the parts of the brain to be mapped and named.

### Superolateral Surface

On the superolateral surface, two sulci, the lateral and the central, can be easily identified. The *lateral (sylvian) sulcus* has a short stem between the orbital surface of the frontal lobe and the temporal pole; in life, the lesser wing of the sphenoid bone projects into it. At its outer end, the stem divides into anterior, ascending and posterior branches. The anterior and ascending rami are each about 2.5 cm long; the former runs horizontally into the inferior frontal gyrus, and the latter, vertically. The posterior ramus is about 7.5 cm long and inclines upward as it extends backward to end in the supramarginal gyrus, which is part of the inferior parietal lobule. These rami separate triangular areas of cortex called opercula, which cover a buried lobe of cortex, the insula.

The *central (rolandic) sulcus* proceeds obliquely downward and forward from a point on the superior border almost halfway between the frontal and occipital poles. It is sinuous and ends above the middle of the posterior ramus of the lateral sulcus. Its upper end usually runs onto the medial surface of the cerebrum and terminates in the paracentral lobule.

The *parietooccipital sulcus* is situated mainly on the medial surface of the cerebrum, but it cuts the superior margin and appears for a short distance on the superolateral surface about 5 cm in front of the occipital pole. At about the same distance from the occipital pole on the inferior margin, there is a shallow indentation, the *preoccipital notch*, produced by a small ridge on the upper surface of the tentorium cerebelli.

The above features divide the cerebrum into frontal, parietal, occipital and temporal lobes. The *frontal lobe* lies in front of the central sulcus and anterosuperior to the lateral sulcus. The *parietal lobe* lies behind the central sulcus, above the

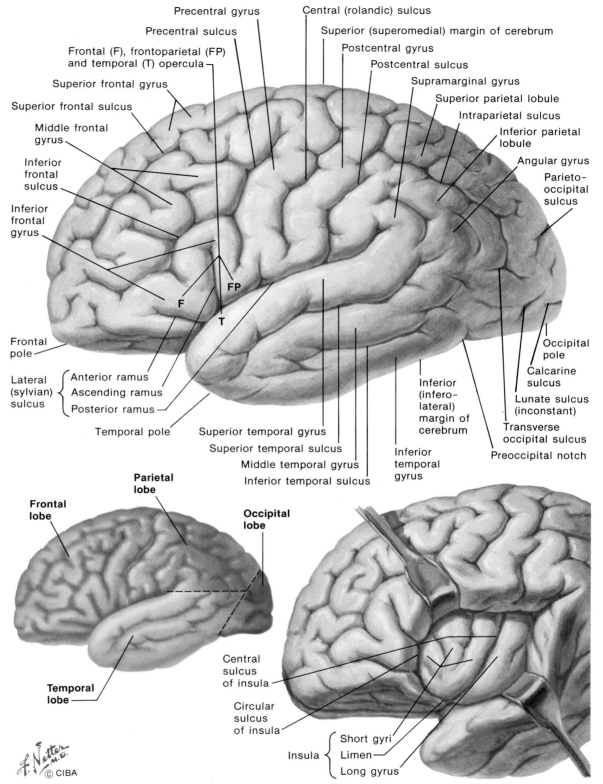

posterior ramus of the lateral sulcus and in front of an imaginary line drawn between the parieto-occipital sulcus and the preoccipital notch. The *occipital lobe* lies behind this same imaginary line. The *temporal lobe* lies below the stem and posterior ramus of the lateral sulcus, and is bounded behind by the lower part of the aforementioned imaginary line.

*Frontal Lobe.* The superolateral surface of the frontal lobe is traversed by three main sulci and thus divided into four gyri. The *precentral sulcus* runs parallel to the central sulcus, separated from it by the *precentral gyrus*, the great cortical somatomotor area. The *superior* and *inferior frontal sulci*

curve across the remaining part of the surface, dividing it into superior, middle and inferior frontal gyri.

*The parietal lobe* shows two main sulci, which divide it into three gyri. The *postcentral sulcus* lies parallel to the central sulcus, separated from it by the *postcentral gyrus*, the great somatic sensory cortical area. The remaining, larger part of the superolateral parietal surface is subdivided into superior and inferior parietal lobules (gyri) by the *intraparietal sulcus*, which runs backward from near the midpoint of the postcentral sulcus and usually extends into the occipital lobe, where it ends by joining the transverse occipital sulcus.

## Medial Surface of Brain

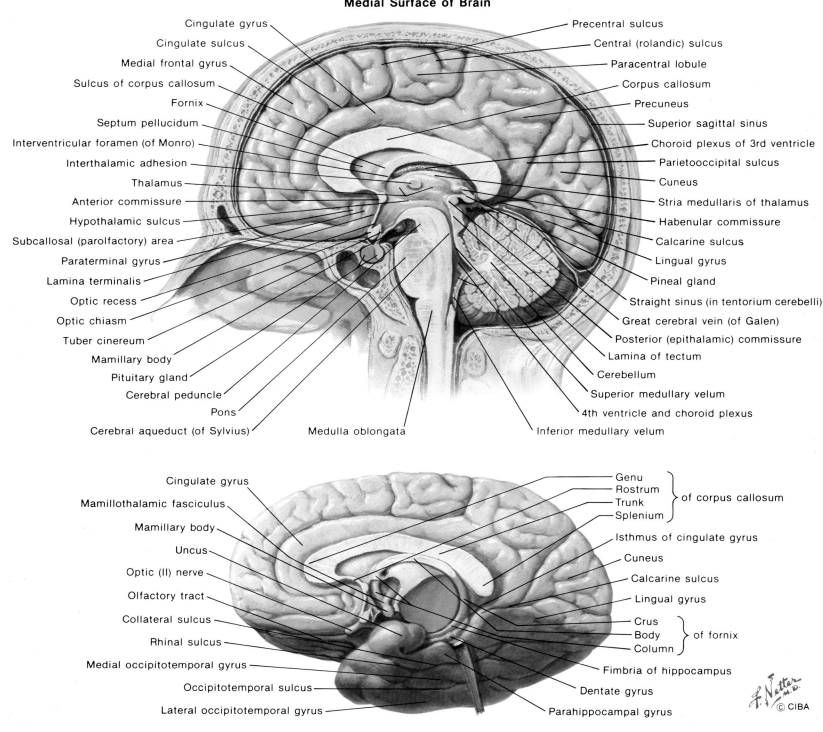

Cingulate gyrus
Cingulate sulcus
Medial frontal gyrus
Sulcus of corpus callosum
Fornix
Septum pellucidum
Interventricular foramen (of Monro)
Interthalamic adhesion
Thalamus
Anterior commissure
Hypothalamic sulcus
Subcallosal (parolfactory) area
Paraterminal gyrus
Lamina terminalis
Optic recess
Optic chiasm
Tuber cinereum
Mamillary body
Pituitary gland
Cerebral peduncle
Pons
Cerebral aqueduct (of Sylvius)
Medulla oblongata

Precentral sulcus
Central (rolandic) sulcus
Paracentral lobule
Corpus callosum
Precuneus
Superior sagittal sinus
Choroid plexus of 3rd ventricle
Parietooccipital sulcus
Cuneus
Stria medullaris of thalamus
Habenular commissure
Calcarine sulcus
Lingual gyrus
Pineal gland
Straight sinus (in tentorium cerebelli)
Great cerebral vein (of Galen)
Posterior (epithalamic) commissure
Lamina of tectum
Cerebellum
Superior medullary velum
4th ventricle and choroid plexus
Inferior medullary velum

Cingulate gyrus
Mamillothalamic fasciculus
Mamillary body
Uncus
Optic (II) nerve
Olfactory tract
Collateral sulcus
Rhinal sulcus
Medial occipitotemporal gyrus
Occipitotemporal sulcus
Lateral occipitotemporal gyrus

Genu
Rostrum
Trunk } of corpus callosum
Splenium
Isthmus of cingulate gyrus
Cuneus
Calcarine sulcus
Lingual gyrus
Crus
Body } of fornix
Column
Fimbria of hippocampus
Dentate gyrus
Parahippocampal gyrus

© CIBA

SECTION II   PLATE 2

## Surfaces of Cerebrum
*(Continued)*

*Occipital Lobe*. The outer surface of the occipital lobe is less extensive than that of the other lobes, and shows a short *transverse occipital sulcus* and a *lunate sulcus*; the latter demarcates the visuosensory and visuopsychic areas of the cortex. The *calcarine sulcus* notches the occipital pole.

**The temporal lobe** is divided by *superior* and *inferior temporal sulci* into superior, middle and inferior temporal gyri. The sulci run backward and slightly upward, in the same general direction as the posterior ramus of the lateral sulcus,

which lies above them. The superior sulcus ends in the lower part of the inferior parietal lobule, and the superjacent cortex is called the angular gyrus. The superior temporal gyrus contains the auditosensory and auditopsychic areas.

**The insula**, or island of Reil, is a sunken lobe of cortex, overlaid by opercula and buried by the exuberant growth of adjoining cortical areas. It is ovoid, or triangular, in shape and is surrounded by a groove, the *circular sulcus* of the insula. The apex is inferior, near the anterior (rostral) perforated substance, and is termed the *limen* of the insula. The insular surface is divided into larger and smaller posterior parts by the *central sulcus* of the insula, which is roughly parallel to the central sulcus of the cerebrum. Each part is further subdivided by minor sulci into short and long insular gyri. The claustrum and lentiform nucleus lie deep to the insula.

**Medial Surface**

The medial surfaces of the cerebral hemispheres are flat, and, although separated for most of their extent by the longitudinal fissure and falx cerebri, they are connected in parts by the cerebral commissures and by the structures bounding the third ventricle (Plates 4 to 8).

**The corpus callosum** is much the largest of the cerebral commissures, and forms most of the roof of the lateral ventricle. In a median sagittal section, it appears as a flattened bridge of white fibers, and its central part, or *trunk*, is convex upward. The anterior end is recurved to form the *genu*, which tapers rapidly into the *rostrum*. The expanded posterior end, or *splenium*, overlies the midbrain and adjacent part of the cerebellum. The corpus callosum is about 10 cm long and 2.5 cm wide between the points where it sinks

**Inferior Surface of Brain**

## Surfaces of Cerebrum
*(Continued)*

into the opposing hemispheres in the depths of the corpus callosal sulcus. Its fibers diverge to all parts of the cerebral cortex.

*Fornix.* Below the splenium and trunk of the corpus callosum are the symmetrical arching bundles (*crura of the fornix*) that meet to form the *body* of the fornix and separate again to become the *columns* of the fornix, curving downward to the mamillary bodies. The body of the fornix lies in the roof of the third ventricle, and the tela choroidea is subjacent; the lateral fringed margins of this double fold of pia mater are the choroid plexuses of the central parts of the lateral ventricles, while an extension from the underside of the fold in the midline forms the choroid plexus of the third ventricle (Plate 9).

*The cingulate sulcus* is easily identified on the medial surface, lying parallel to the corpus callosum. It begins below the genu of the corpus callosum and ends above the posterior part of the trunk by turning upward to cut the superior margin of the hemisphere. Opposite the middle of the trunk is another vertical branch sulcus, and the area of cortex between these ascending sulci is the *paracentral lobule*, which contains parts of the motor and sensory cortical areas. The cingulate sulcus separates the *medial frontal* and *cingulate gyri*, and below the genu and rostrum of the corpus callosum are small *parolfactory sulci* separating the *subcallosal (parolfactory) areas* and *paraterminal gyrus*.

*The posterior part of the medial surface* shows two deep sulci. The upper *parietooccipital sulcus* inclines backward and upward to cut the superior border. The lower *calcarine sulcus* extends forward from the occipital pole to end beneath the splenium of the corpus callosum, and the isthmus of cortex between them connects the cingulate and parahippocampal gyri. The wedge-shaped region between the parietooccipital and calcarine sulci is the *cuneus*, while the area between the parietooccipital sulcus and the paracentral lobule is the *precuneus*. The main visuosensory area is located in the walls of the calcarine sulcus and in the adjacent cortex.

### Inferior Surface

The inferior surface is divided by the stem of the lateral sulcus into smaller, orbital and larger, tentorial surfaces (see Section I, Plates 6 and 7).

*The orbital surface* rests on the roofs of the orbit and nose and is marked by an H-shaped *orbital sulcus*, as well as by a straight groove on the medial side, the *olfactory sulcus*, which lodges

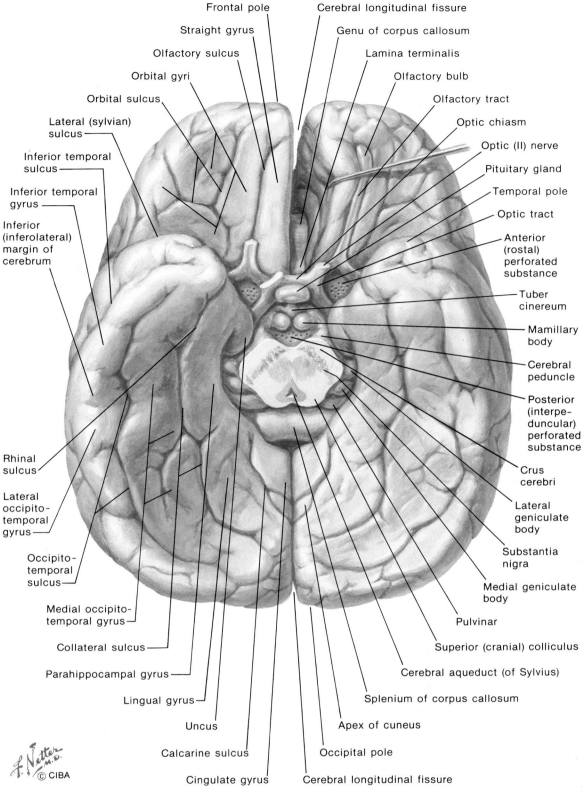

the olfactory bulb and tract. The orbital sulcus demarcates the *orbital gyri*; the small convolution medial to the olfactory sulcus is the *straight gyrus*.

*The tentorial surface* lies partly on the floor of the middle cranial fossa and partly on the tentorium cerebelli. It shows two anteroposterior grooves, the *collateral* and *occipitotemporal sulci*. Both run almost directly forward from the occipital pole to the temporal pole; like other sulci, they may be subdivided, and the anterior end of the collateral sulcus is called the *rhinal sulcus*. The *parahippocampal* and *lingual gyri* lie medial to the collateral sulcus. The *dentate gyrus*, a narrow fringe of cortex with transverse markings, occupies the

groove between the parahippocampal gyrus and the fimbria of the hippocampus. The anterior end of the parahippocampal gyrus becomes recurved to form the *uncus*, which is partly occupied by the cortical olfactory area. The *medial occipitotemporal gyrus* is fusiform in shape, and lies between the collateral and occipitotemporal sulci. The *lateral occipitotemporal gyrus* lies lateral to the occipitotemporal sulcus and is continuous with the *inferior temporal gyrus* around the inferior margin of the hemisphere.

(For detailed information on the actions and connections of the cerebral areas mentioned above, see Section VIII.) ☐

**Labels (clockwise from top):** Frontal pole; Cerebral longitudinal fissure; Straight gyrus; Genu of corpus callosum; Olfactory sulcus; Lamina terminalis; Orbital gyri; Olfactory bulb; Orbital sulcus; Olfactory tract; Lateral (sylvian) sulcus; Optic chiasm; Inferior temporal sulcus; Optic (II) nerve; Inferior temporal gyrus; Pituitary gland; Temporal pole; Inferior (inferolateral) margin of cerebrum; Optic tract; Anterior (rostal) perforated substance; Tuber cinereum; Mamillary body; Cerebral peduncle; Posterior (interpeduncular) perforated substance; Rhinal sulcus; Crus cerebri; Lateral occipito-temporal gyrus; Lateral geniculate body; Substantia nigra; Occipito-temporal sulcus; Medial geniculate body; Medial occipito-temporal gyrus; Pulvinar; Collateral sulcus; Superior (cranial) colliculus; Parahippocampal gyrus; Cerebral aqueduct (of Sylvius); Lingual gyrus; Splenium of corpus callosum; Uncus; Apex of cuneus; Calcarine sulcus; Occipital pole; Cingulate gyrus; Cerebral longitudinal fissure

# Basal Ganglia

Symmetrical subcortical masses of gray matter, the basal ganglia, are embedded in the lower parts of each cerebral hemisphere. Each is composed of the *corpus striatum* formed by the large lentiform (lenticular) and caudate nuclei, a thin sheet of gray matter termed the *claustrum*, and a group of small nuclei combined within the *amygdaloid body*, or *amygdala* (Plates 5 and 6; see also Section VII, Plates 6 and 7 and Section VIII, Plate 40).

***Lentiform Nucleus.*** The biconvex lentiform nucleus is encapsulated in white matter, and the laminae bounding its outer and inner surfaces are known, respectively, as the external and internal capsules. The *external capsule* separates the lentiform nucleus from the claustrum, which is, in turn, separated from the insula by a thin layer of white matter, the extreme capsule. The thicker *internal capsule* is angulated rather than curved and conforms to the shape of the medial surface of the lentiform nucleus. Its anterior part, or limb, is interposed between the lentiform nucleus and the head of the caudate nucleus. The posterior limb of the internal capsule separates the lentiform nucleus from the thalamus, which lies medially. The angle at the junction of the anterior and posterior limbs is termed, rather incongruously, the genu, or knee, of the internal capsule. Above, the lentiform nucleus is covered by white matter containing a mixture of itinerant fibers of the corona radiata, commissural fibers from the corpus callosum and association fibers in the superior longitudinal fasciculus. Below, where it lies above the inferior horn of the lateral ventricle, the lentiform nucleus is in contact with the anterior perforated substance, which gives passage to the striate branches of the middle cerebral artery and is grooved by the anterior commissure. On section, the lentiform nucleus is seen to have a darker lateral portion, the *putamen*, and a smaller, paler medial part, the *globus pallidus*.

***The caudate nucleus*** resembles an elongated and curved exclamation mark. Its main part is an expanded head directly continuous with a smaller and attenuated body that merges into an elongated tail (cauda). The *head* bulges into the anterior horn of the lateral ventricle and forms its sloping floor. The caudate nucleus is separated from the lentiform nucleus by the anterior limb of the internal capsule, but the separation is incomplete because the head of the caudate nucleus and the putamen are connected, especially anteroinferiorly, by bands of gray matter traversing the white matter of the anterior limb. This admixture of gray and white matter produces the striated appearance that justifies the term "corpus striatum" applied to these nuclei. The head tapers into the narrower *body* that lies in

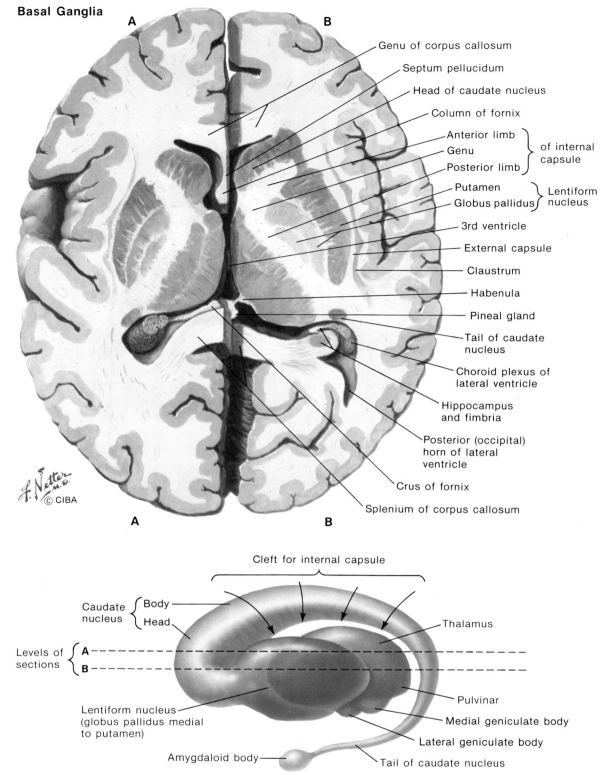

Schematic illustration showing interrelationship of thalamus, lentiform nucleus, caudate nucleus and amygdaloid body (viewed from side)

the floor of the central part of the lateral ventricle, lateral to the superior surface of the thalamus and separated from it by a shallow sulcus lodging the stria terminalis and thalamostriate vein. The *tail* turns downward along the outer margin of the posterior surface of the thalamus, with the stria terminalis still lying in a slight groove between them. It then curves forward into the roof of the inferior horn of the lateral ventricle, where it becomes separated from the thalamus and lentiform nucleus by the inferior part of the internal capsule and by fibers (including some from the anterior commissure) that spread into the temporal lobe.

***Amygdaloid Body***. The tail of the caudate nucleus ends in a small, almond-shaped expansion, the amygdaloid body, which is a complex of several small nuclei located in the forepart of the roof of the inferior horn of the lateral ventricle. The *stria terminalis* issues from the amygdaloid body and runs along the medial side of the caudate nucleus until it reaches the vicinity of the ipsilateral interventricular foramen. Here, some of its fibers join the anterior commissure, others pass to the so-called "septal" cortical areas adjacent to the lamina terminalis, and the remainder descend to the hypothalamus and anterior perforated substance (see Section VIII, Plates 51 to 64). □

# Rhinencephalon and Limbic System

The term "rhinencephalon" is used to describe all those phylogenetically ancient parts of the brain that were once regarded as having primarily olfactory affinities. These parts include the olfactory bulb, tract and striae, the anterior perforated substance, the uncus, the hippocampus, the dentate gyrus, the gyrus fasciolaris, the indusium griseum, the habenular trigone, the subcallosal area, the paraterminal gyrus, the fornix, and, because of its connections with rhinencephalic structures, the amygdaloid body as well.

*Olfactory Pathway.* The *olfactory bulb* receives, through its inferior surface, the delicate *olfactory nerves.* The bulb tapers posteriorly into the slender *olfactory tract,* which extends posteriorly to the anterior perforated substance, where it divides into lateral and medial *olfactory striae* (see Section VIII, Plate 19).

The *lateral olfactory stria,* which contains most of the axons of the mitral cells in the olfactory bulb, runs toward, and becomes attached to, the cortex of the frontal operculum and then crosses the limen of the insula to the uncus of the parahippocampal gyrus. Many of the fibers of the lateral stria end in the cortical areas of gray matter lying immediately adjacent to the stria as it progresses to the uncus. Other fibers end in the anterior part of the superolateral part of the uncus, and a few may reach as far as the amygdaloid body.

The *medial olfactory stria* is smaller than the lateral, and the exact origins and terminations of its fibers are uncertain. It ascends anterolateral to the lamina terminalis and fades away in the so-called parolfactory area of Broca, represented in modern terminology by the paraterminal gyrus and subcallosal area.

*Piriform Area.* The anterior (rostral) perforated substance, the uncus, the anterior end of the dentate gyrus and the anterior part of the parahippocampal gyrus medial to the rhinal sulcus are often referred to as the piriform area. Superiorly, the *anterior perforated substance* is continuous with the paraterminal gyrus and separated from the anterior part of the globus pallidus of the lentiform nucleus by the anterior (rostral) commissure, ansa lenticularis and ansa peduncularis; posteromedially, it blends into the tuber cinereum.

*Hippocampal Formation.* The hippocampus, the posterior part of the dentate gyrus and the indusium griseum are sometimes grouped together as the hippocampal formation. In man, the attenuated gray and white structures of this formation are produced by the enormous enlargement of the corpus callosum, which encroaches upon the parahippocampal and dentate gyri and the hippocampi, thus expanding them.

The *indusium griseum* is a thin layer of gray matter spread over the upper surface of the corpus callosum. Anteriorly, it curves around the genu and rostrum to merge with the paraterminal gyri; laterally, it becomes continuous with the cortex of the cingulate gyrus; and posteriorly, it passes over the splenium to blend with the dentate and parahippocampal gyri through the narrow gyrus fasciolaris. Two slender strands of white fibers, the

**Rhinencephalon and Limbic System**

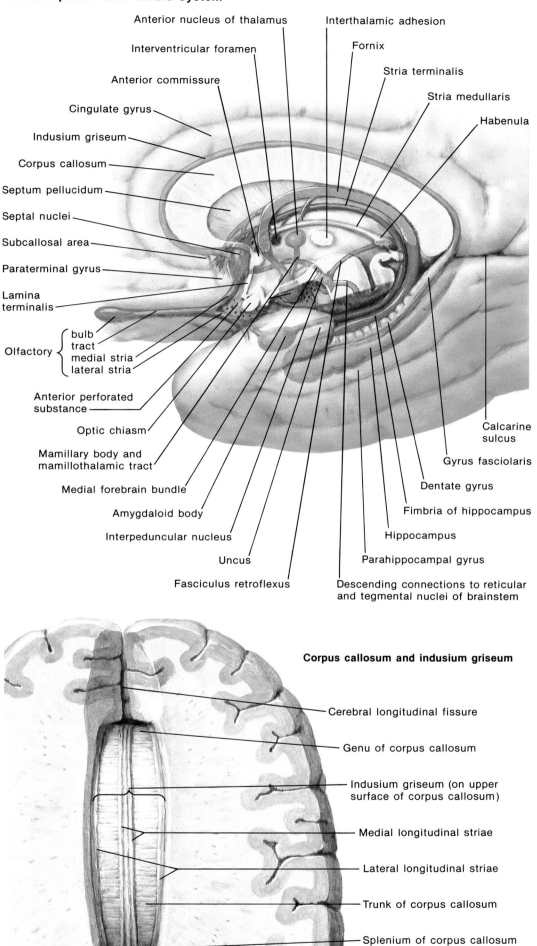

Anterior nucleus of thalamus
Interthalamic adhesion
Interventricular foramen
Fornix
Anterior commissure
Stria terminalis
Cingulate gyrus
Stria medullaris
Indusium griseum
Habenula
Corpus callosum
Septum pellucidum
Septal nuclei
Subcallosal area
Paraterminal gyrus
Lamina terminalis
Olfactory { bulb / tract / medial stria / lateral stria }
Anterior perforated substance
Optic chiasm
Calcarine sulcus
Mamillary body and mamillothalamic tract
Gyrus fasciolaris
Medial forebrain bundle
Dentate gyrus
Amygdaloid body
Fimbria of hippocampus
Interpeduncular nucleus
Hippocampus
Uncus
Parahippocampal gyrus
Fasciculus retroflexus
Descending connections to reticular and tegmental nuclei of brainstem

**Corpus callosum and indusium griseum**

Cerebral longitudinal fissure
Genu of corpus callosum
Indusium griseum (on upper surface of corpus callosum)
Medial longitudinal striae
Lateral longitudinal striae
Trunk of corpus callosum
Splenium of corpus callosum

## Rhinencephalon and Limbic System
*(Continued)*

*medial* and *lateral longitudinal striae*, are embedded in the indusium griseum.

The *hippocampus* is a part of the marginal cortex of the parahippocampal gyrus that has been invaginated, or rolled, into the floor of the inferior horn of the lateral ventricle by the exuberant growth of the nearby temporal cortex. The curved hippocampal eminence is composed mostly of gray matter, and its anterior end is expanded and grooved like a paw, the *pes hippocampi*. Axons conveying efferent impulses from the pyramidal cells of the hippocampus form a white layer on its surface, the *alveus*, and then converge toward its medial edge to form a white strip, the *fimbria*. The hippocampus is an important part of the olfactory apparatus in lower animals; in man, few or no secondary olfactory fibers end in it. However, it possesses substantial connections with the hypothalamus, which regulates many visceral activities that influence emotional behavior, and with temporal lobe areas reputedly associated with memory.

The *dentate gyrus* (dentate fascia) is a crenated fringe of cortex occupying the narrow furrow between the fimbria of the hippocampus and the parahippocampal gyrus. Anteriorly, this fringe fades away on the surface of the uncus, and posteriorly, it becomes continuous with the indusium griseum through the gyrus fasciolaris.

*The fornix* is an almost circular arrangement of white fibers conveying the great majority of the hippocampal efferents to the hypothalamus (see Section VIII, Plate 54) and carrying commissural fibers to the opposite hippocampus and habenular trigone. The fornix rises out of the fimbria of the hippocampus, which turns upward beneath the splenium of the corpus callosum and above the thalamus to form the *crura* (posterior columns) of the fornix. Anterior to the *commissure* of the fornix, the two crura unite for a variable distance in the midline and create the triangular *body* of the fornix. The free lateral edges of the fornix help to bound the choroid fissure, through which the pia mater of the tela choroidea becomes invaginated into the lateral ventricles.

Above the interventricular foramina, the two halves of the body of the fornix separate to become the (anterior) *columns* of the fornix. As each column descends, it sinks into the corresponding lateral wall of the third ventricle; the majority of its fibers end in the *mamillary body*, although some also pass to other hypothalamic nuclei.

The fornix is the main efferent pathway from the hippocampus to the hypothalamus. Fibers ending in the mamillary body form synapses

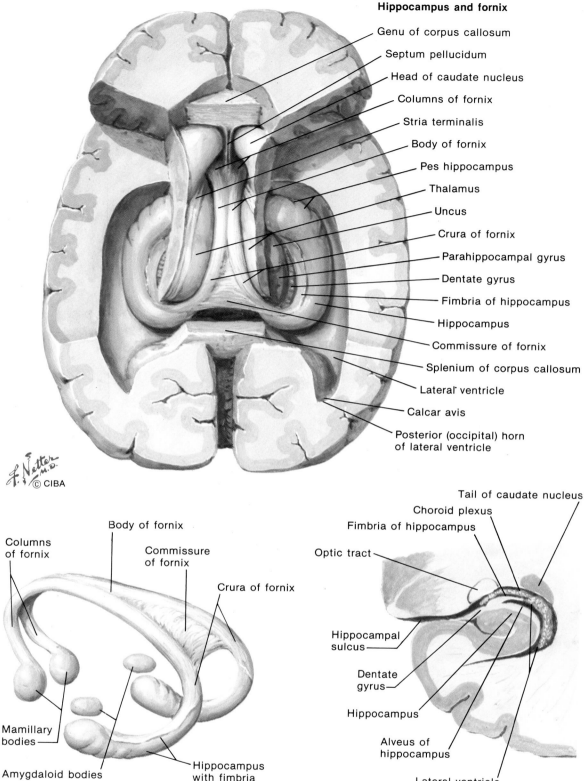

**Hippocampus and fornix**

- Genu of corpus callosum
- Septum pellucidum
- Head of caudate nucleus
- Columns of fornix
- Stria terminalis
- Body of fornix
- Pes hippocampus
- Thalamus
- Uncus
- Crura of fornix
- Parahippocampal gyrus
- Dentate gyrus
- Fimbria of hippocampus
- Hippocampus
- Commissure of fornix
- Splenium of corpus callosum
- Lateral ventricle
- Calcar avis
- Posterior (occipital) horn of lateral ventricle

Columns of fornix
Body of fornix
Commissure of fornix
Crura of fornix
Mamillary bodies
Amygdaloid bodies
Hippocampus with fimbria

Tail of caudate nucleus
Choroid plexus
Fimbria of hippocampus
Optic tract
Hippocampal sulcus
Dentate gyrus
Hippocampus
Alveus of hippocampus
Lateral ventricle

around its cells. The axons of these cells pass upward in the mamillothalamic tract to the homolateral anterior thalamic nucleus, from which they are relayed to the cingulate gyrus.

*Other Structures*. The *habenular trigone* is a small area found bilaterally between the posterior end of the thalamus, the superior (cranial) colliculus and the stalk of the pineal gland. Each trigone overlies a *habenular nucleus*, which receives afferent fibers via the *stria medullaris* of the thalamus (stria habenularis), a fine strand demarcating the superior and medial surfaces of the thalamus. This stria conveys fibers from the anterior perforated substance, the paraterminal gyrus and subcallosal

area, and perhaps other fibers detached from the stria terminalis near the interventricular foramen. Most of these fibers end in the homolateral habenular nucleus, but some decussate in the small habenular commissure lying above the stalk of the pineal gland. The fresh relay of fibers arising in the habenular nucleus passes by way of the fasciculus retroflexus to the *interpeduncular nucleus* in the posterior (interpeduncular) perforated substance. Efferent fibers from the interpeduncular nucleus then descend in or near the medial longitudinal fasciculus to be distributed to tegmental and reticular nuclei in the brainstem. The *amygdaloid body* is described on page 26. □

# Thalamus

The thalami are two symmetrically arranged, large, nuclear masses embedded in the cerebral white matter toward the bases of the hemispheres. Along with the hypothalamus and smaller structures, such as the geniculate bodies, the pineal gland (body) and the habenulae, they are developed from the *diencephalon* (interbrain) between the telencephalon and mesencephalon (see Section VII). The diencephalic cavity becomes the third ventricle.

***Anatomical Relations.*** The thalami are ovoid in shape, with their long axes (about 4 cm) tilted slightly downward posteriorly. They help to form the lateral walls of the third ventricle and project for some distance behind it. Each thalamus has two "ends" and four "surfaces."

The smaller anterior end is near the median plane and forms the posterior boundary of the ipsilateral interventricular foramen. Its upper surface is slightly raised as the *anterior thalamic tubercle*. The larger posterior end projects backward as the rounded *pulvinar* above the ipsilateral superior (cranial) colliculus and habenula.

The superior surface is separated from the medial surface by a slender white strand, the *stria medullaris* of the thalamus (see page 29), and from the lateral thalamic surface and the body of the caudate nucleus by the *stria terminalis* and thalamostriate vein. It has a thin coating of white matter, ·the *stratum zonale*. The outer part of the superior surface lies in the floor of the central part of the lateral ventricle and is partly overlaid by the choroid plexus, which is the frilled edge of the tela choroidea of the third ventricle. The inner part of the superior surface is separated from the body of the fornix by the tela choroidea, but usually shows a shallow impression produced by the overlying fornix.

The inferior surface lies mainly above the tegmentum of the midbrain, which is often termed the *subthalamic tegmental region*, and which contains the subthalamic nucleus, the upper (cranial) ends of the red nuclei and substantia nigra, the zona incerta, and the ansa lenticularis and ansa peduncularis. Many fiber tracts and fasciculi—including the medial, spinal and trigeminal lemnisci, and the rubrothalamic, reticulothalamic, dentatothalamic (cerebellothalamic) tracts—enter the thalamus through this surface. Anteriorly, it is in contact with the posterior part of the hypothalamus.

The medial thalamic surface forms the superior and posterior parts of the lateral wall of the third ventricle. It is demarcated from the hypothalamus by the curved and often indistinct hypothalamic sulcus (Plate 2) that extends from the interventricular foramen to the cerebral (mesencephalic) aqueduct in the midbrain. The medial surfaces are joined by a band (or bands)—the *interthalamic adhesion* (massa intermedia).

The lateral surface is separated from the lentiform nucleus by the posterior limb of the internal capsule (Plate 4). Multiple fibers, the *thalamic radiations*, stream out from this surface en route to the cerebral cortex (see Section VIII, Plate 41). These fibers form the *external medullary lamina*,

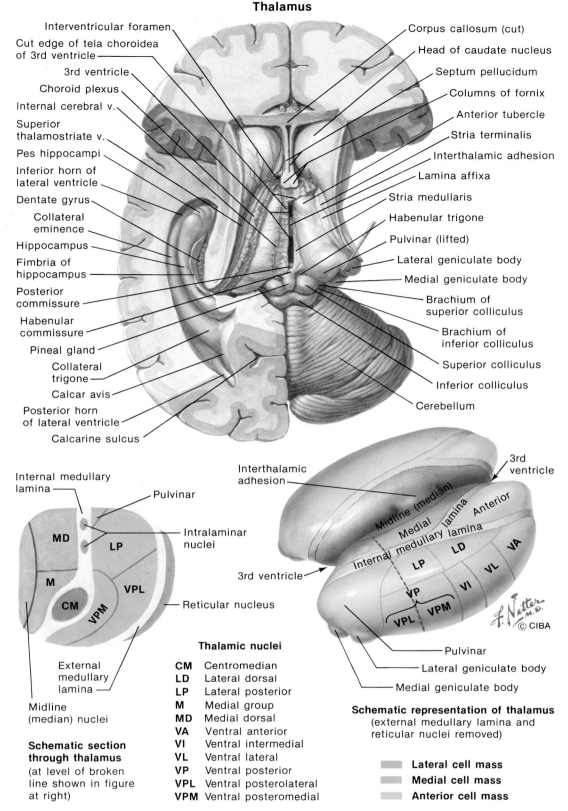

**Thalamus**

Interventricular foramen
Cut edge of tela choroidea of 3rd ventricle
3rd ventricle
Choroid plexus
Internal cerebral v.
Superior thalamostriate v.
Pes hippocampi
Inferior horn of lateral ventricle
Dentate gyrus
Collateral eminence
Hippocampus
Fimbria of hippocampus
Posterior commissure
Habenular commissure
Pineal gland
Collateral trigone
Calcar avis
Posterior horn of lateral ventricle
Calcarine sulcus

Corpus callosum (cut)
Head of caudate nucleus
Septum pellucidum
Columns of fornix
Anterior tubercle
Stria terminalis
Interthalamic adhesion
Lamina affixa
Stria medullaris
Habenular trigone
Pulvinar (lifted)
Lateral geniculate body
Medial geniculate body
Brachium of superior colliculus
Brachium of inferior colliculus
Superior colliculus
Inferior colliculus
Cerebellum

Internal medullary lamina
Pulvinar
MD
LP
M
VPL
CM
VPM
External medullary lamina
Midline (median) nuclei
Intralaminar nuclei
Reticular nucleus

**Schematic section through thalamus**
(at level of broken line shown in figure at right)

**Thalamic nuclei**

| | |
|---|---|
| **CM** | Centromedian |
| **LD** | Lateral dorsal |
| **LP** | Lateral posterior |
| **M** | Medial group |
| **MD** | Medial dorsal |
| **VA** | Ventral anterior |
| **VI** | Ventral intermedial |
| **VL** | Ventral lateral |
| **VP** | Ventral posterior |
| **VPL** | Ventral posterolateral |
| **VPM** | Ventral posteromedial |

Interthalamic adhesion
3rd ventricle
Midline (median)
Medial
Internal medullary lamina
Anterior
LD
VA
LP
VL
VI
VP
VPL
VPM
3rd ventricle
Pulvinar
Lateral geniculate body
Medial geniculate body

**Schematic representation of thalamus**
(external medullary lamina and reticular nuclei removed)

Lateral cell mass
Medial cell mass
Anterior cell mass

coated on its outer surface by an attenuated layer of nerve cells, the thalamic *reticular nucleus*.

***Thalamic Nuclei.*** Each thalamus consists primarily of gray matter, incompletely subdivided into anterior, medial and lateral groups of nuclei by a nearly vertical septum of white matter, the *internal medullary lamina*, which contains small groups of cells, the *intralaminar nuclei*. The septum splits anteriorly in a Y-shaped fashion to demarcate the *anterior thalamic nuclei*, the smallest of the three groups. The *medial thalamic nuclei*—these and the anterior nuclei constitute the older paleothalamus—include the median, or midline, nuclei, eg, the paraventricular, rhomboidal and

reunient. The *lateral nuclei*, which evolved later and have become increasingly important, are the larger group of nuclei and constitute the *neothalamus*. Various classifications and names based on morphological, comparative, experimental and other criteria have been suggested for the multiple constituent nuclei. The relatively small subdivisions of the anterior and medial nuclei are not shown, but the much larger components of the lateral nucleus are illustrated in the lower schematic diagrams.

The thalami are connected with most other parts of the CNS, and thus play a key role in many nervous activities (see Section VIII). □

**Ventricles of Brain**

## Ventricles of Brain

Within the substance of the brain are four communicating cavities—the right and left lateral, third and fourth ventricles (see Section VII, Plates 4 and 5). Each contains a choroid plexus that produces cerebrospinal fluid (Plate 9).

*The lateral ventricles* are extensive, irregular cavities within the cerebral hemispheres. Each consists of a central part, with anterior, posterior and inferior horns. The *central part* extends from the interventricular foramen to the splenium and is bounded above by the corpus callosum; medially, by the posterior part of the septum pellucidum; and below, by parts of the caudate nucleus, thalamus, choroid plexus and fornix. The *anterior (frontal) horn* extends forward and is bounded above by the corpus callosum; medially, by the anterior part of the septum pellucidum; and inferolaterally, by the bulging head of the caudate nucleus; in front, it is limited by the genu of the corpus callosum. The *posterior (occipital) horn* tapers to a blind end (Plate 6). Its roof and lateral wall are formed by fibers of the corpus callosum, and the medial wall shows two elevations—the bulb of the posterior horn and the calcar avis. The *inferior (temporal) horn* curves downward behind the thalamus, passes forward into the temporal lobe, and ends blindly about 2.5 cm behind the temporal pole. Radiating fibers from the corpus callosum form most of its roof and lateral wall. The tail of the caudate nucleus and the amygdaloid body also lie in the roof. The floor is formed by the hippocampus, the fimbria of the hippocampus and the collateral eminence.

The *choroid plexus* of each lateral ventricle extends in an arched fashion from the interventricular foramen to the extremity of the inferior horn (see Section III, Plate 14). The pial vessels forming the plexuses invaginate the ependymal ventricular lining along the choroidal fissure, which lies between the lateral edge of the fornix and the superior and posterior surfaces of the thalamus, and the lining in the inferior horn between the tail of the caudate nucleus and the fimbria of the hippocampus. Between the fornix and thalamus, the pia mater is arranged as a triangular double fold, the *tela choroidea of the third ventricle*. Its apex reaches the contiguous interventricular foramina, and its base is on a level with the posterior surfaces of the thalami, and here the two layers separate. The upper layer ascends to become continuous with the pia over the splenium of the corpus callosum, and the lower layer descends to become continuous with the pia over the tectum. The edges of this tela project as choroid plexuses into the central parts of the lateral ventricles, and the choroid

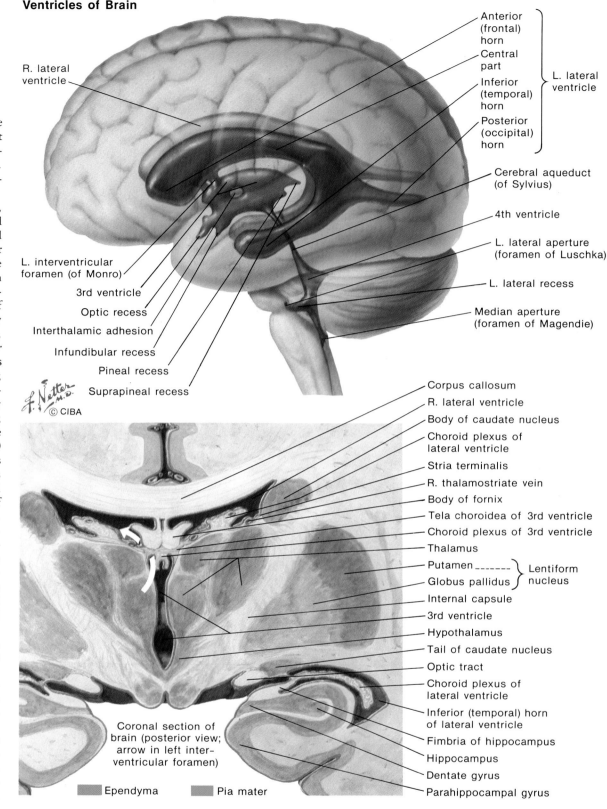

R. lateral ventricle

Anterior (frontal) horn
Central part
Inferior (temporal) horn
Posterior (occipital) horn

L. lateral ventricle

Cerebral aqueduct (of Sylvius)
4th ventricle
L. lateral aperture (foramen of Luschka)
L. lateral recess
Median aperture (foramen of Magendie)

L. interventricular foramen (of Monro)
3rd ventricle
Optic recess
Interthalamic adhesion
Infundibular recess
Pineal recess
Suprapineal recess

Corpus callosum
R. lateral ventricle
Body of caudate nucleus
Choroid plexus of lateral ventricle
Stria terminalis
R. thalamostriate vein
Body of fornix
Tela choroidea of 3rd ventricle
Choroid plexus of 3rd ventricle
Thalamus
Putamen
Globus pallidus
} Lentiform nucleus
Internal capsule
3rd ventricle
Hypothalamus
Tail of caudate nucleus
Optic tract
Choroid plexus of lateral ventricle
Inferior (temporal) horn of lateral ventricle
Fimbria of hippocampus
Hippocampus
Dentate gyrus
Parahippocampal gyrus

Coronal section of brain (posterior view; arrow in left interventricular foramen)

Ependyma          Pia mater

plexus of the third ventricle hangs from it as fringed folds, close to the medial plane.

*The third ventricle* is a median cleft separating the two thalami and the adjacent halves of the hypothalamus (see CIBA COLLECTION, Volume 4, page 36). It possesses a roof, a floor and four walls: anterior, posterior and two lateral. The *roof* is formed by the tela choroidea. The *floor* is made up of the optic chiasm, the tuber cinereum and infundibulum, the mamillary bodies, the posterior perforated substance and the uppermost part of the mesencephalic tegmentum. The *anterior wall* is the delicate lamina terminalis that stretches from the optic chiasm to the rostrum;

near its upper end are the anterior (rostral) commissure and the interventricular foramina. The short *posterior wall* is formed by the stalk of the pineal gland and the posterior (epithalamic) and habenular commissures. *On each side*, the third ventricle is bounded posterosuperiorly by the medial surfaces of the thalami, and anteroinferiorly, by the opposite halves of the hypothalamus. The short *interthalamic adhesion* (massa intermedia) bridges the narrow ventricular space. The third ventricle communicates with the lateral ventricles through the *interventricular foramina* and with the fourth ventricle through the narrow *cerebral (sylvian or mesencephalic) aqueduct* (Plate 10).  □

# Circulation of Cerebrospinal Fluid

The ventricles of the brain, the central canal of the spinal cord and the subarachnoid spaces contain cerebrospinal fluid (CSF), which acts as a liquid buffer to absorb and distribute external or internal forces endangering the brain and cord. By variations in its volume, it regulates the total capacity of the cranium and spinal canal (see Section VII, Plates 5, 7 and 8).

There are no lymphatics in the CNS, and the CSF largely performs the function carried out by lymph in other tissues. It also acts as a medium for the transfer of substances between the blood and nervous tissues, but there is a selective "blood-brain" barrier interposed between the blood and CSF by the endothelial cells of the capillaries and choroid plexuses. This is clinically important because some drugs cannot penetrate the barrier, although its permeability shows regional variations. Thus, interchange of electrolytes occurs more readily in the ventricles than in the subarachnoid cisterns, whereas water exchange is more rapid in the cisterns than in the ventricles.

Most of the CSF is elaborated by the *choroid plexuses*, but whether this is a result of dialysis or secretion, or a combination of both, is uncertain. Experiments with radioisotopes have shown that small amounts of CSF are formed in the subarachnoid and perivascular spaces. In the adult, there is continuous formation, circulation and absorption of about 125 to 150 ml of fluid. It has been calculated that 430 to 450 ml of CSF are produced every day, so the fluid must be changed every 6 to 7 hours.

The choroid plexuses are fringes of capillary tufts from the pia mater invaginating the delicate ependymal walls of the ventricles (Plate 8; see also Section III, Plates 4 and 14). The choroid plexuses of the *lateral ventricles* are the largest and produce most of the CSF. The fluid flows through the *interventricular foramina (of Monro)* into the *third ventricle*, is augmented by fluid formed by the choroid plexus of this ventricle, and passes through the *cerebral (sylvian) aqueduct* to the *fourth ventricle* (Plate 10), which also possesses a choroid plexus. The CSF from all these sources, as well as any formed in the central canal of the spinal cord, escapes from the fourth ventricle into the *subarachnoid space* through the *median aperture (of Magendie)* and *lateral apertures (of Luschka)*.

The CSF then circulates through the freely communicating subarachnoid cisterns at the base of the brain. These are: (1) the *cerebellomedullary cistern (cisterna magna)*, which bridges the medulla oblongata; (2) the *prepontine cistern (cisterna pontis)*,

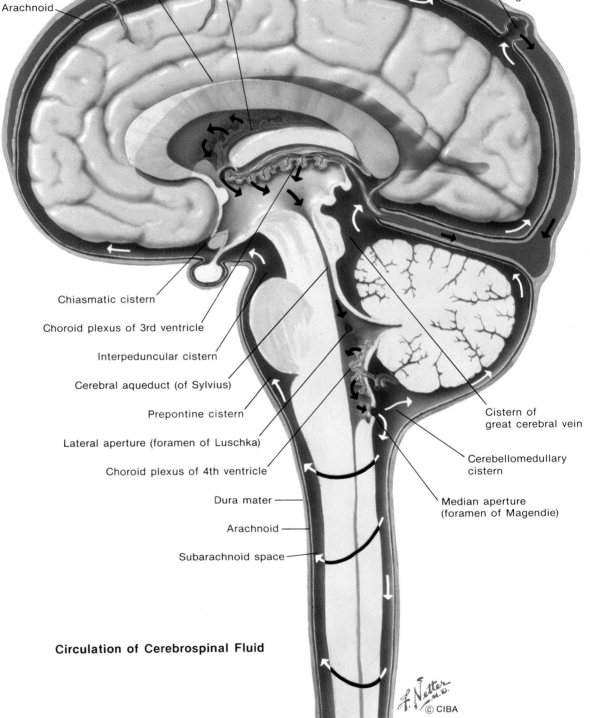

**Circulation of Cerebrospinal Fluid**

Labels (clockwise from top):
Choroid plexus of lateral ventricle
Supracallosal cistern
Dura mater
Arachnoid
Superior sagittal sinus
Subarachnoid space
Arachnoid granulations
Chiasmatic cistern
Choroid plexus of 3rd ventricle
Interpeduncular cistern
Cerebral aqueduct (of Sylvius)
Prepontine cistern
Lateral aperture (foramen of Luschka)
Choroid plexus of 4th ventricle
Dura mater
Arachnoid
Subarachnoid space
Cistern of great cerebral vein
Cerebellomedullary cistern
Median aperture (foramen of Magendie)

which lies on the anterior surface of the pons; (3) the *interpeduncular cistern*, which is located between the medial surfaces of the temporal lobes; (4) the *chiasmatic cistern*, which surrounds the optic chiasm; (5) the *cistern of the lateral fossa*, which bridges the lateral fissure of the temporal lobes; and (6) the *cistern of the great cerebral vein (cisterna ambiens)*, which occupies the space between the corpus callosum and the cerebellum. From the cisterns, most of the CSF is directed upward over the cerebral hemispheres toward the *superior sagittal sinus*, but smaller amounts pass downward around the spinal cord. Because the subarachnoid space in the adult extends to the

level of the second sacral vertebra (Plate 14), CSF can be obtained, without damaging the spinal cord, by a "lumbar puncture" through the interspaces between the spinous processes of the lower lumbar vertebrae.

The CSF is reabsorbed into the blood through the *arachnoid villi* (see Section III, Plates 7 and 11) and through the walls of the capillaries of the CNS and pia mater. Some of the fluid contained within the sheaths of the cranial and spinal nerves finds its way into extradural lymph vessels. If intracranial pressure is abnormally raised, reabsorption may also occur through the choroid plexuses. □

## Fourth Ventricle and Cerebellum

**Posterior view**

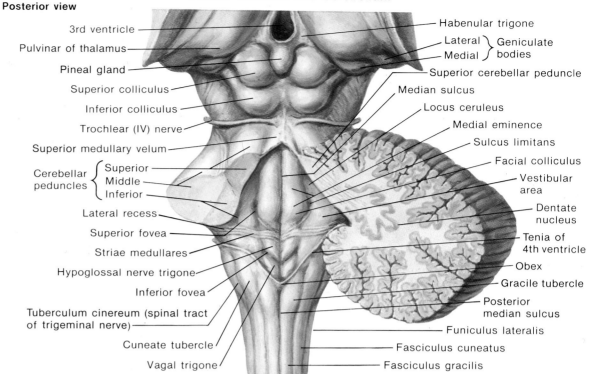

3rd ventricle
Pulvinar of thalamus
Pineal gland
Superior colliculus
Inferior colliculus
Trochlear (IV) nerve
Superior medullary velum
Cerebellar peduncles { Superior / Middle / Inferior }
Lateral recess
Superior fovea
Striae medullares
Hypoglossal nerve trigone
Inferior fovea
Tuberculum cinereum (spinal tract of trigeminal nerve)
Cuneate tubercle
Vagal trigone

Habenular trigone
Lateral } Geniculate
Medial } bodies
Superior cerebellar peduncle
Median sulcus
Locus ceruleus
Medial eminence
Sulcus limitans
Facial colliculus
Vestibular area
Dentate nucleus
Tenia of 4th ventricle
Obex
Gracile tubercle
Posterior median sulcus
Funiculus lateralis
Fasciculus cuneatus
Fasciculus gracilis

# Fourth Ventricle

The fourth ventricle lies posterior to the pons and upper half of the medulla oblongata and anterior to the cerebellum (Plates 8 and 9). Its upper and lower ends become continuous, respectively, with the cerebral (sylvian, or mesencephalic) aqueduct and the central canal of the spinal cord in the lower half of the medulla. On each side, a narrow prolongation, the *lateral recess*, projects outward from its widest part and curves around the brainstem above the corresponding inferior (caudal) cerebellar peduncle; its *lateral aperture* (foramen of Luschka) lies below the cerebellar flocculus and behind the emerging rootlets of the glossopharyngeal (IX) and vagus (X) nerves. The fourth ventricle has lateral boundaries, a roof and a floor.

*The lateral boundaries* are formed on each side from above down by the superior (cranial) cerebellar peduncle, the inferior cerebellar peduncle and the cuneate and gracile tubercles.

*Roof of Fourth Ventricle.* The upper and lower parts of the V-shaped roof are formed by the *superior* and *inferior medullary vela*, which are thin laminae of white matter between the superior and inferior cerebellar peduncles. The lower part of the inferior velum has a *median aperture* (foramen of Magendie); cerebrospinal fluid escapes through this opening and the lateral apertures into the subarachnoid space. Because these are the only communications between the ventricular and subarachnoid spaces, their blockage can produce one type of hydrocephalus.

The lower part of the roof and the posterior walls of the lateral recesses are invaginated by vascular tufts of pia mater, which form the T-shaped *choroid plexus of the fourth ventricle.*

*The floor of the fourth ventricle* is rhomboid-shaped and is divided into symmetrical halves by a vertical *median sulcus*. Its upper (pontine) and lower (medullary) parts are demarcated by delicate transverse strands of fibers, the *striae medullares* of the fourth ventricle.

On each side of the median sulcus is a longitudinal elevation, the *medial eminence*, lateral to which runs the *sulcus limitans*. Its superior part is the *locus ceruleus*, colored bluish-gray from a patch of deeply pigmented nerve cells. Also lateral to the upper part of the medial eminence is a slight depression, the *superior fovea*, and just below and medial to this fovea is a rounded swelling, the

**Median sagittal section**

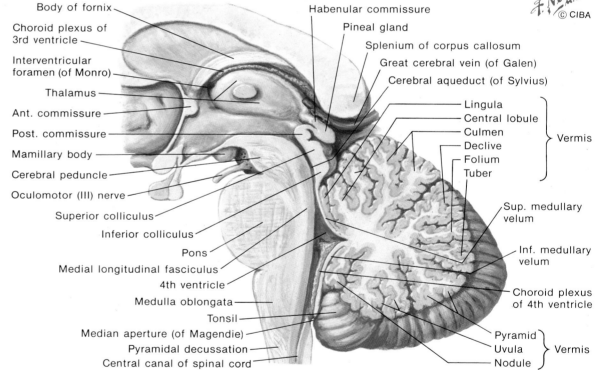

Body of fornix
Choroid plexus of 3rd ventricle
Interventricular foramen (of Monro)
Thalamus
Ant. commissure
Post. commissure
Mamillary body
Cerebral peduncle
Oculomotor (III) nerve
Superior colliculus
Inferior colliculus
Pons
Medial longitudinal fasciculus
4th ventricle
Medulla oblongata
Tonsil
Median aperture (of Magendie)
Pyramidal decussation
Central canal of spinal cord

Habenular commissure
Pineal gland
Splenium of corpus callosum
Great cerebral vein (of Galen)
Cerebral aqueduct (of Sylvius)
Lingula
Central lobule
Culmen
Declive
Folium
Tuber
} Vermis
Sup. medullary velum
Inf. medullary velum
Choroid plexus of 4th ventricle
Pyramid
Uvula
Nodule
} Vermis

*F. Netter M.D.*
© CIBA

*facial colliculus*, which overlies the nucleus of the abducens (VI) nerve and the facial (VII) nerve fibers encircling it; the motor nucleus of the facial nerve lies more deeply in the pons. Inferolateral to the superior fovea is the *upper part of the vestibular area*, which overlies parts of the nuclei of the vestibulocochlear (VIII) nerve.

The lower (medullary) part of the medial eminence overlies the twelfth cranial nerve nucleus, and is termed the *hypoglossal trigone*. Lateral to it is a slight depression, the *inferior fovea*, which, together with the neighboring *vagal trigone*, overlies parts of the dorsal nuclei of the glossopharyngeal and vagus nerves. Lateral to the inferior fovea

is the *lower part of the vestibular area*, overlying parts of the vestibular nuclei of the vestibulocochlear nerve. On a deeper plane, parts of the trigeminal, solitary tract and ambiguus nuclei also underlie the floor of the fourth ventricle. Some of the nuclei mentioned, such as the dorsal vagal and ambiguus nuclei, as well as others located in the nearby reticular formation, are concerned with cardiovascular, respiratory, metabolic and other very important functions, and are known as "vital centers." Any lesion in this relatively small area of the brain may therefore produce disastrous results. (This region is more fully described in Sections V and VIII.) □

# Cerebellum

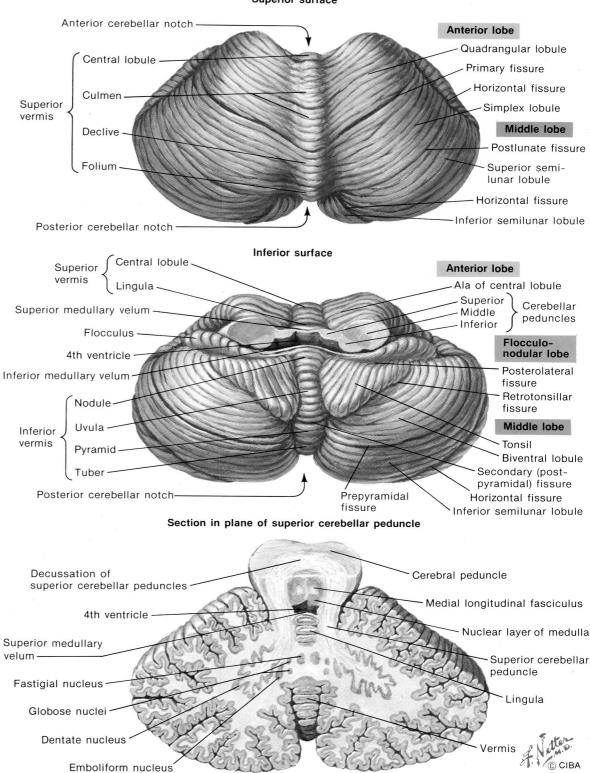

**Superior surface**

Anterior cerebellar notch

Central lobule

Culmen

Superior vermis

Declive

Folium

Posterior cerebellar notch

Anterior lobe
- Quadrangular lobule
- Primary fissure
- Horizontal fissure
- Simplex lobule

Middle lobe
- Postlunate fissure
- Superior semilunar lobule
- Horizontal fissure
- Inferior semilunar lobule

**Inferior surface**

Superior vermis { Central lobule / Lingula

Superior medullary velum

Flocculus

4th ventricle

Inferior medullary velum

Inferior vermis { Nodule / Uvula / Pyramid / Tuber

Posterior cerebellar notch

Prepyramidal fissure

Anterior lobe
- Ala of central lobule
- Superior / Middle / Inferior } Cerebellar peduncles

Flocculonodular lobe
- Posterolateral fissure
- Retrotonsillar fissure

Middle lobe
- Tonsil
- Biventral lobule
- Secondary (postpyramidal) fissure
- Horizontal fissure
- Inferior semilunar lobule

**Section in plane of superior cerebellar peduncle**

Decussation of superior cerebellar peduncles

4th ventricle

Superior medullary velum

Fastigial nucleus

Globose nuclei

Dentate nucleus

Emboliform nucleus

- Cerebral peduncle
- Medial longitudinal fasciculus
- Nuclear layer of medulla
- Superior cerebellar peduncle
- Lingula
- Vermis

The cerebellum is the largest part of the hindbrain and occupies the greater part of the posterior cranial fossa. It is separated from the overlying cerebrum by the tentorium cerebelli and consists of two *hemispheres* united by a median *vermis*, which appears on the superior (cranial) surface as a low ridge and projects below into the *vallecula*, a deep groove separating the hemispheres inferiorly. Anteriorly, there is a wide hollow occupied by the pons, the upper part of the medulla oblongata and the fourth ventricle. Posteriorly, there is a narrow median notch, which lodges the falx cerebelli. A horizontal fissure encircles each hemisphere, demarcating *superior (cranial)* and *inferior (caudal) surfaces.*

*The surfaces of the cerebellum* show numerous parallel curved fissures separating narrow folia. Crossing the superior surface and dividing the *anterior* from the *middle lobe* is a V-shaped *primary fissure,* with its apex backward and limbs that end in front, in the *horizontal fissure.* The primary fissure separates parts of the superior vermis known as the *culmen* and *declive.* About midway between the primary fissure and the posterolateral border of each hemisphere is the *postlunate fissure.* These fissures subdivide the superior surface into *quadrangular, simplex* and *superior semilunar lobules.*

On the inferior surface, the most obvious fissures demarcate the *flocculonodular lobe,* the *tonsil* and the *biventral lobule.* The inferior part of the vermis is subdivided from before backward, into the *nodule, uvula, pyramid* and *tuber.* The prepyramidal and the postpyramidal fissure may seem to be misplaced, unless it is understood that as the developing cerebellum expands backward, its caudal part becomes folded underneath and then passes forward to come into contact with the medullary velum. Thus, parts that were originally posterior on the superior surface become anterior on the definitive inferior surface.

The *posterolateral fissure* lies posterior to the flocculus and becomes continuous with its fellow across the midline by extending between the nodule and uvula. The *flocculus* is a small, semidetached portion of the cerebellum, lying close to the middle (pontine) cerebellar peduncle. Each flocculus is attached to the *nodule* of the median vermis, and together they constitute the *flocculonodular lobe;* this is the oldest part of the cerebellum and has intimate connections with the vestibular nuclei. The *secondary (postpyramidal) fissure* lies between the uvula and pyramid and

extends laterally into the *retrotonsillar fissures* that separate the tonsil and the biventral lobules. The *prepyramidal fissures* intervene between the biventral and inferior semilunar lobules and are continuous across the vermis by a fissure demarcating the pyramid and tuber.

*The interior of the cerebellum* consists of a central mass of white matter surrounded by a gray cortex. Some smaller masses of gray matter, which include the fastigial, globose and emboliform nuclei, exist within the central white core, but only one mass on each side, the *dentate nucleus,* is conspicuous. From the open end of its U-shaped lamina, many fibers emerge to form the major

part of the cerebellorubral tract and the ipsilateral superior (cranial) cerebellar peduncle.

The white matter sends out numerous laminae and secondary laminae, which project into the cortical folia. On section (Plate 10), this branching arrangement has a characteristic appearance termed the *arbor vitae cerebelli.* Some fibers in this "tree" are associative and connect different areas in the same hemisphere; others are commissural and connect similar areas in opposite hemispheres. The remaining fibers are itinerant and are aggregated together on each side into *superior, middle* and *inferior cerebellar peduncles* (described more fully in Section VIII). □

**Brainstem**

# Brainstem

The brainstem comprises the midbrain, pons and medulla oblongata (see Section VII, Plates 6 and 8).

*The midbrain* lies between the cerebrum and the pons and is about 2.5 cm long. The smaller part—dorsal to the cerebral aqueduct—is the *tectum*; it is formed mainly by superior (cranial) and inferior (caudal) pairs of colliculi (corpora quadrigemina). The *superior colliculi* receive some retinal fibers via the optic tracts and superior brachia; others, from the visual (calcarine) cortex; and still others, from the spinotectal tracts. Some fibers reach the *inferior colliculi* from the lateral lemniscus, the acoustic part of the temporal cortex, and the spinotectal tracts. Tectobulbar and tectospinal tracts originating in the colliculi descend to establish connections with cranial and spinal motor nerve cells. They influence movements of the head and neck in response to visual and auditory stimuli.

The larger part of the midbrain—ventral to the aqueduct—forms the *cerebral peduncles*, two rounded columns that ascend and diverge from the upper border of the pons. Each peduncle is subdivided by a pigmented crescent of gray matter, the *substantia nigra*, into a ventral crus cerebri and a dorsal tegmental part.

Each *crus cerebri* is formed almost entirely by descending fibers. The corticospinal and corticonuclear fibers occupy approximately the middle three fifths of each crus; the frontopontine fibers, the medial fifth; and the temporopontine and parietopontine fibers, the lateral fifth.

The *tegmentum* is separated anteriorly from the crura on each side by the substantia nigra. It is subdivided by a median raphe and contains the red, oculomotor, trochlear, subthalamic, tegmental and reticular nuclei, and the mesencephalic and upper ends of the principal sensory nuclei of the trigeminal nerves. Lemniscal fibers and medial and dorsal longitudinal fasciculi run through the tegmentum, while the cerebellorubral fibers, which reach it via the *superior (cranial) cerebellar peduncles*, decussate in the lower half of the midbrain and mostly end by forming synapses in the red nuclei.

*The pons* lies between the midbrain and medulla oblongata and in front of the cerebellum. The pons proper is the part between the emerging trigeminal (V) nerves, lateral to which are the middle cerebellar peduncles. Ventrally, the pyramidal tracts raise up the overlying transverse

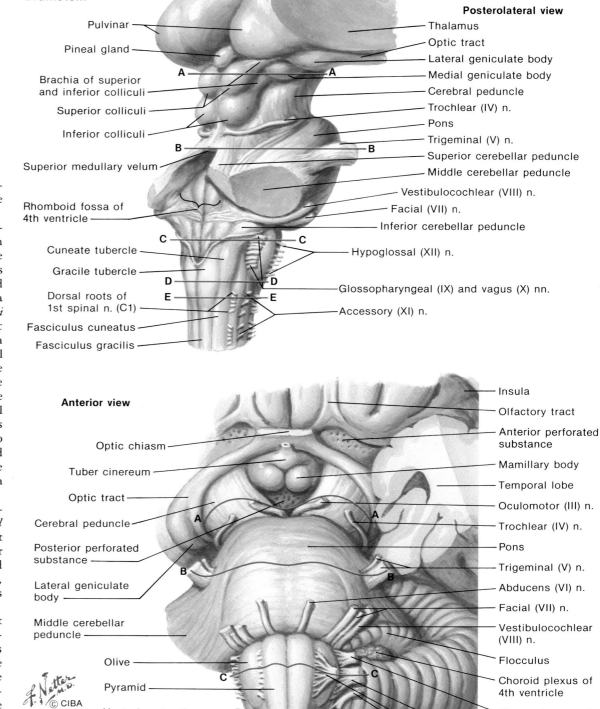

**Posterolateral view**

Pulvinar
Pineal gland
Brachia of superior and inferior colliculi
Superior colliculi
Inferior colliculi
Superior medullary velum
Rhomboid fossa of 4th ventricle
Cuneate tubercle
Gracile tubercle
Dorsal roots of 1st spinal n. (C1)
Fasciculus cuneatus
Fasciculus gracilis

Thalamus
Optic tract
Lateral geniculate body
Medial geniculate body
Cerebral peduncle
Trochlear (IV) n.
Pons
Trigeminal (V) n.
Superior cerebellar peduncle
Middle cerebellar peduncle
Vestibulocochlear (VIII) n.
Facial (VII) n.
Inferior cerebellar peduncle
Hypoglossal (XII) n.
Glossopharyngeal (IX) and vagus (X) nn.
Accessory (XI) n.

**Anterior view**

Optic chiasm
Tuber cinereum
Optic tract
Cerebral peduncle
Posterior perforated substance
Lateral geniculate body
Middle cerebellar peduncle
Olive
Pyramid
Ventral roots of 1st spinal n. (C1)
Pyramidal decussation

Insula
Olfactory tract
Anterior perforated substance
Mamillary body
Temporal lobe
Oculomotor (III) n.
Trochlear (IV) n.
Pons
Trigeminal (V) n.
Abducens (VI) n.
Facial (VII) n.
Vestibulocochlear (VIII) n.
Flocculus
Choroid plexus of 4th ventricle
Glossopharyngeal (IX) n.
Vagus (X) n.
Hypoglossal (XII) n.
Accessory (XI) n.

**A—A to E—E: planes of sections shown in Plate 13**

encephalic and upper ends of the principal sensory nuclei of the trigeminal nerves. Lemniscal fibers and medial and dorsal longitudinal fasciculi run through the tegmentum, while the cerebellorubral fibers, which reach it via the *superior (cranial) cerebellar peduncles*, decussate in the lower half of the midbrain and mostly end by forming synapses in the red nuclei.

fibers to produce a median furrow for the basilar artery. The dorsal surface forms the upper half of the floor of the fourth ventricle.

On transverse section, the pons is seen to consist of ventral and dorsal parts separated by the ascending fibers of the medial, lateral, spinal and trigeminal lemnisci.

The ventral part of the pons contains both longitudinal and transverse fibers intermixed with small masses of gray matter, the *nuclei pontis*. The longitudinal fibers comprise the *pyramidal tracts*, dispersed in this region in discrete bundles, and the *corticopontine fibers*, which form synapses around cells in the nuclei pontis. The axons of

these cells pass transversely across the midline to become aggregated as the *middle cerebellar peduncles*, thus establishing extensive cerebropontine-cerebellar connections.

The dorsal part of the pons contains the *abducens, facial, cochlear* and *trapezoid nuclei*; parts of the *vestibular, motor, mesencephalic* and *sensory trigeminal nuclei*; the *trapezoid body*, a group of fibers forming part of the acoustic pathway that passes from the ventral cochlear nuclei of one side to the heterolateral nuclei of the superior (cranial) olivary complex; and the *reticular formation*, which is continuous above and below with the corresponding areas in the midbrain and medulla.

## Brainstem

*(Continued)*

*The medulla oblongata* is the upward continuation of the spinal cord. It is divided by a median raphe, and each side shows anterolateral and posterolateral sulci, through which emerge the rootlets of the hypoglossal (XII) nerve (anterolateral) and of the glossopharyngeal (IX), vagus (X) and accessory (XI) nerves (posterolateral). The sulci divide the medulla into anterior, lateral and posterior regions, which consist of the pyramids, the olives above and the start of the lateral columns of the cord below, and the lower half of the floor of the fourth ventricle above and the start of the posterior columns of the spinal cord below.

A section through the upper half of the medulla shows convoluted U-shaped laminae of gray matter dorsal to the pyramids, the *inferior olivary nuclei*. Many fibers emerging from the open, medial ends of these nuclei stream across to enter the opposite *inferior (caudal) cerebellar peduncles*. Smaller olivary nuclei give rise to accessory olivocerebellar fibers.

On each side of the median raphe are the *medial lemnisci*, the *tectospinal tracts* and the *medial longitudinal fasciculi*. Subjacent to the lower half of the fourth ventricle on each side are the *hypoglossal, dorsal vagal* and *vestibular nuclei*; deeper still are the *reticular formation*, the *solitary tract* and its *nucleus*, the *nucleus ambiguus*, the *nuclei* and *spinal tract* of the *trigeminal nerve*, and the *spinotectal, anterior (ventral)* and *posterior (dorsal) spinocerebellar, olivospinal, vestibulospinal, rubrospinal, reticulospinal*, and *anterior (ventral)* and *lateral spinothalamic tracts*. The posterolateral margins of the medulla form the inferior cerebellar peduncles.

Other structures appear in the lower half of the medulla, and rearrangements occur in the disposition of the tracts. Near the lower end of the medulla, most of the corticospinal fibers in the pyramidal tracts decussate, incline backward, and become the *lateral corticospinal (crossed pyramidal) tracts*; some 15% to 20% of the fibers continue downward on the ipsilateral side as the *anterior corticospinal (direct pyramidal) tracts*. The fasciculus gracilis and the fasciculus cuneatus terminate in the *gracile* and *cuneate nuclei* located dorsomedially in the lower medulla. The axons of these cells, the *internal arcuate fibers*, cross the midline and turn upward to form the *medial lemnisci*; this great decussation of sensory (lemniscal) fibers is slightly superior to the pyramidal decussation. (See Section VIII for the functional anatomy of the nuclei and tracts discussed above.) □

## Brainstem
**(continued)**

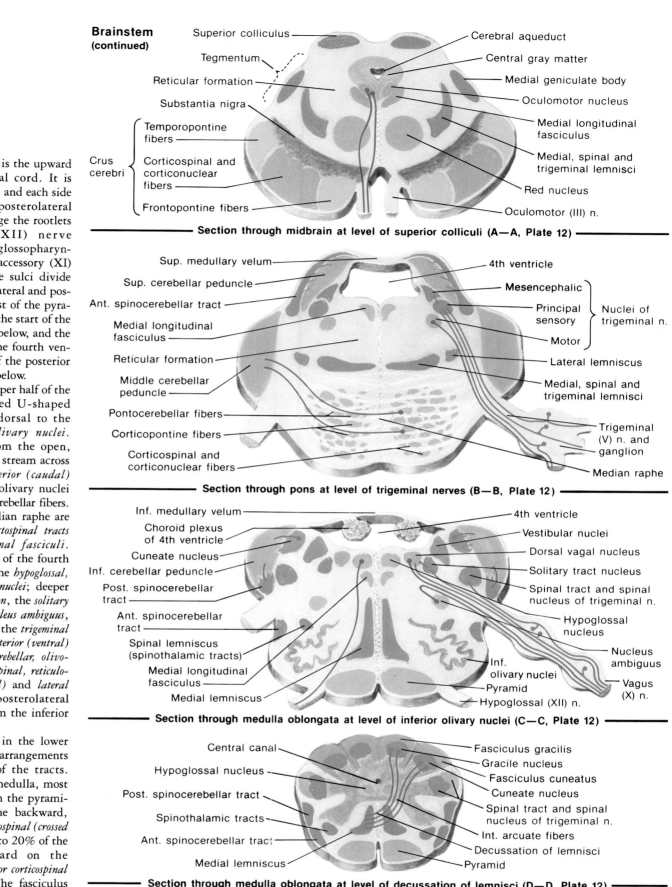

Section through midbrain at level of superior colliculi (A—A, Plate 12)

Section through pons at level of trigeminal nerves (B—B, Plate 12)

Section through medulla oblongata at level of inferior olivary nuclei (C—C, Plate 12)

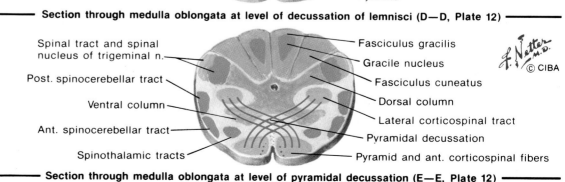

Section through medulla oblongata at level of decussation of lemnisci (D—D, Plate 12)

Section through medulla oblongata at level of pyramidal decussation (E—E, Plate 12)

# Spinal Cord

The spinal cord, or medulla spinalis, is the downward continuation of the medulla oblongata and is about 46 cm long. It extends from the upper border of the atlas to end in a tapering extremity, the *conus medullaris*, opposite the lower border of the first lumbar vertebra, or at the level of the intervertebral disc between the upper two lumbar vertebrae. From the conus, a slender, median, fibrous thread, the *filum terminale*, is prolonged as far as the back of the coccyx. The dura mater and arachnoid (and therefore the subarachnoid space) extend down to the level of the second sacral vertebra. Though generally cylindrical, the cord is slightly flattened anteroposteriorly and shows *cervical* and *lumbar enlargements* that correspond to the segments involved in supplying nerves to the upper and lower limbs. The nerve supply to the upper limb involves the fourth cervical to second thoracic spinal cord segments, and that to the lower limb, the third lumbar to third sacral spinal cord segments (see Section VI, Plates 4 and 10 and Section VII, Plate 4).

*Meninges.* The cord is surrounded by dura, arachnoid and pia mater, which are continuous with the corresponding layers of the cerebral meninges at the foramen magnum (see Section III, Plates 11 and 12). The *spinal dura mater*, unlike the cerebral, consists only of a meningeal layer that is not adherent to the vertebrae; it is separated from the boundaries of the vertebral canal by an epidural space containing fatty areolar tissue and many veins. The spinal and cranial *subarachnoid spaces* are continuous and contain cerebrospinal fluid (Plate 9). The *pia mater* closely invests the cord; on each side, it sends out a series of 22 triangular processes, the *denticulate ligaments*, which are attached to the dura mater and thus anchor the cord (Plate 15). The spinal cord is considerably smaller than the vertebral canal; the meninges, the cerebrospinal fluid and the epidural fatty tissue and veins combine to cushion it against jarring contacts with its bony and ligamentous surroundings.

*Spinal Nerves.* There are 31 pairs (8 cervical, 12 thoracic, 5 lumbar, 5 sacral and 1 coccygeal) of symmetrically arranged *spinal nerves*, attached to the cord in linear series by ventral and dorsal nerve rootlets, or filaments, which coalesce to form the nerve roots. Each dorsal spinal nerve root possesses an oval enlargement, the *spinal (sensory) ganglion* (Plate 16).

In early embryonic life, the cord is as long as the vertebral canal, but as development proceeds, it lags behind the growth of the vertebral column. In consequence, the cord segments move upward

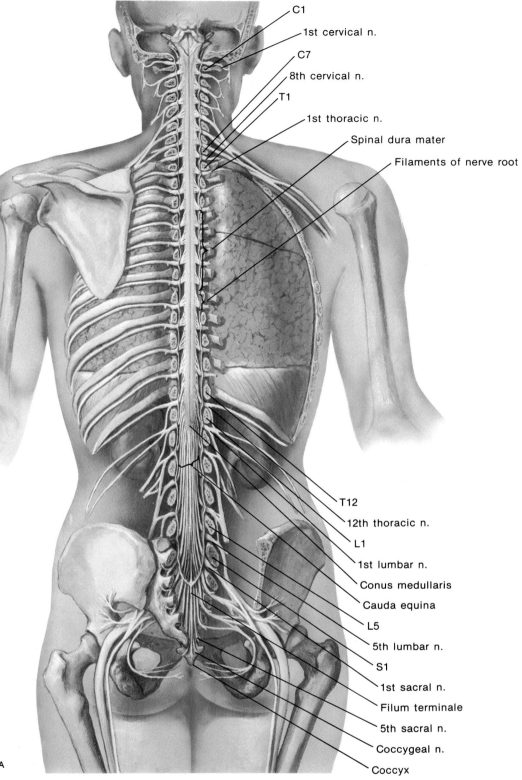

C1
1st cervical n.
C7
8th cervical n.
T1
1st thoracic n.
Spinal dura mater
Filaments of nerve root
T12
12th thoracic n.
L1
1st lumbar n.
Conus medullaris
Cauda equina
L5
5th lumbar n.
S1
1st sacral n.
Filum terminale
5th sacral n.
Coccygeal n.
Coccyx

in relation to the vertebrae, and the nerve roots, originally horizontal, assume an increasingly oblique direction from above downward as they proceed to their foramina of exit. In the adult—except in the upper cervical region—the cord segments lie at varying distances above the corresponding vertebrae. For clinical purposes, it is customary to localize them in relation to the vertebral spinous processes. In the lower cervical region, the vertebral spines are one lower in number than the corresponding cord segments; in the upper thoracic region, two lower in number; and in the lower thoracic region, three lower in number. For example, the fourth thoracic spinous

process is approximately level with the sixth thoracic cord segment. The lumbar, sacral and coccygeal segments of the cord are crowded together and occupy the space approximately opposite the ninth thoracic to the first lumbar vertebra. These alterations of the cord segments relative to the vertebral segments explain why the cervical enlargement (C4 to T2) lies approximately opposite the corresponding vertebrae, whereas the lumbar enlargement (L3 to S3) lies opposite the last three thoracic vertebrae. The nerve roots attached to the lower part of the cord descend to their points of exit as the *cauda equina*, named for their resemblance to the tail of a horse. □

**Spinal Membranes and Nerve Roots**

# Spinal Membranes and Nerve Roots

**Posterior view**

Dura mater

Dorsal root

Spinal ganglion

Arachnoid

Mesothelial septum in posterior median sulcus

Subarachnoid space

Pia mater (overlying spinal cord)

Filaments of dorsal root

Denticulate ligament

**Anterior view**

Gray matter

Filaments of dorsal root

White matter

Dorsal root

Spinal ganglion

Spinal nerve

Ventral root

Filaments of ventral root

Anterior median fissure

*Meninges*. The spinal cord is enveloped by meninges, which, at the level of the foramen magnum, are directly continuous with those surrounding the brain (see Section III, Plates 11 and 12).

The external, tough, fibrous *dura mater* continues downward as far as the second sacral vertebra, where it ends blindly. It is separated from the wall of the vertebral canal by an *epidural space* containing fatty areolar tissue and a plexus of veins. The dura ensheathes the ventral and dorsal spinal nerve roots, which lie close together when they pierce it; then the roots unite almost immediately to form a spinal nerve, and the dural sheath fuses with the epineurium (Plate 16). Between the dura mater and arachnoid is a potential *subdural space*, which normally contains the merest film of lymphlike fluid.

The spinal *arachnoid* is loose and tenuous and also ends at the level of the second sacral vertebra. It is separated from the pia mater by the *subarachnoid space*, which is traversed by delicate mesothelial septa and contains cerebrospinal fluid. The spinal nerve roots, up to the points at which they penetrate the dura mater, are loosely enclosed in arachnoid.

The *pia mater* is a thin layer of vascular connective tissue, which intimately invests the spinal cord and its nerve roots. Below the conus medullaris, it is continuous with the slender *filum terminale* that descends in the midst of the cauda equina, pierces the terminal parts of the dura and arachnoid, and ends by blending with the connective tissue behind the first segment of the coccyx. On each side, the pia is attached to the dura by 22 pointed processes, the *denticulate ligaments*.

*Nerve Roots*. The spinal cord is a segmented structure, and this is indicated by the regular attachments of the pairs of *spinal nerves*. As explained on page 36, the cord and vertebral segments coincide in early embryonic life, but the vertebral canal becomes longer than the cord because of differential rates of growth, so that most of the spinal nerves run obliquely downward to their points of exit.

The nerve filaments, or rootlets, are attached to the cord along its anterolateral and posterolateral regions. The *ventral (anterior) filaments* emerge in two or three irregular rows. They are composed predominantly of efferent fibers, which are the axons of cells in the ventral columns, or horns, of gray matter, and they carry motor impulses to the voluntary muscles. In the thoracic and upper lumbar regions, the filaments also contain preganglionic sympathetic fibers, which are the axons of lateral columnar, or cornual, cells. The *dorsal (posterior) filaments* are attached in a regular series along a shallow groove, the posterolateral sulcus, and are collections of the central processes of pseudounipolar nerve cells located in the spinal ganglia of the related dorsal nerve roots. The lateral cell processes pass on in spinal nerves and their branches to peripheral receptors, and they

convey afferent impulses back to the spinal cord from somatic, visceral and vascular sources (see Section VII, Plate 11 and Section VIII, Plate 2).

The spinal cord shows an *anterior median fissure* and a shallow *posterior median sulcus* from which a *median septum* of neuroglia extends forward for 4 to 6 mm. The cord is divided into symmetrical halves by the fissure, sulcus and septum. The lines of attachment of the ventral and dorsal nerve filaments are used to demarcate the white matter in each half of the cord into *anterior, lateral* and *posterior columns*, or *funiculi*. (The principal tracts and fasciculi are shown in Plate 17 and described in detail in Section VIII.) □

**Spinal Nerves**

## Spinal Nerves

The *ventral (anterior)* and *dorsal (posterior) nerve roots* are closely covered by pia mater and loosely invested by arachnoid. As each pair emerges through an intervertebral foramen, the roots are enclosed in a sheath of dura mater, surrounded by fatty areolar tissue containing a plexus of veins. The roots lie close together as they pierce the dura and unite almost immediately to form a *spinal nerve*, their dural sheaths becoming continuous with the epineurium (Plate 15).

The upper cervical spinal nerves lie horizontally, but all the others assume an increasingly oblique and downward direction as they proceed to their foramina of exit (Plate 14). In the adult, the lumbar, sacral and coccygeal cord segments lie opposite the last three thoracic and first lumbar vertebrae, and their attached nerve roots descend as a sheath around the filum terminale to constitute the *cauda equina*.

The spinal nerves are connected with adjacent sympathetic trunk ganglia by *rami communicantes* (see Section IV, Plates 1 to 3 and Section VII, Plate 11). These rami contribute efferent and afferent sympathetic fibers to the spinal nerves, which consist primarily of efferent and afferent somatic fibers derived from the ventral and dorsal nerve roots.

Shortly after emerging from the intervertebral foramina, the spinal nerves give off small *recurrent meningeal branches*, which supply the meninges and their vessels; they also supply filaments to adjacent articular and ligamentous structures. They then divide into *ventral (anterior)* and *dorsal (posterior primary)* rami, which contain fibers from both nerve roots and a variable number of sympathetic fibers (see Section VI, Plate 3).

***The ventral rami*** supply the anterior and lateral parts of the neck and trunk and make up the nerves of the perineum and limbs. Except in the thoracic region, where they retain their separate identities as intercostal and subcostal nerves, the ventral rami divide and reunite in differing patterns to form the following nerve plexuses: the *cervical plexus*, from the ventral rami of the first four cervical nerves; the *brachial plexus*, from the ventral rami of the lower four cervical and first thoracic nerves; the *lumbar plexus*, from the ventral rami of the first three lumbar nerves and from

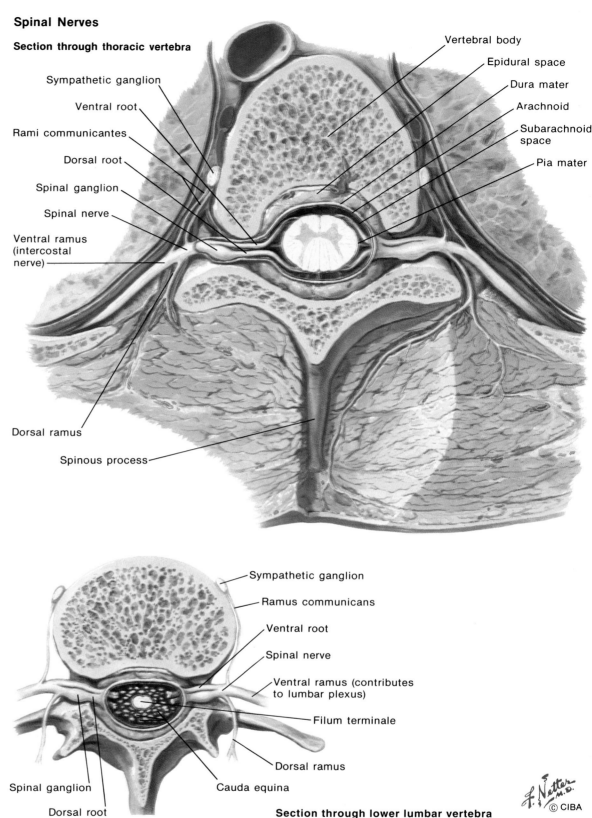

**Section through thoracic vertebra**

Sympathetic ganglion
Ventral root
Rami communicantes
Dorsal root
Spinal ganglion
Spinal nerve
Ventral ramus (intercostal nerve)
Dorsal ramus
Spinous process

Vertebral body
Epidural space
Dura mater
Arachnoid
Subarachnoid space
Pia mater

Sympathetic ganglion
Ramus communicans
Ventral root
Spinal nerve
Ventral ramus (contributes to lumbar plexus)
Filum terminale
Dorsal ramus
Spinal ganglion
Cauda equina
Dorsal root

**Section through lower lumbar vertebra**

most of the ventral ramus of the fourth lumbar nerve; the *sacral plexus*, from the remainder of the ventral ramus of the fourth lumbar nerve and from the ventral rami of the fifth lumbar and first three sacral nerves; and the small *sacrococcygeal plexus*, from the ventral rami of the fourth and fifth sacral nerves and from the coccygeal nerve. (The plexuses and their branches are described in detail in Section VI.)

***The dorsal rami*** turn dorsally and are distributed to cutaneous, muscular and other structures of the back of the neck and trunk. Although some dorsal rami join to form loops, their branches do not form true plexuses as do branches derived

from the ventral rami. Also, the dorsal rami (with the exception of those from the first and second cervical nerves) are generally smaller than the corresponding ventral rami. All the dorsal rami, except those from the first cervical, fourth and fifth sacral and coccygeal nerves, divide into larger *medial* and smaller *lateral branches*. Most medial branches supply the muscles and the skin, while the lateral branches end in the muscles. However, the lateral branches tend to increase in size from above downward, so that those from the last thoracic, five lumbar and five sacral nerves provide both muscular and cutaneous filaments. □

## Principal Fiber Tracts of Spinal Cord

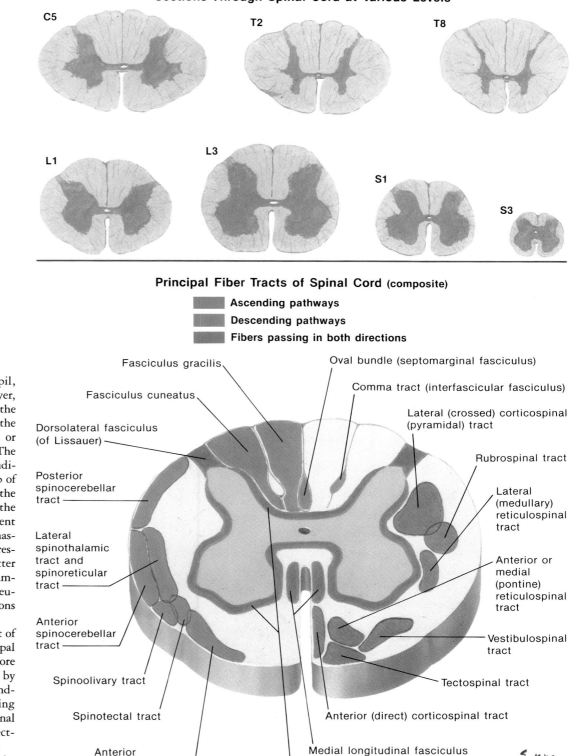

**Sections Through Spinal Cord at Various Levels**

C5    T2    T8

L1    L3    S1    S3

**Principal Fiber Tracts of Spinal Cord (composite)**

- Ascending pathways
- Descending pathways
- Fibers passing in both directions

Fasciculus gracilis

Fasciculus cuneatus

Dorsolateral fasciculus (of Lissauer)

Posterior spinocerebellar tract

Lateral spinothalamic tract and spinoreticular tract

Anterior spinocerebellar tract

Spinoolivary tract

Spinotectal tract

Anterior spinothalamic tract

Fasciculus proprius

Oval bundle (septomarginal fasciculus)

Comma tract (interfascicular fasciculus)

Lateral (crossed) corticospinal (pyramidal) tract

Rubrospinal tract

Lateral (medullary) reticulospinal tract

Anterior or medial (pontine) reticulospinal tract

Vestibulospinal tract

Tectospinal tract

Anterior (direct) corticospinal tract

Medial longitudinal fasciculus

*f. Netter*
© CIBA

The spinal cord consists of a core of neuropil, the *gray matter*, surrounded by an outer fiber layer, the *white matter*. The gray matter consists of the cell bodies and dendrites of spinal neurons and the axons and axon terminals issuing from them or ending upon them (see Section VII, Plate 6). The white matter consists of the axons of longitudinally running fiber tracts. As shown at the top of the illustration and in the cross sections of the medulla oblongata in Plate 13, the outlines of the gray and white matter are different at different spinal levels. The white matter is relatively massive in the cervical region and declines progressively in bulk in the lower levels. The gray matter is most highly developed in the cervical and lumbar enlargements, where it is made up of the neurons involved in the sensory and motor functions of the arms and the legs.

The schematic cross section in the lower part of the illustration shows the location of the principal fiber tracts within the spinal white matter (more fully described in Section VIII). As indicated by the colors, the tracts can be divided into ascending (blue) and descending (red) pathways linking the spinal cord with the brain, and propriospinal (purple) pathways made up of fibers interconnecting different levels within the spinal cord itself.

*The ascending pathways* include the *fasciculus gracilis* and *fasciculus cuneatus* (part of the medial lemniscus system), which convey fine discriminative sensation from the lower and upper parts of the body, respectively. Less discriminative, higher threshold sensations are carried by the *anterior* and *lateral spinothalamic tracts*; the latter is particularly important in conveying the sensations of pain and temperature. Other ascending pathways, which are more closely involved in reflex activity and motor control, include the *posterior* and *anterior spinocerebellar tracts* and the *spinoolivary, spinotectal* and *spinoreticular tracts*.

*The descending pathways* have been usefully divided into two groups. The first group includes the *corticospinal tracts* and the *rubrospinal tract*. It terminates preferentially in the dorsolateral regions of the spinal cord, which contain the

neurons controlling the distal muscles of the limbs. Damage to these pathways results in loss of fine-fractionated control of the extremities. The second group includes the *anterior* and *lateral reticulospinal tracts*, the *tectospinal tract*, the *lateral* and *medial vestibulospinal tracts*, and the *interstitiospinal tract* that runs in the *medial longitudinal fasciculus* and terminates preferentially in the ventromedial regions of the spinal cord. These regions contain the neurons controlling axial and proximal limb muscles. Damage to these pathways results in disorders of posture and righting. In addition to their motor action, both sets of descending pathways also include fibers

that modulate sensory transmission by spinal pathways.

*Propriospinal Pathways.* Some of the propriospinal pathways consist of afferent fibers, which enter the spinal cord via the dorsal roots and then ascend or descend in the *oval bundle, comma tract, dorsolateral fasciculus (of Lissauer), fasciculus gracilis* or *fasciculus cuneatus* to terminate on spinal neurons at other levels of the spinal cord. Other propriospinal fibers originate from interneurons in the spinal gray matter itself. Collectively, propriospinal fibers are important in mediating spinal reflexes and coordinating activity at different levels of the spinal cord. □

Section III

# Blood Vessels of Brain and Spinal Cord

Frank H. Netter, M.D.

*in collaboration with*

**Jerome J. Sheldon, M.D.**   *Plates 1–21*

# Blood Vessels of Scalp

The blood vessels of the scalp lie in the dense subcutaneous tissues superficial to the galea aponeurotica and deep to the skin. The arterial supply is derived from the superficial temporal, posterior auricular and occipital branches of the *external carotid artery*. There is also contribution from the supraorbital and supratrochlear (frontal) branches of the ophthalmic artery, the latter a branch of the *internal carotid arterial system*. The terminal branches of these arteries freely anastomose with each other, as well as with their counterparts on the contralateral side.

*Arteries.* The *superficial temporal artery* is the main blood supply to the scalp and is one of the two terminal branches of the external carotid artery (Plate 8). It arises in the substance of the parotid gland, ascends over the root of the zygomatic arch just anterior to the external auditory canal, and divides 4 to 5 cm above its origin into frontal and parietal branches. These supply the scalp over the frontoparietal convexity, its underlying muscles and the pericranium. The more proximal branches of the superficial temporal artery supply areas other than the scalp —the masseter muscle and the skin— and tiny twigs anastomose with branches of the facial and (internal) maxillary arteries.

The *middle temporal artery* gives branches to the temporalis muscle and anastomoses with the deep temporal branch of the maxillary artery. It also gives rise to a zygomaticoorbital branch, which anastomoses with the lacrimal and palpebral branches of the ophthalmic artery. The anterior auricular branches supply the anterior portion of the ear and anastomose with the posterior auricular artery.

The *posterior auricular artery* originates from the external carotid, above the origin of the occipital artery. It has an auricular, an occipital and a stylomastoid branch; the latter passes through the stylomastoid foramen to supply the tympanic cavity, mastoid air cells and semicircular canals.

The *occipital artery* arises from the external carotid artery, just opposite the origin of the facial artery. It supplies the scalp and the underlying occipitalis muscle in the region of the occiput. It has several meningeal branches, which pass through the hypoglossal canal and the jugular foramen, and a mastoid branch, which passes through the mastoid canal; all these branches supply the meninges of the posterior fossa and dura

mater and anastomose with the middle meningeal artery (Plates 2 and 7).

The *supraorbital artery* arises from the ophthalmic artery as the latter enters the orbit. It passes medially along the border of the superior rectus and levator palpebrae superioris muscles to exit via the supraorbital foramen. It then divides into a superficial and a deep branch to supply the skin, muscles and pericranium of the forehead.

The *supratrochlear (frontal) artery* is one of the terminal branches of the ophthalmic artery. It exits from the medial portion of the orbit to supply the skin, underlying muscles and pericranium of the medial aspect of the forehead.

*The veins* draining the scalp accompany the arteries and have multiple connections with the intracranial venous sinuses and diploic veins.

The multiple *occipital veins* drain via the deep cervical and vertebral venous system. Several tributaries form the *posterior external jugular vein*, which drains into the external jugular vein. The *superficial temporal veins* drain via the retromandibular (posterior facial) veins, which have anterior and posterior divisions. The posterior division and the posterior auricular vein both form the *external jugular vein*. The anterior division joins the (anterior) facial and deep facial veins to drain into the *internal jugular vein*.  □

Blood Vessels of Scalp

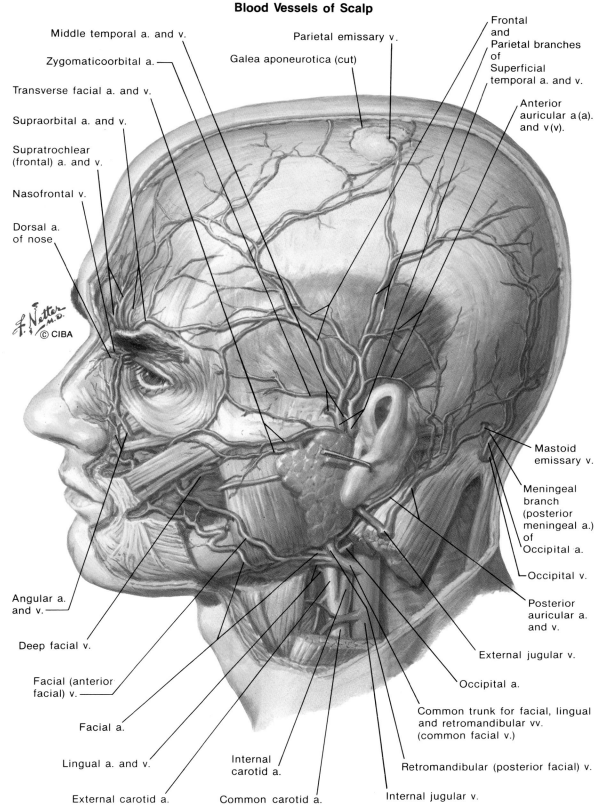

Middle temporal a. and v.
Zygomaticoorbital a.
Transverse facial a. and v.
Supraorbital a. and v.
Supratrochlear (frontal) a. and v.
Nasofrontal v.
Dorsal a. of nose
Parietal emissary v.
Galea aponeurotica (cut)
Frontal and Parietal branches of Superficial temporal a. and v.
Anterior auricular a(a). and v(v).
Mastoid emissary v.
Meningeal branch (posterior meningeal a.) of Occipital a.
Occipital v.
Posterior auricular a. and v.
External jugular v.
Occipital a.
Common trunk for facial, lingual and retromandibular vv. (common facial v.)
Retromandibular (posterior facial) v.
Internal jugular v.
Common carotid a.
Internal carotid a.
External carotid a.
Lingual a. and v.
Facial a.
Facial (anterior facial) v.
Deep facial v.
Angular a. and v.

# Arterial Supply to Brain and Meninges

The brain and meninges are supplied by arteries derived from the internal carotid, the vertebral-basilar and the external carotid arterial systems. These vessels either originate directly from or are branches of the main trunks, which arise from the aortic arch in the superior mediastinum.

### Internal Carotid Artery

The internal carotid artery arises from the common carotid artery at its bifurcation at the level of the upper border of the thyroid cartilage. It has four named segments.

*Segments.* The *cervical segment* ascends vertically in the neck, posterior and slightly medial to the external carotid artery. It lies deep to the sternocleidomastoid muscle, the parotid gland and the digastric and stylohyoid muscles, and is separated from the superior portion of the external carotid artery by the styloglossus and stylopharyngeal muscles. At the base of the skull, it enters the carotid canal of the petrous bone to become the petrous segment.

The *petrous segment* ascends a short distance and bends anteromedially to assume a horizontal course, anterior to the tympanic cavity and the cochlea. It exits anteriorly near the apex of the petrous bone to enter the posterior portion of the foramen lacerum, in which it ascends to a juxtasellar location, piercing the dural layers of the cavernous sinus to become the cavernous segment.

The *cavernous segment* is covered by the vascular membranes lining the sinus and follows a sinuous course, passing anteriorly and then superomedially to exit just medial to the anterior clinoid process. It pierces the dura at this point and becomes the supraclinoid (cerebral) segment.

The *supraclinoid (cerebral) segment* ascends slightly posteriorly and laterally to pass between the oculomotor (III) and optic (II) nerves. The internal carotid terminates just below the anterior perforated substance, where it bifurcates into the anterior and middle cerebral arteries.

*Branches.* The *cervical segment* does not have any branches. The *petrous segment* has two branches: the caroticotympanic branch, which supplies the tympanic cavity, and the pterygoid (vidian) branch, which passes through the pterygoid canal. The *cavernous segment* has many branches,

four of which are main branches: the meningohypophyseal trunk, the anterior meningeal artery, the artery to the inferior portion of the cavernous sinus, and the ophthalmic artery. The latter arises from the internal carotid artery just before it emerges from the cavernous sinus, and passes through the optic canal into the orbit just below and lateral to the optic nerve.

The branches of the *supraclinoid segment* supply the supratentorial portion of the brain, and include the superior hypophyseal branches (which supply the optic chiasm, the anterior lobe of the pituitary and the adjacent pituitary stalk), the posterior communicating artery, the anterior

choroidal artery and the middle and anterior cerebral arteries (Plates 4 to 6).

### Vertebral Artery

*Segments.* The vertebral artery most frequently arises from the subclavian artery. It has four segments. The *first (prevertebral) segment* ascends posterosuperiorly between the longus colli and anterior scalene muscles to enter the transverse foramina of the cervical spine at the level of the sixth cervical vertebra. From this point, the artery ascends as the *second (cervical) segment* through the transverse foramina to become the *third (atlantic) segment* when it exits from the transverse foramen

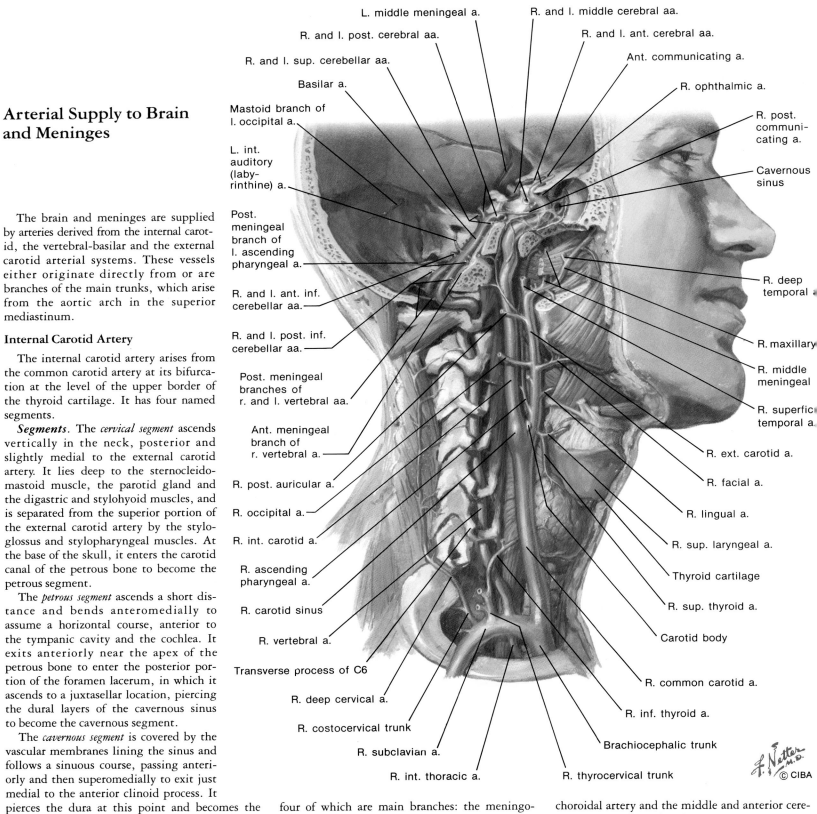

L. middle meningeal a.

R. and l. post. cerebral aa.

R. and l. sup. cerebellar aa.

Basilar a.

Mastoid branch of l. occipital a.

L. int. auditory (labyrinthine) a.

Post. meningeal branch of l. ascending pharyngeal a.

R. and l. ant. inf. cerebellar aa.

R. and l. post. inf. cerebellar aa.

Post. meningeal branches of r. and l. vertebral aa.

Ant. meningeal branch of r. vertebral a.

R. post. auricular a.

R. occipital a.

R. int. carotid a.

R. ascending pharyngeal a.

R. carotid sinus

R. vertebral a.

Transverse process of C6

R. deep cervical a.

R. costocervical trunk

R. subclavian a.

R. int. thoracic a.

R. and l. middle cerebral aa.

R. and l. ant. cerebral aa.

Ant. communicating a.

R. ophthalmic a.

R. post. communicating a.

Cavernous sinus

R. deep temporal a.

R. maxillary

R. middle meningeal

R. superfic. temporal a.

R. ext. carotid a.

R. facial a.

R. lingual a.

R. sup. laryngeal a.

Thyroid cartilage

R. sup. thyroid a.

Carotid body

R. common carotid a.

R. inf. thyroid a.

Brachiocephalic trunk

R. thyrocervical trunk

## Arterial Supply to Brain and Meninges
*(Continued)*

of the atlas. It then passes posteriorly behind the articular process of the atlas, lying in a groove on the superior surface of the posterior arch of the atlas, and enters the cranial cavity by piercing the atlantooccipital membrane and the dura mater to become the *fourth (intradural* or *intracranial) segment*. This segment ascends anteriorly and laterally around the medulla to reach the midline at the pontomedullary junction, where it unites with the vertebral artery of the opposite side to form the *basilar artery*.

*Cervical Branches*. The cervical segment gives rise to multiple muscular and spinal (radicular) branches. The latter pass through the intervertebral foramina to enter the vertebral canal, where they contribute to the blood supply of the cervical portion of the spinal cord and supply the periosteum and bodies of the vertebrae.

*Intracranial Branches*. At the upper end of the second and third segments, respectively, a small anterior and a larger posterior meningeal branch originate (see page 49). The fourth segment gives rise to the anterior and posterior spinal arteries (Plates 19 and 20) and, together with the basilar artery, to the arteries supplying the brain in the posterior fossa. These include the posterior inferior cerebellar artery (occasionally absent), the anterior inferior cerebellar artery, the internal auditory (labyrinthine) artery, the superior cerebellar artery, the posterior cerebral artery and multiple medullary and pontine perforating branches (Plate 10).

### External Carotid Artery

The external carotid artery gives rise to many branches that supply the structures of the face and neck (Plate 1). Some of these arteries have meningeal branches that supply the dura mater surrounding the brain. The maxillary artery gives rise to the middle and accessory meningeal arteries; the ascending pharyngeal artery gives rise to a posterior meningeal branch; and the occipital artery gives rise to perforating meningeal branches, which contribute to the blood supply of the meninges of the posterior fossa (Plate 7).

### Anomalous Origins

There are several morphological variants of the common carotid and vertebral arteries, which usually are not of clinical significance. The *right common carotid artery* can also arise independently from the aortic arch (not shown), in which case the aberrant right subclavian artery originates from the aortic arch distal to the left subclavian artery and crosses to the right side. □

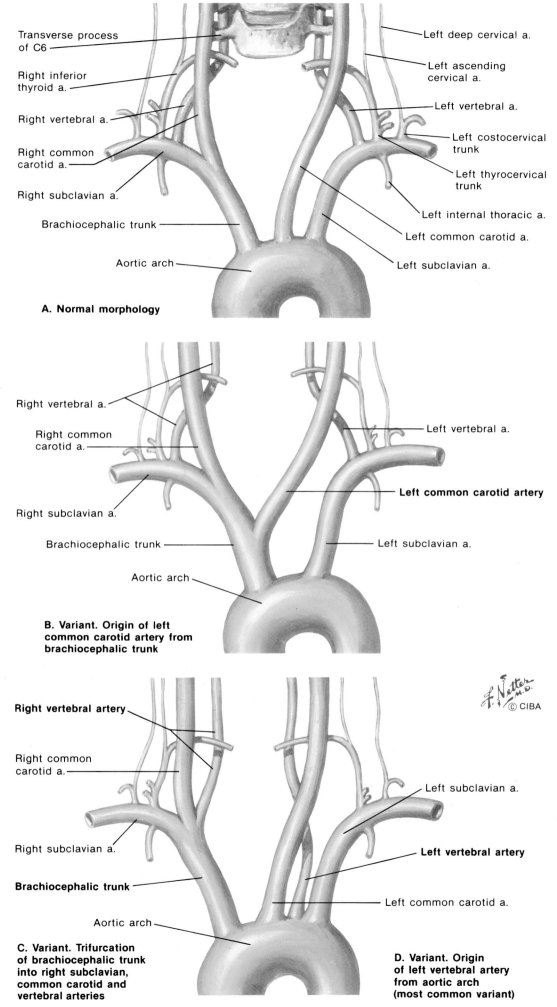

**A. Normal morphology**

Transverse process of C6
Right inferior thyroid a.
Right vertebral a.
Right common carotid a.
Right subclavian a.
Brachiocephalic trunk
Aortic arch
Left deep cervical a.
Left ascending cervical a.
Left vertebral a.
Left costocervical trunk
Left thyrocervical trunk
Left internal thoracic a.
Left common carotid a.
Left subclavian a.

**B. Variant. Origin of left common carotid artery from brachiocephalic trunk**

Right vertebral a.
Right common carotid a.
Right subclavian a.
Brachiocephalic trunk
Aortic arch
Left vertebral a.
**Left common carotid artery**
Left subclavian a.

**C. Variant. Trifurcation of brachiocephalic trunk into right subclavian, common carotid and vertebral arteries**

**Right vertebral artery**
Right common carotid a.
Right subclavian a.
**Brachiocephalic trunk**
Aortic arch
Left subclavian a.
**Left vertebral artery**
Left common carotid a.

**D. Variant. Origin of left vertebral artery from aortic arch (most common variant)**

# Supratentorial Arteries of Brain

The internal carotid arteries supply the anterior portion and the vertebral-basilar system supplies the posterior portion of the brain above the tentorium cerebelli.

*Circle of Willis.* Branches from both arterial systems form an anastomosis at the base of the brain called the circle of Willis. Anteriorly, this circle is formed by the horizontal portions of the anterior cerebral branches of the internal carotid arteries and their interconnection, the anterior communicating artery. Laterally and posteriorly, it is formed by the posterior communicating branches of the internal carotid arteries and their connections with the posterior cerebral branches of the basilar artery.

*The superior hypophyseal artery* is a small vessel that arises as the first branch of the supraclinoid segment of the internal carotid artery. It supplies the optic chiasm and the anterior lobe of the pituitary gland, and anastomoses freely with its counterpart on the contralateral side (see Section VIII, Plate 57).

*The posterior communicating artery* arises from the internal carotid and passes posteriorly just ventral to the optic tract, crossing it to complete the circle of Willis. Several tiny branches arise from the superior and lateral surfaces of the posterior communicating artery (anterior thalamoperforating branches) to supply the optic tract and adjacent posterior portion of the optic chiasm, the posterior hypothalamus, and contribute to the blood supply of the cerebral peduncle. The largest branch is the *premamillary artery*, which supplies the hypothalamus and the anterior and ventral nuclei of the thalamus. Most often, however, the posterior communicating artery is hypoplastic.

*The posterior cerebral artery* usually originates from the terminal bifurcation of the basilar artery in the interpeduncular cistern, and passes above the oculomotor (III) nerve to curve around the midbrain above the level of the tentorium cerebelli. In 15% of normal brains, however, the posterior cerebral artery is a direct continuation of the posterior communicating artery.

The proximal part of the posterior cerebral artery, from which many perforating arteries arise, has *peduncular, ambient* and *quadrigeminal segments* corresponding to the cisterns through which it passes en route to the hippocampal fissure, where it divides into its terminal cortical branches. It lies just ventral to the basal vein (of Rosenthal), and is separated from the superior cerebellar artery by the free margin of the tentorium cerebelli.

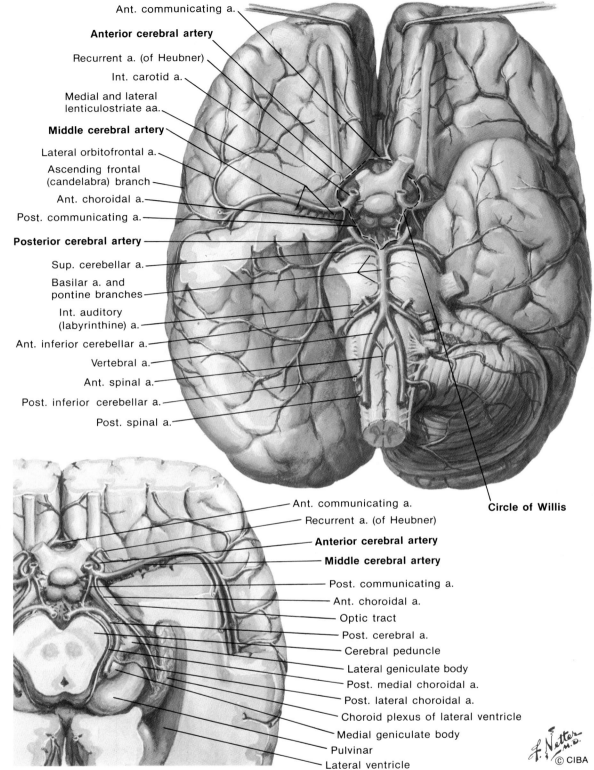

From the peduncular segment, multiple *mesencephalic perforating arteries* arise to supply the tectum and cerebral peduncles of the midbrain, and multiple thalamoperforating branches supply the thalamus. The *posterior thalamoperforating arteries* supply the hypothalamus, subthalamus and midline and medial nuclei of the thalamus. The *thalamogeniculate perforating arteries* arise from the ambient segment and supply the geniculate bodies and adjacent pulvinar.

One or more *posterior medial choroidal arteries* arise from either the peduncular or ambient segment. The main one circles the midbrain parallel to the posterior cerebral artery, contributing perforating branches and supplying the quadrigeminal plate and the pineal gland. It then enters the roof of the third ventricle, continues forward to the level of the interventricular foramen, and supplies the choroid plexus of the third ventricle and the medial dorsal nucleus of the thalamus.

The *posterior lateral choroidal artery* arises from the ambient segment and passes laterally to enter the choroidal fissure. A small anterior branch supplies the choroid plexus of the inferior (temporal) horn of the lateral ventricle and anastomoses with the anterior choroidal artery. The main posterior branch passes posteriorly around the pulvinar,

## Supratentorial Arteries of Brain

*(Continued)*

supplying the choroid plexus of the trigone and lateral ventricle, the fornix, the medial dorsal nucleus of the thalamus, the pulvinar and part of the lateral geniculate body.

The posterior cerebral artery has multiple cortical branches, which arise mainly from the ambient segment. The *anterior temporal artery* passes forward to supply the inferior portion of the temporal lobe and anastomose with the anterior temporal branch of the middle cerebral artery. The *posterior temporal artery* passes backward on the inferior aspect of the posterior temporal and adjacent occipital lobes. The *parietooccipital artery* supplies the medial portion of the parietooccipital lobe from the precuneus to the cuneus. The *calcarine artery* usually arises from the ambient segment in the rostral portion of the calcarine sulcus and passes posteriorly in the sulcus to supply the lingual and cuneate gyri. The *posterior pericallosal artery* arises from the quadrigeminal segment, and passes anteriorly over the splenium of the corpus callosum to run in the supracallosal cistern. It anastomoses with the pericallosal branch of the anterior cerebral artery.

**The anterior choroidal artery** arises from the posterior surface of the internal carotid artery just above the origin of the posterior communicating artery. Occasionally, it arises directly from the latter vessel or from the middle cerebral artery. It has two segments.

The *cisternal segment* courses posteriorly in close relationship to the posterior communicating artery and the basal vein. It crosses from the medial to the lateral side of the optic tract, lying within the ambient cistern, and then passes around the medial portion of the uncus to enter the choroidal fissure, where it becomes the *plexal segment*. The plexal segment enters (and supplies) the choroid plexus just behind the knee of the inferior horn of the lateral ventricle; it anastomoses with the anterior branch of the posterior lateral choroidal artery.

The cisternal segment gives rise to several perforating branches. The *proximal branches* supply the optic tract, the genu of the internal capsule and the medial portion of the globus pallidus. *Lateral branches* supply the piriform cortex and uncus of the temporal lobe, the hippocampal and dentate gyri, the tail of the caudate nucleus and the posteromedial half of the amygdaloid body. *Medial branches* supply the middle third of the cerebral peduncle, the substantia nigra, parts of the red nucleus, a portion of the subthalamus and the ventral anterior and ventral lateral nuclei of the thalamus. *Distal branches* at the level of the choroidal fissure supply the lateral geniculate body,

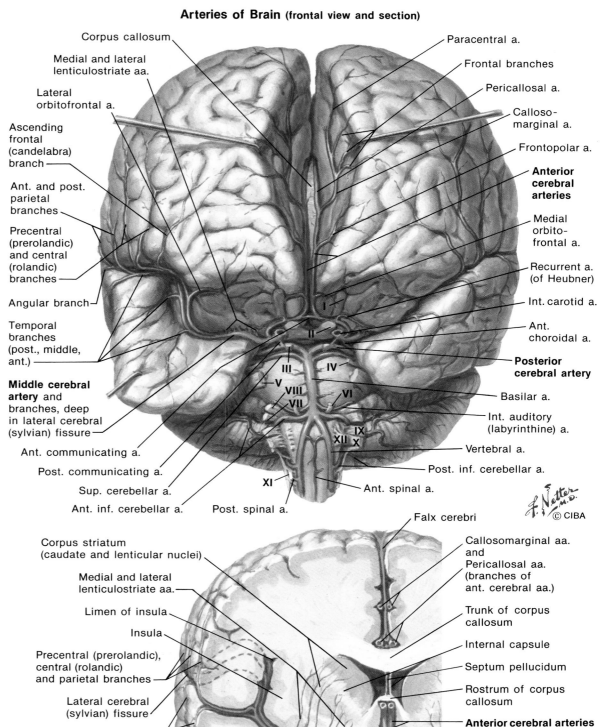

**Arteries of Brain** (frontal view and section)

Corpus callosum

Medial and lateral lenticulostriate aa.

Lateral orbitofrontal a.

Ascending frontal (candelabra) branch

Ant. and post. parietal branches

Precentral (prerolandic) and central (rolandic) branches

Angular branch

Temporal branches (post., middle, ant.)

**Middle cerebral artery** and branches, deep in lateral cerebral (sylvian) fissure

Ant. communicating a.

Post. communicating a.

Sup. cerebellar a.

Ant. inf. cerebellar a.

Post. spinal a.

Paracentral a.

Frontal branches

Pericallosal a.

Callosomarginal a.

Frontopolar a.

**Anterior cerebral arteries**

Medial orbitofrontal a.

Recurrent a. (of Heubner)

Int. carotid a.

Ant. choroidal a.

**Posterior cerebral artery**

Basilar a.

Int. auditory (labyrinthine) a.

Vertebral a.

Post. inf. cerebellar a.

Ant. spinal a.

Corpus striatum (caudate and lenticular nuclei)

Medial and lateral lenticulostriate aa.

Limen of insula

Insula

Precentral (prerolandic), central (rolandic) and parietal branches

Lateral cerebral (sylvian) fissure

Temporal branches

Temporal lobe

**Middle cerebral artery**

Int. carotid a.

Falx cerebri

Callosomarginal aa. and Pericallosal aa. (branches of ant. cerebral aa.)

Trunk of corpus callosum

Internal capsule

Septum pellucidum

Rostrum of corpus callosum

**Anterior cerebral arteries**

Recurrent a. (of Heubner)

Ant. communicating a.

Optic chiasm

the origin of the optic radiations, and the retrolenticular fibers of the posterior limb of the internal capsule.

**The anterior cerebral artery** is the smaller of the two terminal branches of the internal carotid artery. Its origin on one side may be hypoplastic, in which case the contralateral anterior cerebral artery supplies the distal branches via the *anterior communicating artery*. More often, the anterior communicating artery itself is hypoplastic.

The horizontal part of the anterior cerebral artery gives rise to several small inferior and superior branches. The *inferior branches* supply the superior surface of the optic nerves and adjacent

chiasm. The *superior branches* penetrate the brain to supply the anterior part of the hypothalamus, the septum pellucidum, the medial portion of the anterior commissure, the columns of the fornix and the anteroinferior part of the corpus striatum. The largest of the striatal arteries is the *recurrent artery (of Heubner)*, which supplies the anteroinferior portion of the head of the caudate nucleus, the putamen and the anterior limb of the internal capsule.

The interhemispheric part of the anterior cerebral artery is first convex anteriorly, then concave anteriorly (in the cistern of the lamina terminalis), and again convex anteriorly as it passes around

## Supratentorial Arteries of Brain

*(Continued)*

the genu of the corpus callosum. The anterior cerebral artery has several prominent branches. The *medial orbitofrontal artery* courses anteriorly along the gyrus rectus to supply the medial part of the orbital gyrus and the olfactory bulb and tract. The *frontopolar artery*, which may arise separately or from a common trunk with the medial orbitofrontal artery, supplies the medial and lateral portions of the anterior part of the superior frontal gyrus.

Near the genu of the corpus callosum, the anterior cerebral artery usually divides into callosomarginal and pericallosal branches. The *callosomarginal artery* passes over the cingulate gyrus to enter the cingulate sulcus. It gives off *anterior, middle* and *posterior internal frontal (interhemispheric) branches*, which supply the posterior part of the superior frontal gyrus and the medial surface of the frontal lobe as far as the precentral gyrus. The callosomarginal artery may terminate as the *paracentral artery*, which supplies the superior portions of the precentral and postcentral gyri and the paracentral lobule. Some or all of the above branches can arise from the *pericallosal artery*, which runs in a sulcus between the corpus callosum and the cingulate gyrus, and is considered to be the continuation of the anterior cerebral artery. It anastomoses with the pericallosal branch of the posterior cerebral artery. Its main branch is the *precuneal artery*, which supplies the anterior portion of the precuneus and then passes over the convexity of the hemisphere to supply the superior parietal lobule.

***The middle cerebral artery*** is the largest branch of the internal carotid artery. It arises from the internal carotid bifurcation just lateral to the optic chiasm, and passes ventral to the anterior perforated substance in a horizontal lateral direction, bowing slightly anteriorly, to enter the lateral cerebral (sylvian) fissure, where it divides into two, three or four branches.

The branches range superiorly and posteriorly over the insula, make a hairpin turn at its upper border, then descend over the inner surface of the operculum, and exit from the lateral cerebral fissure to spread out superiorly over the frontal, parietal and occipital convexities, and inferiorly over the temporal convexity. The branches to the cerebral convexities vary, but *anterior temporal, ascending frontal (candelabra), precentral (prerolandic), central (rolandic), anterior parietal (postrolandic), posterior parietal, angular* and *posterior temporal branches* are fairly common.

The cortical area supplied by the middle cerebral artery includes the insula, the claustrum, the lateral portion of the hemisphere (except for the superior convexity extending from the frontal

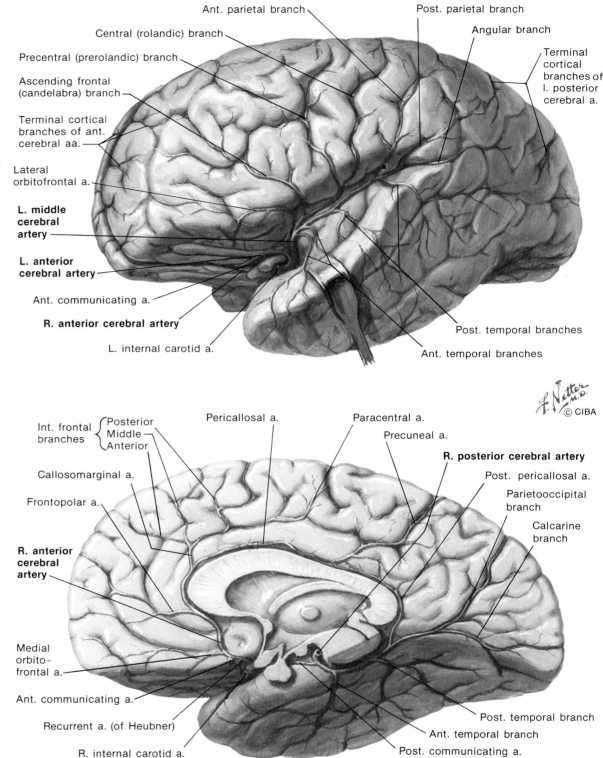

to the occipital pole), and the inferior convexity extending from the occipital to the temporal pole. The terminal branches of the middle cerebral artery anastomose at the convexities with the terminal branches of the anterior cerebral and posterior cerebral arteries.

The middle cerebral artery has other, smaller branches. Three to six *medial* and the same number of *lateral lenticulostriate arteries* arise from the upper surface of the horizontal segment. These make a right angle at their point of origin and pass superiorly and posteriorly to penetrate the anterior perforated substance, forming a gentle convex bend laterally. The vessels have a gentle

"S" shape on the right side of the brain and a gentle reverse "S" shape on the left. The *medial lenticulostriate arteries* supply the outer segment of the globus pallidus; the *lateral lenticulostriate arteries* supply the putamen, the superior half of the internal capsule, the adjacent corona radiata and much of the caudate nucleus. One of the lenticulostriate arteries may be slightly larger and is the artery most likely to rupture and cause a stroke—"the artery of cerebral hemorrhage." The *lateral orbitofrontal artery* arises from the anterior surface of the horizontal segment of the middle cerebral artery and passes forward and laterally to supply the lateral orbital and inferior frontal gyri. □

# Meningeal Arteries

The meningeal arteries, as well as the veins, are located in the outer portion of the dura, grooving the inner table of the calvaria. They supply the dura, help supply the adjacent bones, and form free anastomoses across both sides of the skull and with the cerebral arteries.

*Branches of the External Carotid System.* The *middle meningeal artery* is the largest of the meningeal arteries, and provides the major blood supply to the dura mater (Plate 8). It arises from the maxillary artery and ascends just lateral to the external pterygoid muscle to enter the calvaria through the foramen spinosum. It then passes forward and laterally across the floor of the middle fossa and divides into two branches below the pterion. The *frontal (anterior) branch* climbs across the greater wing of the sphenoid and the parietal bone, forming a groove on the inner table of the calvaria, and divides into branches that supply the outer surface of the dura from the fronto-parietal convexity to the vertex and as far posterior as the occiput. The smaller *parietal (posterior) branch* curves backward over the temporal squama to supply the posterior part of the dura.

The *accessory meningeal artery* may arise from the maxillary artery or the middle meningeal artery. It ascends through the foramen ovale to supply the trigeminal ganglion and adjacent dura.

The bone and dura of the posterior fossa are supplied by: (1) the *meningeal branches* of the *ascending pharyngeal artery*, which pass through the jugular foramen, foramen lacerum and hypoglossal canal; (2) the *meningeal branches* of the *occipital artery*, which pass through the jugular foramen and condylar canal; and (3) the small *mastoid branch* of the *occipital artery*, which passes through the mastoid foramen.

*Branches of the Internal Carotid System.* The *meningohypophyseal trunk* has three main branches. The *tentorial branch* enters the tentorium cerebelli at the apex of the petrous bone, and supplies the anterolateral free margin of the incisura and the base of the tentorium near its attachment to the petrous bone. A *dorsal branch* supplies the dura of the dorsum sella and clivus, sending several small twigs to supply the dura around the internal auditory canal. The *artery to the inferior portion of the cavernous sinus* arises from the lateral aspect of the cavernous segment.

An *anterior meningeal artery* arises from the anterior aspect of the cavernous segment, and passes over the top of the lesser sphenoid wing to supply the dura of the floor of the anterior fossa.

As the *ophthalmic artery* passes medially and then above the optic (II) nerve, it gives off a *lacrimal branch.* The *recurrent meningeal artery* arises from this lacrimal branch and passes through the

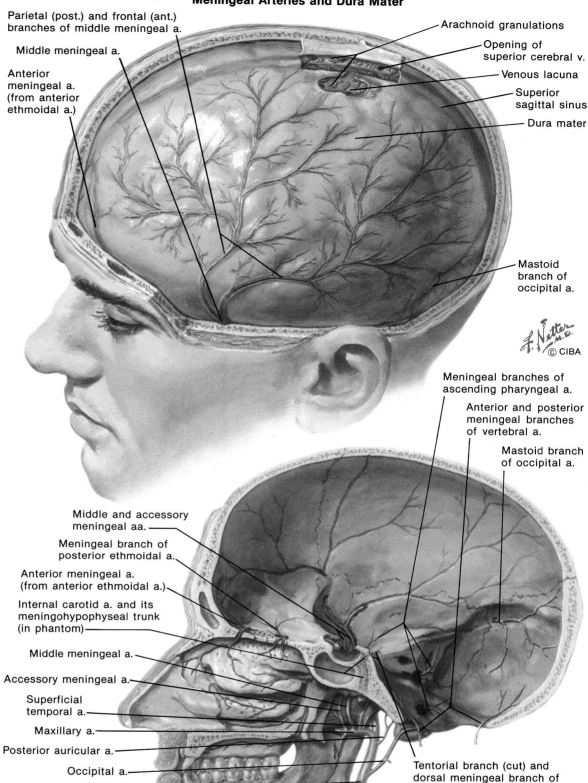

superior orbital fissure to supply the dura of the anterior wall of the middle fossa.

The ophthalmic artery also gives rise to several ethmoidal branches. The *posterior ethmoidal artery* leaves the orbit to supply the posterior ethmoid air cells and the dura of the planum sphenoidale and posterior half of the cribriform plate. The *anterior ethmoidal artery* passes through the anterior ethmoidal canal, supplying the mucosa of the anterior and middle ethmoidal air cells and the frontal sinus. It then enters the cranium, where it gives off an *anterior meningeal branch (anterior falx artery)* to the dura mater and the anterior portion of the falx cerebri.

*The meningeal branches of the vertebral artery* enter the skull through the foramen magnum. The *anterior meningeal branch* arises from the distal portion of the second segment of the vertebral artery, just proximal to its lateral bend at the level of the atlas. It ascends and passes antero-medially to supply the dura of the anterior margin of the foramen magnum. The *posterior meningeal branch* arises from the third segment of the vertebral artery, between the atlas and the foramen magnum. It passes between the dura and the calvaria, supplying the posterior rim of the foramen magnum, the falx cerebelli and the posteromedial portion of the dura of the posterior fossa. ☐

**Image labels (top figure):**
Parietal (post.) and frontal (ant.) branches of middle meningeal a.
Middle meningeal a.
Anterior meningeal a. (from anterior ethmoidal a.)
Arachnoid granulations
Opening of superior cerebral v.
Venous lacuna
Superior sagittal sinus
Dura mater
Mastoid branch of occipital a.

**Image labels (bottom figure):**
Meningeal branches of ascending pharyngeal a.
Anterior and posterior meningeal branches of vertebral a.
Mastoid branch of occipital a.
Middle and accessory meningeal aa.
Meningeal branch of posterior ethmoidal a.
Anterior meningeal a. (from anterior ethmoidal a.)
Internal carotid a. and its meningohypophyseal trunk (in phantom)
Middle meningeal a.
Accessory meningeal a.
Superficial temporal a.
Maxillary a.
Posterior auricular a.
Occipital a.
External carotid a.
Tentorial branch (cut) and dorsal meningeal branch of meningohypophyseal trunk

# Femorocerebral Angiography

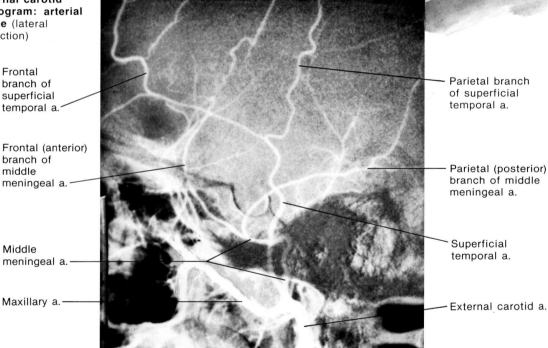

Catheter introduced via femoral artery may be directed selectively to left subclavian, left common carotid or brachiocephalic arteries and thence to vertebral and external or internal carotid arteries

Catheter in aorta

Femoral a.

Pressure injector

**External carotid angiogram: arterial phase** (lateral projection)

Frontal branch of superficial temporal a.

Frontal (anterior) branch of middle meningeal a.

Middle meningeal a.

Maxillary a.

Parietal branch of superficial temporal a.

Parietal (posterior) branch of middle meningeal a.

Superficial temporal a.

External carotid a.

## Femorocerebral Angiography

### Technique

Femorocerebral angiography, using the transcutaneous technique for arterial catheter introduction described by Seldinger in 1953, has become a common method for evaluating the brachiocephalic vessels in most clinical situations.

With fluoroscopic x-ray control and television monitoring of the fluoroscopic image, a preshaped, semirigid catheter is passed through a needle inserted into the femoral artery and is guided up through the iliac vessels and the aorta as far as the aortic arch. The catheter tip can then be maneuvered selectively into either the brachiocephalic, left common carotid or left subclavian artery (all of which arise from the aortic arch), and thence into the vertebral and external or internal carotid arteries. After the catheter tip is positioned, an iodinated contrast agent is injected through it by an automatic injector or a hand-held syringe. Rapid serial x-rays are taken in the frontal and lateral projections simultaneously, providing visualization of the injected vessel and its many intracranial branches. Serial x-ray exposures over an interval of 8 to 10 seconds reveal in sequence the morphological and physiological states of the arterial, capillary and venous phases of the cerebral circulation.

Femorocerebral catheterization is safe, provides great flexibility to the radiologist, and causes little discomfort to the patient. It allows evaluation of all the brachiocephalic vessels from the puncture of a single artery, and the selective catheterization of individual brachiocephalic arteries, which enables the operator to demonstrate the circulatory bed of interest, thus providing maximum radiographic detail for the diagnosis of intracerebral lesions.

### Representative Angiograms

*External Carotid Artery Injection.* The angiogram shown in Plate 8 is a representative lateral radiograph, in the arterial phase, from a serialogram of a selective external carotid artery injection. The examination, which in this case revealed normal vascular anatomy, was performed to determine whether the middle meningeal artery contributed to the blood supply of a benign tumor of the meninges (meningioma). The *middle meningeal artery* can be seen to arise from the maxillary artery, and then ascend vertically in the infratemporal fossa. It then enters the calvaria through the foramen spinosum and turns forward to run anteriorly along the floor of the middle fossa, with a gentle posterosuperior concavity, to terminate as two major branches. The *parietal (posterior) branch* arises as the middle meningeal artery reaches the lateral wall of the middle fossa, from where it extends posteriorly in a curve along the inner table of the skull to cross the temporal squama and posterior part of the parietal bone. The larger *frontal (anterior) branch* crosses the greater wing of the sphenoid bone, passes close to the pterion, and then gives a branch that ascends along the inner table of the parietal bone just posterior to the coronal suture. The frontal and parietal branches of the superficial temporal artery, which supplies the scalp (Plate 1), are also demonstrated in the angiogram.

*Internal and Common Carotid Artery Injection.* The angiogram at the top of Plate 9 is a representative lateral radiograph, in the arterial

## Femorocerebral Angiography
*(Continued)*

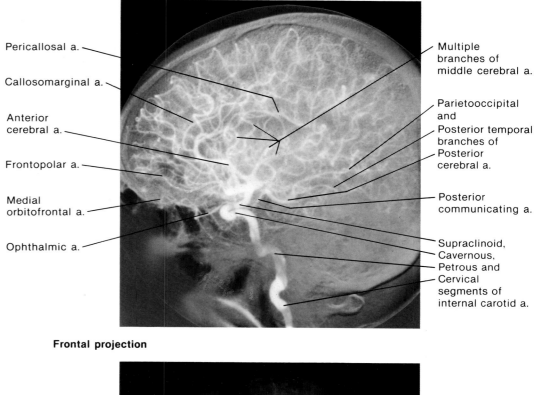

**Lateral projection**

Pericallosal a.

Callosomarginal a.

Anterior cerebral a.

Frontopolar a.

Medial orbitofrontal a.

Ophthalmic a.

Multiple branches of middle cerebral a.

Parietooccipital and Posterior temporal branches of Posterior cerebral a.

Posterior communicating a.

Supraclinoid, Cavernous, Petrous and Cervical segments of internal carotid a.

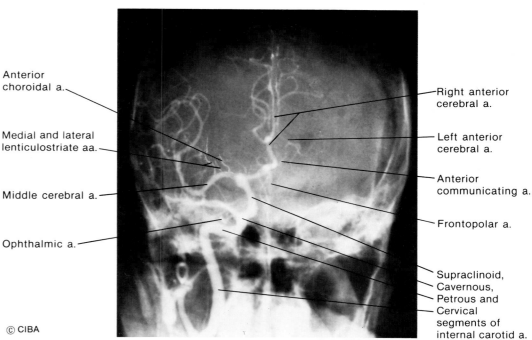

**Frontal projection**

Anterior choroidal a.

Medial and lateral lenticulostriate aa.

Middle cerebral a.

Ophthalmic a.

Right anterior cerebral a.

Left anterior cerebral a.

Anterior communicating a.

Frontopolar a.

Supraclinoid, Cavernous, Petrous and Cervical segments of internal carotid a.

© CIBA

phase, from a serialogram after selective internal carotid artery injection, while that at the bottom is a representative frontal film, also in the arterial phase, from a serialogram after a common carotid artery injection. Both demonstrate normal vascular anatomy (Plates 4 to 6).

The *cervical segment* of the *internal carotid artery* is tortuous and ascends behind and slightly medial to the external carotid artery. At the level of the petrous pyramid, the cervical segment enters the carotid canal to become the *petrous segment*, passing medially and slightly forward. The artery leaves the petrous tip to enter the cavernous sinus as the *cavernous segment*, which passes anteriorly with a sinuous course in a juxtasellar location. (The cavernous segment is superimposed upon itself in the frontal projection, although its posterior portion is slightly more medially placed than its anterior portion.) Leaving the cavernous sinus, the artery pierces the dura mater just medial to the anterior clinoid process to become the *supraclinoid (cerebral) segment*. This segment then passes posteriorly and slightly laterally to bifurcate into the *anterior* and *middle cerebral arteries*, usually just above the cavernous segment. The cavernous and supraclinoid segments are known together as the "carotid siphon" because of their sinuous appearance on the lateral projection.

The multiple, tiny branches of the petrous and cavernous segments of the internal carotid artery (see page 44) are usually not visualized in a normal arteriographic examination. The *ophthalmic artery*, however, can be seen to arise from the anterior portion of the carotid siphon as it pierces the dura mater. It immediately enters the orbit through the optic canal. The *posterior communicating artery* (seen on the lateral projection) will be demonstrated on a carotid serialogram in 20% to 33% of patients. It arises from the posterior wall of the supraclinoid segment and passes posteriorly with a gentle superior concavity. The artery can be seen to join the peduncular segment of the *posterior cerebral artery*, filling its parietooccipital and posterior temporal branches.

The *anterior choroidal artery* is the next branch from the supraclinoid segment of the internal

carotid artery. It arises from the posterior wall and extends posteriorly and laterally around the uncus to enter the choroidal fissure, terminating as a capillary "blush" within the choroid plexus of the inferior (temporal) horn of the lateral ventricle. The artery is convex superiorly and medially.

The *anterior cerebral artery* is the medial terminal branch of the internal carotid artery. It passes horizontally from the internal carotid bifurcation to enter the interhemispheric fissure. On the lateral projection, the artery at first is convex anteriorly, then convex posteriorly, and finally convex anteriorly again. Its larger branches can be identified—the *medial orbitofrontal, frontopolar, pericallosal* and *callosomarginal arteries*—as well as the multiple *interhemispheric branches* ramifying in the midline on the inner aspect of the hemisphere. Occasionally, the contralateral anterior

cerebral artery will fill with contrast medium via the *anterior communicating artery*, best seen in the frontal projection.

The *middle cerebral artery* is the largest terminal branch of the internal carotid artery (frontal projection). It passes laterally in a horizontal and then downward direction to enter the lateral cerebral fissure. At this point, the artery divides into two or more branches, which ascend over the insula, reach the top, make a hairpin turn, descend along the inner surface of the operculum, and leave the lateral cerebral fissure to ramify along the convexities of the hemisphere. The horizontal portion of the middle cerebral artery gives rise to the *medial* and *lateral lenticulostriate arteries*. These originate from the middle cerebral artery at a right angle, and have a slight lateral convexity as they ascend to supply the basal ganglia. □

# Arteries of Posterior Cranial Fossa

The portion of the brain lying in the posterior cranial fossa is supplied by arteries arising from the vertebral-basilar system.

The *vertebral artery*, after leaving the transverse foramen of the atlas, wraps posteriorly around the atlantooccipital joint and penetrates the atlanto-occipital membrane and the dura mater to enter the intracranial cavity through the foramen magnum. The artery courses anteriorly, at first lateral to the medulla and then ventral to the hypoglossal (XII) nerve to reach the midline at the pontomedullary junction, where–between the two abducens (VI) nerves–it joins the vertebral artery of the opposite side to form the *basilar artery*. The basilar artery ascends superiorly along the ventral surface of the pons to terminate as the two *posterior cerebral arteries*. This usually occurs at the level of the pontomesencephalic junction.

*Vertebral Artery.* Some branches of the vertebral artery, although they either originate or terminate intracranially, do not supply the brain of the posterior fossa. These include the anterior and posterior spinal arteries (Plate 19), and the anterior and posterior meningeal arteries, which contribute to the blood supply of the meninges of the posterior fossa (Plate 7).

The branches of the vertebral artery supplying the brain include the small *medullary (bulbar) arteries* and the larger *posterior inferior cerebellar artery*, which can arise from the basilar artery.

*The posterior inferior cerebellar artery* has four segments. The *anterior medullary segment* passes laterally and slightly inferiorly in the anterior medullary cistern to reach the inferior end of the olive. It then becomes the *lateral medullary segment*, coursing posteriorly between the biventral lobule of the cerebellum and the lateral medulla in the cerebellomedullary fissure. This segment appears as the "caudal loop" on angiography. On reaching the posterior margin of the medulla, the lateral medullary segment becomes the *posterior medullary segment* and ascends in the tonsillomedullary fissure, posterior to the glossopharyngeal (IX) and vagus (X) nerves, to reach the level of the superior pole of the tonsil. It then leaves the posterior surface of the medulla, loops over the superior pole of the tonsil, and becomes the *supratonsillar segment*. This "cranial loop" is close to (and supplies) the choroid plexus of the fourth ventricle, and is called the choroidal point. The artery then descends in the retrotonsillar vallecular fissure, and bifurcates into medial and lateral terminal branches.

The *inferior vermian branch* of the posterior inferior cerebellar artery runs between the inferior cerebellar vermis and adjacent cerebellar hemisphere. The *tonsillohemispheric (tonsillocerebellar) branches* continue on the medial surface of the tonsil, sending branches to that structure and

to the occipital surface of the cerebellar hemisphere. Multiple perforating *medullary branches* arise from the first three segments of the artery to supply the lateral and posterior part of the medulla.

There are many variations in the configuration, size and origin of the branches of the posterior inferior cerebellar artery. If the artery is small or altogether absent, an enlarged ipsilateral anterior inferior cerebellar artery or contralateral posterior inferior cerebellar artery will contribute to its vascular distribution.

*The basilar artery* originates at the confluence of the two vertebral arteries. It terminates in the interpeduncular (crural) cistern by dividing into the two posterior cerebral arteries just superior to the two oculomotor (III) nerves.

The *pontine arteries* are numerous, small, penetrating branches of the basilar artery, and can be divided into medial and lateral groups. The lateral group supplies not only the pons, but also the ventrolateral aspect of the cerebellar cortex. Toward its upper end, the basilar artery sends penetrating branches to the inferior portion of the midbrain.

The *internal auditory (labyrinthine) artery* can arise either from the basilar artery or (more often) as a branch of the anterior inferior cerebellar artery. It passes along in company with the facial (VII) and vestibulocochlear (VIII) nerves to enter the internal auditory canal, contributing to the blood supply of the dura of the canal and sending branches to the cochlea, labyrinth and horizontal portion of the facial nerve.

The *anterior inferior cerebellar artery* arises from the basilar artery at the junction of its inferior and middle thirds. It passes first ventrally, then horizontally across the inferior portion of the pons, and then through the cerebellar pontine angle cistern, along with the seventh and eighth cranial nerves, to reach the internal auditory meatus. The internal auditory artery may arise from it at this point. The anterior inferior cerebellar artery then loops onto the anteroinferior surface of the cerebellum, supplying the middle cerebellar peduncle and adjacent areas of the cerebellar hemisphere. In its pontine course, the vessel gives rise to many pontine perforating arteries.

The *superior cerebellar artery* arises from the basilar artery, just proximal to its termination, and passes laterally just below the oculomotor nerve to circle the cerebral peduncles or upper pons just below the trochlear (IV) nerve. It sends multiple perforating branches to the midbrain and adjacent pons. On the upper surface of the cerebellum, it divides into two branches. Alternatively, each branch can have an independent origin from the basilar artery.

The lateral marginal branch of the superior cerebellar artery passes anterior to the brachium pontis and on to the anterosuperior portion of the cerebellar hemisphere. It supplies the superior cerebellar peduncle, the upper portion of the middle cerebral peduncle, the dentate nucleus, the roof nuclei and the anterolateral portion of the superior half of the cerebellar hemisphere.

The more medial superior vermian branch continues around the brainstem, passing over the superior cerebellar peduncle and superior cerebellar vermis to anastomose with the inferior vermian branch of the posterior inferior cerebellar artery. It sends multiple hemispheric branches to supply the tentorial and incisural surface of the cerebellar

hemisphere. It also sends tiny branches to the inferior colliculi, the superior cerebellar peduncle and the dentate nucleus.

The terminal branches of all the cerebellar arteries freely anastomose with each other over the convexity of the cerebellar hemispheres.

*The posterior cerebral artery* arises from the terminal bifurcation of the basilar artery (Plates 4 and 5). While this artery supplies predominantly supratentorial structures, it also contributes to the blood supply of the upper part of the midbrain.

*Vertebral-Basilar Angiograms.* The illustration shows representative films, in the arterial phase, from a lateral and frontal serialogram of a normal vertebral-basilar injection arteriogram. The catheter has been selectively positioned into the left vertebral artery, where the iodinated contrast agent was injected.

On the lateral projection, the *vertebral artery* can be seen to pass from the transverse foramen of the atlas, backward around the atlantooccipital articulation, and then forward and upward to form the basilar artery. The *basilar artery* ascends 2 to 3 mm posterior to the clivus with a gentle anterior convexity to match the configuration of the belly of the pons.

On the frontal projection, the *basilar artery* is convex to the right, a normal variation. The artery may be straight or convex in either direction, and is usually convex away from the side of the larger (dominant) vertebral artery, in this case the one on the left. Both *posterior inferior cerebellar arteries* are visualized. The lateral projection shows the cranial and caudal loops. The *inferior vermian* and *tonsillohemispheric branches* are also demonstrated, and the former branches usually serve as a guide to the midline of the posterior fossa on the frontal projection. The *anterior inferior cerebellar arteries* arise from the basilar artery, and their sinuous courses through the cisterns at the cerebellopontine angles near the internal auditory canals are demonstrated on the frontal projection.

The *superior cerebellar arteries* arise from the basilar artery, just proximal to its termination. Their mesencephalic segments have a gentle convex inferior course. The hemispheric and vermian branches may be difficult to identify angiographically due to the superimposition of the branches of the posterior cerebral artery on the film.

The basilar artery terminates as the *posterior cerebral arteries*. The lateral projection shows that their mesencephalic segments are slightly convex in an inferior direction and run parallel to the mesencephalic segments of the superior cerebellar arteries. This projection shows reflux of contrast fluid into the *posterior communicating arteries*, with filling of their *thalamoperforating branches*. The origins and mesencephalic portions of the *posterior medial* and *posterior lateral choroidal arteries* run parallel to the mesencephalic segments of the posterior cerebral arteries and are obscured by those vessels. Their distal segments can be identified on the lateral projection. The double curve of the posterior medial choroidal artery is slightly anterior to the smoother concave curve of the posterior lateral choroidal artery. The major cortical branches of the posterior cerebral arteries can also be identified. These include the *posterior pericallosal*, the *parietooccipital*, the *calcarine* and the *posterior temporal branches*. □

# Arteries of Posterior Cranial Fossa

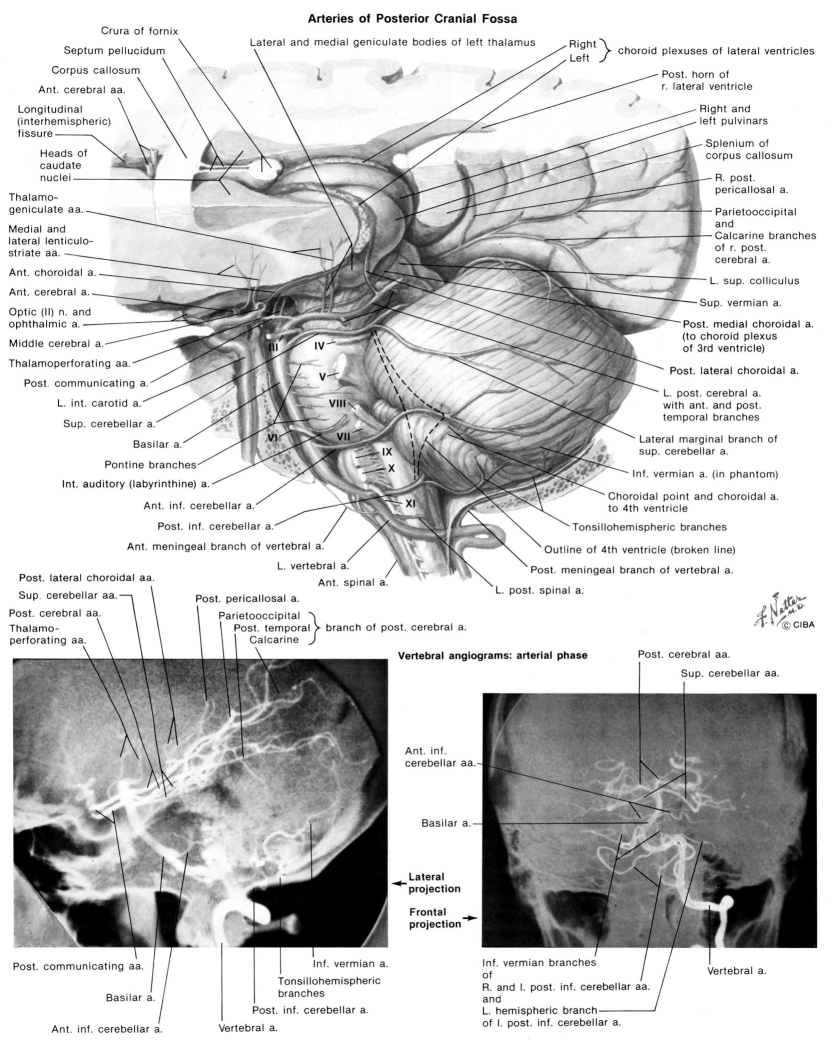

Crura of fornix
Septum pellucidum
Corpus callosum
Ant. cerebral aa.
Longitudinal (interhemispheric) fissure
Heads of caudate nuclei
Thalamogeniculate aa.
Medial and lateral lenticulostriate aa.
Ant. choroidal a.
Ant. cerebral a.
Optic (II) n. and ophthalmic a.
Middle cerebral a.
Thalamoperforating aa.
Post. communicating a.
L. int. carotid a.
Sup. cerebellar a.
Basilar a.
Pontine branches
Int. auditory (labyrinthine) a.
Ant. inf. cerebellar a.
Post. inf. cerebellar a.
Ant. meningeal branch of vertebral a.
L. vertebral a.
Ant. spinal a.

Lateral and medial geniculate bodies of left thalamus

Right
Left } choroid plexuses of lateral ventricles

Post. horn of r. lateral ventricle
Right and left pulvinars
Splenium of corpus callosum
R. post. pericallosal a.
Parietooccipital and Calcarine branches of r. post. cerebral a.
L. sup. colliculus
Sup. vermian a.
Post. medial choroidal a. (to choroid plexus of 3rd ventricle)
Post. lateral choroidal a.
L. post. cerebral a. with ant. and post. temporal branches
Lateral marginal branch of sup. cerebellar a.
Inf. vermian a. (in phantom)
Choroidal point and choroidal a. to 4th ventricle
Tonsillohemispheric branches
Outline of 4th ventricle (broken line)
Post. meningeal branch of vertebral a.
L. post. spinal a.

III  IV  V  VIII  VI  VII  IX  X  XI

Post. lateral choroidal aa.
Sup. cerebellar aa.
Post. cerebral aa.
Thalamoperforating aa.
Post. pericallosal a.
Parietooccipital
Post. temporal } branch of post. cerebral a.
Calcarine

## Vertebral angiograms: arterial phase

Post. cerebral aa.
Sup. cerebellar aa.
Ant. inf. cerebellar aa.
Basilar a.

Post. communicating aa.
Basilar a.
Ant. inf. cerebellar a.
Inf. vermian a.
Tonsillohemispheric branches
Post. inf. cerebellar a.
Vertebral a.

← Lateral projection

Frontal projection →

Inf. vermian branches of R. and l. post. inf. cerebellar aa. and L. hemispheric branch of l. post. inf. cerebellar a.
Vertebral a.

## Meninges and Superficial Cerebral, Meningeal, Diploic and Emissary Veins

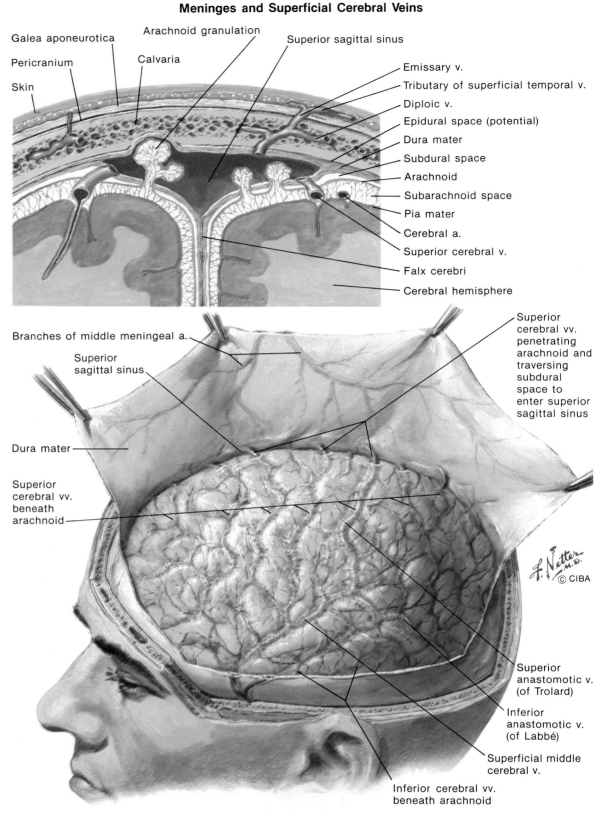

Galea aponeurotica

Pericranium

Skin

Arachnoid granulation

Calvaria

Superior sagittal sinus

Emissary v.

Tributary of superficial temporal v.

Diploic v.

Epidural space (potential)

Dura mater

Subdural space

Arachnoid

Subarachnoid space

Pia mater

Cerebral a.

Superior cerebral v.

Falx cerebri

Cerebral hemisphere

Branches of middle meningeal a.

Superior sagittal sinus

Dura mater

Superior cerebral vv. beneath arachnoid

Superior cerebral vv. penetrating arachnoid and traversing subdural space to enter superior sagittal sinus

Superior anastomotic v. (of Trolard)

Inferior anastomotic v. (of Labbé)

Superficial middle cerebral v.

Inferior cerebral vv. beneath arachnoid

*The meninges* of the brain are composed of three layers (see Section II, Plates 14 and 15). The innermost layer, the *pia mater*, is closely adherent to the brain and follows its folds and fissures; the major arteries and veins of the brain lie within this layer. By its various invaginations, the pia forms the main substance of the tela choroidea and the choroid plexuses of the lateral, third and fourth ventricles (see Section II, Plate 9). External to the pia mater is the lacelike *arachnoid*, which bridges over the folds and fissures. Between these two layers is the *subarachnoid space*, which contains the cerebrospinal fluid. The subarachnoid space communicates with the fourth ventricle through the *median aperture (of Magendie)* and the *lateral apertures (of Luschka)*.

The outermost meningeal covering is the *dura mater*, a tough, inelastic membrane consisting of an outer endosteal layer and an inner meningeal layer. The endosteal layer is adherent to the inner surface of the skull, and corresponds to the periosteum on the outer surface. The meningeal arteries and veins are located in the outer portion of the dura, and groove the inner table of the calvaria (Plate 7). The potential space between the two dural layers is called the *epidural space*. The meningeal layer is smooth on its inner surface and envelops the brain closely, following the arachnoid; the potential space between the dura and the arachnoid is the *subdural space*. Cerebral veins crossing this space have little supporting structure and are therefore most vulnerable to injury. Hemorrhaging blood accumulating here has no pathway of escape. Cuffs of dura surround the cranial nerves at their points of exit from the skull; at the foramen magnum, the cerebral dura becomes continuous with the spinal dura mater. The dura mater is relatively insensitive, except in the vicinity of its blood vessels and over the basal areas of the skull.

*Dural Infoldings.* The calvaria is divided into various compartments by four infoldings of the dura mater (Plate 13). Along the base of the skull, there is the *tentorium cerebelli*, which divides the cranial cavity into supratentorial and subtentorial (posterior fossa) compartments, connected via the tentorial incisura at its free concave anterior border. Its outer convex border is attached posteriorly to the lips of the transverse sulci of the occipital

bone and the mastoid angles of the parietal bones, and its margins enclose the transverse sinuses. More anteriorly, the tentorium is fixed to the superior borders of the petrous parts of the temporal bones, where its layers are separated by the superior petrosal sinuses. The supratentorial compartment is divided into a right and a left side by the *falx cerebri*, which extends between the hemispheres from the cranial vault to a level just above the corpus callosum. It attaches anteriorly to the crista galli, and posteriorly, to the tentorium cerebelli behind the incisura. The upper convex margin of the falx cerebri is attached to the inner surface of the calvaria, and lodges the superior

sagittal sinus; the concave inferior margin is free, and contains the inferior sagittal sinus. The *falx cerebelli* is a similar, but much smaller, dural reflection that extends between the posterosuperior portions of the cerebellar hemispheres. It attaches to the posterior portion of the inferior surface of the tentorium cerebelli and internal occipital protuberance above, and to the foramen magnum below. It encloses the occipital sinus. The *diaphragma sellae* roofs over the sella turcica and separates the pituitary gland from the hypothalamus and optic chiasm. It is a horizontal, circular fold and contains a central aperture for the infundibulum.

## Meninges and Superficial Cerebral, Meningeal, Diploic and Emissary Veins
*(Continued)*

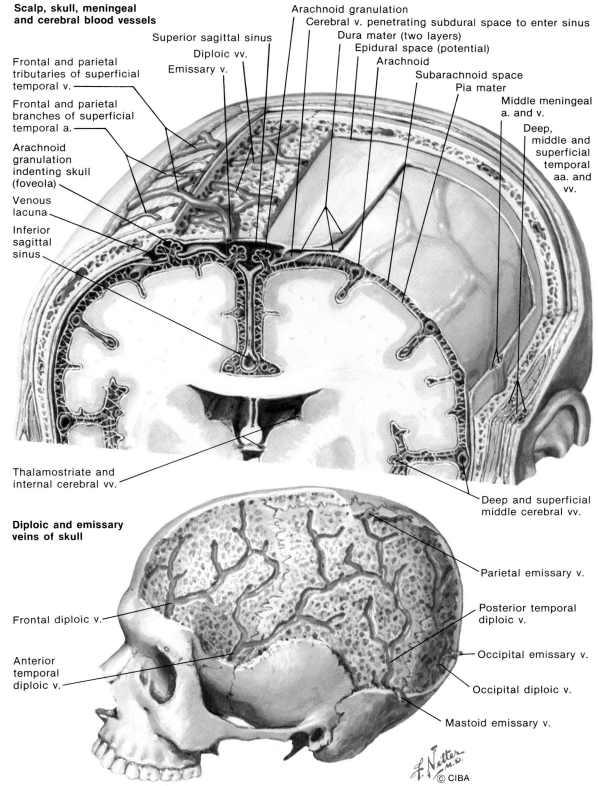

**Scalp, skull, meningeal and cerebral blood vessels**

Frontal and parietal tributaries of superficial temporal v.

Frontal and parietal branches of superficial temporal a.

Arachnoid granulation indenting skull (foveola)

Venous lacuna

Inferior sagittal sinus

Superior sagittal sinus

Diploic vv.

Emissary v.

Arachnoid granulation

Cerebral v. penetrating subdural space to enter sinus

Dura mater (two layers)

Epidural space (potential)

Arachnoid

Subarachnoid space

Pia mater

Middle meningeal a. and v.

Deep, middle and superficial temporal aa. and vv.

Deep and superficial middle cerebral vv.

Thalamostriate and internal cerebral vv.

**Diploic and emissary veins of skull**

Frontal diploic v.

Anterior temporal diploic v.

Parietal emissary v.

Posterior temporal diploic v.

Occipital emissary v.

Occipital diploic v.

Mastoid emissary v.

*The superficial cerebral veins* arise in the substance of the brain and are at first located within the pia mater. They drain toward the *superior sagittal* and *transverse sinuses*, crossing the subarachnoid and subdural spaces near their termination to pierce the dura. They enter the sinuses in the opposite direction to that of the blood flow within. Hence, the superior cerebral veins join the superior sagittal sinus in an anterior direction, and the transverse sinus in a posterior direction.

In some places, the superior cerebral veins empty first into irregularly shaped *venous lacunae*, or lakes, on either side of the superior sagittal sinus, or into smaller lacunae. These lacunae and those in the transverse sinus are invaginated by *arachnoid granulations* or villi—cauliflowerlike projections of the arachnoid through the dura. They first appear at about age 7, and increase in number and size until adult life. They thin out the dura and neighboring inner table of the skull as they grow, forming *foveolae*, and serve as the pathway through which the subarachnoid cerebrospinal fluid enters the venous circulation.

*The meningeal veins* are small and follow the arteries, and are located between the dura and the skull. They communicate with emissary, diploic and cerebral veins and end in various dural sinuses.

Small veins in the *falx cerebri* drain into the superior and inferior sagittal sinuses, while the *tentorium cerebelli* is drained by veins that join the transverse and the superior sagittal sinuses. The veins of the *falx cerebelli* drain into the straight sinus, the confluence of the sinuses and the occipital sinus. The *major meningeal veins* drain the dura covering the convexity of the cerebral hemispheres and follow the branches of the middle meningeal artery. They empty into the *transverse, cavernous* and *sphenoparietal dural sinuses* and the *meningeal sinus* (a large sinus that reaches from the bregma to the sphenoparietal sinus, running parallel to the anterior branch of the middle meningeal artery), and drain into the *pterygoid venous plexus* through the floor of the middle fossa via the foramina spinosum, ovale and lacerum.

*Diploic and Emissary Veins.* The *diploic veins* are endothelium-lined channels located between the inner and outer tables of the calvaria. The *emissary veins* pass through the foramina in the cranial bones to link the venous sinuses and the diploic veins with the veins on the surface of the skull. Some are constant, but others are occasionally absent.

There are four main diploic veins on each side. The *frontal diploic vein* drains the anterior portion of the frontal bone into the supraorbital vein and the superior sagittal sinus. The *anterior temporal diploic vein* drains the posterior portion of the frontal bone and the anterior portion of the parietal and temporal bones into the sphenoparietal sinus and through emissary veins in the greater wing of the sphenoid into the temporal veins. The *posterior temporal diploic veins* drain the posterior temporal parietal bones into the transverse sinus and the mastoid emissary vein. The *occipital diploic veins* drain the occiput into the confluence of the sinuses and the inconstant occipital emissary vein.

The dural venous sinuses, the meningeal, diploic and emissary veins and the veins of the scalp do not have valves, and there is free communication between these venous systems—a significant factor in the possible spread of infection from foci outside the cranium to the venous sinuses within. ☐

# Venous Sinuses of Dura Mater

The endosteal and meningeal layers of the dura mater are separated in places to form the *dural venous sinuses*. They receive blood from the brain, meninges and diploë, and communicate through emissary channels with veins outside the skull (Plates 11 and 12).

***The posterosuperior group*** consists of six dural sinuses:

1. The *superior sagittal sinus* originates at the foramen cecum, usually with a tributary from the nasal cavity. It continues posteriorly in a groove in the skull, encased within the superior margin of the falx cerebri, receiving the superior cerebral veins and terminating near the occipital protuberance at the confluence of the sinuses.

2. The *inferior sagittal sinus* runs along the lower crescentic margin of the falx cerebri. It increases in size as it runs backward to join the straight sinus, receiving several veins from the falx and small veins from the cerebral hemispheres.

3. The *straight sinus*, formed by the union of the inferior sagittal sinus with the great cerebral vein, runs in a dural fold at the junction of the falx cerebri and tentorium cerebelli toward the occipital protuberance, where it empties into the confluence of the sinuses.

4. Of the two *transverse sinuses*, the larger (usually the right) is the continuation of the superior sagittal sinus, and the smaller, of the straight sinus. Each curves within a groove on the occipital bone in the attached margin of the tentorium cerebelli and then passes anteriorly to become the sigmoid sinus. Each transverse sinus receives blood from the superior petrosal sinuses, mastoid and condyloid emissary veins, inferior cerebral and cerebellar veins (anchoring veins) and diploic veins.

5. The *sigmoid sinuses* are the continuations of the transverse sinuses and end at the jugular foramina to become the internal jugular veins.

6. The *occipital sinus* lies in the falx cerebelli and arises by small veins near the foramen magnum. It also empties into the confluence of the sinuses.

***The anteroinferior group*** consists of five paired sinuses and one plexus:

1. The *cavernous sinuses*, on each side of the sphenoid bone, are trabeculated structures, beginning at the superior orbital fissure and stretching as far as the apex of the petrous parts of the temporal bones (see Section VIII, Plate 57 and CIBA COLLECTION, Volume 4, page 7). The internal carotid artery and the divisions of the trigeminal (V) nerve pass forward in its walls (see Section V, Plate 5). Tributaries to the cavernous sinuses include the superior and inferior ophthalmic veins, superior middle cerebral vein, inferior cerebral veins and the sphenoparietal sinus. The cavernous

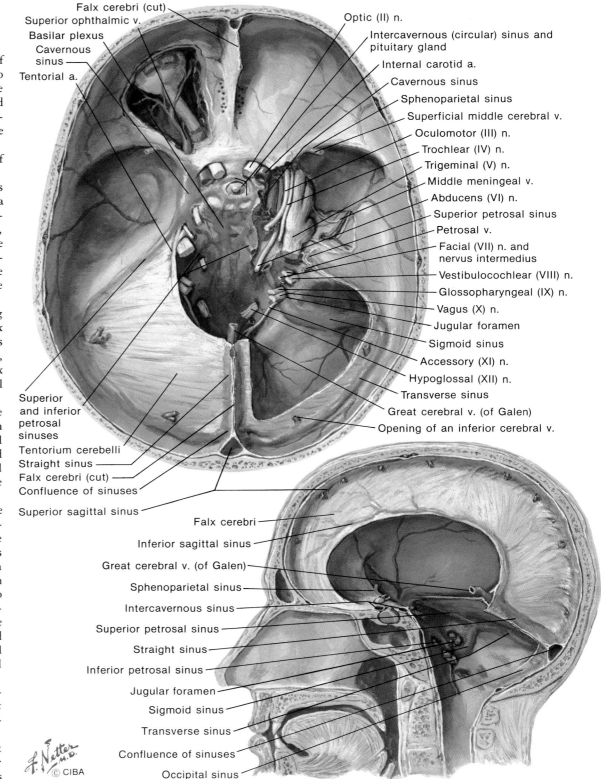

sinuses drain chiefly into the transverse sinuses via the superior petrosal sinuses, into the internal jugular veins via the inferior petrosal sinuses, and into the pterygoid plexuses via several small emissary veins.

2. The *sphenopalatine sinuses*, situated below the lesser wings of the sphenoid bone, drain the dura mater into the cavernous sinuses.

3. The *intercavernous sinus* (circular sinus) forms a venous collar around the stalk of the pituitary gland and connects the two cavernous sinuses.

4. The *superior petrosal sinus* connects the cavernous with the transverse sinus and runs in the margin of the tentorium cerebelli, crossing the

fifth cranial nerve. It receives veins from the tympanic cavity, cerebellum and inferior parts of the cerebrum.

5. *The inferior petrosal* sinus begins at the cavernous sinus, passes through the jugular foramen, and joins the internal jugular vein. It receives the internal auditory (labyrinthine) veins and veins from the medulla oblongata, pons and cerebellum.

6. The *basilar plexus* lies over the basilar portion of the occipital bone. It consists of interlacing venous channels, communicates with the two inferior petrosal sinuses, and drains blood from the anterior vertebral plexuses. □

## Deep and Subependymal Veins of Brain

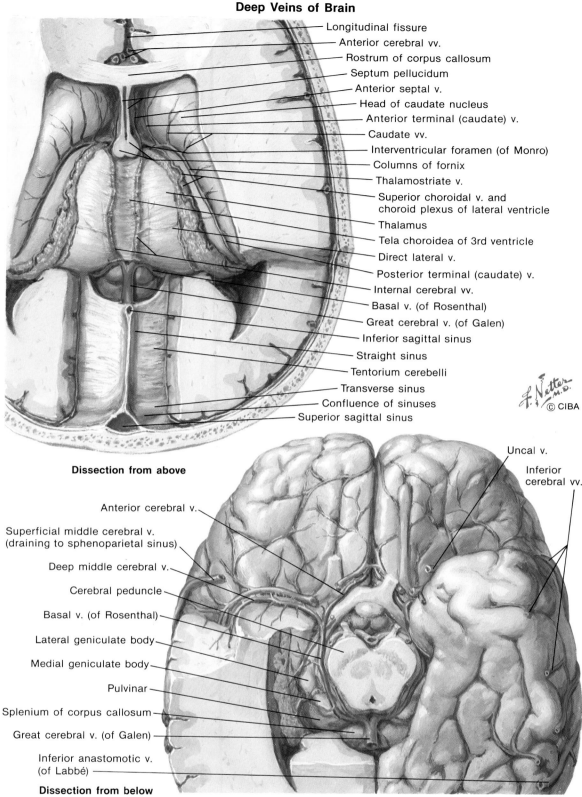

**Deep Veins of Brain**

Longitudinal fissure
Anterior cerebral vv.
Rostrum of corpus callosum
Septum pellucidum
Anterior septal v.
Head of caudate nucleus
Anterior terminal (caudate) v.
Caudate vv.
Interventricular foramen (of Monro)
Columns of fornix
Thalamostriate v.
Superior choroidal v. and choroid plexus of lateral ventricle
Thalamus
Tela choroidea of 3rd ventricle
Direct lateral v.
Posterior terminal (caudate) v.
Internal cerebral vv.
Basal v. (of Rosenthal)
Great cerebral v. (of Galen)
Inferior sagittal sinus
Straight sinus
Tentorium cerebelli
Transverse sinus
Confluence of sinuses
Superior sagittal sinus

**Dissection from above**

Uncal v.
Inferior cerebral vv.

Anterior cerebral v.
Superficial middle cerebral v. (draining to sphenoparietal sinus)
Deep middle cerebral v.
Cerebral peduncle
Basal v. (of Rosenthal)
Lateral geniculate body
Medial geniculate body
Pulvinar
Splenium of corpus callosum
Great cerebral v. (of Galen)
Inferior anastomotic v. (of Labbé)

**Dissection from below**

*The great cerebral vein (of Galen)* receives the deep veins of the brain. It is a short vessel, about 2 cm in length, and originates under splenium of the corpus callosum from the union of the two *internal cerebral veins*. It passes through the upper portion of the cistern of the great cerebral vein to join the inferior sagittal sinus at a right angle and form the straight sinus (Plate 13). It receives the two *basal veins*, as well as the *posterior pericallosal, internal occipital, posterior mesencephalic, precentral* and *superior vermian* (or, if present, *superior cerebellar*) *veins*.

*The internal cerebral veins* (right and left) are formed at the level of the interventricular foramen by the union of the *anterior septal* and the *thalamostriate veins*. The internal cerebral veins run backward, parallel to each other, and immediately enter the tela choroidea of the third ventricle. From here, they pass through the velum interpositum to the level of the splenium of the corpus callosum, where they join with the two basal veins to form the great cerebral vein. Each is at first concave inferiorly and then concave superiorly as it passes backward. The internal cerebral veins receive the *superior choroidal veins*, the *roof veins* of the *lateral ventricle*, the *veins* of the *posterior horn* of the *lateral ventricle* and the *thalamic veins*.

The *thalamostriate vein*, also known as the superior thalamostriate, or terminal, vein, drains the caudate nucleus, the internal capsule and the deep white matter of the posterior frontal and anterior parietal lobes. It is formed by the *anterior terminal (caudate)* and *posterior terminal (caudate) veins*. The latter originates at the level of the atrium, passes anteriorly between the body of the caudate nucleus and the thalamus, and receives *transverse caudate veins* from the body of the caudate nucleus, *intramedullary veins* from the deep superior white matter of the posterior frontal and anterior parietal lobes, and *striate veins* from the lentiform nuclei. The anterior portion of

the thalamostriate vein passes through the interventricular foramen and forms an important angiographic landmark called the *venous angle* (see page 58). Occasionally, the thalamostriate vein will drain into one of the superior thalamic veins, draining directly into the internal cerebral vein. On angiography, this produces a false venous angle, which lies behind the interventricular foramen.

The *anterior septal vein* is formed by the union of multiple *intramedullary veins*, which drain the deep white matter of the anterior portion of the frontal lobe. These unite in the anterior portion of the anterior (frontal) horn of the lateral ventricle,

## Deep and Subependymal Veins of Brain
*(Continued)*

anterior to the head of the caudate nucleus, and form one or, sometimes, two veins. The anterior septal vein runs medially, curving posteriorly along the septum pellucidum and passing lateral to the columns of the fornix, to join with the ipsilateral thalamostriate vein and form the internal cerebral vein.

The *superior choroidal vein* courses over the top of the thalamus in the anterior portion of the choroid plexus of the lateral ventricle, and terminates in the anterior portion of the internal cerebral vein or the thalamostriate vein. The superior choroidal vein provides the main venous drainage of the choroid plexus in this location.

The *roof veins of the lateral ventricle*, of which the principal one is the *direct lateral vein*, drain the deep white matter of the anterior frontal and posterior parietal lobes. After reaching the lateral angle of the lateral ventricle, these veins either pass across the roof of the lateral ventricle and down the septum pellucidum or cross its floor to reach the internal cerebral vein.

The *veins of the posterior horn of the lateral ventricle* pass along the medial and lateral walls of the posterior (occipital) horn and atria to drain into the internal cerebral vein. These veins drain the white matter of the posterior temporal and occipital lobes, the fimbria of the fornix and the choroid plexus of the atrium.

The *veins of the thalamus* drain into the internal cerebral vein via several small *superior thalamostriate veins*. Several surface veins drain into the

superior aspect of the internal cerebral vein, and an *anterior thalamic vein* drains into its anterior portion. Several small *midthalamic veins* coalesce to form a *major thalamic vein*, which drains into the inferior aspect of the midportion of the internal cerebral vein.

*The basal vein* (of Rosenthal) arises on the ventral surface of the brain, just lateral to the optic chiasm and inferior to the anterior perforated substance. It is formed by the union of the *deep middle cerebral vein* and the *anterior cerebral vein*, and courses posteriorly around the cerebral peduncle, just superior and medial to the posterior cerebral artery. The basal vein joins the two internal cerebral veins and the basal vein of the opposite side, just under the splenium of the corpus callosum, at the origin of the great cerebral vein. It receives several large and small veins during its course.

The *anterior cerebral vein* follows the course of the anterior cerebral artery, and drains the anterior third of the corpus callosum, the anterior portion of the medial surface of the frontal lobe and the medial orbital frontal gyri. Just anterior to the optic chiasm and the lamina terminalis, it communicates with the contralateral anterior cerebral vein via the *anterior communicating vein*; just lateral to the optic chiasm, it joins the deep middle cerebral vein to form the basal vein.

The *deep middle cerebral vein* originates on the insula and drains that structure. It passes medially through the anterior part of the interpeduncular cistern ventral to the anterior perforated substance, and drains the inferior portion of the corpus striatum. It then joins the anterior cerebral vein just lateral to the optic chiasm to form the basal vein.

Among the many other venous tributaries to the basal vein are those draining the optic chiasm, the optic tract, the hypothalamus and the medial aspect of the cerebral peduncles. The *peduncular veins* coalesce to form the *interpeduncular vein*, which drains the anterior midbrain, the subthalamus and posterior perforated substance; it connects with the corresponding tributary vein to the contralateral basal vein. The anastomosis between the basal veins posteriorly, and the anterior communicating anastomosis between the anterior cerebral veins anteriorly, form a venous circle similar to the circle of Willis.

Midway in its passage around the mesencephalon, the basal vein receives *temporal veins* and an *inferior ventricular vein* from the inferior horn of the lateral ventricle. These drain the deep white matter of the superior and lateral portions of the temporal lobe, the hippocampus, the dentate gyrus and the choroid plexus. The hindmost portion of the basal vein receives the *lateral mesencephalic vein* from the mesencephalon (Plate 16).

*Internal Occipital Vein*. Multiple veins on the inferior and medial surface of the occipital lobe coalesce to form the internal occipital vein, which drains into the great cerebral vein and provides the venous drainage for the inferior and medial surfaces of the occipital lobe. These coalescing veins also drain to the superior sagittal and the transverse sinuses, and provide an anastomotic pathway between the great cerebral vein and the sinuses.

*The posterior pericallosal vein* can be single or double. It passes posteriorly, curving around the splenium of the corpus callosum to enter the great cerebral vein, and provides the venous drainage

for the posterosuperior surface of the corpus callosum and splenium.

*Posterior Fossa Veins*. The *precentral cerebellar veins*, the *posterior mesencephalic vein* and the *superior vermian vein* (or *superior cerebellar vein*, if present) drain into the great cerebral vein. They drain the posterior mesencephalon and the superior cerebellum (Plate 16).

### Angiography

*Venous Landmarks*. The *dural sinuses*, the *superficial cerebral veins* and the *deep cerebral venous system* are visualized during the venous phase of a cerebral angiogram. The inferior sagittal, straight and superior sagittal sinuses are well visualized on the lateral projection, but are superimposed on each other in the frontal view. Both the frontal and lateral projections demonstrate drainage from the confluence of the sinuses via the transverse and sigmoid sinuses into the jugular vein (Plate 13). The *great cerebral vein* and its main tributaries are constant angiographic features. Inasmuch as there are no large arteries in the depth of the brain, the neuroradiologist can use the deep venous system to evaluate the deep structures of the hemispheres.

*The superficial veins* on the convexity of the cerebral hemispheres bridge the subarachnoid and subdural spaces near their sites of entrance into the superior sagittal and transverse sinuses (Plates 11 and 12). The largest vein draining into the superior sagittal sinus is the *superior anastomotic vein (of Trolard)*, which links the middle cerebral vein (and hence the cavernous sinus) with the superior sagittal sinus. The largest vein draining into the transverse sinus is the *inferior anastomotic vein (of Labbé)*, which thus forms a connection between the middle cerebral vein and the transverse sinus. The superficial veins vary in size and location, and are not of great value to the neuroradiologist in the angiographic localization of space-occupying intracranial lesions.

*On the lateral projection*, the *anterior septal vein* can be seen joining the *thalamostriate vein* to form the *internal cerebral vein*. The latter at first is concave inferiorly and then concave superiorly as it joins the *basal vein* to form the *great cerebral vein*. The junction of the thalamostriate vein with the internal cerebral vein is the *venous angle*, at the level of the interventricular foramen. The course of the internal cerebral vein gives a rough approximation of the upper medial aspect of the thalamus, while the basal vein approximately follows the ventrolateral aspect of the thalamus. The courses of the *anterior* and *posterior terminal veins* outline the caudate nucleus; together with the course of the anterior septal vein, they roughly outline the anterior (frontal) horn and body of the lateral ventricle. The *superior choroidal vein* can be seen running parallel to the posterior terminal vein as it drains anteriorly into the thalamostriate vein.

*On the frontal projection*, the course of the *internal cerebral vein* can be used to fix the midline of the brain. The *thalamostriate* and *posterior terminal veins* have a slightly convex inferolateral configuration, and this provides an approximate outline of the body of the lateral ventricle. The *basal vein*, curving to reach the midline with a slight medial (and posterior) concavity, provides an outline of the lateral portion of the mesencephalon. □

# Subependymal Veins

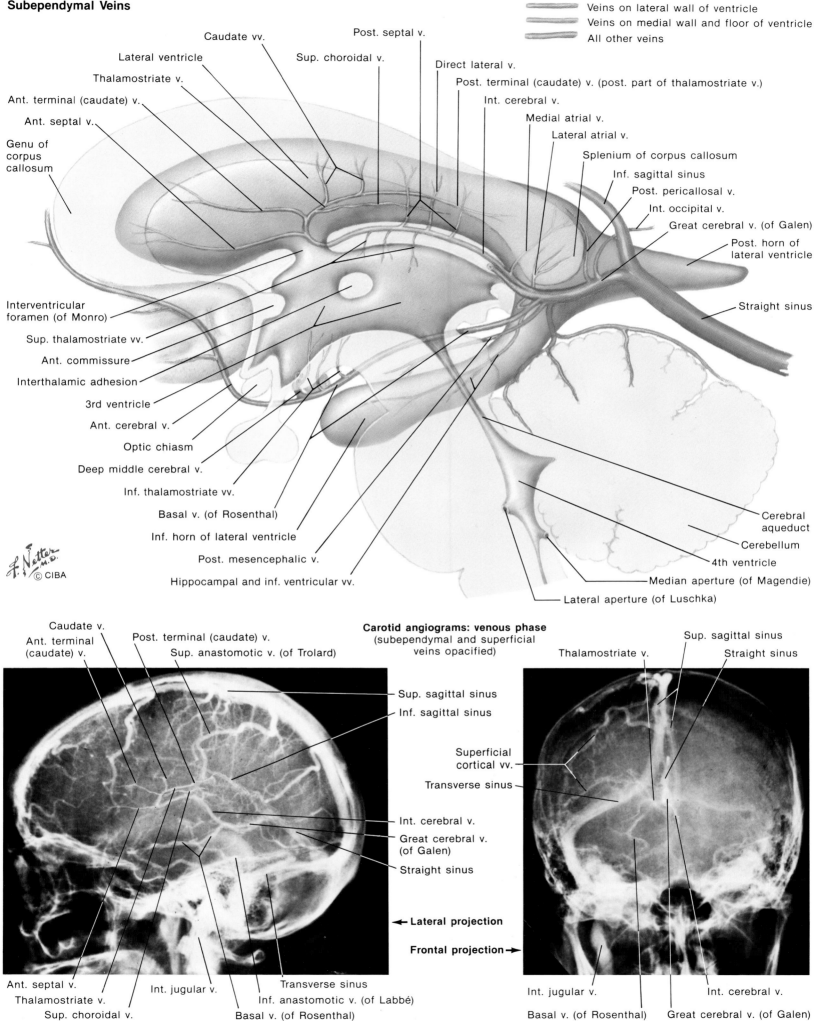

Veins on lateral wall of ventricle
Veins on medial wall and floor of ventricle
All other veins

Caudate vv.
Lateral ventricle
Thalamostriate v.
Ant. terminal (caudate) v.
Ant. septal v.
Genu of corpus callosum
Post. septal v.
Sup. choroidal v.
Direct lateral v.
Post. terminal (caudate) v. (post. part of thalamostriate v.)
Int. cerebral v.
Medial atrial v.
Lateral atrial v.
Splenium of corpus callosum
Inf. sagittal sinus
Post. pericallosal v.
Int. occipital v.
Great cerebral v. (of Galen)
Post. horn of lateral ventricle
Straight sinus
Interventricular foramen (of Monro)
Sup. thalamostriate vv.
Ant. commissure
Interthalamic adhesion
3rd ventricle
Ant. cerebral v.
Optic chiasm
Deep middle cerebral v.
Inf. thalamostriate vv.
Basal v. (of Rosenthal)
Inf. horn of lateral ventricle
Post. mesencephalic v.
Hippocampal and inf. ventricular vv.
Lateral aperture (of Luschka)
Median aperture (of Magendie)
4th ventricle
Cerebellum
Cerebral aqueduct

**Carotid angiograms: venous phase**
(subependymal and superficial veins opacified)

Caudate v.
Ant. terminal (caudate) v.
Post. terminal (caudate) v.
Sup. anastomotic v. (of Trolard)
Sup. sagittal sinus
Inf. sagittal sinus
Int. cerebral v.
Great cerebral v. (of Galen)
Straight sinus
Ant. septal v.
Thalamostriate v.
Sup. choroidal v.
Int. jugular v.
Basal v. (of Rosenthal)
Inf. anastomotic v. (of Labbé)
Transverse sinus

← Lateral projection

Frontal projection →

Sup. sagittal sinus
Thalamostriate v.
Straight sinus
Superficial cortical vv.
Transverse sinus
Int. jugular v.
Basal v. (of Rosenthal)
Great cerebral v. (of Galen)
Int. cerebral v.

# Veins of Posterior Cranial Fossa

The veins of the posterior fossa drain the cerebellum and brainstem, and are classified from their direction of drainage into the *superior (galenic) group*, the *anterior (petrosal) group* and the *posterior (tentorial) group*.

## Superior Group

These veins drain the superior portion of the cerebellum and upper part of the brainstem.

The midline *precentral vein* is a major vessel that originates in the primary fissure between the lingula and central lobule of the anterior superior cerebellar vermis. Within the fissure, the precentral vein runs parallel to the roof of the fourth ventricle, but as it passes out of the fissure and between the inferior colliculi and the central lobule of the cerebellum, it angles upward and backward around the culmen. This angle, which is clearly visible on the lateral projection of the angiogram, is called the *colliculocentral point*. The vein leaves the culmen to enter the superior portion of the quadrigeminal cistern and join the great cerebral vein. On leaving the primary fissure, it is joined by the right and left lateral brachial veins, which are anastomotic connections via the lateral mesencephalic vein with the basal vein, and via the brachial veins with the petrosal vein.

The *superior vermian vein* is formed by the union of tiny preculminate, intraculminate and supraculminate tributaries that drain the culmen of the cerebellar vermis. As it ascends toward the apex of the cerebellum to join the great cerebral vein, the superior vermian vein arches over the culmen. Occasionally, it unites with the precentral vein to form a common trunk called the *superior cerebellar vein*, which then drains into the great cerebral vein.

The *superior cerebellar hemispheric veins* vary in number and location. Some run medially and anteriorly across the superior aspect of the cerebellum to join one of the culminate tributaries, the stem of the superior vermian vein or the precentral vein, and hence drain into the great cerebral vein or the straight sinus; others run laterally to end in the transverse and superior petrosal sinuses.

The *posterior mesencephalic vein*, which can be single or multiple, originates in the interpeduncular fossa or on the lateral aspect of the mesencephalon. Its size is inversely proportional to that of the basal vein; it may be present in addition to the basal vein, or replace its posterior portion. It courses backward and upward around the midbrain to join the posterior portion of the great cerebral vein.

The *anterior pontomesencephalic vein* may drain into the superior group via its anastomoses with the basal vein, or into the petrosal group.

The *lateral mesencephalic vein* is a relatively constant anastomotic vein that runs within, or adjacent to, the lateral mesencephalic sulcus. It connects with the basal or posterior mesencephalic veins above, and with the brachial tributary of the petrosal vein below, and occasionally, with the brachial tributaries of the precentral vein.

The *quadrigeminal veins* (not shown in the illustration) are small veins that drain the corpora quadrigemina and then pass upward and backward to join the great cerebral vein.

## Anterior or Petrosal Group

The *petrosal vein* receives venous drainage from the anterior aspect of the brainstem, the superior and inferior surfaces of the cerebellar hemispheres, the region of the cerebellomedullary fissure and the lateral recess of the fourth ventricle. It drains into the superior petrosal sinus and has several named tributaries.

The *anterior medullary vein* courses anterior to the medulla in or near the midline. It is a direct continuation of the anterior spinal veins and drains into the anterior pontomesencephalic vein. The *anterior pontomesencephalic vein* is a longitudinal venous plexus that has a tortuous course in or near the midline. It is the continuation of the anterior medullary vein, and ascends anterior to the belly of the pons to terminate in the interpeduncular fossa by sending anastomotic branches to the great cerebral vein or to the petrosal vein. The *transverse pontine veins* are connecting veins that run anterior to the medulla, pons and mesencephalon. They connect the anterior medullary and anterior pontomesencephalic veins with the petrosal vein. The *peduncular vein* (a transverse mesencephalic vein) courses in front of the cerebral peduncle and connects the termination of the anterior pontomesencephalic vein with the basal vein. Consequently, the anterior pontomesencephalic vein may drain into the great cerebral vein via the basal vein, or into the petrosal vein via transverse pontine veins.

There are numerous other small vessels in this region. The *lateral pontomesencephalic veins* are longitudinal veins on the lateral aspect of the cerebral peduncle that drain inferiorly to the petrosal vein. The *lateral pontine vein* courses superiorly in the lateral pontine sulcus between the pons and the brachium pontis to join the petrosal vein. The *anterolateral marginal vein* passes medially parallel to the anterolateral margin of the cerebellar hemisphere to join the petrosal vein. The *brachial veins* pass along the lateral aspect of the brachium pontis and brachium conjunctivum, and anastomose with the lateral mesencephalic vein and the lateral brachial tributaries of the precentral vein. As they pass to the petrosal vein, the brachial veins receive venous drainage from the anterior superior margin of the cerebellum, and thus outline the cerebellar notch on angiography.

The *vein of the great horizontal fissure of the cerebellum* originates in the depth of the horizontal fissure and courses anterolaterally to reach the petrosal cerebellar surface. It passes medially between the inferior semilunar and quadrangular lobules to drain into the petrosal vein.

Some *superior cerebellar hemispheric veins* pass forward and down to join the vein of the great horizontal fissure or the anterolateral marginal vein.

Occasionally, they drain directly into the inferior petrosal sinus, precentral vein, culminate veins or lateral mesencephalic vein.

The *inferior cerebellar hemispheric veins* also vary in number and course. They run anteriorly and superiorly on the ventral surface of the inferior semilunar and biventral lobules to drain into the vein of the great horizontal fissure, anterolateral marginal vein, vein of the lateral recess of the fourth ventricle or lateral pontine vein.

The *retroolivary (lateral medullary) vein* runs in the retroolivary sulcus to drain into the lateral pontine vein or directly into the inferior petrosal sinus. Among its tributaries is the *vein of the restiform body* (the superior continuation of the median posterior spinal vein), which ascends parallel to the lower border of the fourth ventricle, posterior to the restiform body, and drains into either the retroolivary vein or the vein of the lateral recess of the fourth ventricle. The *medial tonsillar veins* are also tributaries, draining the medial surface of the tonsil and joining the retroolivary vein, the vein of the restiform body or the vein of the lateral recess of the fourth ventricle.

The *vein of the lateral recess of the fourth ventricle* originates in the region of the dentate impression on the superior surface of the cerebellar tonsil. It receives tributaries from the dentate nucleus and adjacent cerebellar white matter and from the subependymal and tonsillar veins, and runs parallel to, and slightly below, the lateral recess of the fourth ventricle. At the level of the flocculus, the vein ascends and runs anteromedially to join the petrosal vein.

## Posterior or Tentorial Group

This group of veins drains the inferior portion of the cerebellar vermis and the medial portion of the superior and inferior cerebellar hemispheres.

The *inferior vermian vein* is formed in the region of the copula pyramis by the union of superior and inferior retrotonsillar tributaries from the corresponding poles of the tonsil. It ascends in the paravermian sulcus and drains into the straight sinus 1.5 to 2.0 cm anterior to the confluence of the sinuses, as well as anastomosing with the superior vermian vein. During its course, it receives the suprapyramidal vein from the suprapyramidal fissure and the declival vein from the primary fissure in the clival sulcus.

The posterior group also includes those *superior cerebellar hemispheric veins* that drain the superomedial surface of the cerebellar hemisphere, via a tentorial venous sinus, into the lateral sinus or straight sinus near the torcular, and those *inferior cerebellar hemispheric veins* that drain the inferomedial surface of the cerebellar hemisphere into the transverse sinus.

## Angiography

The venous phase of a selective vertebral-basilar arteriogram shows many of the veins of the posterior cranial fossa.

**On the lateral projection**, the veins most useful for localizing space-occupying lesions, because they are always visualized, are the *precentral vein*, the *superior* and *inferior vermian veins*, the *anterior pontomesencephalic vein* and the *posterior* and *lateral mesencephalic veins*.

**On the frontal projection**, the veins constantly visualized are the *inferior vermian, petrosal, lateral mesencephalic* and *lateral brachial veins*. □

# Veins of Posterior Cranial Fossa

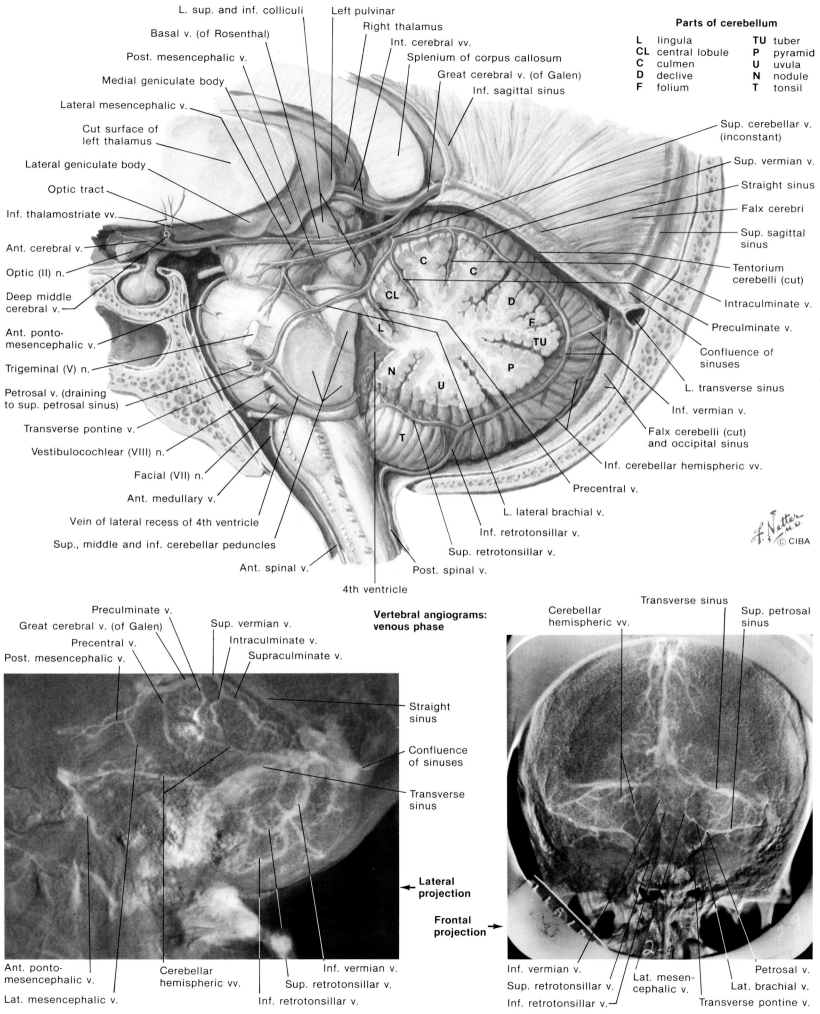

**Parts of cerebellum**

| | | | |
|---|---|---|---|
| **L** | lingula | **TU** | tuber |
| **CL** | central lobule | **P** | pyramid |
| **C** | culmen | **U** | uvula |
| **D** | declive | **N** | nodule |
| **F** | folium | **T** | tonsil |

L. sup. and inf. colliculi

Basal v. (of Rosenthal)

Post. mesencephalic v.

Medial geniculate body

Lateral mesencephalic v.

Cut surface of left thalamus

Lateral geniculate body

Optic tract

Inf. thalamostriate vv.

Ant. cerebral v.

Optic (II) n.

Deep middle cerebral v.

Ant. ponto-mesencephalic v.

Trigeminal (V) n.

Petrosal v. (draining to sup. petrosal sinus)

Transverse pontine v.

Vestibulocochlear (VIII) n.

Facial (VII) n.

Ant. medullary v.

Vein of lateral recess of 4th ventricle

Sup., middle and inf. cerebellar peduncles

Ant. spinal v.

Left pulvinar

Right thalamus

Int. cerebral vv.

Splenium of corpus callosum

Great cerebral v. (of Galen)

Inf. sagittal sinus

Sup. cerebellar v. (inconstant)

Sup. vermian v.

Straight sinus

Falx cerebri

Sup. sagittal sinus

Tentorium cerebelli (cut)

Intraculminate v.

Preculminate v.

Confluence of sinuses

L. transverse sinus

Inf. vermian v.

Falx cerebelli (cut) and occipital sinus

Inf. cerebellar hemispheric vv.

Precentral v.

L. lateral brachial v.

Inf. retrotonsillar v.

Sup. retrotonsillar v.

Post. spinal v.

4th ventricle

## Vertebral angiograms: venous phase

Preculminate v.

Great cerebral v. (of Galen)

Precentral v.

Post. mesencephalic v.

Sup. vermian v.

Intraculminate v.

Supraculminate v.

Straight sinus

Confluence of sinuses

Transverse sinus

Ant. ponto-mesencephalic v.

Cerebellar hemispheric vv.

Sup. retrotonsillar v.

Inf. retrotonsillar v.

Inf. vermian v.

Lat. mesencephalic v.

← **Lateral projection**

**Frontal projection** →

Cerebellar hemispheric vv.

Transverse sinus

Sup. petrosal sinus

Inf. vermian v.

Sup. retrotonsillar v.

Inf. retrotonsillar v.

Lat. mesencephalic v.

Petrosal v.

Lat. brachial v.

Transverse pontine v.

# Computerized Tomography (CT Scanning)

Computerized axial tomography (CT scanning) is a specialized x-ray examination in which a transaxial image is obtained from multiple angular projections. The x-ray tube within the scanning gantry is rotated 180° to 360° around the area to be examined—in this case, the brain. The multiple angular projections thus obtained are detected by an array of either solid state scintillation detectors or xenon gas ionization detectors, which are also located within the gantry. These detectors either rotate in conjunction with the x-ray tube or are stationary in a 360° circle around the patient. They are more sensitive than x-ray film, and are able to detect variations of as little as 1% in the density of soft tissue (x-ray film detects differences of 10% to 15%). The information obtained by these detectors is analyzed by a computer which, using a technique called "filtered back-projection," constructs an image of the cross section of the region within the plane of the x-ray beam. The section may be 13, 10, 7 or 2 mm thick (depending upon the type of CT scanner and the preselected image thickness), and it reveals the organs in an aspect which, until the development of the CT scanner, could be seen only in the anatomy department.

*Technique.* For CT scanning of the brain, the patient's head is placed in the center of the scanning gantry and then positioned so that the plane of the gantry, and consequently of the axial image, makes a 20° angle to the canthomeatal plane (an imaginary plane passing through the lateral canthus of the eye and the center of the external auditory canal). This angle is selected so that the air-containing paranasal sinuses (which can form disturbing low-density artifacts that reduce the quality of the image) will be excluded as much as possible from the axial cross section chosen.

The first image selected is usually at a level passing through the floor of the anterior fossa and, because of the 20° angle, the foramen magnum. Multiple sequential contiguous images are then obtained up to the vertex of the calvaria. These images directly reveal the subarachnoid space, ventricles, basal ganglia, thalamus, internal and external capsules, gray and white matter of the hemispheres and bony calvaria.

If an iodinated contrast agent is injected intravenously (as shown in the films in Plate 18), the tentorium cerebelli, falx cerebri, choroid plexus of the lateral ventricles, dural venous sinuses, major deep veins and major blood vessels at the base of the brain will also be evident. Under normal circumstances, the contrast agent does not enter the brain, but if the blood-brain barrier is disrupted by a lesion, the contrast agent will leak into that area and produce better visualization ("enhancement"). Using CT scanning, the neuroradiologist can precisely locate an intracerebral lesion and assess its relationship to the intrinsic anatomy of the brain and the bony calvaria, without resorting to invasive techniques. □

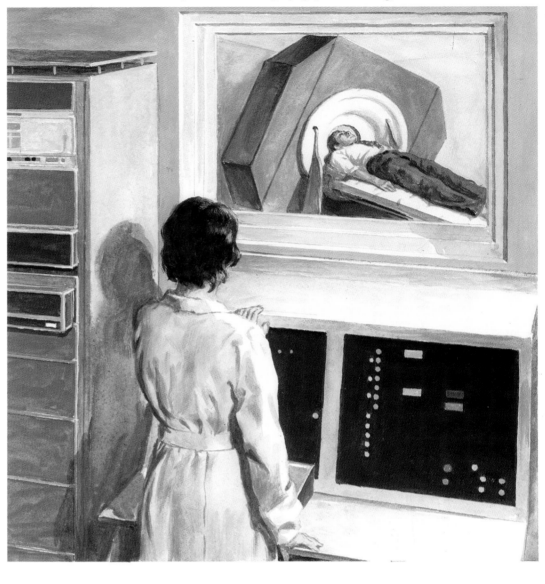

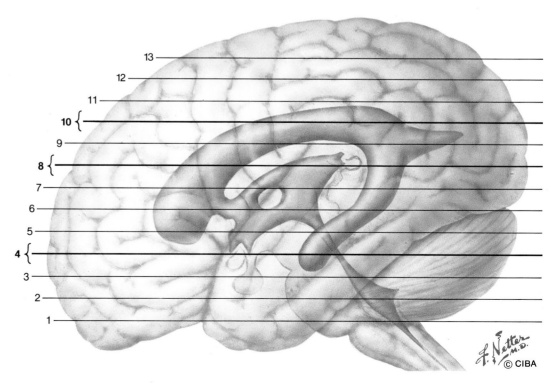

**Planes of CT scan sections**

Sections 10, 8 and 4 are shown in Plate 18; brackets indicate thickness of sections

**Section 10**

Frontal lobe

Parietal lobe

Temporal lobe

Occipital lobe

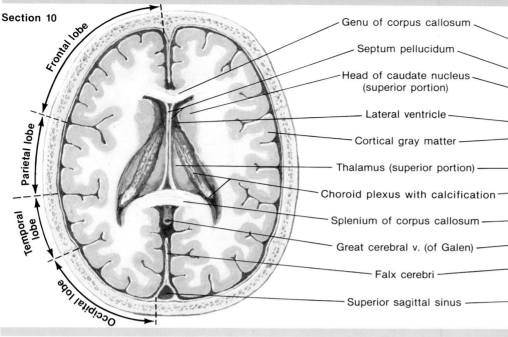

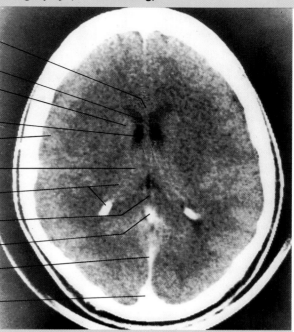

Genu of corpus callosum

Septum pellucidum

Head of caudate nucleus (superior portion)

Lateral ventricle

Cortical gray matter

Thalamus (superior portion)

Choroid plexus with calcification

Splenium of corpus callosum

Great cerebral v. (of Galen)

Falx cerebri

Superior sagittal sinus

---

**Section 8**

Frontal lobe

Temporal lobe

Occipital lobe

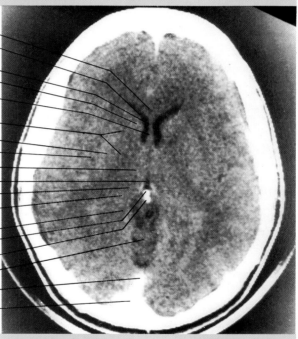

Rostrum of corpus callosum

Anterior horn of lateral ventricle

Septum pellucidum

Head of caudate nucleus

Column of fornix

Anterior and posterior limbs of internal capsule

Lentiform nucleus

External capsule

Thalamus

3rd ventricle

Pulvinar

Choroidal fissure

Retrosplenial parahippocampal gyrus

Calcified pineal gland

Great cerebral v. (of Galen)

Superior cerebellar vermis

Straight sinus

Confluence of sinuses

---

**Section 4**

Frontal lobe

Temporal lobe

Posterior fossa

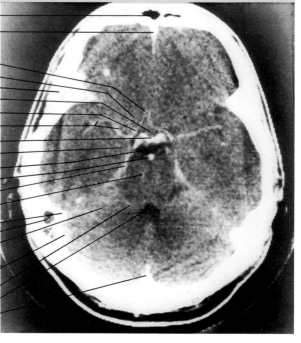

Frontal sinus

Bony frontal crest

Anterior cerebral a.

Parolfactory area

Pterion

Suprasellar cistern

Internal carotid a.

Middle cerebral a.

Dorsum sellae

Uncus

Prepontine cistern

Basilar a.

Posterior cerebral a.

Pons

Petrous pyramid

Mastoid air cells

Tentorium cerebelli

Sigmoid sinus going to internal jugular v.

Middle cerebellar peduncle

4th ventricle

Internal occipital crest

*F. Netter M.D.*
© CIBA

# Arteries of Spinal Cord

The spinal cord is supplied by multiple *radicular arteries*, which form the *anterior spinal* and two *posterior spinal arteries*.

*The radicular arteries* arise from neighboring arteries at the level of each vertebral segment. Regardless of their origin, the many small radicular arteries pass medially through the intervertebral foramina, together with the nerve roots. Most do not reach the spinal cord, being principally concerned with supplying the exiting nerve roots. However, some of the larger arteries reach the dura mater, where they give off small *meningeal branches*, and then divide into *ascending* and *descending branches* to form the spinal arteries. The larger radicular arteries, which supply both the nerve roots and the spinal cord, are called *radiculomedullary arteries* to distinguish them from those radicular arteries that supply only the nerve roots.

*The anterior spinal artery* runs the entire length of the spinal cord in the midline. It usually originates in the upper cervical region at the junction of the two *anterior spinal branches* that arise from the *fourth segment of each vertebral artery*. Six to ten *anterior radicular arteries* contribute to it throughout its length, branching upward and downward. As a result, there is a point between two anterior radicular arteries where, because of the opposing blood flow, there will be no flow in either direction. Occasionally, in the thoracic region, the anterior spinal artery narrows to such a degree that it will not function as an adequate anastomosis. Blood from the anterior spinal artery is distributed to the anterior two thirds of the substance of the spinal cord via *central branches* and *penetrating branches* from the *pial plexus*.

The *cervical* and *first two thoracic segments of the spinal cord* are supplied by radicular arteries that arise from branches of the *subclavian artery*. Variability is the rule, and the branches can arise from either the right or the left (usually alternately) to join the anterior spinal artery at an angle of 60° to 80°. Not uncommonly, one anterior radicular branch arises from the vertebral artery and accompanies the C3 nerve root, one branch arises from the deep cervical artery and accompanies the C6 root, and one branch arises from the superior intercostal artery and accompanies the C8 root.

The *middorsal region of the spinal cord* (T3 to T7) usually receives only one radicular artery, which accompanies the T4 or T5 nerve root. Consequently, this

## Arteries of Spinal Cord

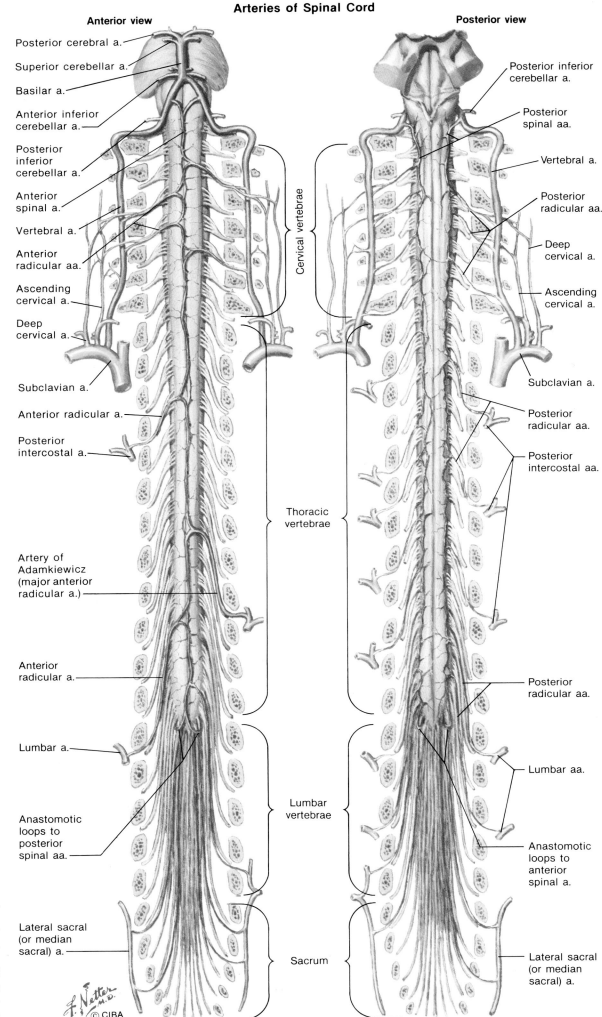

**Anterior view**

- Posterior cerebral a.
- Superior cerebellar a.
- Basilar a.
- Anterior inferior cerebellar a.
- Posterior inferior cerebellar a.
- Anterior spinal a.
- Vertebral a.
- Anterior radicular aa.
- Ascending cervical a.
- Deep cervical a.
- Subclavian a.
- Anterior radicular a.
- Posterior intercostal a.
- Artery of Adamkiewicz (major anterior radicular a.)
- Anterior radicular a.
- Lumbar a.
- Anastomotic loops to posterior spinal aa.
- Lateral sacral (or median sacral) a.

**Posterior view**

- Posterior inferior cerebellar a.
- Posterior spinal aa.
- Vertebral a.
- Posterior radicular aa.
- Deep cervical a.
- Ascending cervical a.
- Subclavian a.
- Posterior radicular aa.
- Posterior intercostal aa.
- Posterior radicular aa.
- Lumbar aa.
- Anastomotic loops to anterior spinal a.
- Lateral sacral (or median sacral) a.

- Cervical vertebrae
- Thoracic vertebrae
- Lumbar vertebrae
- Sacrum

## Arteries of Spinal Cord
*(Continued)*

section of the cord is characterized by its poor afferent blood supply, and the anterior spinal artery may not be continuous at this level.

The *dorsolumbosacral part of the spinal cord* (T8 to the conus medullaris) derives its main arterial supply from the artery of Adamkiewicz, which arises from a left-sided *intercostal (lumbar) artery* in 80% of individuals. In 85% of instances, it reaches the cord with a nerve root between T9 and L2; in the 15% of cases in which it reaches the cord between T5 and T8, it is supplemented by a radicular artery arising more inferiorly. The *artery of Adamkiewicz* (the major anterior radicular artery) has a large anterior and a smaller posterior radicular branch. On reaching the anterior aspect of the spinal cord, the *anterior radicular branch* ascends a short distance and then makes a hairpin turn to give off a small ascending branch and a larger descending branch, which drops to the level of the conus medullaris where it forms an anastomotic circle with the terminal branches of the two posterior spinal arteries.

The *cauda equina* is accompanied and supplied by one or two branches from the *lumbar, iliolumbar,* and *lateral* and *median sacral arteries*. These branches also ascend to contribute to the anastomotic arterial circle around the conus medullaris.

**The central branches** of the anterior spinal artery pass back into the anterior median fissure to supply the central parts of the substance of the spinal cord. At the anterior commissure, the branches turn alternately right and left to supply the corresponding halves of the cord, except in the lumbar enlargement, where the left and right branches arise from a common trunk. The terminal branches ascend and descend within the cord, supplying overlapping territories. There are 5 to 8 central arteries for each centimeter length of the spinal cord in the cervical region, 2 to 6 in the thoracic region and 5 to 12 in the lumbosacral area. The central arteries supply the anterior commissure and adjacent white matter of the ventral columns, anterior horns, bases of the posterior horns, Clarke's columns, corticospinal tracts, spinothalamic tracts, ventral parts of the gracile and cuneate fasciculi and the region around the central canal.

**The posterior spinal arteries** are paired arteries coursing on the posterolateral aspects of the entire length of the spinal cord, although they may become discontinuous at times. Each originates

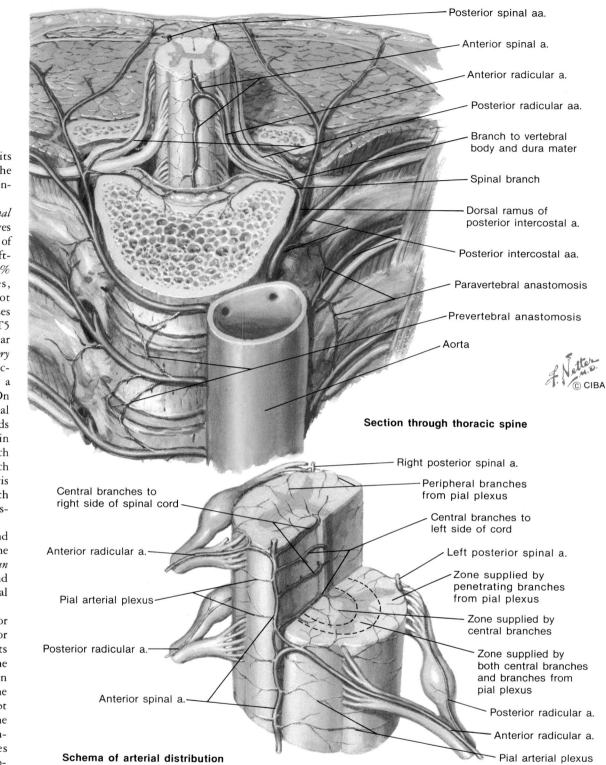

**Section through thoracic spine**

Posterior spinal aa.
Anterior spinal a.
Anterior radicular a.
Posterior radicular aa.
Branch to vertebral body and dura mater
Spinal branch
Dorsal ramus of posterior intercostal a.
Posterior intercostal aa.
Paravertebral anastomosis
Prevertebral anastomosis
Aorta

Central branches to right side of spinal cord
Anterior radicular a.
Pial arterial plexus
Posterior radicular a.
Anterior spinal a.

Right posterior spinal a.
Peripheral branches from pial plexus
Central branches to left side of cord
Left posterior spinal a.
Zone supplied by penetrating branches from pial plexus
Zone supplied by central branches
Zone supplied by both central branches and branches from pial plexus
Posterior radicular a.
Anterior radicular a.
Pial arterial plexus

**Schema of arterial distribution**

from the *fourth segment* of the corresponding *vertebral artery*, and receives contributions from 10 to 23 *posterior radicular arteries*. The posterior spinal arteries distribute blood to the posterior third of their respective sides of the cord.

In the *cervicodorsal region*, the posterior spinal arteries receive one, and sometimes two, tributaries at each segment. *Below the T4 or T5 level*, there is, on the average, one posterior radicular branch every other segment, including the *posterior radicular branch of the artery of Adamkiewicz*.

**Pial Arterial Plexus**. Small pial branches arise from the spinal arteries, and ramify and interconnect on the surface of the cord to form a *pial*

*plexus*. Penetrating branches of the plexus supply the outer part of the substance of the cord; they follow the principal sulci of the cord (the posterior median sulcus and the posterior intermedian sulcus) to reach the anterior and posterior horns. The peripheral pial branches supply the outer portions of the posterior horns, most of the posterior columns, and the outer portion of the white matter of the periphery of the spinal cord.

There is some degree of overlap in the distribution of the peripheral and central arteries at the capillary level, but they do not anastomose at the arterial level, and hence both types are, in effect, *end arteries*. ☐

# Veins of Spinal Cord and Vertebrae

Two plexuses of veins, external and internal, extend along the entire length of the vertebral column and form a series of moderately distinct rings around each vertebra. The plexuses anastomose freely with each other, receive tributaries from the vertebrae, ligaments and spinal cord, and are relatively devoid of valves. Consequently, changes in the pressure of intrathoracic or cerebrospinal fluid may produce variations in the volume of blood, especially in the internal vertebral venous plexuses.

*The external vertebral plexus* consists of anterior and posterior parts, which anastomose freely. The veins forming the *anterior external plexus* lie in front of the vertebral bodies, from which they receive venous tributaries and through which they communicate with the basivertebral veins. The *posterior external plexus* is a network located over the vertebral laminae and extending around the spinous, transverse and articular processes. In the upper cervical region, the posterior plexus communicates with the occipital veins and, via these, with the mastoid and occipital emissary veins. The posterior plexus also communicates with the vertebral and deep cervical veins, and a few channels pass through the foramen magnum to the dural sinuses in the posterior cranial fossa.

*The internal vertebral plexus* is formed by networks of veins lying in the epidural space within the vertebral canal. The networks are arranged in anterior and posterior groups, which are interconnected by many smaller oblique and transverse channels. The *anterior internal plexus* consists of longitudinal veins lying on the posterior surfaces of the vertebral bodies and intervertebral discs found on each side of the posterior longitudinal ligament. Interconnecting branches lie between the ligament and the vertebral bodies, and receive the basivertebral veins. The longitudinal veins in the *posterior internal plexus* are smaller than their anterior counterparts. They are located on each side of the median plane, in front of the vertebral arches and ligamenta flava. They anastomose with the veins of the posterior external vertebral plexus via small veins that pierce the ligaments and pass between them.

*The basivertebral veins* resemble the cranial diploë, and tunnel through the cancellous tissue of the vertebral bodies. They converge to form a comparatively large, single (occasionally, double) vein, which emerges through the posterior surface of the vertebral body to end, via openings guarded by valves, in the transverse interconnections of the

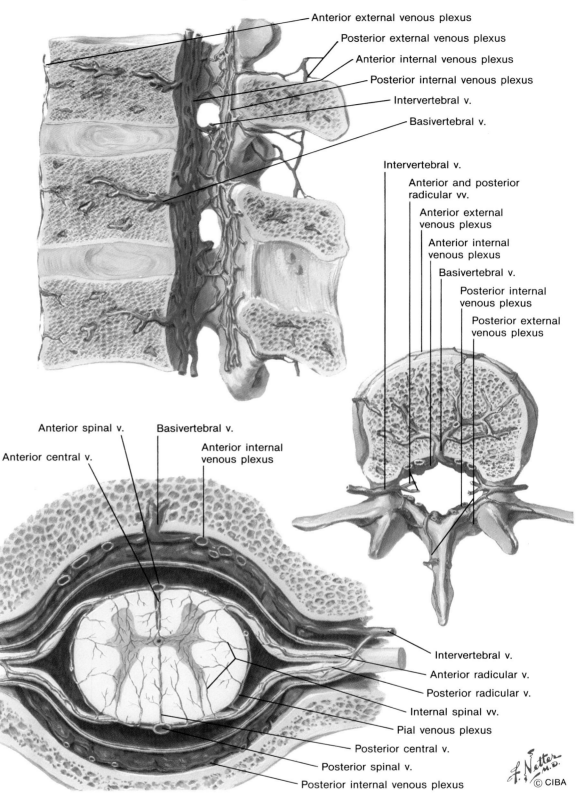

Anterior external venous plexus
Posterior external venous plexus
Anterior internal venous plexus
Posterior internal venous plexus
Intervertebral v.
Basivertebral v.

Intervertebral v.
Anterior and posterior radicular vv.
Anterior external venous plexus
Anterior internal venous plexus
Basivertebral v.
Posterior internal venous plexus
Posterior external venous plexus

Anterior spinal v.    Basivertebral v.
Anterior central v.    Anterior internal venous plexus

Intervertebral v.
Anterior radicular v.
Posterior radicular v.
Internal spinal vv.
Pial venous plexus
Posterior central v.
Posterior spinal v.
Posterior internal venous plexus

anterior internal vertebral plexus. The basivertebral veins also drain into the anterior external plexus through openings in the front and sides of the vertebral body.

*The veins of the spinal cord* resemble the related arteries in their distribution, and form a tortuous plexus in the pia mater (Plates 19 and 20). The venules empty into *anterior* and *posterior central veins*, which drain into two *median longitudinal veins*, and into two pairs of *anterolateral* and *posterolateral longitudinal veins* lying adjacent to the ventral and dorsal nerve roots. Above, the spinal veins communicate with veins draining the medulla oblongata and the inferior surface of the cerebellum through the foramen magnum. *Anterior* and *posterior radicular veins*, associated with the spinal nerve roots and radicular arteries, unite with branches from the anterior and posterior internal vertebral plexuses to form the *intervertebral veins*.

*The intervertebral veins* drain most of the blood from the spinal cord and from the internal and external vertebral venous plexuses. They accompany the spinal nerves through the intervertebral foramina, and end in the vertebral, posterior intercostal, subcostal, lumbar and lateral sacral veins. Their orifices are usually protected by valves. □

Section IV

# Autonomic Nervous System

Frank H. Netter, M.D.

*in collaboration with*

G.A.G. Mitchell, Ch.M., D.Sc., F.R.C.S.   *Plates 1–21*

Barry W. Peterson, Ph.D. and Alexander Mauro, Ph.D.   *Plate 22*

## Schema of Autonomic Nervous System

The nervous system is divided into somatic and autonomic components chiefly on functional grounds: the former controls predominantly voluntary activities, while the latter regulates involuntary functions. The two divisions are not disparate entities; they develop from the same primordial cells, they comprise closely associated central and peripheral parts, and they are both built up from afferent, efferent and internuncial neurons linked to produce ascending and descending nerve pathways and to form similar reflex arcs.

*The central autonomic components* are intrinsic parts of the CNS. They are located in the frontal premotor and other areas of the cerebral cortex, thalamus, hypothalamus, hippocampus, cerebellum, brainstem and spinal cord; these higher and lower levels of representation are interconnected by ascending and descending tracts, or pathways (see Section VIII). For example, efferent autonomic impulses originating in the frontal premotor cortical areas descend through fiber tracts, or fasciculi, usually via synaptic relays in the thalamus, hypothalamus and reticular formation, to end in certain *cranial nerve nuclei* and thus influence the involuntary muscles, vessels and glands supplied by them (see Section V and Section VIII, Plate 12). Other fibers descend still farther to end by forming synapses with lateral cornual neurons in the *thoracic* and *upper two lumbar spinal cord segments*, and around neurons located in similar positions in the gray matter of the *second to fourth sacral cord segments*. The axons of these neurons leave the cord in the ventral roots of the corresponding spinal nerves (see Section VI, Plates 3 and 10).

*The peripheral parts of the autonomic nervous system* include: *two chains* of *sympathetic ganglia*; paravertebral *sympathetic trunks*, which extend from the cranial base to the coccyx; *ganglia* in the *head region*, such as the ciliary, pterygopalatine, otic, submandibular and carotid; *prevertebral plexuses* and *ganglia*, such as the cardiac, celiac, mesenteric, intermesenteric (abdominal aortic) and hypogastric; *plexuses* located on or in the *walls of hollow viscera* and vessels; *ganglia associated* with *glands* (hepatic and adrenal); the myriad of *interconnections* and *branches* of these trunks, ganglia and plexuses; and the *autonomic efferent* and *afferent fibers* that are constituents of most cranial and spinal nerves.

Experimental and clinical evidence has established that the axons of autonomic neurons in cranial nerve nuclei and sacral spinal segments convey impulses that usually produce effects opposite to those produced when impulses are

### General Topography of Autonomic Nervous System

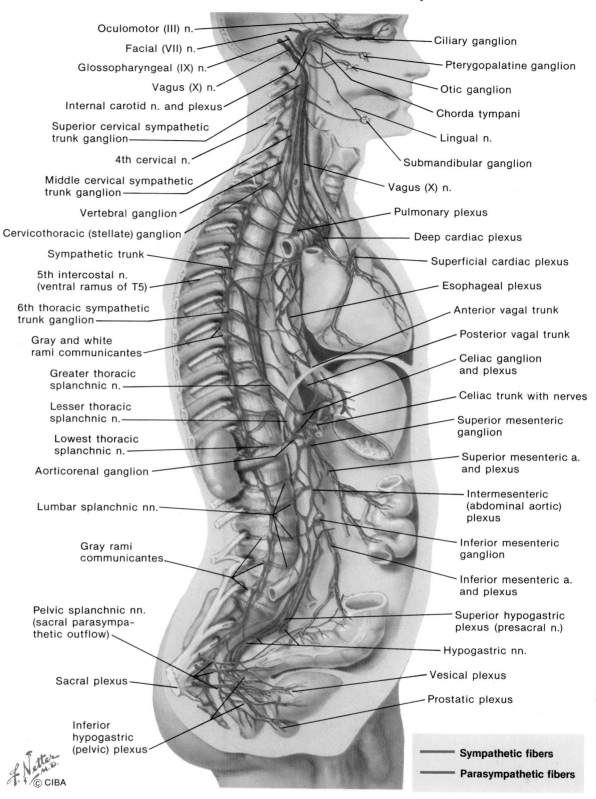

Oculomotor (III) n.
Facial (VII) n.
Glossopharyngeal (IX) n.
Vagus (X) n.
Internal carotid n. and plexus
Superior cervical sympathetic trunk ganglion
4th cervical n.
Middle cervical sympathetic trunk ganglion
Vertebral ganglion
Cervicothoracic (stellate) ganglion
Sympathetic trunk
5th intercostal n. (ventral ramus of T5)
6th thoracic sympathetic trunk ganglion
Gray and white rami communicantes
Greater thoracic splanchnic n.
Lesser thoracic splanchnic n.
Lowest thoracic splanchnic n.
Aorticorenal ganglion
Lumbar splanchnic nn.
Gray rami communicantes
Pelvic splanchnic nn. (sacral parasympathetic outflow)
Sacral plexus
Inferior hypogastric (pelvic) plexus

Ciliary ganglion
Pterygopalatine ganglion
Otic ganglion
Chorda tympani
Lingual n.
Submandibular ganglion
Vagus (X) n.
Pulmonary plexus
Deep cardiac plexus
Superficial cardiac plexus
Esophageal plexus
Anterior vagal trunk
Posterior vagal trunk
Celiac ganglion and plexus
Celiac trunk with nerves
Superior mesenteric ganglion
Superior mesenteric a. and plexus
Intermesenteric (abdominal aortic) plexus
Inferior mesenteric ganglion
Inferior mesenteric a. and plexus
Superior hypogastric plexus (presacral n.)
Hypogastric nn.
Vesical plexus
Prostatic plexus

F. Netter M.D.
© CIBA

━━━ **Sympathetic fibers**
━━━ **Parasympathetic fibers**

transmitted by the axons of the thoracolumbar lateral cornual neurons. The cranial and sacral groups are called *parasympathetic*, and the more numerous thoracolumbar groups, *sympathetic*.

Although sympathetic and parasympathetic fibers (axons) transmit impulses producing different effects, their neurons are morphologically similar (see Section VII, Plates 10 to 13 and Section VIII, Plate 2). They are smallish, ovoid, multipolar cells with myelinated axons and a variable number of dendrites. All the axons form synapses in peripheral ganglia, and the unmyelinated axons of the ganglionic neurons convey impulses to the viscera, vessels and other structures

innervated. Because of this arrangement, the axons of the autonomic nerve cells in the nuclei of the cranial nerves, in the thoracolumbar lateral cornual cells, and in the gray matter of the sacral spinal segments are termed *preganglionic fibers*, while those of the ganglion cells are called *postganglionic fibers* (see page 71).

The cranial *parasympathetic preganglionic fibers* form synapses in the ciliary, pterygopalatine, otic, submandibular, cardiac and celiac ganglia, or in much smaller ganglia in the walls of the trachea, bronchi and gastrointestinal tract. The corresponding sacral fibers form synapses in the inferior hypogastric (pelvic) plexuses, in minute

## Schema of Autonomic Nervous System

*(Continued)*

ganglia within the enteric plexuses of the distal colon and rectum, or in the walls of the urinary bladder or other pelvic viscera. Most of the thoracolumbar *sympathetic preganglionic fibers* end by forming synapses in sympathetic trunk ganglia, but other fibers pass through them to form synapses in such ganglia as the celiac, mesenteric and renal.

The *parasympathetic relay ganglia* are located near the structures innervated or are actually within the walls of hollow organs or the substance of solid viscera, so that the *parasympathetic postganglionic fibers* are relatively short. The *sympathetic relay ganglia* are generally more distant from the structures innervated, so that the *sympathetic postganglionic fibers* are often much longer than their parasympathetic counterparts. (This is one reason why sympathetic effects are usually more diffuse than parasympathetic effects.) Plate 2 illustrates the arrangement of the preganglionic and postganglionic fibers to all the important viscera, the positions of the ganglia in which the synaptic relays occur, and the consequent disparities in the lengths of the postganglionic fibers. Take the heart, perhaps the most important example: its sympathetic preganglionic fibers relay mainly in sympathetic trunk ganglia, from the superior cervical to the fourth or fifth thoracic, and the relatively long postganglionic fibers are conveyed to the heart in the cervical and thoracic sympathetic cardiac nerves. The parasympathetic preganglionic fibers reach the heart in the cardiac branches of the vagus nerves and relay in ganglia of the cardiac plexus or in small subendocardial ganglia, so that their postganglionic fibers are relatively short (see pages 76 and 77).

The concept that the autonomic nervous system is purely efferent has been discarded. Large numbers of afferent autonomic fibers from the heart, vessels, lungs, gastrointestinal tract, genitourinary tract and other vascular and visceral structures transmit essential information to the CNS.

*Autonomic Afferent Neurons.* The *first neurons*, or lowest autonomic sensory neurons, like the somatic afferent neurons, are pseudounipolar cells located in dorsal spinal nerve root ganglia and in the ganglia of certain cranial nerves (eg, the facial, glossopharyngeal and vagal). The peripheral processes of the first neurons convey impulses from various types of free and specialized nerve endings and from fine nerve networks in viscera and vessels. Their central processes enter the spinal cord, and thereafter some take part in the formation of reflex

arcs, for example, by forming synapses with cells in the lateral columns of spinal gray matter. The *second neurons* in the autonomic afferent pathways form synapses with cells in the posterior gray columns or in the substantia intermedia centralis of the cord at about the level of their entry. Most second neurons carry the impulses upward, mainly through tracts in the lateral and anterior white columns of the cord, although some neurons

ascend in the posterior white columns. Some fibers may reach the thalamus, while others—perhaps the majority—may reach the hypothalamus through the mamillary peduncles and other ascending afferent hypothalamic pathways. After relaying, the impulses ultimately attain cortical levels in the premotor and orbital areas of the cerebral frontal lobes; these represent the *third (highest) neurons* in somatic afferent pathways. ☐

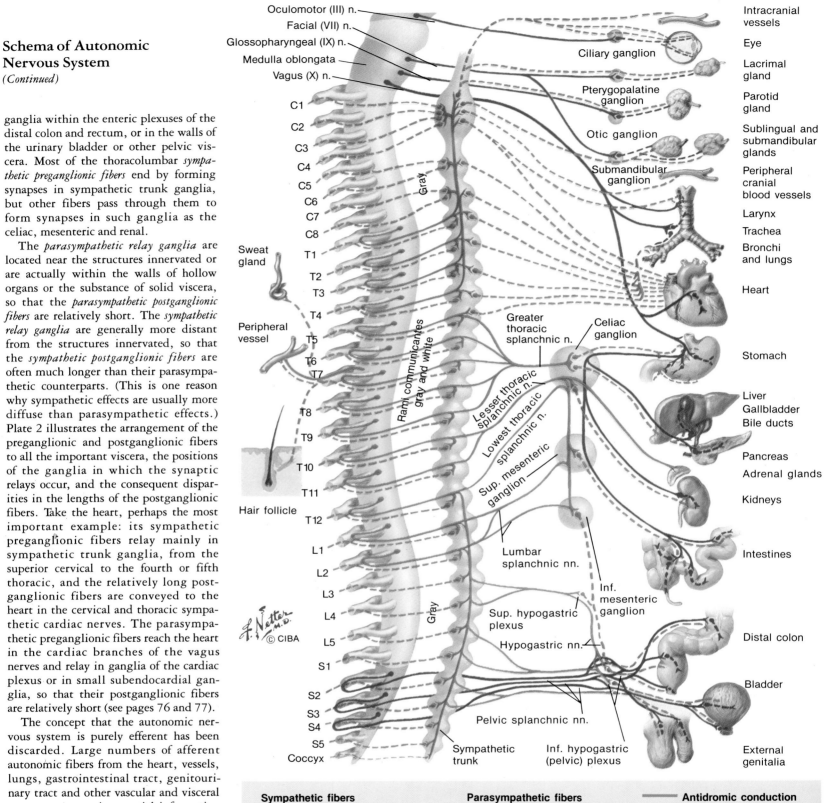

| Sympathetic fibers | Parasympathetic fibers | Antidromic conduction |
|---|---|---|
| —— preganglionic | —— preganglionic | |
| --- - postganglionic | --- - postganglionic | |

# Autonomic Reflex Pathways

The illustration shows the arrangement of a typical spinal autonomic reflex arc, in this example involving the enteric plexus in the gut. Similar reflex arcs exist in the brainstem.

The basic similarity of autonomic and somatic reflex arcs is apparent from comparing this illustration with Plate 32 in Section VIII, although in the somatic arcs, the internuncial neurons lie entirely within the CNS. In the autonomic arcs, the internuncial cell bodies lie within the CNS, but their axons travel outside to reach the ganglia in which they terminate. Initially, the autonomic and somatic components of the nervous system develop together, but during the embryonic and fetal phases, groups of nerve cells migrate outward along the spinal nerve roots and form ganglia, such as those of the sympathetic trunks, and more peripheral ganglia, such as the celiac and mesenteric (see Section VII, Plate 11). These migrant cells are efferent autonomic neurons, and in order to maintain their synaptic relationships, the axons of the internuncial cells must follow them, so they, too, wander outside the CNS to reach the autonomic ganglion cells with which they form synapses. Because they precede the ganglia, these axons are termed *preganglionic fibers*, whereas the axons of ganglionic neurons lie beyond the ganglia and are called *postganglionic* fibers. The preganglionic fibers are myelinated. When seen in mass, as in the large groups of sympathetic preganglionic fibers passing from all the thoracic and the upper two lumbar spinal nerves to nearby sympathetic trunk ganglia, they are almost white in color and constitute the *white rami communicantes*. Afferent myelinated fibers pass through these rami to the spinal nerves and contribute to their whitish appearance. The postganglionic fibers are unmyelinated and appear grayish-pink in color when seen in mass. They form the *gray rami communicantes* connecting each sympathetic trunk ganglion to the adjoining spinal nerves.

Only part of a *parasympathetic arc (vagal)* is illustrated, and it should be understood that the cell bodies of the afferent pseudounipolar neurons are located in vagal nerve ganglia, that their central axonal processes enter the brainstem to end in the dorsal vagal nuclei, and that the axons of these nuclear cells form synapses with cells in ganglia of the enteric plexus.

The illustration also shows that sympathetic preganglionic fibers emerging through the thoracic or upper lumbar spinal nerves behave in various ways. They all pass through white rami communicantes to adjacent sympathetic trunk

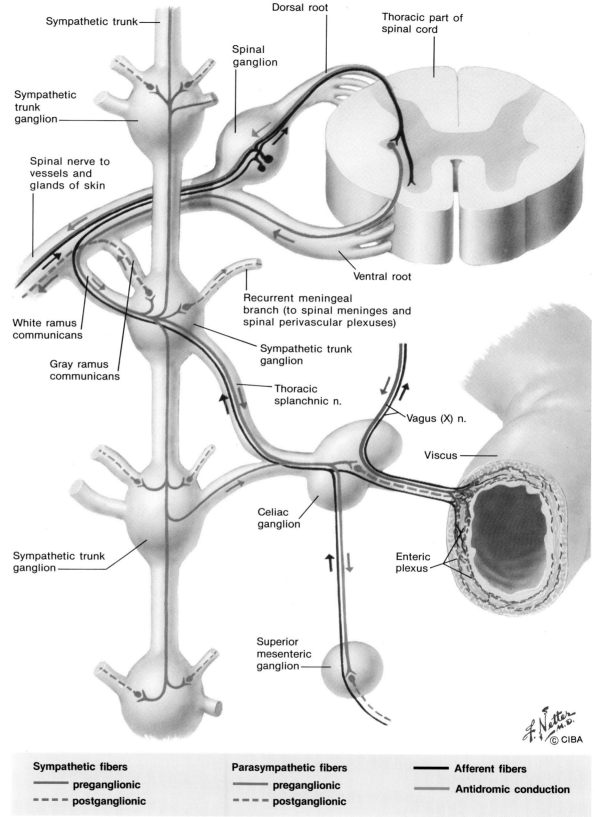

ganglia, and many end in synapses around the cells of the ganglia. Others pass upward or downward in the sympathetic trunks to form synapses with neurons in cervical, lower lumbar and sacral trunk ganglia, and the axons of these cells (postganglionic fibers) again behave in various ways. Many fibers pass to adjacent spinal nerves as gray rami communicantes, which explains why all spinal nerves have such connections, whereas white rami communicantes are limited to the thoracolumbar region. Still other preganglionic fibers pass through the sympathetic trunk ganglia without relaying, and run in splanchnic nerves to end in ganglia such as the celiac and mesenteric.

Also shown is a recurrent meningeal sympathetic branch carrying postganglionic fibers to the spinal meninges and the spinal perivascular plexuses. □

# Cholinergic and Adrenergic Nerves

The terms "adrenergic" and "cholinergic," introduced by Dale in 1933, are based on the concept that the transmission of nerve impulses across the microscopic gaps between autonomic nerve fibers and the structures they innervate is effected by chemical mediation.

*Epinephrine* (adrenaline), and especially the closely related *norepinephrine* (noradrenaline), are the chief "neurotransmitters" at peripheral sympathetic, or *adrenergic*, terminations, whereas *acetylcholine* is generally associated with parasympathetic, or *cholinergic*, effects. However, acetylcholine is also an important, or probably the most important, neurotransmitter at synapses in both sympathetic and parasympathetic pathways. If it is appreciated that Dale's terms were initially applied only to *postganglionic fibers*, the fact that acetylcholine may be the chief neurotransmitter at synapses between *preganglionic fibers* and ganglionic neurons should cause no misconception.

The illustration shows the sites at which acetylcholine (C) and norepinephrine (A) are the chief neurotransmitters. Other chemical substances, for example adenosine triphosphate (ATP), gamma-aminobutyric acid (GABA), a polypeptide called Substance P, histamine, glutamic acid and prostaglandins have also been implicated as transmitter agents.

Impulses conducted by sympathetic, or adrenergic, nerve fibers usually elicit active reactions in effector structures, such as smooth (unstriated) muscle or glands, which are the reverse of the diminished activity produced by parasympathetic, or cholinergic, fibers. Thus, stimulation of the sympathetic and parasympathetic cardiac nerves produces cardiac acceleration and deceleration. However, these effects are not universal. For example, activity of the alimentary adrenergic nerves produces retardation of gastrointestinal motility; conversely, activity in the cholinergic supply results in acceleration of gastric and intestinal movements. Similar reactions occur in other structures. Thus, in the urinary tract, the sympathetic nerves produce relaxation of the bladder wall, and the parasympathetic nerves cause contraction, so that the former have been aptly described as "filling" and the latter, as "emptying" nerves.

Claims that some peripheral arteries and sweat glands are innervated by "sympathetic cholinergic fibers" must be accepted with reservation. Although stimulation of these vascular nerves leads to the release of acetylcholine (Plate 10) in the areas of distribution of cranial and sacral parasympathetic outflows (Plates 1 and 2), the viscera and vessels have cholinergic and adrenergic supplies, so that the structures served actually receive fibers from both sympathetic and parasympathetic sources.

Vessels and sweat glands in the limbs and body wall also reputedly receive only adrenergic innervation, and the nerves involved are supposed to contain a proportion of "sympathetic cholinergic fibers," which release acetylcholine, with consequent vasodilator and secretomotor effects. There is another possible explanation for such effects: these vessels and glands may receive a supply through parasympathetic fibers in the putative dorsal spinal nerve root efferent fibers. Incidentally, if these efferent fibers exist, their presence casts doubts on the hypothesis that "antidromic" conduction along afferent fibers causes the peripheral vasodilatation that follows stimulation of the distal ends of divided dorsal spinal nerve roots. □

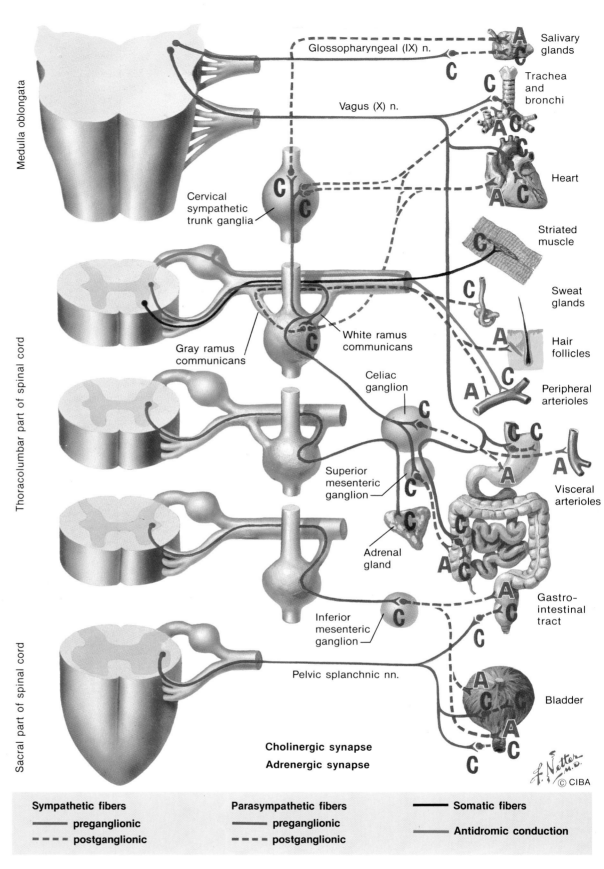

Medulla oblongata

Thoracolumbar part of spinal cord

Sacral part of spinal cord

Glossopharyngeal (IX) n.

Vagus (X) n.

Cervical sympathetic trunk ganglia

Gray ramus communicans

White ramus communicans

Celiac ganglion

Superior mesenteric ganglion

Adrenal gland

Inferior mesenteric ganglion

Pelvic splanchnic nn.

Salivary glands

Trachea and bronchi

Heart

Striated muscle

Sweat glands

Hair follicles

Peripheral arterioles

Visceral arterioles

Gastro-intestinal tract

Bladder

Cholinergic synapse
Adrenergic synapse

| Sympathetic fibers | Parasympathetic fibers | Somatic fibers |
|---|---|---|
| preganglionic | preganglionic | |
| postganglionic | postganglionic | Antidromic conduction |

# Autonomic Nerves in Head and Neck

The cervical part of each sympathetic trunk generally incorporates four ganglia –*superior* and *middle cervical, vertebral* and *cervicothoracic*. The superior and middle cervical ganglia are usually connected by a single cord, but the middle cervical, vertebral and cervicothoracic ganglia are connected by several cords, one or more of which form a loop, the ansa subclavia, around the subclavian artery and sometimes also around the vertebral artery. A true inferior cervical ganglion is present only in about 20% of individuals; in the majority, the lowest cervical and uppermost thoracic ganglia are fused to form the cervicothoracic (stellate) ganglion.

*The superior cervical ganglion is* elongated and waisted, or fusiform, in shape. It is produced by the coalescence of the upper three or four cervical ganglia. The preganglionic fibers forming synapses there mostly emerge through the uppermost thoracic spinal nerves and ascend to it in the cervical sympathetic trunk, but a relatively small number of these fibers may reach it from adjacent cervical nerve roots. An unknown proportion of the preganglionic fibers pass through it without interruption and relay at higher levels in the internal carotid ganglia.

The superior cervical ganglion receives or supplies communicating, visceral, vascular, muscular, osseous and articular rami. It *communicates* with the last four cranial nerves or their branches, with the vertebral arterial plexus and, occasionally, with the phrenic nerve. It supplies gray rami to the upper three or four cervical spinal nerves, and the contained postganglionic fibers are distributed with the branches of the cervical nerves they join. *Visceral filaments* pass to the larynx, pharynx and heart, and other fibers are carried in vascular plexuses to the salivary, lacrimal, pituitary, pineal, thyroid and other glands. *Vascular filaments* are supplied to the internal and external carotid arteries and form plexuses around them; prolongations from these form subsidiary plexuses around all their branches. From the internal carotid plexus, minute caroticotympanic offshoots join the tympanic branch of the glossopharyngeal nerve and thus reach the tympanic plexus (see Section V, Plate 10). A deep petrosal branch unites with the greater petrosal nerve to form the *nerve of the pterygoid canal*, which constitutes the so-called *sympathetic root of the pterygopalatine ganglion* (see Section V, Plate 4). Actually, sympathetic fibers are already postganglionic and run through the ganglion without relaying, to be distributed to vessels and glands in the nose, palate, nasopharynx and orbit. The *sympathetic root of the ciliary ganglion* arises from the cranial end of the

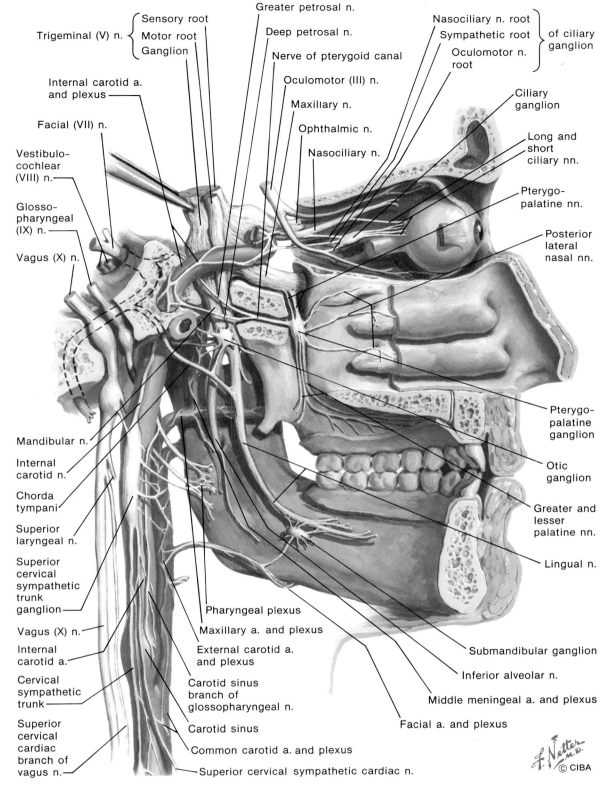

Trigeminal (V) n. { Sensory root / Motor root / Ganglion }
Greater petrosal n.
Deep petrosal n.
Nerve of pterygoid canal
Nasociliary n. root / Sympathetic root / Oculomotor n. root } of ciliary ganglion
Internal carotid a. and plexus
Facial (VII) n.
Oculomotor (III) n.
Maxillary n.
Ophthalmic n.
Nasociliary n.
Ciliary ganglion
Vestibulo-cochlear (VIII) n.
Long and short ciliary nn.
Pterygo-palatine nn.
Glosso-pharyngeal (IX) n.
Vagus (X) n.
Posterior lateral nasal nn.
Mandibular n.
Internal carotid n.
Chorda tympani
Superior laryngeal n.
Superior cervical sympathetic trunk ganglion
Vagus (X) n.
Internal carotid a.
Cervical sympathetic trunk
Superior cervical cardiac branch of vagus n.
Pharyngeal plexus
Maxillary a. and plexus
External carotid a. and plexus
Carotid sinus branch of glossopharyngeal n.
Carotid sinus
Common carotid a. and plexus
Superior cervical sympathetic cardiac n.
Pterygo-palatine ganglion
Otic ganglion
Greater and lesser palatine nn.
Lingual n.
Submandibular ganglion
Inferior alveolar n.
Middle meningeal a. and plexus
Facial a. and plexus

homolateral internal carotid nerves or plexus; its fibers are postganglionic, having relayed in the superior cervical or internal carotid ganglia; they pass through the ganglion and run onward in the ciliary nerves to supply the ocular vessels and the dilator pupillae (see Section V, Plates 5 and 6). In addition to postganglionic efferent fibers, many *visceral efferent* and *afferent fibers* are also present in the vascular plexuses. They convey sympathetic impulses to the pituitary, lacrimal, salivary, thyroid and other smaller glands in the territories supplied by the carotid arteries, and they also transmit sensory information from the same structures. In a similar fashion, sympathetic fibers are

carried to adjacent *osseous, articular* and *muscular* structures.

*The middle cervical ganglion is* much smaller than the superior ganglion and usually represents fused fifth and sixth cervical ganglia. It contributes gray rami communicantes to the fifth and sixth cervical nerves and sends filaments to the vertebral periarterial plexus. Inconstant strands form interconnections with the vagus, phrenic and recurrent laryngeal nerves, and *visceral branches* are supplied to the thyroid and parathyroid glands. The ganglion may give off the middle cervical sympathetic cardiac nerve, and contributes several twigs to the esophagus and

## Autonomic Nerves in Head and Neck

*(Continued)*

trachea. *Vascular branches* help in the innervation of the common carotid, inferior thyroid and vertebral arteries and the jugular veins. Filaments pass to adjacent muscular, osseous and articular structures, usually alongside the arteries supplying them.

*The vertebral ganglion* is small and is located anterior to the vertebral artery, near its point of entry into the transverse foramen of the sixth cervical vertebra. It may receive gray rami communicantes from the sixth and/or seventh cervical nerves, and may thus represent a lower detached element of the middle cervical ganglion or an upper disjoined portion of the cervicothoracic ganglion. It gives off *vascular branches* that accompany the vertebral artery; it may be connected by filaments to the vagus and phrenic nerves; and it supplies tiny *visceral branches* to the thyroid gland, trachea and esophagus.

*The cervicothoracic (stellate) ganglion* is formed by the fusion of the seventh and eighth cervical ganglia with the first and/or second thoracic ganglia. It is an irregularly fusiform structure with many radiating branches.

The cervicothoracic ganglion is situated posterior to the first part of the subclavian artery, the origin of the vertebral artery, the vertebral vein and the apex of the lung. It lies anterior to the last cervical transverse process, the neck of the first rib and the anterior primary ramus of the eighth cervical nerve as it passes outward to unite with the corresponding ramus of the first thoracic nerve and form the inferior trunk of the brachial plexus. The vertebral vessels run over the upper pole of the ganglion, and the superior intercostal vessels run lateral to it at the level of the neck of the first rib. An aponeurotic slip from the scalene muscles spreads out to become attached to the suprapleural membrane and may veil the ganglion during the anterior operative approach. If a scalenus minimus is present, it may also obscure the ganglion.

The cervicothoracic ganglion receives white rami communicantes from the first and second thoracic nerves and sends gray rami communicantes to the eighth cervical and first thoracic nerves and, occasionally, to the seventh cervical and second thoracic nerves. These rami carry efferent and afferent sympathetic fibers to and from the brachial plexus and the uppermost intercostal nerves, thus helping to innervate *vessels, sweat glands, arrectores pilorum, bones* and *joints* in the upper limbs and superior parts of the chest wall. The ganglion or the ansa subclavia invariably communicate with the homolateral phrenic

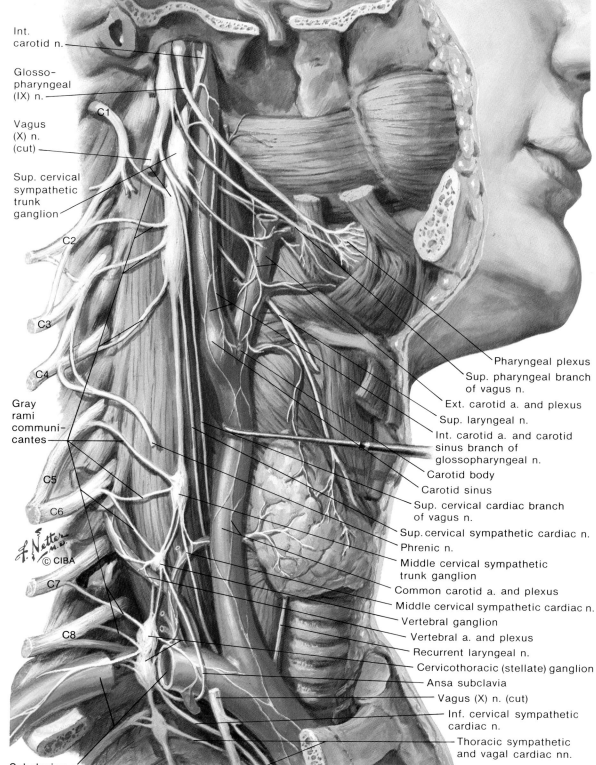

Int. carotid n.

Glossopharyngeal (IX) n.

Vagus (X) n. (cut)

Sup. cervical sympathetic trunk ganglion

C1

C2

C3

C4

Gray rami communicantes

C5

C6

C7

C8

Subclavian a.

Pharyngeal plexus

Sup. pharyngeal branch of vagus n.

Ext. carotid a. and plexus

Sup. laryngeal n.

Int. carotid a. and carotid sinus branch of glossopharyngeal n.

Carotid body

Carotid sinus

Sup. cervical cardiac branch of vagus n.

Sup. cervical sympathetic cardiac n.

Phrenic n.

Middle cervical sympathetic trunk ganglion

Common carotid a. and plexus

Middle cervical sympathetic cardiac n.

Vertebral ganglion

Vertebral a. and plexus

Recurrent laryngeal n.

Cervicothoracic (stellate) ganglion

Ansa subclavia

Vagus (X) n. (cut)

Inf. cervical sympathetic cardiac n.

Thoracic sympathetic and vagal cardiac nn.

nerve, and almost constantly with the vagus or the recurrent laryngeal nerve. Filaments are supplied to the heart, esophagus, trachea and thymus. Some vascular filaments from the ganglion pass directly to the large vessels in the cervicothoracic inlet, but most of the sympathetic fibers for the upper limb structures enter the inferior trunk of the brachial plexus. They pass mainly into the medial cord of the plexus and then into the median and ulnar nerves and, to a lesser extent, into the axillary, radial, musculocutaneous and other branches of the plexus (see Section VI, Plate 4). Vasomotor and sudomotor disturbances, or causalgia, are therefore

most likely to follow irritation or injury to the inferior trunk of the brachial plexus or to the ulnar or median nerves.

Most of the preganglionic fibers for the upper limbs emerge through the ventral rami of the second to sixth or seventh thoracic nerves, and the second and third nerves probably contain the majority of the fibers. Consequently, complete or almost complete sympathetic denervation of the upper limb can be produced by Telford's operation, which involves cutting the rami communicantes attached to the second and third thoracic ganglia and dividing the trunk below the third ganglion. □

**Autonomic Innervation of Eye**

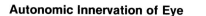

# Autonomic Innervation of Eye

*Sympathetic Fibers*. The sympathetic *preganglionic fibers* for the eye emerge in the homolateral first and second, and occasionally in the third, thoracic spinal nerves. They pass through white or mixed rami communicantes to the sympathetic trunks in which the fibers ascend to the superior cervical ganglion where they relay, although a proportion may form synapses higher up in the internal carotid ganglia. The *postganglionic fibers* run either in the internal carotid plexus and reach the eye in filaments that enter the orbit through its superior fissure, or else they run alongside the ophthalmic artery in its periarterial plexus. Some of the ocular sympathetic fibers (at least in some animals) make a curious detour through the caroticotympanic nerves and tympanic plexus before rejoining the cavernous part of the internal carotid plexus by means of a filament that emerges from the anterior surface of the petrous part of the temporal bone near the greater petrosal nerve; thereafter, they accompany the other ocular fibers.

Some of the filaments passing through the superior orbital fissure form the *sympathetic root of the ciliary ganglion*; their contained fibers pass through it without relaying, to become incorporated in the 8 to 10 *short ciliary nerves*. Other filaments join the ophthalmic nerve or its nasociliary branch and reach the eye in the two to three *long ciliary nerves* that supply the radial musculature in the iris (dilator pupillae). Both long and short ciliary nerves also contain afferent fibers from the cornea, iris and choroid. Fibers conveyed in the short ciliary nerves pass through a communicating ramus from the ciliary ganglion to the nasociliary nerve; this ramus is called the *sensory root of the ciliary ganglion*. The parent cells of these sensory fibers are located in the trigeminal (semilunar) ganglion, and their central processes end in the *sensory trigeminal nuclei* in the brainstem. The sensory trigeminal nuclei have multiple interconnections with other somatic and autonomic centers and thus influence many reflex reactions. Other sympathetic fibers from the internal carotid plexus reach the eye through the ophthalmic periarterial plexus, and along its subsidiary plexuses around the central retinal, ciliary, scleral and conjunctival arteries (Plate 5; see also Section V, Plates 5 and 6).

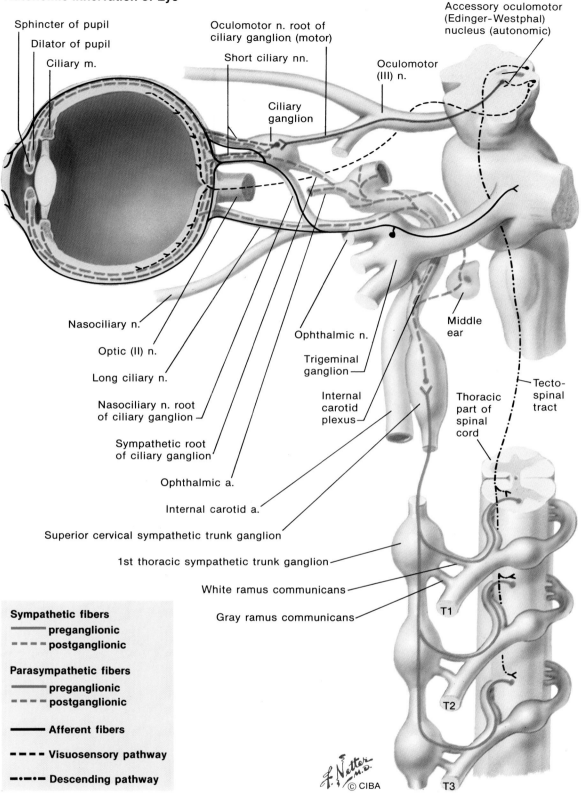

Legend:

**Sympathetic fibers**
—— preganglionic
- - - postganglionic

**Parasympathetic fibers**
—— preganglionic
- - - postganglionic

—— Afferent fibers
- - - Visuosensory pathway
—·—· Descending pathway

*Parasympathetic Fibers*. The parasympathetic preganglionic fibers for the eye are the axons of cells in the *accessory, or autonomic, (Edinger-Westphal) oculomotor nucleus*. They run in the third cranial nerve and exit in the *motor root of the ciliary ganglion*, where they relay. The axons of these ganglionic cells are postganglionic parasympathetic fibers, which reach the eye in the *short ciliary nerves* and are distributed to the constrictor fibers of the iris (sphincter pupillae), to the ciliary muscle, and to the blood vessels in the coats of the eyeball.

*Visual Centers*. The visual reflex centers are located in the tectal and pretectal areas of the mesencephalon. They are connected to the lateral geniculate bodies (lower visual centers) and to the superior colliculi in which the *tectospinal tracts* originate; these connections provide the anatomical basis for the reflex movements of the head and eyes in response to visual stimuli. The light and accommodation reflexes are effected through pretectal connections. Fibers from the lateral geniculate bodies are connected, through synapses in pretectal nuclei, to the accessory oculomotor nucleus, which controls the sphincter pupillae and the ciliary muscle (see Section VIII, Plates 21, 22 and 30). (The nerves supplying the extrinsic eye muscles are illustrated in Section V, Plates 5 and 6.) □

# Autonomic Nerves in Thorax

The thoracic parts of the sympathetic trunks lie anterior to the junctions between the heads and necks of the ribs, and posterior to the pleura. There are usually 10 or 11 ganglia on each side, because the first is often incorporated into the cervicothoracic (stellate) ganglion (Plate 6), and the last thoracic and first lumbar ganglia may also be united. The interganglionic cords are usually single, but double or triple cords between some adjacent ganglia are not uncommon. The thoracic trunks supply or receive communicating, visceral, vascular, muscular, osseous and articular branches.

Each ganglion receives at least one white ramus communicans and contributes at least one gray ramus to the adjacent spinal nerve, although several white and gray rami communicantes may be attached to each ganglion. Visceral branches are supplied to the heart and pericardium, lungs, trachea and bronchi, esophagus and thymus.

*Sympathetic Cardiac Nerves.* Three pairs of sympathetic cardiac nerves arise from the cervical trunk ganglia, and the others emerge from the upper thoracic ganglia.

The *superior cervical sympathetic cardiac nerves* originate from the corresponding trunk ganglia. On the right, the nerve passes posterolateral to the brachiocephalic artery and aortic arch; on the left, it curves downward over the left side of the aortic arch to reach the cardiac plexus.

The *middle cervical sympathetic cardiac nerves* are usually larger than the corresponding superior and inferior nerves. They arise from the middle cervical and vertebral ganglia of the sympathetic trunks, and usually run independently to the cardiac plexus.

The *inferior cervical sympathetic cardiac nerves* consist of filaments arising from the cervicothoracic ganglia and subclavian ansae.

The *thoracic sympathetic cardiac nerves* are four or five slender branches, which run forward and medially from the thoracic trunk ganglia to the cardiac plexus.

*Parasympathetic Cardiac Nerves.* Three pairs of parasympathetic (vagal) cardiac nerves are usually present. The *superior cervical vagal cardiac branches* leave the vagus nerves in the upper part of the neck. The *inferior cervical vagal cardiac branches* arise in the lower third of the neck and descend posterolateral to the brachiocephalic artery and aortic arch on the right side; on the left side, they descend lateral to the left common carotid artery and aortic arch. The *thoracic vagal cardiac branches* arise at or below the level of the thoracic inlet (see Section V, Plate 11).

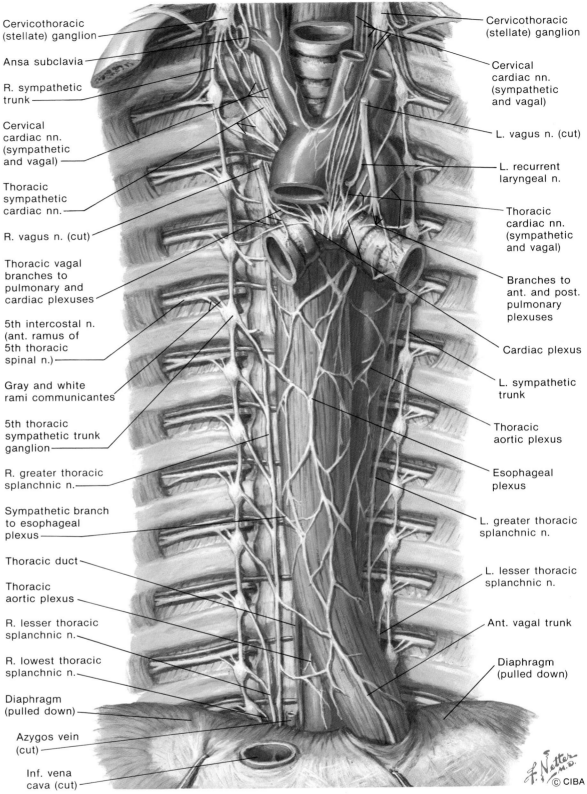

Multiple interconnections exist between all the sympathetic and parasympathetic cardiac nerves (see page 77) and between the cardiac and other visceral branches of the sympathetic trunks.

*Other thoracic sympathetic branches* supply the thoracic viscera from the paired greater, lesser and lowest thoracic splanchnic nerves, althoughthese are mainly destined to supply abdominal structures and contain a mixture of preganglionic, postganglionic and afferent fibers (Plates 11 to 13). The *greater (major) splanchnic nerve* lies medial to the homolateral sympathetic trunk and enters the abdomen by piercing the crus of the diaphragm. The *lesser (minor) splanchnic*

*nerve* lies slightly lateral to the greater splanchnic nerve and also usually pierces the diaphragmatic crus. The *lowest (imus) splanchnic nerve* is inconstant.

Minute twigs from the sympathetic trunks join and innervate the intercostal arteries. Other sympathetic postganglionic fibers reach these vessels in fascicles from adjacent intercostal nerves or their branches, and these also carry sudomotor and pilomotor fibers.

The muscular, osseous and articular filaments from the thoracic sympathetic trunks and their branches supply the adjacent structures concerned; their exact functions are uncertain. ☐

**Innervation of Heart**

# Innervation of Heart

The heart is supplied by sympathetic nerves arising mainly in the neck, because the heart develops initially in the cervical region and later migrates into the thorax, taking its nerves down with it (Plates 5 and 6). The parasympathetic supply is conveyed in cardiac branches of the vagus nerves (see Section V, Plate 11; see also CIBA COLLECTION, Volume 5, pages 18 and 19.)

The *sympathetic preganglionic cardiac fibers* leave the spinal cord in the ventral roots of the upper four to five thoracic spinal nerves and enter the white or mixed rami communicantes passing to adjacent thoracic sympathetic trunk ganglia. Some of the fibers relay here; others ascend in the trunks to form synapses in the cervical ganglia, giving rise to the *cardiac nerves* (see page 76). Most cardiac fibers are postganglionic and pass onward through the cardiac plexus without relaying, to be distributed to the heart wall and its vessels via the *coronary plexuses*.

The *parasympathetic preganglionic (vagal) fibers* are the axons of dorsal vagal nuclear cells. From the vagal cardiac nerves, they relay in ganglia of the *cardiac plexus* or in *intrinsic cardiac ganglia*, which are located mainly in the atrial subepicardial tissue along the coronary sulcus and around the roots of the great vessels. Many nerve cells and fibers are always present in or near the sinoatrial node and the atrioventricular node and bundle. Ventricular ganglia are scanty, but enough of them exist to cast doubts on the hypothesis that ventricular innervation is purely sympathetic.

The more important afferent and efferent pathways in cardiac innervation are shown in the illustration. The peripheral processes of the afferent pseudounipolar neurons in the dorsal root ganglia transmit impulses from cardiac receptors of various types, and from terminal nerve networks in reflexogenic zones, such as those in and around the large cardiac venous openings, the interatrial septum and the ascending aorta. Some of their central processes are implicated in spinal reflex arcs, while others ascend to the dorsal vagal nuclei in the medulla oblongata, the nearby reticular formation, or the hypothalamus and frontal cortex.

The thoracic sympathetic cardiac nerves carry many *afferent pain fibers* from the heart and great vessels, and this endows them with a clinical interest disproportionate to their small size, since their surgical or chemical destruction produces alleviation of angina pectoris. Other cardiac pain afferents run in the middle and inferior cervical sympathetic cardiac nerves; however, after entering the corresponding cervical ganglia, they descend within the sympathetic trunks to the thoracic region

before passing through rami communicantes to the upper four or five thoracic spinal nerves.

*Afferent vagal fibers* from the heart and vessels appear to be mainly concerned with modifying efferent impulses in order to restrain the rate and strength of the heartbeat; in other words, they depress cardiac activity. In some animals, these fibers are aggregated in a separate "depressor

nerve." In man, they may pass through cardiac branches of the recurrent laryngeal nerves to the main vagus nerves, and thus to the brainstem.

*Afferent pericardial fibers* from the fibrous and parietal serous pericardium are carried mainly in the phrenic nerves (see Section VI, Plate 2), but those from the visceral serous pericardium join the coronary arterial plexuses. □

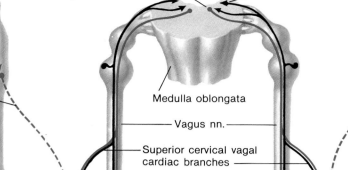

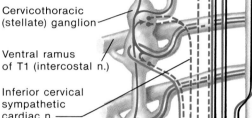

Superior cervical sympathetic trunk ganglion
Superior cervical sympathetic cardiac n.
Middle cervical sympathetic trunk ganglion
Middle cervical sympathetic cardiac n.
Vertebral ganglion
Ansa subclavia
Cervicothoracic (stellate) ganglion
Ventral ramus of T1 (intercostal n.)
Inferior cervical sympathetic cardiac n.
2nd thoracic sympathetic trunk ganglion
Thoracic vagal cardiac branch
White rami communicantes
Gray ramus communicans
4th thoracic sympathetic trunk ganglion
Thoracic sympathetic cardiac nn.
Cardiac plexus

Dorsal vagal nucleus
Solitary tract nucleus
Medulla oblongata
Vagus nn.
Superior cervical vagal cardiac branches
Inferior cervical vagal cardiac branches
Ascending connections
T1
T2
T3
T4

| Sympathetic fibers | Vagal fibers |
|---|---|
| —— preganglionic | —— preganglionic |
| - - - postganglionic | - - - postganglionic |
| —— afferent | —— afferent |

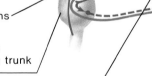

# Innervation of Blood Vessels

The blood vessels are innervated by afferent and efferent autonomic nerves. All receive sympathetic fibers, but some may not have a parasympathetic supply.

The great vessels near the midline in the neck and body cavities receive direct filaments from adjacent parts of the sympathetic trunks. Some of these vessels and their branches also obtain supplies from nearby autonomic plexuses, which contain both sympathetic and parasympathetic elements. Thus, the ascending aorta, the aortic arch and its branches and the superior vena cava receive offshoots from the cardiac plexus; the pulmonary vessels, from the pulmonary plexuses; the celiac, hepatic, gastric, splenic, superior mesenteric, renal and adrenal vessels and the portal and inferior caval veins, from the celiac and superior mesenteric plexuses; the inferior mesenteric vessels, from the corresponding plexus; and the pelvic vessels, from the superior and inferior hypogastric plexuses.

The chief outflow of sympathetic preganglionic fibers is through the ventral roots of spinal nerves T1 to L2 (see Section VI, Plate 3). The fibers pass in white rami communicantes to adjacent sympathetic trunk ganglia, where many relay. The axons of these ganglionic cells (postganglionic fibers) may pass in nerves or filaments to nearby structures, such as midline vessels and prevertebral plexuses (cardiac, celiac, mesenteric), or they may join the lowest cervical, thoracic and upper lumbar spinal nerves through gray rami communicantes, to be distributed with them to vessels and glands in the parietes and limbs.

Other preganglionic fibers, however, do not relay in adjacent trunk ganglia, but ascend or descend in the sympathetic trunks to form synapses in the cervical or lower lumbar and sacral ganglia. The axons (postganglionic fibers) of the cervical ganglionic cells supply the vessels and glands in the head and neck, while others contribute to the sympathetic cervical cardiac nerves. Some of the postganglionic fibers arising in the lumbar and sacral ganglia run in lumbar and sacral splanchnic nerves to the mesenteric and hypogastric plexuses, but others pass through gray rami communicantes to the lumbar, sacral and coccygeal spinal nerves, to be distributed with them and their branches to vessels, sweat glands and arrectores pilorum muscles in the loin, lower abdominal wall, buttocks, perineum and lower limbs (see Section VI, Plate 10).

The vascular nerves and filaments from the diverse sources indicated become united around individual vessels in wide-meshed *perivascular adventitial plexuses*. Fascicles arising from these sink inward to form more delicate plexuses between the adventitial and medial coats, from

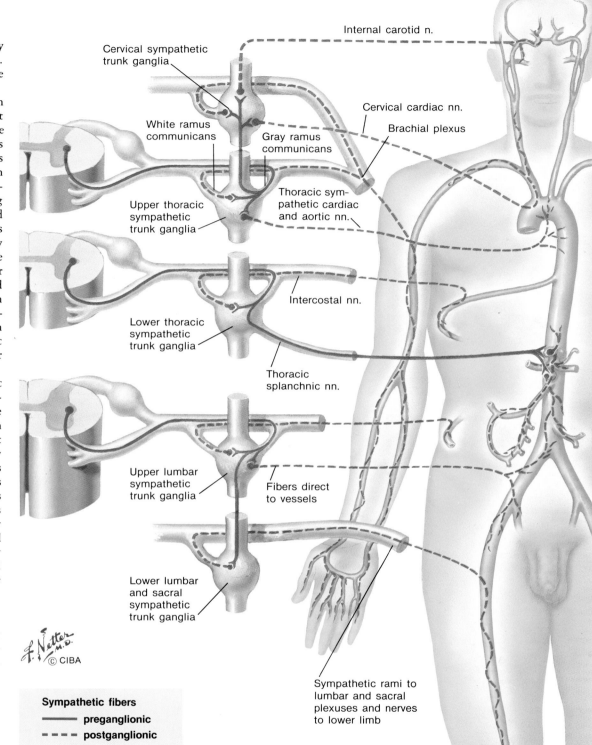

Cervical sympathetic trunk ganglia

Internal carotid n.

White ramus communicans

Gray ramus communicans

Cervical cardiac nn.

Brachial plexus

Upper thoracic sympathetic trunk ganglia

Thoracic sympathetic cardiac and aortic nn.

Intercostal nn.

Lower thoracic sympathetic trunk ganglia

Thoracic splanchnic nn.

Upper lumbar sympathetic trunk ganglia

Fibers direct to vessels

Lower lumbar and sacral sympathetic trunk ganglia

Sympathetic rami to lumbar and sacral plexuses and nerves to lower limb

**Sympathetic fibers**
——— preganglionic
- - - - postganglionic

which filaments originate to ramify in the media and in the zone between the media and intima. Subsidiary perivascular plexuses extend along the vessel branches and are augmented at intervals by branchlets from nearby cranial or spinal nerves, which contain autonomic fibers. Thus, innervation is segmental rather than longitudinal, and only relatively short lengths of arteries can be denervated by the removal of adventitial cuffs.

Most cranial and spinal nerves contain efferent and afferent vascular fibers. The oculomotor (III), trigeminal (V), facial (VII), vagus (X), glossopharyngeal (XI), phrenic, ulnar, median, pudendal and tibial nerves contain relatively large numbers of vascular fibers. Accordingly, lesions involving these nerves are more likely to produce vasomotor and other autonomic disturbances. Vascular disorders are usually more evident in peripheral arteries and arterioles (like those in the fingers and toes), and in arteriovenous anastomoses, because they have thicker muscular layers and a richer innervation than larger arteries, which have more elastic tissue in their walls. Arteries supplying erectile tissues and the skin are also richly innervated, whereas the nerve supply to veins and venules is comparatively sparse. Nerve fibers are often associated with capillaries, but their functions are unknown. □

# Autonomic Nerves and Ganglia in Abdomen

There are more sympathetic nerves in the abdomen and pelvis than anywhere else, because these cavities contain the major parts of the digestive and urogenital systems and their associated glands and vessels, the adrenal glands and the extensive peritoneum.

The abdominal sympathetic nerves include the lumbar parts of the sympathetic trunks and their branches and contribute to the celiac, mesenteric, intermesenteric (abdominal aortic), hepatic, renal, adrenal, superior hypogastric and other plexuses, including all subsidiary plexuses. Apart from the lumbar sympathetic trunks and branches, however, all the autonomic plexuses mentioned contain both sympathetic and parasympathetic elements.

The lumbar parts of the sympathetic trunks are directly continuous above with their thoracic counterparts behind the medial arcuate ligaments (Plate 8), while below, they pass over the pelvic brim and behind the common iliac vessels to become the sacral parts of the sympathetic trunks (Plate 17). The trunks lie in the retroperitoneal connective tissue on the anterolateral aspect of the lumbar vertebrae, along the medial margins of the psoas muscles; the right trunk is partly overlapped by the inferior vena cava and the cisterna chyli, and the left trunk is just lateral to the abdominal aorta. There are usually four lumbar ganglia on each side; the intervening cords may be single or split into two or even three strands. Each trunk supplies or receives communicating, visceral, vascular, muscular, osseous and articular branches.

Only the upper two or, occasionally, three lumbar spinal nerves contribute white rami communicantes to the adjacent lumbar trunk ganglia, but every lumbar spinal nerve receives one or more gray communicating rami from adjacent trunk ganglia (Plate 17; see also Section VI, Plate 10). White rami contain preganglionic and visceral afferent fibers, while gray rami contain vasomotor, sudomotor and pilomotor fibers, which are distributed with the lumbar spinal nerves.

Three or four lumbar splanchnic nerves arise on each side and are seldom arranged symmetrically. The *first lumbar splanchnic nerve* arises from the first lumbar ganglion and ends in the renal, celiac and/or intermesenteric plexuses, but some filaments may end directly in the duodenum, pancreas and gastroesophageal junction. The *second lumbar splanchnic nerve* arises from the second lumbar ganglion and ends mainly in the intermesenteric plexus, although it may give direct contributions to the renal plexus, duodenum and pancreas. The *third lumbar splanchnic nerve* usually originates

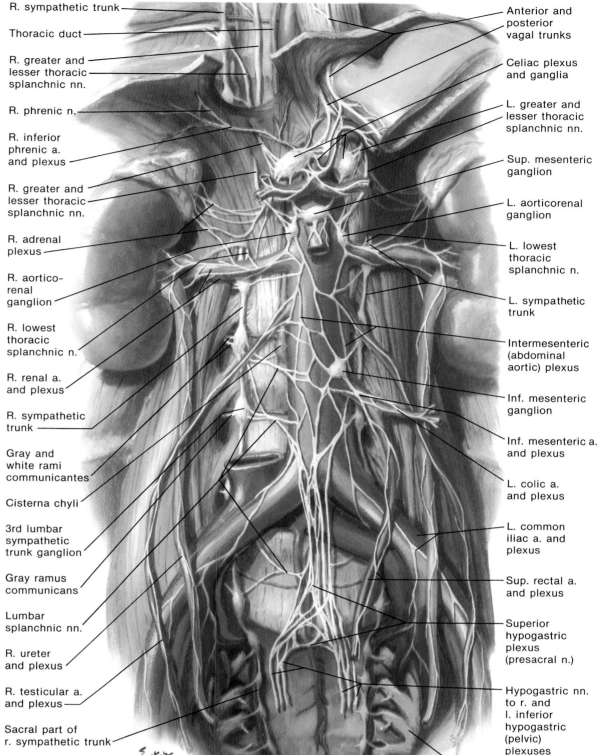

R. sympathetic trunk
Thoracic duct
R. greater and lesser thoracic splanchnic nn.
R. phrenic n.
R. inferior phrenic a. and plexus
R. greater and lesser thoracic splanchnic nn.
R. adrenal plexus
R. aortico-renal ganglion
R. lowest thoracic splanchnic n.
R. renal a. and plexus
R. sympathetic trunk
Gray and white rami communicantes
Cisterna chyli
3rd lumbar sympathetic trunk ganglion
Gray ramus communicans
Lumbar splanchnic nn.
R. ureter and plexus
R. testicular a. and plexus
Sacral part of r. sympathetic trunk

Anterior and posterior vagal trunks
Celiac plexus and ganglia
L. greater and lesser thoracic splanchnic nn.
Sup. mesenteric ganglion
L. aorticorenal ganglion
L. lowest thoracic splanchnic n.
L. sympathetic trunk
Intermesenteric (abdominal aortic) plexus
Inf. mesenteric ganglion
Inf. mesenteric a. and plexus
L. colic a. and plexus
L. common iliac a. and plexus
Sup. rectal a. and plexus
Superior hypogastric plexus (presacral n.)
Hypogastric nn. to r. and l. inferior hypogastric (pelvic) plexuses
L. sacral plexus

from the third and fourth ganglia and ends in the upper part of the superior hypogastric plexus. The *fourth lumbar splanchnic nerve,* when present, arises from the fourth and/or the inconstant fifth lumbar ganglion and joins the lower part of the superior hypogastric plexus or the homolateral hypogastric nerve; it communicates with the ureteric and testicular plexuses.

Vascular filaments from the lumbar sympathetic trunks and their lumbar splanchnic branches pass to the abdominal aorta and the inferior vena cava, where they form the delicate intermesenteric and caval plexuses (Plate 10). All the aortic branches and vena caval tributaries are

surrounded by subsidiary plexuses continuous with those around the parent vessels. Twigs from the right sympathetic trunk also supply the cisterna chyli and the commencement of the thoracic duct. Filaments from the renal plexus, sometimes reinforced by fascicles from the second and third lumbar splanchnic nerves, usually join the plexus around the common or external iliac arteries.

Muscular, osseous and articular filaments supply the adjacent muscles, vertebrae and joints in the lumbar region. They contain postganglionic (efferent) fibers, which are possibly vasomotor, and afferent fibers conveying impulses from meningeal, bony and articular structures. ☐

# Innervation of Stomach and Proximal Duodenum

*Sympathetic Fibers.* The gastric sympathetic preganglionic fibers are the axons of lateral cornual cells located in the sixth to ninth or tenth thoracic spinal segments. They reach the celiac plexus via the *sympathetic trunk ganglia* and the *greater (major)* and *lesser (minor) thoracic splanchnic nerves.* Some of the fibers form synapses in trunk ganglia, but most continue through them to end in synapses within the *celiac* and *superior mesenteric ganglia.* The resulting postganglionic fibers may run in fascicles ending directly in the stomach and duodenum, but the majority are conveyed to their destinations in the *perivascular plexuses* along the various branches and subbranches of the celiac trunk. These plexuses are composed mainly of sympathetic fibers, but they also contain parasympathetic fibers derived from the celiac branches of the vagal trunks. The sympathetic postganglionic fibers traverse the intramural enteric ganglia without relaying, and are distributed mainly to the gastric musculature and blood vessels.

*Parasympathetic Fibers.* The two *vagus nerves* form an *esophageal plexus* around the lower esophagus, which is reinforced by twigs from the *thoracic parts* of the *sympathetic trunks* and from the *greater (major)* and *lesser (minor) thoracic splanchnic nerves.* Before reaching the diaphragm, the meshes of the esophageal plexus are reconstituted to form *anterior* and *posterior vagal trunks.* In general, more fibers from the left vagus enter the anterior trunk, while the posterior trunk contains more fibers from the right vagus, although the anatomical relationships are highly variable. The vagal trunks give off gastric, pyloric, hepatic and celiac branches (see Section V, Plate 11).

*Anterior* and *posterior gastric branches* supply the corresponding surfaces of the stomach. They run between the layers of the lesser omentum and give off branches that radiate over the surfaces of the stomach and can be traced for some distance in the subperitoneal tissue before they sink into muscle coats; no definite anterior or posterior gastric plexuses exist. Often, one branch on both the anterior and posterior aspects is larger than the others— the *greater anterior* and *greater posterior gastric nerves.* *Pyloric branches* arise from the anterior vagal trunk or its greater anterior gastric branch and supply the pyloric antrum, pylorus and superior (first) part of the duodenum. *Hepatic branches* are provided by both vagal trunks; that from the anterior trunk arises near the gastric cardiac ostium and is called the *hepatogastric nerve* because it supplies offshoots to the hepatic plexus and stomach (there may be more than one hepatogastric nerve). The hepatic contribution from the

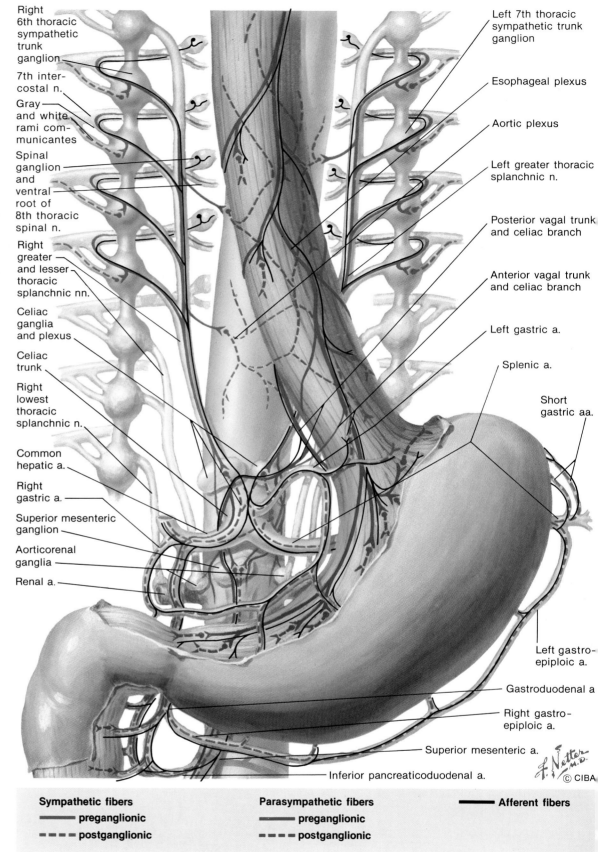

posterior vagal trunk usually reaches the hepatic plexus through its celiac branch. Both vagal trunks give off *celiac branches,* and the posterior branch is larger than the anterior. All efferent (preganglionic) vagal fibers ending in the stomach make synaptic contacts with ganglionic neurons in the gastric parts of the *myenteric* and *submucous plexuses;* the resulting postganglionic fibers are distributed to the gastric musculature, glands and

vessels, where they exert both motor and secretory effects (Plate 14).

*Afferent Fibers.* Afferent parasympathetic and sympathetic fibers pursue reverse routes to those described for vagal and sympathetic efferent fibers. (For greater detail on the innervation of the esophagus, stomach and upper intestines, see CIBA COLLECTION, Volume 3/I, pages 44 to 46, 64 and 65.) □

**Labels (figure):**
Right 6th thoracic sympathetic trunk ganglion
7th intercostal n.
Gray and white rami communicantes
Spinal ganglion and ventral root of 8th thoracic spinal n.
Right greater and lesser thoracic splanchnic nn.
Celiac ganglia and plexus
Celiac trunk
Right lowest thoracic splanchnic n.
Common hepatic a.
Right gastric a.
Superior mesenteric ganglion
Aorticorenal ganglia
Renal a.
Left 7th thoracic sympathetic trunk ganglion
Esophageal plexus
Aortic plexus
Left greater thoracic splanchnic n.
Posterior vagal trunk and celiac branch
Anterior vagal trunk and celiac branch
Left gastric a.
Splenic a.
Short gastric aa.
Left gastro-epiploic a.
Gastroduodenal a
Right gastro-epiploic a.
Superior mesenteric a.
Inferior pancreaticoduodenal a.

| Sympathetic fibers | Parasympathetic fibers | ━━ Afferent fibers |
|---|---|---|
| ── preganglionic | ── preganglionic | |
| ─ ─ ─ postganglionic | ─ ─ ─ postganglionic | |

# Innervation of Intestines

*Sympathetic Fibers*. The preganglionic sympathetic fibers to the intestines are the axons of lateral cornual cells located in the lowest four or five thoracic and upper two lumbar spinal segments. Some form synapses in the *sympathetic trunk ganglia*, but most are conveyed in the *thoracic, lumbar* and *sacral splanchnic nerves* to the celiac, mesenteric and hypogastric plexuses, where they relay. From the celiac and superior mesenteric plexuses, an unknown proportion of fibers descends in the *intermesenteric* and *hypogastric nerves* to the inferior mesenteric and hypogastric plexuses. Postganglionic fibers resulting from ganglionic synapses, along with afferent and preganglionic parasympathetic fibers, are carried to the intestines in branches of the various plexuses.

*The parasympathetic supply* to the intestines is derived from the vagus and pelvic splanchnic nerves.

The *vagal* contributions pass to the celiac plexus in the *larger* and *smaller celiac branches* arising, respectively, from the *posterior* and *anterior vagal trunks*. Some fibers are distributed with branches of the *celiac plexus* to the stomach and duodenum (Plate 12), but others descend to the *superior mesenteric plexus*. They comprise efferent (preganglionic) and afferent fibers, and innervate the small intestines and the colon almost to the left colic flexure. Parasympathetic fibers follow the same routes to the intestines as sympathetic postganglionic fibers, but are still preganglionic and end by forming synapses in the enteric plexuses (Plate 14).

The *pelvic splanchnic nerves* arise from the second, third and fourth sacral nerves. They contain parasympathetic preganglionic and afferent fibers, which include those supplying the distal end of the transverse colon and left colic flexure, the descending and sigmoid colons and the rectum. They join the *inferior hypogastric (pelvic) plexuses* and are distributed with their branches. The preganglionic intestinal fibers pass through the ganglia in these plexuses without relaying; like their vagal counterparts, they end by making synaptic contacts in the *enteric plexuses*. Some branches pass directly to the rectum and lower end of the sigmoid colon, others accompany rectal and colic vessels, and still others may ascend in the *hypogastric nerves* to the *superior hypogastric plexus* and thence to the *inferior mesenteric plexus*, to be distributed with its branches to the distal parts of the colon. However, the majority of the parasympathetic fibers for these parts of the colon pursue a different course: they arise by several filaments from the *pelvic splanchnic nerves* or the *inferior hypogastric plexuses* and run upward across the sigmoid

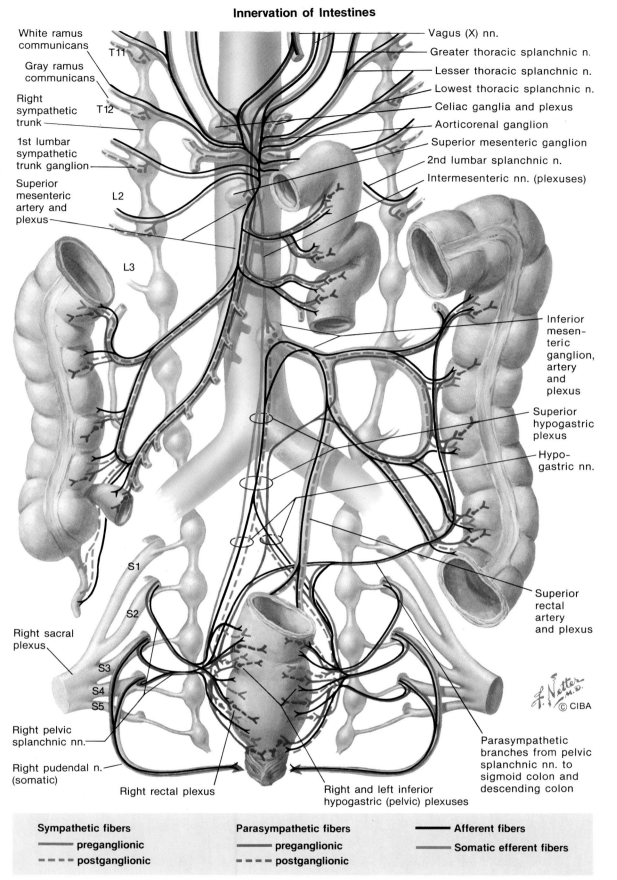

and left colic vessels. They can be traced as far as the left colic flexure, and they supply offshoots to the adjacent parts of the sigmoid and descending colons and communicate with branches of the inferior mesenteric plexus.

*Afferent pathways*, in general, follow (in reverse direction) both the sympathetic and the parasympathetic supplies to the small and large bowel. The afferent components of the vagus and

pelvic nerves and of the sympathetic pathways subserve reflex activity, but most localized sensations referable to the gastrointestinal tract appear to be mediated through the sympathetic afferents. At the anorectal junction, the autonomic type of innervation gives way to the somatic. (For greater detail on the innervation of the small and large intestines, see CIBA COLLECTION, Volume 3/II, pages 76 to 81.) □

**Enteric Plexuses**

## Enteric Plexuses

Enteric plexuses exist within the walls of the alimentary tract, from the esophagus to the rectum. They form microscopic networks and consist of bundles of nerve fibers (axons) and dendrites, which link ganglia located chiefly at nodal points in the meshes. These networks are most evident between the layers of the muscle coats (myenteric, or Auerbach's, plexus) and in the submucosa (submucous, or Meissner's, plexus). Tenuous subserous plexuses with sparsely disposed nerve cells are present in those parts of the gastrointestinal tract that possess peritoneal coverings.

The *myenteric (Auerbach's) plexus* is relatively coarse, with thicker meshes and larger ganglia. The main, or primary, meshes give off fascicles that form secondary networks in the interstices of the primary networks. These, in turn, split into minute bundles of fibers that ramify between the muscle tunics and supply them. The *submucous (Meissner's) plexus* is more delicate and its meshes are more irregular. Its delicate offshoots mostly end in relation to cells forming the muscularis mucosae or form rarefied periglandular plexuses, while other offshoots end in almost invisible subepithelial plexuses.

The patterns and densities of these plexuses vary in different parts of the alimentary tract. They are less well defined in the upper part of the esophagus but are well developed from the stomach to the lower end of the rectum. The ganglia are not uniformly distributed. The density of ganglionic cells in the plexuses is lowest in the esophagus, rises steeply in the stomach until it reaches a peak at the pylorus, falls to an intermediate level throughout the small intestines, and gradually increases along the colon to reach another, lesser peak in the rectum.

The extrinsic nerves involved contain *efferent* and *afferent sympathetic* and *parasympathetic fibers* derived from thoracic, lumbar and sacral branches of the sympathetic trunks and from the vagus and pelvic splanchnic nerves. Most of the sympathetic efferent fibers entering the enteric plexuses are postganglionic, while parasympathetic efferent fibers are still preganglionic. The vagal fibers form synapses with ganglion cells located in the enteric plexuses, from the esophagus to the distal third of the transverse colon; below this level, the preganglionic parasympathetic fibers are carried in branches of the pelvic splanchnic

nerves. Thus, in this as in other situations, the parasympathetic postganglionic fibers are very much shorter than their sympathetic counterparts.

Many interconnections exist between the myenteric and submucous plexuses. In general, the former are mainly concerned with the innervation of the muscle layers in the visceral walls, whereas the latter are chiefly involved with supplying the glands and muscularis mucosae and in forming delicate subepithelial plexuses. The enteric plexuses and their subdivisions are also responsible for supplying adjacent vessels and

transmitting sensory impulses. The sympathetic innervation is primarily inhibitory to peristalsis and stimulatory to the sphincters, while the parasympathetic innervation is the opposite.

Afferent fibers from the alimentary tract are conveyed to the CNS through the same sympathetic and parasympathetic nerves that carry the corresponding efferent fibers. There is also evidence that local reflex arcs exist. (For greater detail on the intrinsic innervation of the intestines, see CIBA COLLECTION, Volume 3/I, page 46 and Volume 3/II, pages 77 and 78.) □

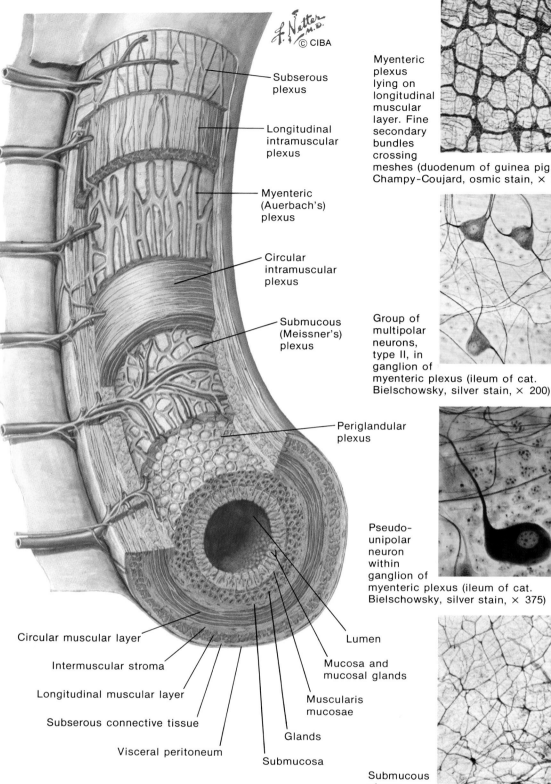

Circular muscular layer
Intermuscular stroma
Longitudinal muscular layer
Subserous connective tissue
Visceral peritoneum

Subserous plexus
Longitudinal intramuscular plexus
Myenteric (Auerbach's) plexus
Circular intramuscular plexus
Submucous (Meissner's) plexus
Periglandular plexus

Lumen
Mucosa and mucosal glands
Muscularis mucosae
Glands
Submucosa

*Modification from schematic drawing supplied by M.D. Thomas BSc (Hons), Anatomy Department, The University, Manchester, England*

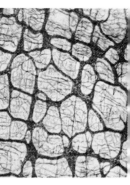

Myenteric plexus lying on longitudinal muscular layer. Fine secondary bundles crossing meshes (duodenum of guinea pig. Champy-Coujard, osmic stain, × 20)

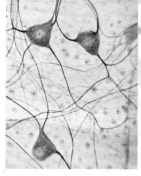

Group of multipolar neurons, type II, in ganglion of myenteric plexus (ileum of cat. Bielschowsky, silver stain, × 200)

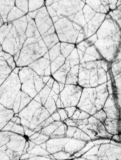

Pseudo-unipolar neuron within ganglion of myenteric plexus (ileum of cat. Bielschowsky, silver stain, × 375)

Submucous plexus (ascending colon of guinea pig. Stained by gold impregnation, × 20)

# Innervation of Liver and Biliary Tract

The liver, biliary tract and gallbladder receive their nerve supplies from sympathetic and parasympathetic sources. The *preganglionic sympathetic fibers* originate mainly in the seventh to tenth thoracic segments and pass to the celiac plexus via the sympathetic trunk ganglia and the greater and lesser thoracic splanchnic nerves (Plates 11 and 12). Most of the fibers form synapses in the celiac ganglia, although some may relay in small ganglia located in the porta hepatis. The *postganglionic sympathetic fibers* reach the liver in the hepatic plexuses, which also contain parasympathetic and afferent fibers. The *parasympathetic supply* is provided by branches of the vagal trunks (see Section V, Plate 11).

Afferent fibers from the liver and biliary tract are conveyed through the hepatic and celiac plexuses to the *thoracic splanchnic nerves* or to branches of the *vagus nerves*. The sympathetic afferents reach the seventh to twelfth thoracic spinal cord segments through the corresponding dorsal spinal nerve roots, while the vagal afferents are carried upward to the brainstem. The right, and possibly the left, phrenic nerve also conveys afferents from receptors in the peritoneal lining over the liver and biliary tract, which can be stimulated by stretching—as by acute hepatic enlargement or distention of the gallbladder (see Section VI, Plate 2). The resultant pain in the right shoulder region associated with liver and biliary tract disorders is an example of referred pain.

*Liver.* The *hepatic plexuses* lie in the right free margin of the lesser omentum anterior to the epiploic (omental) foramen. They are formed mainly by offshoots from the *celiac plexus*, which contain sympathetic and parasympathetic efferent and afferent fibers, supplemented by direct contributions from the *anterior vagal trunk* and by indirect contributions from the *right phrenic nerve*. They are arranged in two interconnected groups, one of which lies along the anterior and lateral sides of the hepatic artery, and the other, posterior to the common bile duct and portal vein.

*Subsidiary plexuses* surround and accompany the branches of the hepatic artery, portal vein and right and left hepatic ducts as they enter and ramify within the liver; their offshoots penetrate between the cells of the liver lobules to form a widespread *parenchymal plexus*. Histochemical studies reveal that the nerve fibers in relation to the hepatocytes and sinusoids are parasympathetic, whereas sympathetic fibers remain mainly or entirely associated with vessels in the interlobular spaces. Direct contacts between the terminations of nerve fibers and liver cells have been observed in electron micrographs.

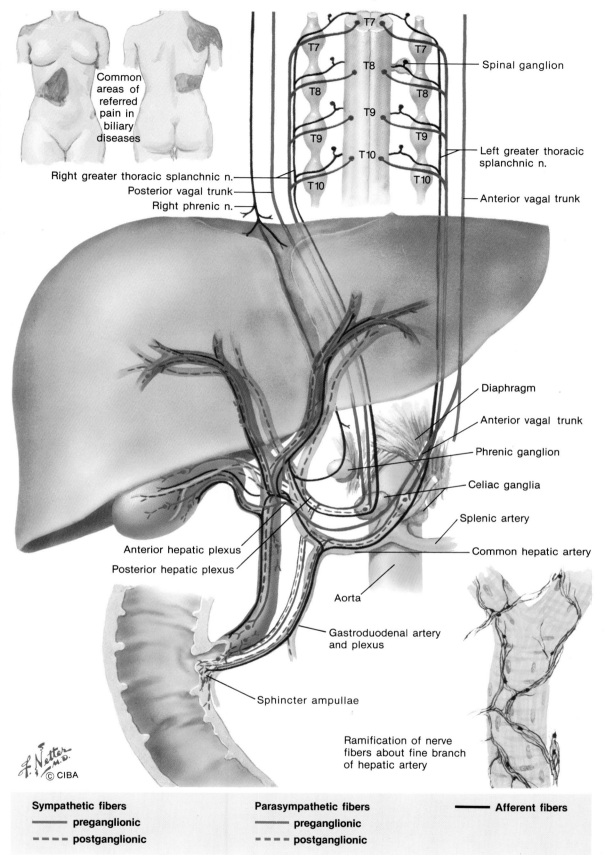

Common areas of referred pain in biliary diseases

Right greater thoracic splanchnic n.
Posterior vagal trunk
Right phrenic n.

T7
T8
T9
T10

Spinal ganglion

Left greater thoracic splanchnic n.

Anterior vagal trunk

Diaphragm

Anterior vagal trunk

Phrenic ganglion

Celiac ganglia

Splenic artery

Common hepatic artery

Anterior hepatic plexus
Posterior hepatic plexus

Aorta

Gastroduodenal artery and plexus

Sphincter ampullae

Ramification of nerve fibers about fine branch of hepatic artery

| Sympathetic fibers | Parasympathetic fibers | —— Afferent fibers |
|---|---|---|
| —— preganglionic | —— preganglionic | |
| - - - postganglionic | - - - postganglionic | |

*The gallbladder* is supplied by perivascular nerve filaments accompanying the right hepatic and cystic arteries from the *anterior hepatic plexus*, and by other nerve filaments extending along the cystic duct from the *posterior hepatic plexus*. The common bile duct (choledochal duct) is supplied by twigs from both anterior and posterior hepatic plexuses and by offshoots from the plexus around the gastroduodenal artery and its retroduodenal

branches. The arrangement of the nerves within the walls of these structures resembles that in the enteric plexuses.

Both the sphincter ampullae and the sphincter of the choledochal duct are supplied by sympathetic and parasympathetic fibers. The former normally cause contraction of the sphincters and dilatation of the gallbladder, while the latter produce the opposite effects. □

## Innervation of Adrenal Glands

The adrenal (suprarenal) glands show a high degree of species variation, and this also applies to their nerve supplies. The cortex and medulla differ in their development (see CIBA COLLECTION, Volume 4, page 77). The *medullary (chromaffin) cells* are modified migrant neuroblasts from the neural tube or crest and are homologous with ganglion cells in the sympathetic trunks. Accordingly, they are innervated directly by preganglionic fibers. Relative to their size, the adrenal medullae are more richly innervated than any other viscus.

The *preganglionic sympathetic fibers* are the axons of cells located in the lateral gray columns of the lower three or four thoracic and upper one or two lumbar segments of the spinal cord. They emerge in the anterior rootlets of the corresponding spinal nerves, pass in white rami communicantes to the sympathetic trunks, and leave them in the thoracic and first lumbar splanchnic nerves that run to the celiac, aorticorenal and renal ganglia. Some of the fibers conveying impulses for the adrenal vessels may relay in these ganglia, but the majority continue onward to enter the adrenal branches of the celiac plexus.

Some of the *parasympathetic fibers* reaching the celiac plexus through the vagal trunks may be concerned with adrenal innervation and may relay in small ganglia near or in the glands, but as yet no definite proof of this hypothesis exists. The adrenal parasympathetic supply may well emerge via dorsal spinal nerve root efferents, which enter the thoracic splanchnic nerves and thereafter follow the same routes as the sympathetic preganglionic fibers; however, the existence of such dorsal root efferents is still unproven. A proportion of the fibers in the adrenal nerves may be afferent and enter the spinal cord through the ninth to eleventh thoracic spinal nerves.

*Adrenal Nerves.* Numerous fine nerves pass outward to each gland from the *celiac plexus and ganglia*. They are joined by contributions from the terminations of the *greater* and *lesser thoracic splanchnic nerves*, and they communicate with the ipsilateral *phrenic nerve* and *renal plexus*. According to Swinyard, the adrenal nerves in man contain myelinated and unmyelinated fibers in about equal numbers, but Coupland cites evidence that in small animals, such as rats, the majority of fibers are unmyelinated.

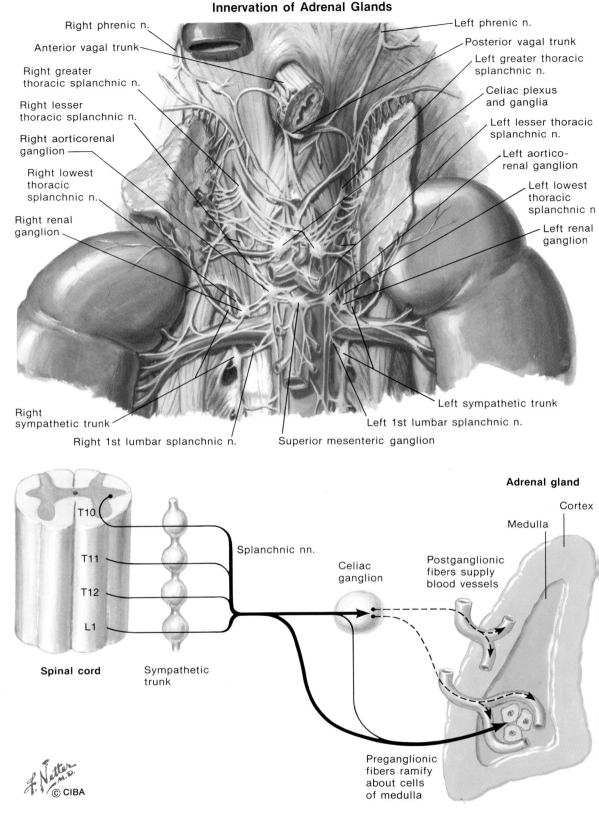

**Innervation of Adrenal Glands**

Right phrenic n.
Anterior vagal trunk
Right greater thoracic splanchnic n.
Right lesser thoracic splanchnic n.
Right aorticorenal ganglion
Right lowest thoracic splanchnic n.
Right renal ganglion
Right sympathetic trunk
Right 1st lumbar splanchnic n.
Left phrenic n.
Posterior vagal trunk
Left greater thoracic splanchnic n.
Celiac plexus and ganglia
Left lesser thoracic splanchnic n.
Left aortico-renal ganglion
Left lowest thoracic splanchnic n
Left renal ganglion
Left sympathetic trunk
Left 1st lumbar splanchnic n.
Superior mesenteric ganglion

Spinal cord
Sympathetic trunk
T10
T11
T12
L1
Splanchnic nn.
Celiac ganglion
**Adrenal gland**
Cortex
Medulla
Postganglionic fibers supply blood vessels
Preganglionic fibers ramify about cells of medulla

Many filaments from the adrenal nerves enter the gland through its hilus and medial margin. Other filaments associated with occasional nerve cells spread out over the gland to form a delicate *subcapsular plexus* from which fascicles penetrate the cortex to run alongside arterioles in the trabeculae to the medulla. Stöhr claims that the cortex is richly innervated, but Hollinshead and Lever state that the nerves traversing the cortex mainly supply its vessels, and that most of their fibers end in the medulla.

However, there is now general agreement that the majority of nerve filaments entering the gland end in the medulla, where they ramify profusely and give off fibers which mostly terminate in synaptic-type contacts with the chromaffin cells. As already stated, these are the homologues of ganglion cells in the sympathetic trunks. Some fibers invaginate the cell membranes deeply but do not penetrate them. A minority of fibers innervate the medullary arterioles and the central vein, which has an unusually thick muscle coat.

Multipolar or bipolar neurons, singly or in small groups, have been noted within the adrenal medullae. Their significance and the destinations of their axons have not yet been determined, although it is assumed that the cells are the final relay stations in the parasympathetic pathways. □

# Autonomic Nerves and Ganglia in Pelvis

*Sympathetic fibers* reach the pelvis through the sympathetic trunks and the superior hypogastric plexus, and in visceral and vascular nerves accompanying and supplying such structures as the colon, ureters and the inferior mesenteric and common iliac vessels. *Parasympathetic fibers* emerge in the ventral roots of the second, third and, sometimes, fourth sacral spinal nerves, and leave them in the slender right and left groups of pelvic splanchnic nerves (nervi erigentes) that join the corresponding inferior hypogastric (pelvic) plexuses and are distributed with their branches.

*Sympathetic Fibers.* The lumbar and sacral parts of the sympathetic trunks are directly continuous at the level of the pelvic brim (Plate 11). The sacral trunks lie in the parietal pelvic fascia behind the parietal peritoneum and rectum, and on the ventral surface of the sacrum, just medial to its anterior foramina and the nerves and vessels passing through them. Below, they converge and unite in a single tiny "ganglion impar" anterior to the coccyx. Generally, four or sometimes three sacral trunk ganglia exist on each side. No white rami communicantes are present in this region, but each ganglion supplies one or more gray rami communicantes containing postganglionic sympathetic fibers to the adjoining sacral and coccygeal spinal nerves; these fibers are conveyed in branches of the sacral and coccygeal plexuses to vessels, sweat glands, arrectores pilorum muscles, striated muscles, bones and joints.

The pelvic sympathetic trunk ganglia also supply slender rami, the *sacral splanchnic nerves*, which pass to the inferior hypogastric plexuses. The majority of sympathetic fibers, however, reach these plexuses through the *right* and *left hypogastric nerves*, formed just below the level of the lumbosacral junction by the splitting of the median superior hypogastric plexus (often misleadingly referred to as the "presacral nerve"—a single nerve is very rare). Similarly, the right and left hypogastric nerves are more often elongated plexuses consisting of several nerves interconnected by oblique strands, which incline downward on each side, behind the peritoneum and lateral to the sigmoid colon and rectosigmoid junction, to end in the upper parts of the homolateral inferior hypogastric plexus.

The *inferior hypogastric plexuses* are situated on each side of the rectum, lower part of the bladder, prostate and seminal vesicles. In females, the cervix of the uterus and vaginal fornices replace the prostate gland and seminal vesicles as medial relations. The plexuses supply branches to the pelvic

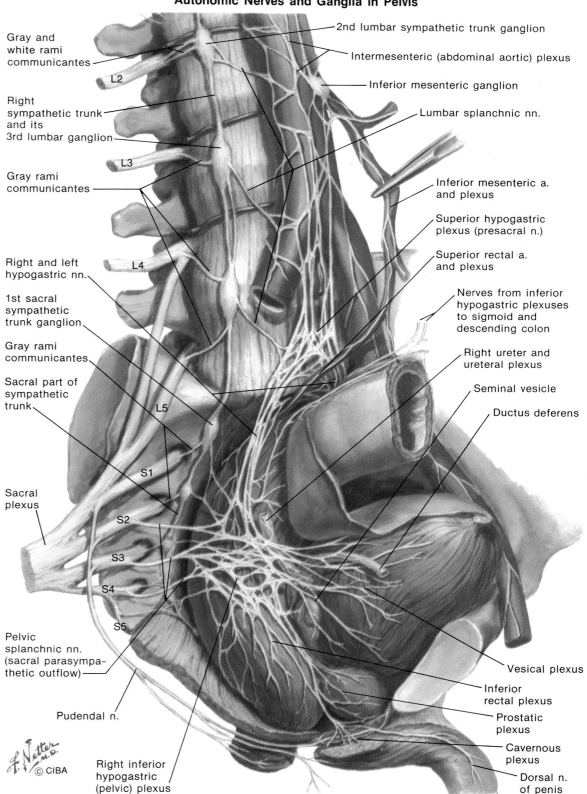

Gray and white rami communicantes

L2

Right sympathetic trunk and its 3rd lumbar ganglion

Gray rami communicantes

L3

Right and left hypogastric nn.

L4

1st sacral sympathetic trunk ganglion

Gray rami communicantes

Sacral part of sympathetic trunk

L5

Sacral plexus

S1

S2

S3

S4

S5

Pelvic splanchnic nn. (sacral parasympathetic outflow)

Pudendal n.

Right inferior hypogastric (pelvic) plexus

2nd lumbar sympathetic trunk ganglion

Intermesenteric (abdominal aortic) plexus

Inferior mesenteric ganglion

Lumbar splanchnic nn.

Inferior mesenteric a. and plexus

Superior hypogastric plexus (presacral n.)

Superior rectal a. and plexus

Nerves from inferior hypogastric plexuses to sigmoid and descending colon

Right ureter and ureteral plexus

Seminal vesicle

Ductus deferens

Vesical plexus

Inferior rectal plexus

Prostatic plexus

Cavernous plexus

Dorsal n. of penis

viscera and genitalia and often form subsidiary plexuses (rectal, prostatic, vesical, etc). The branches contain visceral, glandular, vascular and afferent fibers, often combined in the nerve fascicles supplying the various structures concerned (Plates 18 to 21). The *sympathetic efferent fibers* in these branches, like those in the gray rami communicantes connecting the ganglia of the pelvic sympathetic trunks to the sacral and coccygeal spinal nerves, are almost entirely postganglionic, because most or all of the sympathetic preganglionic fibers involved in the supply of pelvic, perineal, gluteal and lower limb structures relay in lumbar and sacral trunk ganglia; a minority

may form synapses in ganglia within the inferior hypogastric plexuses.

*The parasympathetic fibers* in the *pelvic splanchnic nerves*, which arise from the sacral nerves and end in the *inferior hypogastric plexuses*, are preganglionic. Some relay in ganglia within the plexuses, but many more form synapses in ganglia located near or within the walls of the viscera and vessels innervated.

Other branches from the inferior hypogastric plexuses ascend to assist in the innervation of the distal colon and the renal pelvises (see CIBA COLLECTION, Volume 3/II, pages 79 to 81 and Volume 6, pages 27 to 29). □

# Innervation of Kidneys, Ureters and Urinary Bladder

***Kidney and Upper Ureter.*** The *preganglionic sympathetic fibers* for the kidneys and upper ureters emerge from the spinal cord through the ventral nerve roots of the eleventh and twelfth thoracic spinal nerves, and usually of the tenth thoracic and first lumbar spinal nerves as well. The fibers then pass in white rami communicantes to adjacent ganglia in the sympathetic trunks. They leave the ganglia in the lesser and lowest thoracic and first and second lumbar splanchnic nerves. The lesser thoracic splanchnic nerve usually ends in the ipsilateral celiac or aorticorenal ganglia, and the other nerves mentioned may do the same, although they usually end directly in the renal plexus or in the small renal ganglion lying posterior or posterosuperior to the renal artery. Most of the preganglionic fibers form synaptic relays in the aorticorenal or posterior renal ganglia or in other, even smaller ganglia incorporated into the renal plexuses. The *postganglionic sympathetic fibers* form fascicles that surround and accompany the upper ureteric, renal, pelvic, calyceal and segmental branches of the renal vessels.

Some *parasympathetic fibers* are carried through the vagal contributions to the celiac plexus and are conveyed onward to the kidneys in the renal branches of this plexus; others emerge through the pelvic splanchnic nerves and may reach the renal collecting tubules, renal calyces and renal pelvis and upper ureter by a more indirect route. Such an arrangement is understandable on embryological grounds, since the structures mentioned are all derived from buds developed from the cloacal ends of the mesonephric (Wolffian) ducts. These pelvic parasympathetic fibers join the inferior hypogastric plexuses, ascend in the hypogastric nerves to the superior hypogastric plexus, and exit in fine branches that ascend retroperitoneally to enter the inferolateral parts of the homolateral renal plexus.

*Afferent fibers* from the kidneys and upper ureter follow similar routes in the reverse direction, but they do not form relays in peripheral ganglia; their cell bodies are located in dorsal spinal nerve root ganglia. The central processes of these ganglion cells enter the spinal cord mainly through the dorsal nerve roots of the tenth to twelfth thoracic spinal nerves, and then ascend in or alongside the spinothalamic tracts and also in the posterior white columns of the cord.

Within the renal hilus and sinus, the *renal plexus* supplies filaments to the renal pelvis, calyces and upper ureter. Other filaments form rich plexuses around the renal vessels and their branches and accompany them into the kidney. They contain mostly unmyelinated fibers, and

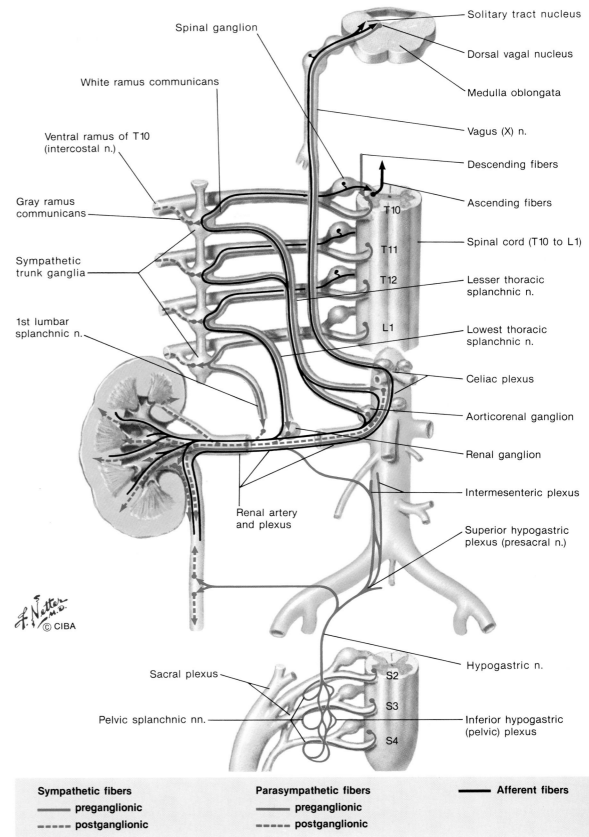

**Innervation of Kidney and Upper Ureter**

- Spinal ganglion
- White ramus communicans
- Ventral ramus of T10 (intercostal n.)
- Gray ramus communicans
- Sympathetic trunk ganglia
- 1st lumbar splanchnic n.
- Renal artery and plexus
- Sacral plexus
- Pelvic splanchnic nn.

- Solitary tract nucleus
- Dorsal vagal nucleus
- Medulla oblongata
- Vagus (X) n.
- Descending fibers
- Ascending fibers
- T10
- T11
- T12
- L1
- Spinal cord (T10 to L1)
- Lesser thoracic splanchnic n.
- Lowest thoracic splanchnic n.
- Celiac plexus
- Aorticorenal ganglion
- Renal ganglion
- Intermesenteric plexus
- Superior hypogastric plexus (presacral n.)
- S2
- S3
- S4
- Hypogastric n.
- Inferior hypogastric (pelvic) plexus

| Sympathetic fibers | Parasympathetic fibers | Afferent fibers |
|---|---|---|
| preganglionic | preganglionic | |
| postganglionic | postganglionic | |

relatively few of the myelinated type. The *sympathetic fibers* are distributed to the smooth muscle in the renal pelvis and calyces, to the vascular musculature, and possibly to the juxtaglomerular cells and glomeruli. The *parasympathetic fibers* supply the muscle in the pelvis, calyces and upper ureter, but it is uncertain whether they supply the vessels and tubules. *Sensory nerve endings* have reputedly been detected in the pelvis and ureter,

in the adventitia of the larger vessels, and near the glomeruli.

***Urinary Bladder and Lower Ureter.*** The *preganglionic sympathetic cells* concerned with vesical innervation are located in the upper two lumbar segments and perhaps also in the lowest thoracic segment of the spinal cord. The sites where the preganglionic fibers form synapses with the ganglionic neurons that give off the postganglionic

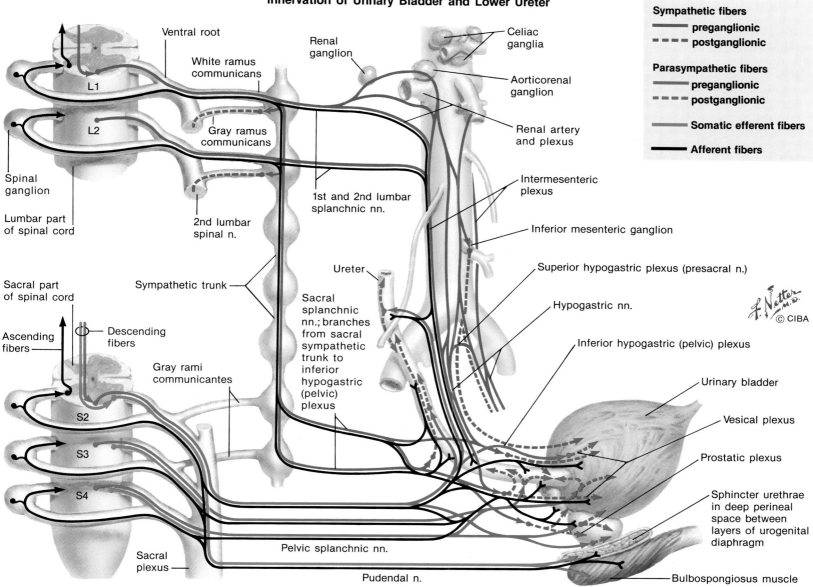

**Innervation of Urinary Bladder and Lower Ureter**

Sympathetic fibers
—— preganglionic
----- postganglionic

Parasympathetic fibers
—— preganglionic
----- postganglionic

—— Somatic efferent fibers

—— Afferent fibers

Ventral root

White ramus communicans

L1

Gray ramus communicans

L2

2nd lumbar spinal n.

Spinal ganglion

Lumbar part of spinal cord

Sympathetic trunk

Renal ganglion

Celiac ganglia

Aorticorenal ganglion

Renal artery and plexus

1st and 2nd lumbar splanchnic nn.

Intermesenteric plexus

Inferior mesenteric ganglion

Ureter

Superior hypogastric plexus (presacral n.)

Hypogastric nn.

Inferior hypogastric (pelvic) plexus

Urinary bladder

Sacral part of spinal cord

Ascending fibers

Descending fibers

Gray rami communicantes

Sacral splanchnic nn.; branches from sacral sympathetic trunk to inferior hypogastric (pelvic) plexus

S2

S3

S4

Sacral plexus

Pelvic splanchnic nn.

Pudendal n.

Vesical plexus

Prostatic plexus

Sphincter urethrae in deep perineal space between layers of urogenital diaphragm

Bulbospongiosus muscle

F. Netter M.D. © CIBA

SECTION IV PLATE 19

## Innervation of Kidneys, Ureters and Urinary Bladder

*(Continued)*

fibers have not been determined accurately. The *preganglionic parasympathetic cells* are located in the second to fourth sacral segments of the spinal cord, and their axons relay in ganglia close to or within the wall of the urinary bladder. *Afferent fibers* pursue similar pathways, but in the reverse direction; thus, some vesical sensory impulses enter the cord through the upper lumbar and last thoracic dorsal nerve roots, while others from the neck of the bladder and the lowest parts of the ureters reach the cord via the pelvic splanchnic nerves and the dorsal nerve roots of the second to fourth sacral nerve segments.

Many fascicles from the *extrinsic vesical plexuses* enter the bladder wall, mainly alongside its blood vessels. They divide and subdivide and are ultimately carried to all parts, forming a widespread *intramural*, or *intrinsic, vesical plexus*. The nerve fasciculi are most conspicuous in the trigonal and neighboring regions, becoming more scattered and attenuated toward the fundus. Many small ganglia are present on the surface or are buried

more deeply between the muscular bundles, and these are more numerous in the trigonal region. Many fibers enter the submucosa and penetrate between the mucosal cells, where they apparently end in small boutons.

Most of the nerve fasciculi in the urinary bladder wall contain unmyelinated or finely myelinated fibers. A small proportion of larger myelinated and, presumably, sensory fibers are connected with terminal arborizations regarded as stretch receptors. Many other putative sensory endings have been described in the submucosa and mucous membrane. The parasympathetic nerves may transmit many or most of the afferent fibers from the trigonal area of the urinary bladder and from the lowest parts of the ureters, including those conveying painful impulses. However, some afferents from the neck of the bladder and prostatic urethra may reach the spinal cord via the pudendal nerves.

Sensations associated with vesical distention may be mediated through sympathetic pathways, because vague discomfort may still be experienced by patients with transverse lesions of the cord below the level of the uppermost lumbar segments. This suggests that there is an afferent inflow from the bladder through the upper lumbar or lowest thoracic dorsal spinal nerve roots. Alternatively, such sensations may be produced by the

stimulation of nerve endings in the peritoneum over a distended bladder. However, since "presacral neurectomy" (removal of the superior hypogastric plexus) alleviates discomfort in patients with painful and intractable cystitis, a proportion of the vesical afferent fibers may traverse the hypogastric nerves and superior hypogastric plexus. Other afferent fibers traveling in the perivascular plexuses of the vesical and iliac arteries may also reach the superior hypogastric plexus. Beyond the plexus, the fibers run in lumbar splanchnic nerves to the sympathetic trunks, pass through rami communicantes to the upper lumbar and lowest thoracic spinal nerves, and enter the spinal cord through the dorsal roots of these nerves.

The parasympathetic supply to the bladder produces contraction of the walls and relaxation of the sphincteric mechanism, and is thus actively involved in micturition (see page 72). Most investigators associate the sympathetic supply with opposing effects, such as relaxation of the vesical walls and contraction of the sphincter, but a minority claim that the sympathetic effects are predominantly vasomotor and that the parasympathetic nerves are of paramount importance in controlling both the filling and emptying of the urinary bladder. (For greater details on the innervation of the kidneys, ureters and bladder, see CIBA COLLECTION, Volume 6, pages 27 to 29.) □

# Innervation of Reproductive Organs

The nerves supplying the male and female genital organs are autonomic and contain sympathetic and parasympathetic efferent and afferent fibers; their origins are similar in both sexes.

*Sympathetic preganglionic fibers* are the axons of lateral cornual cells located in the lowest two or three thoracic and upper one or two lumbar segments of the spinal cord. They emerge in the ventral nerve roots of the corresponding spinal nerves and leave them in white rami communicantes passing to adjacent sympathetic trunk ganglia. They course via the thoracic and the upper lumbar splanchnic nerve, the celiac, intermesenteric (aortic) and superior hypogastric plexuses and the hypogastric nerves to the *inferior hypogastric (pelvic) plexuses.* Many of these fibers relay in the lowest thoracic and upper lumbar sympathetic trunk ganglia or within the celiac plexus, but others do not relay until they reach ganglia in the inferior hypogastric plexuses. Consequently, the postganglionic fibers to the pelvic organs may be either long or relatively short. A minority of the sympathetic fibers for the pelvic viscera descend in the sympathetic trunks to emerge in the tiny *sacral splanchnic nerves* and thus join the inferior hypogastric plexuses.

*Preganglionic parasympathetic fibers* reach the inferior hypogastric plexuses in *pelvic splanchnic nerves* arising from the second, third and fourth sacral spinal nerves. Filaments from the *inferior hypogastric plexuses* supply the genital organs, and most of them relay in ganglia close to the prostate gland, neck of the bladder, cervix of the uterus and upper vagina. Others relay in microscopic ganglia in or near the walls of seminal vesicles, deferent ducts, epididymis and uterine tubes. There are no ganglia within the substance of the testes and ovaries. Inconclusive evidence suggests that parasympathetic fibers reach the outer parts of the uterine tubes by passing through the celiac plexus into the superior ovarian nerves that help to supply the oviducts. Histochemical studies indicate that parasympathetic innervation of the genital systems in both sexes is less abundant than sympathetic innervation.

*Afferent fibers* exist in both the sympathetic and parasympathetic pathways and follow the same routes as the efferent fibers, but in the reverse direction. Their parent pseudounipolar cells are situated in the dorsal root ganglia of the lower thoracic, upper lumbar and midsacral spinal nerves. The peripheral processes of these cells transmit impulses from the genital organs, ducts and vessels. Their central processes carry the impulses into the cord, where many are carried to the brain in ascending pathways in the lateral and

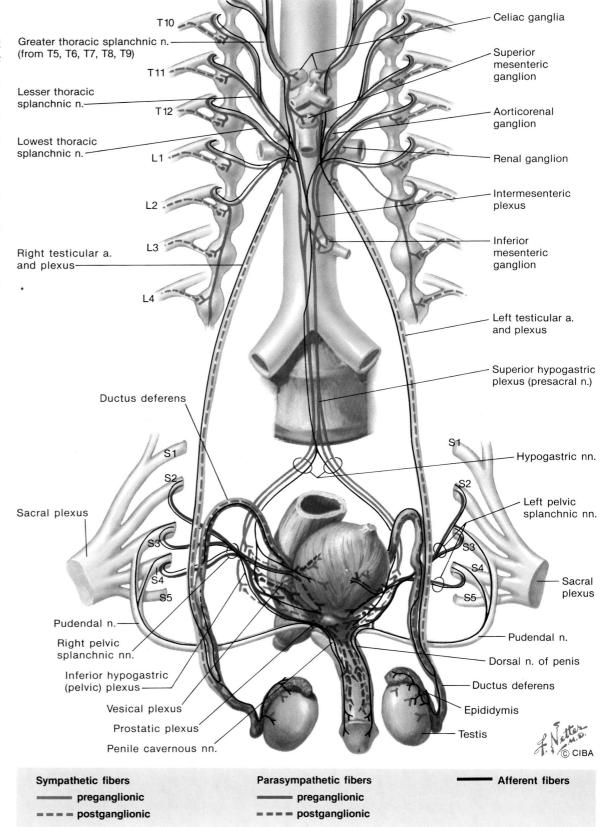

posterior white columns, while others form synapses with lateral cornual cells in the related cord segments and are thus involved in spinal reflex arcs.

### Male Reproductive Organs

The nerves supplying the testis, epididymis and ductus (vas) deferens are derived from three bilateral sources.

*A superior group* arises by rootlets from the *renal* and *intermesenteric plexuses*, with inconstant contributions from the *lumbar splanchnic nerves* and the origin of the *superior mesenteric plexus*. One or two small ganglia are associated with these rootlets. They communicate with the superior ureteric nerves and, on the right side, with branches supplying the duodenum and pancreas. The rootlets coalesce to form two or three slender nerves,

## Innervation of Reproductive Organs
*(Continued)*

which descend on the testicular artery to the *testis*.

*A middle group* arises by rootlets from the *superior hypogastric plexus* and from the ipsilateral *hypogastric nerve*, and often communicates with the *middle ureteric* and *genitofemoral nerves*. The resultant nerves are mostly or entirely distributed to the *epididymis* and the *ampulla* of the *ductus deferens*.

*An inferior group* of a few small nerves arises from the *inferior hypogastric plexus* and from the nerve loops around the *lower end of the ureter* (see page 87). This third group is closely associated with small nerves given off from the anterior part of the inferior hypogastric plexus to the seminal vesicles, prostate gland, ejaculatory ducts and the base of the urinary bladder. The *prostatic* and *urethral filaments* communicate with branchlets of the *pudendal nerves*, and offshoots from these united nervelets innervate the corpora cavernosa, the corpus spongiosum and the part of the urethra within it, and the bulbourethral glands. The filaments supplying the cavernous structures and their vessels are termed the *penile cavernous nerves*, while their ramifications are often called the *cavernous plexuses*.

### Female Reproductive Organs

The autonomic nerves supplying the female genital organs have similar origins to those supplying the male genital organs.

*The superior group* coalesces to form two or three slender nerves, which accompany the ovarian artery and supply filaments to it and to the *ovary* and outer parts of the *uterine tube*. Their terminal fibers communicate with *uterine fibers* innervating the inner end of the uterine tube. Most of the afferent fibers in these nerves enter the spinal cord through the dorsal roots of the tenth and the eleventh thoracic nerve, although a number may enter through the ninth or twelfth nerves.

*The middle group* helps to supply the *ovary* and the *uterine tube* and vessels, and gives off fascicles to the common and external iliac arteries.

*The inferior group* consists of nerves that enter the *cervix* of the *uterus* and the *vagina* directly, often alongside branches of the uterine and vaginal vessels, and other nerves that ascend with or near the uterine artery, supplying filaments to the *body* and *fundus* of the *uterus*, as well as to the artery and its branches. The terminal filaments supply the uterine end and isthmus of the *uterine tube*, where they communicate with corresponding filaments from the superior and middle groups of nerves.

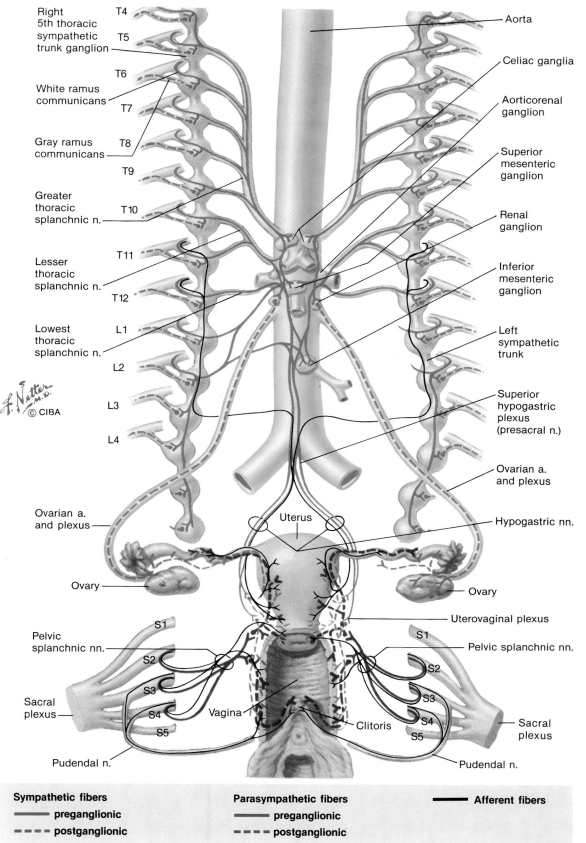

**Innervation of Female Reproductive Organs**

Right 5th thoracic sympathetic trunk ganglion — T4, T5

White ramus communicans — T6, T7

Gray ramus communicans — T8

T9

Greater thoracic splanchnic n. — T10

Lesser thoracic splanchnic n. — T11, T12

Lowest thoracic splanchnic n. — L1, L2, L3, L4

Ovarian a. and plexus

Ovary

Pelvic splanchnic nn. — S1, S2, S3, S4, S5

Sacral plexus

Pudendal n.

Aorta
Celiac ganglia
Aorticorenal ganglion
Superior mesenteric ganglion
Renal ganglion
Inferior mesenteric ganglion
Left sympathetic trunk
Superior hypogastric plexus (presacral n.)
Ovarian a. and plexus
Uterus
Hypogastric nn.
Ovary
Uterovaginal plexus
Pelvic splanchnic nn. — S1, S2, S3, S4, S5
Sacral plexus
Vagina
Clitoris
Pudendal n.

| Sympathetic fibers | Parasympathetic fibers | Afferent fibers |
|---|---|---|
| —— preganglionic | —— preganglionic | —— |
| - - - postganglionic | - - - postganglionic | |

The *uterine nerves* ramify throughout the myometrium. The fibers, which are predominantly unmyelinated and adrenergic in type, are most plentiful around the uterine end of the uterine tube, in the cervix, and near the arterial branches.

The nerves entering the upper part of the *vagina* contain tiny ganglia. They break up into filaments that supply the vaginal arteries and give off fascicles to the muscular and mucous coats of the vagina and urethra, the erectile tissue of the vestibular bulb and corpora cavernosa clitoridis, and the greater and lesser vestibular glands. These nerves contain a mixture of sympathetic and parasympathetic efferent and afferent fibers. (For more details, see CIBA COLLECTION, Volume 2, pages 18, 19 and 103 to 105 and Volume 3/II, pages 40 to 44.) □

## Pharmacology of Autonomic Nervous System

| | Sympathetic | | Parasympathetic |
|---|---|---|---|
| | $\alpha$-adrenergic receptors | $\beta$-adrenergic receptors | muscarinic cholinergic receptors |
| **Natural agonists** | | | |
| **Norepinephrine (released by sympathetic nerve endings)** | + + + | + | − |
| **Epinephrine (released by adrenal medulla)** | + | + + + | − |
| **Acetylcholine (released by parasympathetic nerve endings)** | − | − | + + + |
| **Other (artificial) agonists** | Methoxamine Phenylephrine | Isoproterenol Methoxyphenamine | Muscarine Pilocarpine Carbachol |
| **Direct effects of agonists on:** | | | |
| **Heart** | − | Increased rate and force of contraction | Decreased rate and force of contraction |
| **Blood vessels** | Vasoconstriction | Vasodilatation | Vasodilatation |
| **Intestines** | Decreased motility | Decreased motility | Increased motility |
| **Antagonists (blocking agents)** | Phentolamine Phenoxybenzamine Ergot alkaloids | Propranolol Pindolol Alprenolol | Atropine Scopolamine 3-quinuclidinyl benzylate |
| **Agents that block enzymatic degradation of transmitter** | Monoamine Oxidase (MAO) inhibitors Catechol-O-methyltransferase (CCMT) inhibitors | | Anticholinesterase |

© CIBA

Section V

# Cranial Nerves

Frank H. Netter, M.D.

*in collaboration with*

G.A.G. Mitchell, Ch.M., D.Sc., F.R.C.S.   *Plates 1–13*

# Cranial Nerves

| Name, Number and Type | Origin, Course and Distribution | Chief Functions |
|---|---|---|
| **Olfactory (I)**<br><br>*Special sensory* | • Olfactory cells in nasal mucosa.<br>• Through cribriform plate to olfactory bulb and tract (Plate 4). Tract divides into *medial branch*, which fades away in parolfactory and subcallosal areas, and *lateral branch*, which ends in uncus of parahippocampal gyrus. | *Nerve of smell.* |
| **Optic (II)**<br><br>*Special sensory* | • Retinal ganglion cells.<br>• Optic nerve (Plates 5 and 6) through optic canal to optic chiasm, where fibers from medial halves of retinae decussate. Fibers then pass in optic tracts to lateral geniculate bodies, where they relay, giving rise to optic radiations, which end in striate area of occipital cortex. | *Nerve of vision.* |
| **Oculomotor (III)**<br><br>*Motor* | • Complicated nucleus ventral to cerebral aqueduct, including *accessory (autonomic: Edinger-Westphal) nucleus.*<br>• Fibers emerge on medial side of cerebral peduncle. Nerve passes lateral to posterior clinoid process into lateral wall of cavernous sinus and enters orbit through superior orbital fissure. Supplies all orbital muscles except lateral rectus and superior oblique (Plates 5 and 6). Also conveys parasympathetic root to ciliary ganglion, in which fibers form synapses; postganglionic fibers reach eye in short ciliary nerves and supply pupillary sphincter and ciliary muscles. | Muscles supplied turn eye upward, downward and medially, produce constriction of pupil, participate in accommodation reflexes, and raise upper eyelid (some fibers end in levator palpebrae superioris muscle). |
| **Trochlear (IV)**<br><br>*Motor* | • Nucleus of origin ventral to cerebral aqueduct.<br>• Fibers decussate in superior medullary velum and emerge just below superior colliculus as slender nerve that curves around homolateral cerebral peduncle above upper border of pons, runs in lateral wall of cavernous sinus, and enters orbit through superior orbital fissure to end in superior oblique muscle (Plates 5 and 6). | Supplies superior oblique muscle, which assists in turning eye downward and outward. |
| **Trigeminal (V)**<br><br>*Sensory and motor* | • Sensory receptors in eye and surroundings, face, forehead, upper and lower jaws, sinuses, teeth and nasopharynx; proprioceptive receptors in orbital and masticatory muscles; *trigeminal motor nucleus* in upper part of pons is origin of motor fibers. Pain, touch and temperature fibers end in *principal (pontine) sensory nucleus* and *spinal nucleus of trigeminal nerve*; proprioceptive fibers from orbital and masticatory muscles end in *mesencephalic nucleus.*<br>• Large sensory and smaller motor roots enter and emerge through lateral part of pons; former expands over apex of petrous temporal bone into *trigeminal (semilunar) ganglion*, which gives off ophthalmic, maxillary and mandibular nerves; they pass through superior orbital fissure, foramen rotundum and foramen ovale. *Ophthalmic nerve* divides into lacrimal, frontal and nasociliary branches, which participate in innervating eye, nose and scalp. *Maxillary nerve* traverses pterygopalatine fossa, enters infra-orbital groove (canal) and emerges as *infraorbital nerve* through infraorbital foramen; supplies meningeal, zygomatic, superior alveolar, inferior palpebral, nasal and superior labial branches, and is connected with pterygopalatine ganglion through which it supplies orbital, nasal, palatine and pharyngeal branches. *Mandibular nerve* is joined by entire motor root of trigeminal nerve in foramen ovale, and gives off meningeal, buccal, auriculotemporal, lingual and inferior alveolar branches, and nerves supplying masticatory muscles and tensors of soft palate and tympanic membrane (Plate 7). | *Ophthalmic nerve* carries sensory fibers from cornea, conjunctiva, iris, lacrimal gland, upper eyelid, brow and front of scalp, nasal mucosa and vessels.<br>*Maxillary nerve* conveys sensation from lower eyelid, side of nose, upper lip, palate, upper jaw and teeth, part of buccal mucosa, nasal sinuses, nasopharynx, and from vessels and glands in its area of supply.<br>*Mandibular nerve* carries sensory fibers from lower jaw, teeth and overlying skin and mucosa, part of skin and mucosa of cheek, from auricle and part of external auditory meatus, from temporal region, temporomandibular joint and masticatory muscles, from salivary glands, from vessels in its area of supply and from anterior two thirds of tongue. Its *motor component* supplies muscles of mastication and tensors of soft palate and tympanic membrane. |
| **Abducens (VI)**<br><br>*Motor* | • Fibers arise from nucleus in pons, near midline and beneath upper part of floor of fourth ventricle.<br>• Nerve emerges in groove between pons and pyramid, and runs upward and laterally before bending forward over apex of petrous temporal bone. It then traverses cavernous sinus, and reaches orbit through its superior fissure (Plates 5 and 6). | Supplies lateral rectus muscle, which rotates eye outward. |
| **Facial (VII)**<br><br>*Motor, secretomotor and special sensory* | • Motor fibers arise in *facial nucleus* in pons and loop around abducens nucleus; secretomotor fibers originate in *superior salivatory nucleus*, located near caudal end of motor nucleus; special sensory fibers arise from receptors in anterior two thirds of tongue and soft palate, and end in *nucleus of solitary tract.*<br>• Nerve emerges through recess between inferior cerebellar peduncle and olive as two parts: larger *motor root* and smaller *nervus intermedius* containing secretomotor and special sensory fibers. Most of latter are conveyed to peripheral destinations in chorda tympani and lingual nerve; lacrimal fibers are carried in greater petrosal nerve. Both parts enter internal acoustic meatus alongside vestibulocochlear nerve, and run through angulated facial canal. At angle, two parts of nerve unite and expand into *geniculate ganglion*, which contains cell bodies of sensory fibers. Most special sensory and secretomotor fibers branch off in chorda tympani, and main part of the nerve emerges through stylomastoid foramen. It soon enters parotid gland, where it divides into diverging branches (Plate 8). | *Motor supply* to muscles of face, scalp, auricle, buccinator, stapedius, stylohyoid and posterior belly of digastric: controls facial expression, and assists in regulating movements required in speech and mastication.<br>*Secretomotor* to submandibular and sublingual salivary glands, to lacrimal glands and to glands of nasal and palatine mucosae.<br>*Special sensory* taste fibers from anterior two thirds of tongue (via chorda tympani) and soft palate (via greater petrosal nerve). |

# Cranial Nerves: Distribution of Motor and Sensory Fibers

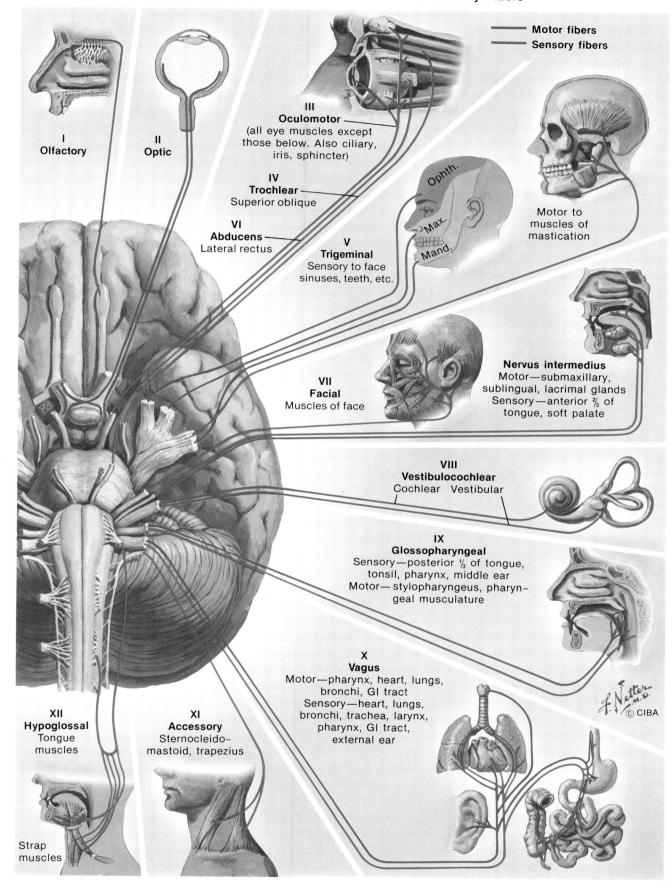

Motor fibers
Sensory fibers

**III**
**Oculomotor**
(all eye muscles except
those below. Also ciliary,
iris, sphincter)

**IV**
**Trochlear**
Superior oblique

**VI**
**Abducens**
Lateral rectus

Ophth.
Max.
Mand.

Motor to
muscles of
mastication

**V**
**Trigeminal**
Sensory to face
sinuses, teeth, etc.

**I**
Olfactory

**II**
Optic

**VII**
**Facial**
Muscles of face

**Nervus intermedius**
Motor—submaxillary,
sublingual, lacrimal glands
Sensory—anterior ⅔ of
tongue, soft palate

**VIII**
**Vestibulocochlear**
Cochlear   Vestibular

**IX**
**Glossopharyngeal**
Sensory—posterior ⅓ of tongue,
tonsil, pharynx, middle ear
Motor—stylopharyngeus, pharyn-
geal musculature

**X**
**Vagus**
Motor—pharynx, heart, lungs,
bronchi, GI tract
Sensory—heart, lungs,
bronchi, trachea, larynx,
pharynx, GI tract,
external ear

**XII**
**Hypoglossal**
Tongue
muscles

**XI**
**Accessory**
Sternocleido-
mastoid, trapezius

Strap
muscles

_F. Netter_ M.D.
© CIBA

**Vestibulocochlear (VIII)**

**Special sensory**

• Fibers arise from bipolar cells in vestibular and spiral cochlear ganglia.
• Nerve appears in groove between pons and medulla posterolateral to facial nerve (Plate 9). Peripheral processes pass to special receptors in vestibular apparatus and cochlea, and central processes pass to nuclei in brainstem. _Vestibular nucleus_ comprises superior, inferior, medial and lateral parts located deep to floor of fourth ventricle; they are connected with cerebellum (and through medial longitudinal fasciculus) with cranial motor nerve nuclei and spinal ventral horn cells controlling some muscles of

_Vestibular_ component conveys impulses concerned with equilibration and position and with movements of head and neck.

_(Continued)_

# Cranial Nerves: Nerves and Nuclei Viewed in Phantom From Behind

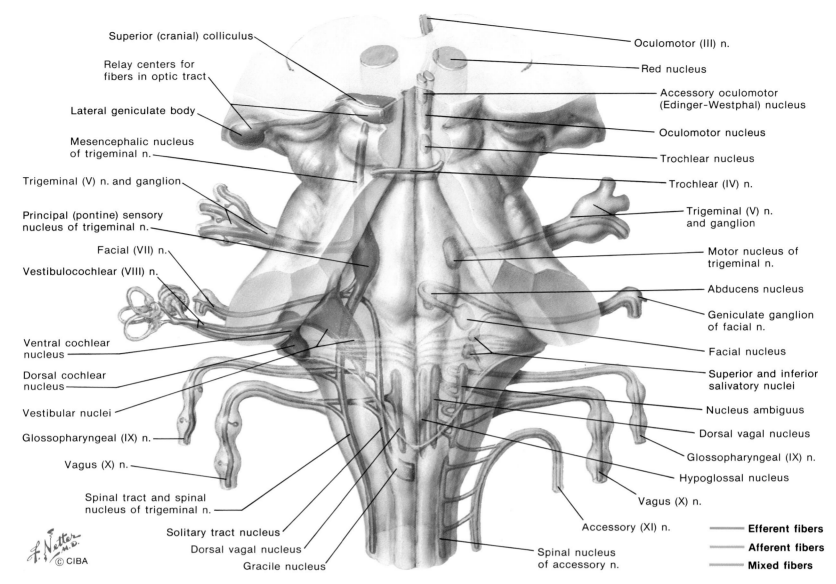

Superior (cranial) colliculus

Relay centers for fibers in optic tract

Lateral geniculate body

Mesencephalic nucleus of trigeminal n.

Trigeminal (V) n. and ganglion

Principal (pontine) sensory nucleus of trigeminal n.

Facial (VII) n.

Vestibulocochlear (VIII) n.

Ventral cochlear nucleus

Dorsal cochlear nucleus

Vestibular nuclei

Glossopharyngeal (IX) n.

Vagus (X) n.

Spinal tract and spinal nucleus of trigeminal n.

Solitary tract nucleus

Dorsal vagal nucleus

Gracile nucleus

Oculomotor (III) n.

Red nucleus

Accessory oculomotor (Edinger-Westphal) nucleus

Oculomotor nucleus

Trochlear nucleus

Trochlear (IV) n.

Trigeminal (V) n. and ganglion

Motor nucleus of trigeminal n.

Abducens nucleus

Geniculate ganglion of facial n.

Facial nucleus

Superior and inferior salivatory nuclei

Nucleus ambiguus

Dorsal vagal nucleus

Glossopharyngeal (IX) n.

Hypoglossal nucleus

Vagus (X) n.

Accessory (XI) n.

Spinal nucleus of accessory n.

Efferent fibers
Afferent fibers
Mixed fibers

**Vestibulocochlear (VIII)**
*(Continued)*

head and neck. Vestibulospinal tract originates in lateral vestibular nucleus. *Cochlear nucleus* consists of ventral and dorsal parts lying on corresponding aspects of inferior cerebellar peduncle. Most cochlear nuclear fibers decussate in trapezoid body; some may cross in striae medullares of fourth ventricle to form lateral lemniscus of opposite side, but some ascend homolaterally. Some lateral lemniscal fibers may relay in nuclei in trapezoid body, olivary complex or lateral lemniscus before reaching inferior colliculus, where a proportion relay and enter tectospinal tract; most pass through inferior colliculus into inferior brachium and on to medial geniculate body, where they form synapses. Resulting acoustic radiations pass to auditory cortex in superior temporal gyrus.

*Cochlear* component is nerve of hearing.

**Glossopharyngeal (IX)**

*Motor, secretomotor, special sensory and sensory*

• Motor fibers arise from cranial ends of *ambiguus* and *dorsal vagal nuclei*; secretomotor fibers arise from *inferior salivatory nucleus*, lying in reticular formation below its superior counterpart; special sensory fibers arise from posterior third of tongue, as do sensory fibers, which also arise from pharynx, fauces, tonsil, tympanic cavity, auditory tube and mastoid cells. "Visceral" sensory fibers end in combined *dorsal glossopharyngeal-vagal nucleus*; ordinary sensory fibers probably end in *spinal tract* and *nucleus of trigeminal nerve*, and those concerned with special sensation, in *solitary tract nucleus*.
• Nerve emerges from medulla above vagus, leaves skull through jugular foramen, runs forward between internal carotid artery and internal jugular vein, curves over stylopharyngeus muscle, and usually passes between adjoining margins of superior and middle pharyngeal constrictor muscles to end in branches for tonsils and mucous membrane and glands of pharynx and pharyngeal part of tongue (Plate 10). In addition, it gives off tympanic, carotid and stylopharyngeal twigs, and contributes to pharyngeal plexus. *Tympanic branch* forms main part of tympanic plexus, which supplies tympanic cavity, and lesser petrosal nerve, which carries secretomotor fibers for parotid gland.

*Motor supply* to stylopharyngeus; may help innervate pharyngeal muscles.
*Secretomotor* fibers promote parotid secretion and activity of mucous glands in territory of supply.
*Special sensory* is nerve of taste for posterior third of tongue, including numerous taste buds in vallate papillae.
*Sensory* fibers convey ordinary sensation from pharynx, pharyngeal part of tongue, fauces, tonsil, tympanic cavity, auditory tube and mastoid cells. Chief nerve supply of carotid body and sinus.

**Vagus (X)**

*Motor, sensory and special sensory*

• Motor fibers for cardiac and unstriated muscle arise in *dorsal vagal nucleus*, which is mixture of visceral efferent and afferent cells forming elongated column on each side of midline, lying lateral to hypoglossal nuclei, and extending throughout length of medulla oblongata. Motor fibers for striated muscles of larynx and pharynx originate in *nucleus ambiguus*, an ill-defined column of large cells located in reticular formation.

*Motor fibers* innervate intrinsic laryngeal muscles and help to supply pharyngeal constrictors. Provide parasympathetic supply to heart and its vessels, to trachea and bronchi, to alimentary canal from

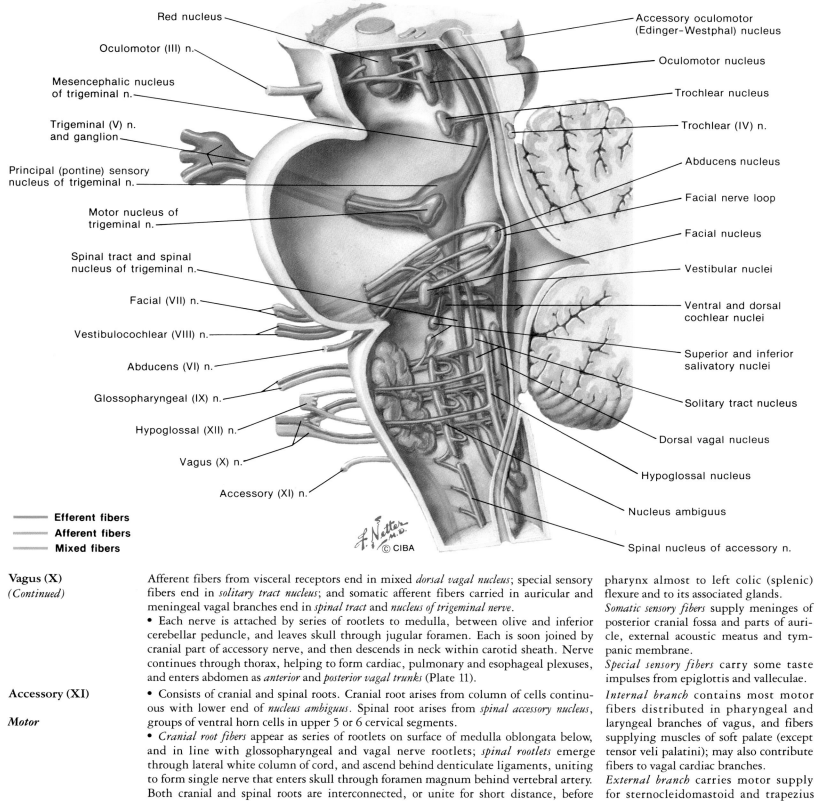

## Cranial Nerves: Schema of Nerves and Nuclei in Lateral Dissection

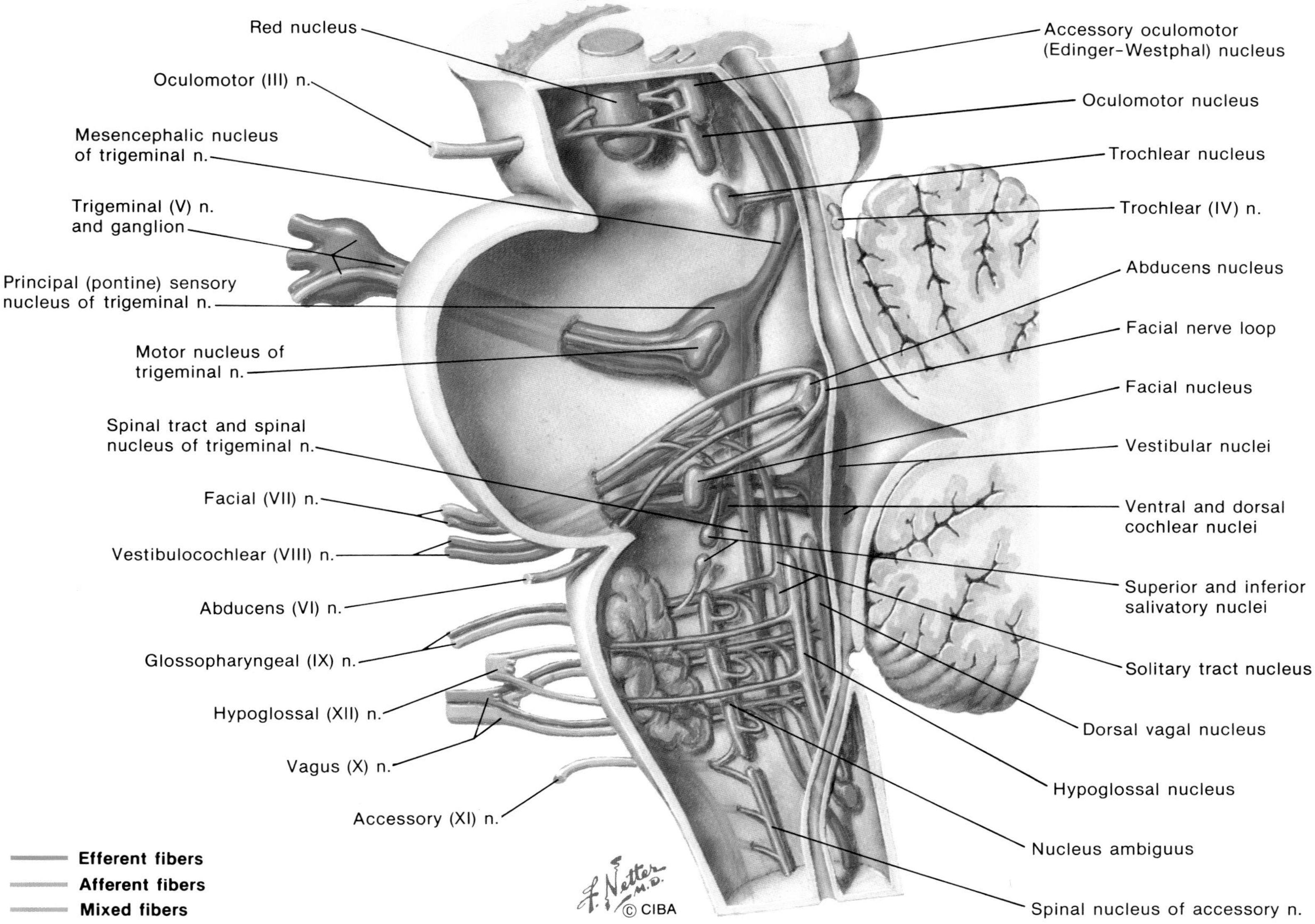

Red nucleus
Oculomotor (III) n.
Mesencephalic nucleus of trigeminal n.
Trigeminal (V) n. and ganglion
Principal (pontine) sensory nucleus of trigeminal n.
Motor nucleus of trigeminal n.
Spinal tract and spinal nucleus of trigeminal n.
Facial (VII) n.
Vestibulocochlear (VIII) n.
Abducens (VI) n.
Glossopharyngeal (IX) n.
Hypoglossal (XII) n.
Vagus (X) n.
Accessory (XI) n.
Accessory oculomotor (Edinger-Westphal) nucleus
Oculomotor nucleus
Trochlear nucleus
Trochlear (IV) n.
Abducens nucleus
Facial nerve loop
Facial nucleus
Vestibular nuclei
Ventral and dorsal cochlear nuclei
Superior and inferior salivatory nuclei
Solitary tract nucleus
Dorsal vagal nucleus
Hypoglossal nucleus
Nucleus ambiguus
Spinal nucleus of accessory n.
Efferent fibers
Afferent fibers
Mixed fibers
F. Netter M.D.
© CIBA


**Vagus (X)**
*(Continued)*

Afferent fibers from visceral receptors end in mixed *dorsal vagal nucleus*; special sensory fibers end in *solitary tract nucleus*; and somatic afferent fibers carried in auricular and meningeal vagal branches end in *spinal tract* and *nucleus of trigeminal nerve*.

• Each nerve is attached by series of rootlets to medulla, between olive and inferior cerebellar peduncle, and leaves skull through jugular foramen. Each is soon joined by cranial part of accessory nerve, and then descends in neck within carotid sheath. Nerve continues through thorax, helping to form cardiac, pulmonary and esophageal plexuses, and enters abdomen as *anterior* and *posterior vagal trunks* (Plate 11).

pharynx almost to left colic (splenic) flexure and to its associated glands.
*Somatic sensory fibers* supply meninges of posterior cranial fossa and parts of auricle, external acoustic meatus and tympanic membrane.
*Special sensory fibers* carry some taste impulses from epiglottis and valleculae.

**Accessory (XI)**
***Motor***

• Consists of cranial and spinal roots. Cranial root arises from column of cells continuous with lower end of *nucleus ambiguus*. Spinal root arises from *spinal accessory nucleus*, groups of ventral horn cells in upper 5 or 6 cervical segments.

• *Cranial root fibers* appear as series of rootlets on surface of medulla oblongata below, and in line with glossopharyngeal and vagal nerve rootlets; *spinal rootlets* emerge through lateral white column of cord, and ascend behind denticulate ligaments, uniting to form single nerve that enters skull through foramen magnum behind vertebral artery. Both cranial and spinal roots are interconnected, or unite for short distance, before leaving skull through jugular foramen. Thereafter, nerve divides into internal and external branches containing, respectively, cranial and spinal fibers. *Internal branch* joins vagus nerve. *External branch* runs downward and backward through sternocleidomastoid muscle, crosses posterior triangle of neck, and ends in trapezius muscle; it communicates with branches of spinal nerves C2, C3 and C4 (Plate 12).

*Internal branch* contains most motor fibers distributed in pharyngeal and laryngeal branches of vagus, and fibers supplying muscles of soft palate (except tensor veli palatini); may also contribute fibers to vagal cardiac branches.
*External branch* carries motor supply for sternocleidomastoid and trapezius muscles.

**Hypoglossal (XII)**
***Motor***

• *Hypoglossal nucleus* is column of cells near median plane, situated deep to lower half of floor of fourth ventricle, and extending inferiorly ventral to central canal in "closed" part of medulla oblongata.

• Fibers emerge as rootlets between pyramid and olive, and fuse to form two bundles, which unite as they pass through hypoglossal canal of occipital bone. Nerve then runs forward between internal carotid artery and internal jugular vein and inclines upward into tongue. It is joined by a filament from spinal nerve C1, which soon leaves to form *superior root (descendens hypoglossi)* of *ansa cervicalis* (Plate 13).

*Motor nerve* of tongue muscles. Descending branch (not connected to hypoglossal nucleus) consists of fibers from C1, which join fibers from C2 and C3 to form ansa cervicalis; ansa supplies twigs to sternohyoid, sternothyroid and omohyoid muscles.

# Olfactory (I) Nerves, Nerves of Nose and Pterygopalatine Ganglion

*The olfactory nerves* are concerned with the special sense of smell. Their fibers are the central processes of bipolar nerve cells located in the olfactory epithelium, which covers most of the superior nasal conchae and the opposed surfaces of the nasal septum.

The olfactory nerve cells are unique in that they retain their primitive superficial position. The majority develop from dorsomedian ectodermal thickenings (neural plate, tube and crests—see Section VII, Plate 2), and only a minority arise from the small ectodermal plaques, the *olfactory placodes*. At about the fifth week of embryonic life, these superficial placodes appear on the ventrolateral surface of the head; during nasal development (see Section VII, Plates 3 to 5 and 7), the nerve cells formed in them ultimately become located in the olfactory epithelium.

On each side, the unmyelinated peripheral olfactory fibers become aggregated into about 20 slender olfactory nerves, which traverse the ethmoidal cribriform plate in bundles surrounded by fingerlike extensions from the dura mater and arachnoid to end in the "glomeruli" of the homolateral olfactory bulb (see Section I, Plate 7, Section II, Plate 5 and Section VIII, Plates 18 and 19). These nerves and their meningeal coverings may be torn by fractures involving the cribriform plate, with consequent partial or complete anosmia, cerebrospinal fluid rhinorrhea and possible meningeal infection.

Ordinary sensations such as touch, pain and temperature are conveyed from the nasal cavities through the *maxillary* and *ophthalmic nerves*, which are major branches of the trigeminal (V) nerve (Plate 7).

*Nerves of Nose*. The *anterior ethmoidal nerve*, a branch of the nasociliary nerve (itself a branch of the ophthalmic nerve), enters the roof of the nose through the corresponding foramen and divides into internal and external nasal branches. The *internal nasal branch* gives off medial and lateral rami; the former supplies the mucous membrane over the anterosuperior part of the nasal septum; the latter supplies the mucous membrane of the anterior parts of the lateral nasal wall, including that which covers the anterior ends of the middle and inferior nasal conchae and lines the anterior and middle ethmoidal sinuses. The *external nasal branch* runs between the nasal bone and lateral nasal cartilage to supply the skin over the lower anterolateral surfaces of the external nose.

The *infraorbital nerve*, a continuation of the maxillary nerve, gives off alveolar branches that end in the superior dental plexuses (see page 100). In addition, its branches supply the parts of the lateral nasal wall not supplied by the anterior ethmoidal nerve nor by branches of the pterygopalatine (sphenopalatine) ganglion. The tiny, inconstant *posterior ethmoidal branch* of the nasociliary nerve helps to supply the posterior ethmoidal and sphenoidal sinuses, and filaments from the *nerve of the pterygoid canal* may assist in supplying the posterosuperior parts of the nasal septum. The maxillary nerves, however, are the major sources

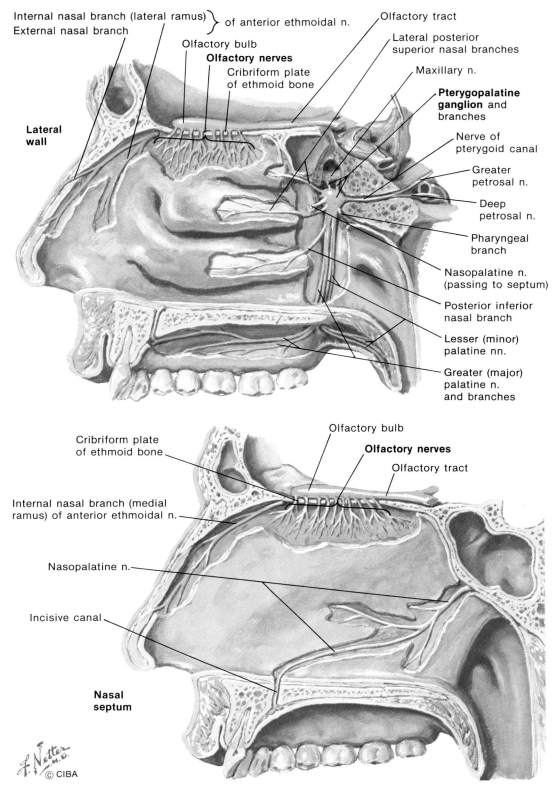

### Olfactory (I) Nerve, Pterygopalatine Ganglion and Nerves of Nose

Internal nasal branch (lateral ramus) } of anterior ethmoidal n.
External nasal branch
Olfactory bulb
**Olfactory nerves**
Cribriform plate of ethmoid bone
Lateral wall
Olfactory tract
Lateral posterior superior nasal branches
Maxillary n.
**Pterygopalatine ganglion** and branches
Nerve of pterygoid canal
Greater petrosal n.
Deep petrosal n.
Pharyngeal branch
Nasopalatine n. (passing to septum)
Posterior inferior nasal branch
Lesser (minor) palatine nn.
Greater (major) palatine n. and branches

Cribriform plate of ethmoid bone
Olfactory bulb
**Olfactory nerves**
Olfactory tract
Internal nasal branch (medial ramus) of anterior ethmoidal n.
Nasopalatine n.
Incisive canal
**Nasal septum**

of nasal sensory fibers. All the nasal nerves are accompanied by sympathetic and parasympathetic fibers, which transmit vasomotor, secretomotor and other impulses (see Section IV, Plate 5).

***Pterygopalatine Ganglion***. Among the nerves supplying the lateral nasal wall are the *lateral posterior superior* and *inferior posterior nasal branches* of the *pterygopalatine ganglion*; the latter usually arise from the *greater (major) palatine branch* of the ganglion. These ganglionic branches innervate extensive areas of mucosa over the nasal conchae and lateral nasal walls, and also the linings of the maxillary sinus and posterior ethmoidal cells. The fibers involved pass through the ganglion without

relaying, continue centrally in the pterygopalatine branches of the maxillary nerve, and end in the trigeminal nuclei in the brainstem.

The *nasopalatine (long sphenopalatine) nerve*, another branch of the pterygopalatine ganglion and the largest of the *medial posterior superior nasal nerves*, enters the nose through the sphenopalatine foramen. It supplies the posterior part of the nasal roof and then runs anteroinferiorly over the nasal septum, giving off twigs to most of its mucosal covering, before passing through the incisive canal to end in the mucoperiosteum over the anterior part of the hard palate and the adjacent gums. □

# Nerves of Orbit and Ciliary Ganglion

The greater parts of the optic (II), oculomotor (III), trochlear (IV), ophthalmic division of the trigeminal (V) and abducens (VI) nerves, and the ciliary ganglion with its roots and branches are located in the orbit. The nerves are closely interrelated as they pass through the cavernous sinus (see Section III, Plate 13).

### Ophthalmic Nerve

The *ophthalmic nerve* is the superior and smallest division of the trigeminal nerve (Plate 7). It transmits sensory impulses from the eye, conjunctiva, lacrimal gland, eyelids, forehead, scalp and parts of the nose (see page 96), and also conveys vasomotor, secretomotor and sensory autonomic fibers to and from orbital and nasal vessels and glands (see Section IV, Plate 5). It arises from the anteromedial part of the trigeminal ganglion and runs forward in the lateral wall of the cavernous sinus below the oculomotor and trochlear nerves to enter the orbit through the medial end of the superior orbital fissure (see Section I, Plate 7). At about this level, the ophthalmic nerve gives off a *tentorial (meningeal) branch* and divides into the frontal, nasociliary and lacrimal nerves.

*The frontal nerve*, the largest branch, continues forward between the orbital roof and the levator palpebrae superioris muscle, and splits into larger supraorbital and smaller supratrochlear nerves. The *supraorbital nerve* leaves the orbit through the supraorbital notch and divides into medial and lateral branches (the division may occur within the orbit), which ascend to supply the forehead and the scalp almost to the level of the lambdoid suture; the branches subdivide to supply the skin and conjunctiva of the upper eyelid, the subjacent pericranium and the mucous membrane of the homolateral frontal sinus. The *supratrochlear nerve* passes above the trochlea of the superior oblique muscle, leaves the orbit medial to the supraorbital nerve, ascends to supply the inferomedial part of the forehead, and gives off small descending branches to the skin and conjunctiva of the medial end of the upper eyelid.

*The nasociliary nerve* is intermediate in size between the frontal and lacrimal branches of the ophthalmic nerve, and enters the orbit through the common annular tendon. It lies at first between the superior and inferior divisions of the oculomotor nerve, then crosses over the optic nerve to run between the superior oblique and medial rectus muscles, and ends by dividing into the small *anterior ethmoidal* and *infratrochlear nerves*; the former supplies internal nasal branches (Plate 4), and the latter gives off twigs to the skin and conjunctiva of the lower eyelid, the lacrimal sac and the skin over the upper part of the anterolateral surface of the external nose. An inconstant *posterior ethmoidal branch* passes through the corresponding foramen to supply the mucosa of the posterior ethmoidal and sphenoidal sinuses. Near its origin, the nasociliary nerve gives off the *sensory root to the ciliary ganglion* and two or three slender *long ciliary nerves*, which pierce the sclera

## Nerves of Orbit, Ciliary Ganglion and Cavernous Sinus

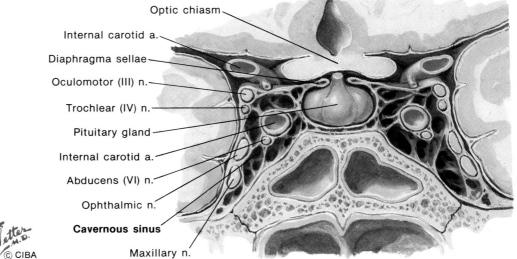

Supratrochlear n.
Medial rectus m.
Superior oblique m.
Nasociliary n.
Cribriform plate of ethmoid bone
Common annular tendon
Optic (II) n.
Optic chiasm
Pituitary stalk (infundibulum)
Oculomotor (III) n.
Trochlear (IV) n.
Abducens (VI) n.
Tentorial (meningeal) branch of ophthalmic n.

Medial branch ⎫ of supraorbital n.
Lateral branch ⎭
Levator palpebrae superioris m.
Superior rectus m.
Eyeball
Lacrimal gland
Supraorbital n.
Lacrimal n.
Lateral rectus m.
Frontal n.
Ophthalmic n.
Maxillary n.
Meningeal branch of maxillary n.
Mandibular n.
Meningeal branch (nervus spinosus) of mandibular n.
Lesser petrosal n.
Greater petrosal n.
Trigeminal ganglion
Tentorium cerebelli

Supratrochlear n. (cut)
Medial and lateral branches of supraorbital n. (cut)
Infratrochlear n.
Anterior ethmoidal n.
Long ciliary nn.
Optic (II) n.
Posterior ethmoidal n.
Nasociliary n.
Ophthalmic n. (cut and turned back)
Trochlear (IV) n. (cut)
Oculomotor (III) n.
Abducens (VI) n.

Levator palpebrae superioris m. (cut)
Superior rectus m. (cut)
Lacrimal n. (cut)
Short ciliary nn.
Branch of oculomotor n. to inferior oblique m.
**Ciliary ganglion:**
Motor (parasympathetic) root from oculomotor n.
Sympathetic root from internal carotid plexus
Sensory root from nasociliary n.
Branches to medial and inferior rectus mm.
Abducens (VI) n. (to lateral rectus m.)
Inferior division of oculomotor n.
Superior division of oculomotor n.

Optic chiasm
Internal carotid a.
Diaphragma sellae
Oculomotor (III) n.
Trochlear (IV) n.
Pituitary gland
Internal carotid a.
Abducens (VI) n.
Ophthalmic n.
**Cavernous sinus**
Maxillary n.

# Nerves of Orbit and Ciliary Ganglion
*(Continued)*

near the optic nerve and run forward in the perichoroidal space to supply the ciliary body, iris and cornea; the nerves may be joined by the sympathetic postganglionic fibers proceeding to the dilator pupillae (see Section IV, Plate 7).

*The lacrimal nerve*, the smallest branch of the ophthalmic nerve, runs with the lacrimal artery to the lacrimal gland, above the upper border of the lateral rectus muscle. It supplies several branchlets to the lacrimal gland and to the adjacent conjunctiva; its terminal filaments pierce the orbital septum, communicate with branches of the facial and infraorbital nerves, and end in the subcutaneous tissue and skin of the upper eyelid. Its communication with the zygomaticotemporal branch of the maxillary nerve is thought to carry secretomotor parasympathetic fibers from the pterygopalatine ganglion to the lacrimal nerve and gland (see Section IV, Plate 5).

## Oculomotor Nerve

The oculomotor nerve carries somatic motor fibers to the levator palpebrae superioris muscle and to all the extraocular muscles of the eyeball, except the lateral rectus and the superior oblique. It also conveys important parasympathetic fibers to intraocular structures, such as the sphincter pupillae and ciliary muscles, and is joined by sympathetic fibers from the internal carotid plexus, which are distributed with its branches (see Section IV, Plate 7 and Section VIII, Plate 64). Some oculomotor proprioceptive fibers may reach the midbrain through the oculomotor nerve; most of them join the ophthalmic branch of the trigeminal nerve via its communications with the oculomotor nerve.

*Oculomotor Nuclei.* The somatic and parasympathetic efferent fibers in the oculomotor nerve are the axons of cells located in the complex oculomotor nuclei situated ventrolateral to the upper end of the cerebral aqueduct (Plates 2 and 3; see also Section II, Plate 13). The nuclei are composed of groups of large and small multipolar cells. The main groups of large cells are arranged in two columns of *dorsolateral, intermediate* and *ventromedial nuclei*, one on each side of the midline, which control the rectus and oblique extraocular muscles. A single *median nucleus*, composed of similar cells and partly overlying the caudal and dorsal aspects of the bilateral columns, controls the levator muscles of the upper eyelids. Cranial to the median nucleus, and also partially overlying the dorsal aspects of the main bilateral columns, are two narrow, wing-shaped nuclei, which are interconnected across the midline at their cranial ends— the *accessory (autonomic) nuclei (Edinger-Westphal)*. They are the source of parasympathetic preganglionic fibers for the ciliary ganglion.

*Oculomotor Nerve.* The axons from the bilateral oculomotor nuclear cells form minute bundles, which run through the mesencephalic tegmentum, traversing the red nuclei to emerge from the mesencephalic oculomotor sulcus as the oculomotor nerve rootlets.

Each *oculomotor nerve* runs forward between the posterior cerebral and superior cerebellar arteries

and lateral to the posterior communicating artery in the interpeduncular subarachnoid cistern (see Section II, Plate 10). It pierces the arachnoid and dura mater in the angle between the free and attached margins of the tentorium cerebelli to enter first the roof of the cavernous sinus and then its lateral wall. Continuing forward above the trochlear nerve, the oculomotor nerve divides into superior and inferior rami as it enters the orbit through the superior orbital fissure.

The smaller *superior division* gives branches to the superior rectus muscle and to the main superficial (voluntary, or striated, muscular) lamina of the levator palpebrae superioris. (The deep lamina is a tenuous layer of involuntary, or unstriated, fibers—the superior tarsal muscle; a similar but even more tenuous inferior tarsal muscle is present in the lower eyelid, and both these tarsal muscles are innervated by sympathetic fibers.) The larger *inferior division* supplies the medial and inferior recti and the inferior oblique muscles.

*Extrinsic Eye Muscles.* Movements produced by the extraocular muscles are shown in Plate 6. The *medial* and *lateral rectus muscles* turn the eyeball in a horizontal arc on an imaginary vertical axis, causing the cornea to look medially or laterally. The actions of the superior and inferior rectus muscles and those of the oblique muscles are more complicated. The *superior* and *inferior rectus muscles* turn the eyeball upward and downward. Because they are disposed at an angle of about 20° to the sagittal plane (due to the long axis of each orbit being directed slightly outward), they also impart a minor degree of inward rotation to the eyeball. The *superior oblique muscle* turns the eyeball so that the cornea looks downward and outward, while the *inferior oblique muscle* turns it so that the cornea looks upward and outward. However, an exact idea of the actions of the extrinsic eye muscles cannot be obtained by considering each muscle separately, because, under normal circumstances, none of the six extraocular muscles acts alone. Consequently, all eye movements are the result of highly integrated and delicately controlled agonist and antagonist activities. The actions of individual muscles have been determined from studies of congenital defects or from functional disturbances caused by disease or injury to the nerve supply (see Section VIII, Plates 22, 30, 31 and 45).

## Ciliary Ganglion

The ciliary ganglion is tiny and lies in the posterior part of the orbit between the optic nerve and the lateral rectus muscle. Only the first of its three roots is constant, because the sensory and/or sympathetic roots may bypass the ganglion (see Section IV, Plate 7).

*Motor Root.* The ciliary ganglion is the relay station for preganglionic *parasympathetic fibers*, which originate in the accessory (autonomic) oculomotor nucleus and reach the ganglion through a short offshoot from the oculomotor branch to the inferior oblique muscle. The postganglionic fibers form the 12 to 20 delicate *short ciliary nerves* that penetrate the sclera around the optic nerve and continue forward in the perichoroidal space to supply the ciliaris and sphincter pupillae muscles and the intraocular vessels.

*The sensory and sympathetic roots* of the ciliary ganglion are derived from the nasociliary nerve and the internal carotid vascular nerve plexus, but they do not always join the ganglion.

Instead, their fibers may reach the eye by joining the ciliary nerves directly, while the *sympathetic fibers* (already postganglionic after relaying in the superior cervical trunk ganglia) may follow the ophthalmic artery and its branches to their destinations. The *sensory fibers* convey impulses from the cornea, iris and choroid and the intraocular muscles.

## Trochlear Nerve

The trochlear nerve is slender and its nucleus of origin is located in the midbrain, just caudal to the oculomotor nuclei (Plates 2 and 3). The trochlear fibers curve posterolaterally and slightly caudally around the cerebral aqueduct to reach the upper part of the superior medullary velum; here, the nerve fibers from opposite sides decussate before emerging on either side of the frenulum veli, below the inferior colliculi (see Section II, Plate 12). No other cranial nerves emerge from the dorsal aspect of the brainstem.

Each trochlear nerve winds forward around the midbrain below the free edge of the tentorium cerebelli, passes between the superior cerebellar and posterior cerebral arteries and above the trigeminal nerve, and pierces the inferior surface of the tentorium near its attachment to the posterior clinoid process to run forward in the lateral wall of the cavernous sinus between the oculomotor and ophthalmic nerves. The nerve enters the orbit through its superior fissure, immediately lateral to the common annular tendon, and passes medially between the orbital roof and the levator palpebrae superioris to supply the *superior oblique muscle*. Through a communication with the ophthalmic nerve, proprioceptive fibers are transferred to the trigeminal nerve. The trochlear nerve usually receives sympathetic filaments from the internal carotid nerve plexus.

## Abducens Nerve

The abducens nerve arises from the abducens nucleus, which is located in the pons, subjacent to the facial colliculus in the upper half of the floor of the fourth ventricle. The nucleus is encircled by fibers of the homolateral facial nerve (Plates 2 and 3). The abducens nerve fibers pass forward to emerge near the midline through the groove between the pons and the pyramid of the medulla oblongata. Each abducens nerve then inclines upward in front of the pons, usually behind the inferior cerebellar artery. Near the apex of the petrous part of the temporal bone, the nerve bends sharply forward above the superior petrosal sinus to enter the lateral wall of the cavernous sinus, where it lies between the internal carotid artery and the ophthalmic nerve. In this situation, the abducens may transfer proprioceptive fibers to the ophthalmic nerve and receive sympathetic filaments from the internal carotid nerve plexus. The abducens nerve enters the orbit through the superior orbital fissure, within the common annular tendon, and ends by supplying the *lateral rectus muscle*.

The abducens, like the trochlear nerve, has a relatively long intracranial route in the posterior cranial fossa and cavernous sinus. Consequently, it is vulnerable to increases in intracranial pressure and to pathological or traumatic lesions affecting nearby parts of the brain, skull or sinus, which produce characteristic disturbances in ocular movements. □

# Oculomotor (III), Trochlear (IV) and Abducens (VI) Nerves and Ciliary Ganglion

**Motor fibers**
**Sensory fibers**
**Sympathetic fibers**
**Parasympathetic fibers**

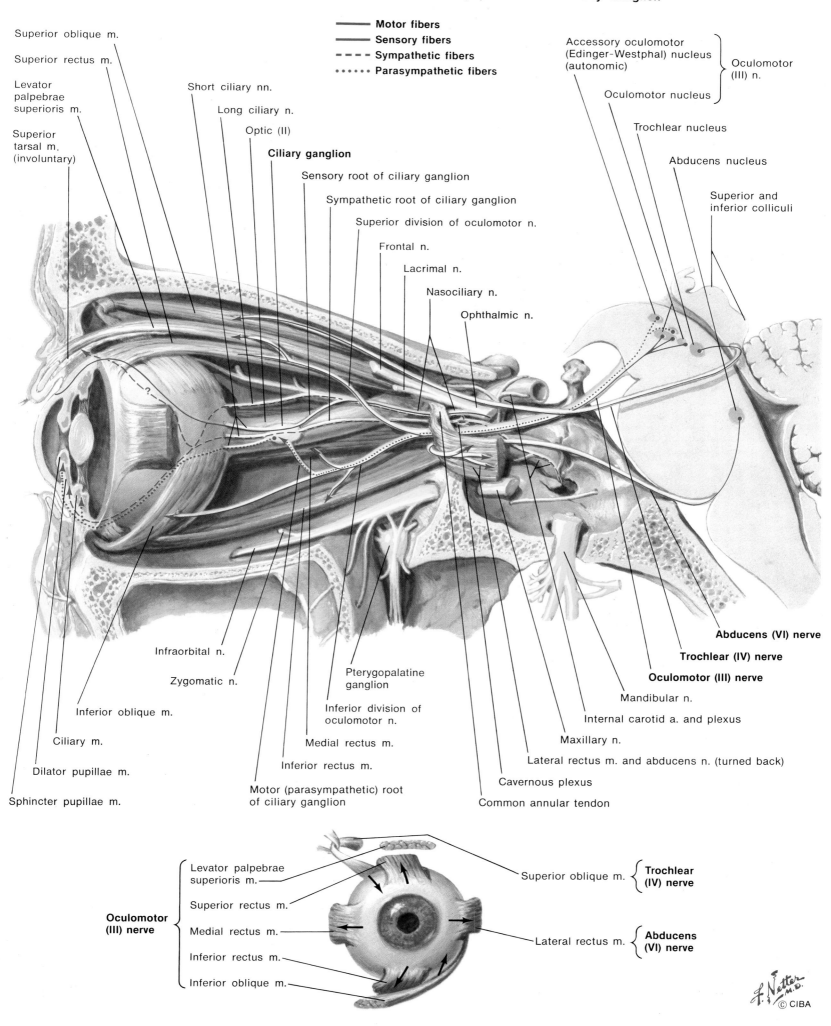

Superior oblique m.

Superior rectus m.

Levator palpebrae superioris m.

Superior tarsal m. (involuntary)

Short ciliary nn.

Long ciliary n.

Optic (II)

**Ciliary ganglion**

Sensory root of ciliary ganglion

Sympathetic root of ciliary ganglion

Superior division of oculomotor n.

Frontal n.

Lacrimal n.

Nasociliary n.

Ophthalmic n.

Accessory oculomotor (Edinger-Westphal) nucleus (autonomic)

Oculomotor (III) n.

Oculomotor nucleus

Trochlear nucleus

Abducens nucleus

Superior and inferior colliculi

Infraorbital n.

Zygomatic n.

Inferior oblique m.

Ciliary m.

Dilator pupillae m.

Sphincter pupillae m.

Pterygopalatine ganglion

Inferior division of oculomotor n.

Medial rectus m.

Inferior rectus m.

Motor (parasympathetic) root of ciliary ganglion

Cavernous plexus

Common annular tendon

Maxillary n.

Lateral rectus m. and abducens n. (turned back)

Internal carotid a. and plexus

Mandibular n.

**Abducens (VI) nerve**

**Trochlear (IV) nerve**

**Oculomotor (III) nerve**

Levator palpebrae superioris m.

Superior rectus m.

Medial rectus m.

Inferior rectus m.

Inferior oblique m.

**Oculomotor (III) nerve**

Superior oblique m. **Trochlear (IV) nerve**

Lateral rectus m. **Abducens (VI) nerve**

F. Netter
© CIBA

# Trigeminal (V) Nerve

The trigeminal nerve is the largest cranial nerve and gives origin to three major, named branches—the *ophthalmic, maxillary* and *mandibular nerves*.

The trigeminal nerve is attached to the ventrolateral aspect of the pons near its upper border, and consists of a larger sensory root and a much smaller, medial motor root. It conveys *sensory impulses* from most of the face and scalp, parts of the auricle and the external acoustic (auditory) meatus, the nasal and oral cavities, the teeth, the temporomandibular joint, the nasopharynx and most of the meninges in the anterior and middle cranial fossae. It also carries *proprioceptive impulses* from the masticatory and, perhaps, from the extraocular and facial muscles. Its *motor root fibers* supply muscles derived from the first branchial (mandibular) arch—the masticatory muscles, the mylohyoid, the anterior belly of the digastric, and the tensor veli palatini and tensor tympani (see Section VIII, Plate 45). Numerous *parasympathetic* and *sympathetic fibers* join branches of the trigeminal nerve through interconnections with the oculomotor (III), trochlear (IV), facial (VII) and glossopharyngeal (IX) nerves, and with sympathetic plexuses around branches of the carotid arteries (see Section IV, Plate 5).

From their attachments to the pons, the sensory and motor roots pass outward and forward over the superior border of the petrous temporal bone near its apex. The sensory root expands into the semilunar-shaped *trigeminal ganglion*, which contains pseudounipolar cells. The processes of these cells divide into a peripheral and a central part; the former constitutes the majority of sensory fibers in the ophthalmic and maxillary nerves and in the larger part of the mandibular nerve; the latter coalesces to form the trigeminal sensory root, which enters the brainstem and either ends in the *principal sensory (pontine) trigeminal nucleus* or descends in the *trigeminal spinal tract* to end in the *spinal (inferior) trigeminal nucleus*. The proprioceptive fibers are the peripheral processes of unipolar cells located in the *trigeminal mesencephalic nucleus*. They are unique in being the only primary sensory neurons whose cell bodies lie within the CNS. The motor fibers originate in the *trigeminal motor nucleus*, which is embedded in the upper pons on the medial side of the principal sensory motor nucleus. (Plates 2 and 3; see also Section II, Plates 12 and 13 and Section VIII, Plates 16, 44 and 47.)

The ophthalmic, maxillary and mandibular nerves arise from the convex margin of the trigeminal ganglion; the small motor root passes under the ganglion to join the mandibular nerve.

**The ophthalmic nerve** is sensory, but is joined by filaments from the internal carotid sympathetic plexus (see Section IV, Plate 6) and communicates with the oculomotor, trochlear and abducens nerves as it runs forward in the lateral wall of the cavernous sinus (Plate 5; see also Section III, Plate 13). Near its origin, it gives off a small *recurrent tentorial (meningeal) branch*

to the tentorium cerebelli and soon divides into *lacrimal, frontal* and *nasociliary branches*, which enter the orbit through the superior orbital fissure (see page 97).

**The maxillary nerve** is larger than the ophthalmic and is also sensory. Like the other branches of the trigeminal nerve, it acts as a vehicle for the distribution of sympathetic and parasympathetic fibers.

The maxillary nerve gives off a small *meningeal branch* to the meninges of the middle cranial fossa before passing forward in the lower part of the lateral wall of the cavernous sinus (Plate 5). It then leaves the skull through the foramen rotundum (see Section I, Plate 7), enters the pterygopalatine fossa, where it communicates with the corresponding ganglion (Plate 4), and curves anterolaterally across the upper part of the posterior surface of the maxilla to enter the orbit through the inferior orbital fissure. Finally, the maxillary nerve traverses the infraorbital groove as the *infraorbital nerve* and emerges on the face, where it divides into *inferior palpebral, external* and *internal nasal* and *superior labial branches*, which supply the lower eyelid, nasal alae and upper lip (skin and mucous membrane), respectively.

In the pterygopalatine fossa, the maxillary nerve gives off the *zygomatic nerve*, which divides into zygomaticotemporal and zygomaticofacial branches, and the *superior posterior alveolar nerves*. The *superior middle* and *superior anterior alveolar nerves* arise from the infraorbital part of the nerve, descend in the wall of the maxillary sinus between the bone and the mucous membrane, and split into delicate dental and gingival rami, which unite to form the *superior dental plexus* that supplies the upper teeth and gums.

**The mandibular nerve** is the largest branch of the trigeminal nerve and consists of a large *sensory root* issuing from the lateral half of the trigeminal ganglion and the entire, small trigeminal *motor root*. The two parts leave the skull through the foramen ovale and unite almost immediately to form a short, thick nerve lying between the lateral pterygoid and tensor veli palatini muscles, anterior to the middle meningeal artery. A small otic ganglion is closely applied to the medial side of the nerve (see Section IV, Plate 5). Just below the foramen, the mandibular nerve gives off a *meningeal branch (nervus spinosus)*, which enters the skull through the foramen spinosum, alongside the middle meningeal artery (see Section I, Plate 7); it helps to supply the meninges of the middle and anterior cranial fossae and calvaria, and the mucous membrane of the mastoid air cells. The *nerve to the medial pterygoid muscle* also arises at this level; it sends filaments to the otic ganglia, which pass through them without relaying, to supply the tensor veli palatini and tensor tympani muscles. The main mandibular nerve then divides into small anterior and large posterior parts.

The *anterior part* of the mandibular nerve contains mostly motor fibers, but it has one sensory branch, the *buccal nerve*, which runs forward to innervate the areas of skin overlying the buccinator muscle and the mucous membrane beneath it. The other motor branches are: the *nerve to the lateral pterygoid muscle*, which enters its deep surface; the *masseteric nerve(s)*, which reaches the muscle by passing outward above the lateral pterygoid, anterior to the temporomandibular

joint (supplying it with a filament); and two or three *deep temporal nerves*, which curve upward in the deep surface of the temporalis muscle.

The *posterior part* of the mandibular nerve is mainly sensory, but also contains motor fibers that are distributed in the *mylohyoid branch* of the *inferior alveolar nerve*. It divides into auriculotemporal, lingual and inferior alveolar nerves.

At its origin, the *auriculotemporal nerve* often splits in two around the middle meningeal artery. Beyond the artery, the single nerve runs posteriorly between the sphenomandibular ligament and the neck of the mandible before turning laterally behind the temporomandibular joint and passing through (or over) the upper part of the parotid gland. It then ascends over the posterior part of the zygomatic arch, behind the superficial temporal artery, and ends in *superficial temporal branches*, which supply the skin and fascia of the temple and adjoining areas of the scalp. The auriculotemporal nerve also gives *branches* to the *temporomandibular joint*, the *external acoustic meatus* and the *tympanic membrane*, and an *anterior auricular branch* to the skin of the tragus and part of the helix. It contributes filaments containing secretomotor and vasomotor fibers to the parotid gland (Plate 10), which reach the nerve through the otic ganglion.

The *lingual nerve* carries general sensory fibers from the anterior two thirds of the tongue and the floor of the mouth. It is joined near its origin by a branch of the facial nerve, the *chorda tympani*, which conveys special sensory (taste) fibers from the anterior two thirds of the tongue or, more accurately, from the part anterior to the V-shaped sulcus terminalis. The lingual nerve descends for a short distance anterior to the inferior alveolar nerve before curving forward between the medial pterygoid muscle and mandibular ramus to reach the space between the hyoglossus and mylohyoid muscles, where the *submandibular ganglion* is suspended from the nerve by several filaments. It then loops under the submandibular duct and turns upward on its medial side to divide into its *terminal branches*, which supply the mucous membrane of the anterior two thirds of the tongue, the lower part of the isthmus of the fauces, and the floor of the mouth, including the lingual surfaces of the lower gums. The branches communicate with terminal branches of the glossopharyngeal and hypoglossal nerves (Plates 10 and 13).

The *inferior alveolar nerve* is mainly sensory, but it does carry some motor fibers. It descends behind the lingual nerve and runs between the sphenomandibular ligament and the ramus of the mandible to the mandibular foramen, through which it enters the mandibular canal. Before entering this canal, it gives off its only motor branch, the *mylohyoid nerve*, which supplies the mylohyoid muscle and anterior belly of the digastric. The other branches of the inferior alveolar nerve are the *mental nerve* and the *inferior dental* and *gingival rami*, which arise from the nerve as it runs in the mandibular canal. The latter are fine nerves that unite to form the *inferior dental plexuses* supplying the lower teeth and gums. They may be joined by branches of the lingual and buccal nerves or by filaments from nerves supplying the muscles attached to the mandible. The branches may carry some sensory fibers, which explains why blocking of the inferior alveolar nerve alone does not always anesthetize the lower teeth, especially the molars and premolars. □

# Trigeminal (V) Nerve

| | |
|---|---|
| —————— | Motor fibers |
| —————— | Sensory fibers |
| • • • • • | Proprioceptive fibers |
| • • • • • | Parasympathetic fibers |
| – – – – – | Sympathetic fibers |

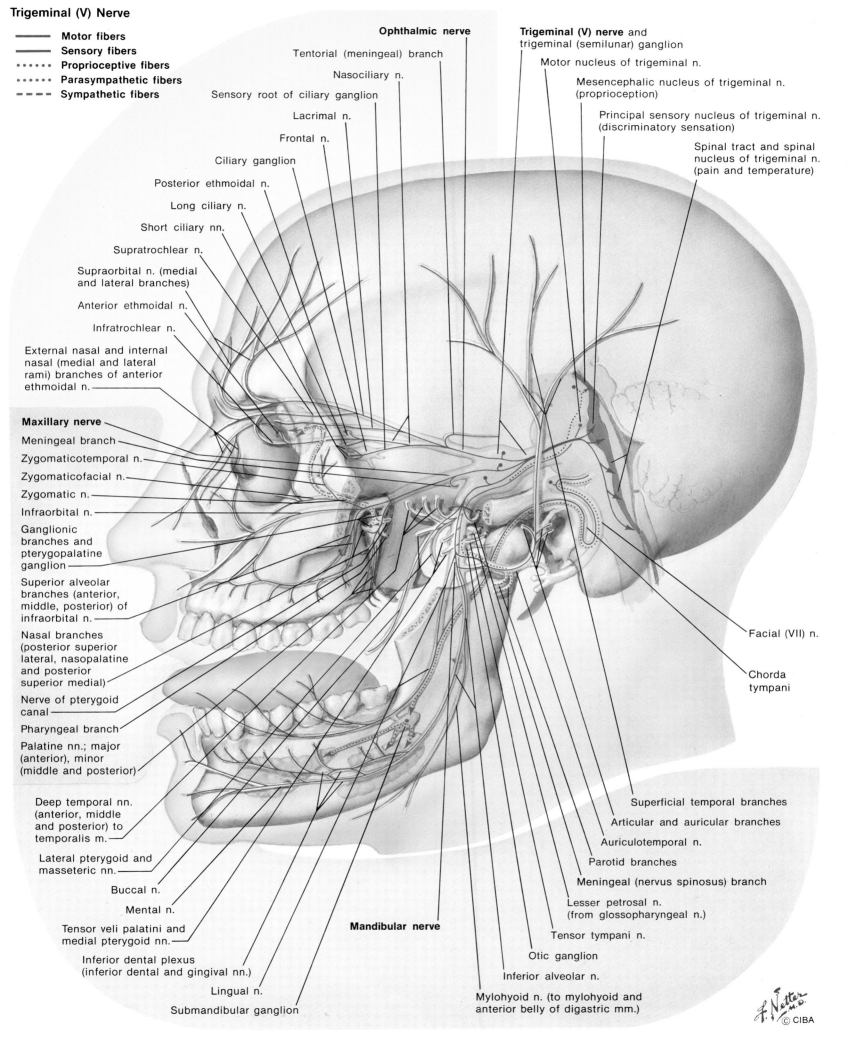

**Ophthalmic nerve**

Tentorial (meningeal) branch

Nasociliary n.

Sensory root of ciliary ganglion

Lacrimal n.

Frontal n.

Ciliary ganglion

Posterior ethmoidal n.

Long ciliary n.

Short ciliary nn.

Supratrochlear n.

Supraorbital n. (medial and lateral branches)

Anterior ethmoidal n.

Infratrochlear n.

External nasal and internal nasal (medial and lateral rami) branches of anterior ethmoidal n.

**Maxillary nerve**

Meningeal branch

Zygomaticotemporal n.

Zygomaticofacial n.

Zygomatic n.

Infraorbital n.

Ganglionic branches and pterygopalatine ganglion

Superior alveolar branches (anterior, middle, posterior) of infraorbital n.

Nasal branches (posterior superior lateral, nasopalatine and posterior superior medial)

Nerve of pterygoid canal

Pharyngeal branch

Palatine nn.; major (anterior), minor (middle and posterior)

Deep temporal nn. (anterior, middle and posterior) to temporalis m.

Lateral pterygoid and masseteric nn.

Buccal n.

Mental n.

Tensor veli palatini and medial pterygoid nn.

Inferior dental plexus (inferior dental and gingival nn.)

Lingual n.

Submandibular ganglion

**Mandibular nerve**

**Trigeminal (V) nerve** and trigeminal (semilunar) ganglion

Motor nucleus of trigeminal n.

Mesencephalic nucleus of trigeminal n. (proprioception)

Principal sensory nucleus of trigeminal n. (discriminatory sensation)

Spinal tract and spinal nucleus of trigeminal n. (pain and temperature)

Facial (VII) n.

Chorda tympani

Superficial temporal branches

Articular and auricular branches

Auriculotemporal n.

Parotid branches

Meningeal (nervus spinosus) branch

Lesser petrosal n. (from glossopharyngeal n.)

Tensor tympani n.

Otic ganglion

Inferior alveolar n.

Mylohyoid n. (to mylohyoid and anterior belly of digastric mm.)

# Facial (VII) Nerve

The facial nerve is a mixed nerve containing motor, sensory and parasympathetic fibers, all of which arise or end in nuclei in the pons (Plates 2 and 3).

## Facial Nerve Nuclei

*The motor nucleus* is located in the reticular formation of the lowest part of the pons; it lies dorsal to the trapezoid body and ventromedial to the spinal tract of the trigeminal (V) nerve. Corticonuclear fibers from the motor cortex of both sides end there, and, while the upper facial muscles are controlled bilaterally, those of the lower face are controlled only by the contralateral corticonuclear fibers (see Section VIII, Plates 45 to 47). The efferent fibers arising in the motor nucleus form the large *motor root* and loop around the abducens nucleus en route to their exit from the brainstem in the cerebellopontine angle.

*The superior salivatory nucleus* lies near the motor nucleus and is the source of *secretomotor* (*parasympathetic efferent*) *fibers* for the submandibular and sublingual salivary glands, the lacrimal gland and some of the palatine, pharyngeal and nasal mucosal glands. These fibers emerge as the small *nervus intermedius*, which lies between the facial motor root and the vestibulocochlear (VIII) nerve and is often called the "sensory root" of the facial nerve. This is a misnomer, however, because the sensory root contains many secretomotor fibers and also carries many parasympathetic efferent (vasodilator) fibers for vessels in the areas supplied by the facial nerve.

*The sensory nucleus* is the upper part of the *solitary tract nucleus*. The fibers ending there transmit *taste* sensations from the oral part of the tongue and palate, which are first carried in the chorda tympani and greater petrosal nerves and then in the nervus intermedius. Apart from these special sensory fibers, some fibers conveying *general sensations* from the external acoustic meatus and the adjacent part of the auricular concha are carried in the facial nerve; these fibers probably come through interconnections between the facial or chorda tympani nerves and the auricular branch of the vagus (X) nerve and terminate in the *spinal nucleus* of the *trigeminal nerve* (see Section VIII, Plate 16). Proprioceptive afferents from the facial muscles run in the facial nerves, and, like those from ocular and masticatory muscles, end in the *trigeminal mesencephalic nucleus*. Possibly, afferents from the meninges and their arteries in the middle cranial fossa also reach the facial nerve through its greater petrosal branch.

## Course and Branches

*Facial Canal.* The facial nerve (motor root and nervus intermedius) and the vestibulocochlear nerve appear at the bulbopontine sulcus in the cerebellopontine angle, and pass outward and forward to enter the internal acoustic meatus in the same meningeal sheath (Plate 9; see also Section I, Plate 7 and Section III, Plate 13). Piercing the sheath at the outer end of the meatus, the facial nerve enters the sinuous *facial canal*, which traverses the petrous part of the temporal bone. The nerve then continues laterally, above and between the bony vestibule and cochlea and toward the medial wall of the epitympanic recess, where it bends backward at almost a right angle to form the *facial geniculum*, or knee. From this point, the nerve curves downward within the bony septum that separates the tympanic cavity from the mastoid antrum and air cells to its exit from the facial canal through the *stylomastoid foramen*.

In the *internal acoustic meatus*, the nervus intermedius is connected to the vestibulocochlear nerve by several fascicles. Most of the fibers in these fascicles probably rejoin the facial nerve, but some may be carried through the vestibulocochlear nerve to the tympanic plexus. The *chorda tympani* arises from the facial nerve about 6 to 8 mm above the stylomastoid foramen, below the minute *nerve to the stapedius muscle*.

*Geniculate Ganglion.* The geniculum is expanded to accommodate the geniculate ganglion, and the facial motor and sensory (nervus intermedius) roots fuse at or near this ganglion. The ganglion contains pseudounipolar cells, with single processes bifurcating in a T-shaped fashion into peripheral and central parts. The majority of the peripheral processes are the *taste fibers* conveyed to the facial nerve in the chorda tympani and greater petrosal nerves. Their central processes are carried in the nervus intermedius to the solitary tract nucleus in the brainstem (see Section VIII, Plate 24). Other ganglion cells and their processes are concerned with transmitting *afferent vascular, glandular* and *meningeal impulses*; a small minority are the *somatic afferents* conducting general sensations from the external acoustic meatus and adjacent part of the auricular concha. The *parasympathetic efferent fibers* in the nervus intermedius pass through the geniculate ganglion without relaying. They enter such branches as the greater petrosal and chorda tympani nerves and are carried in them to more peripheral ganglia (pterygopalatine and submandibular), where they do relay (see Section III, Plate 5); the postganglionic fibers arising from synapses in these ganglia innervate the various glandular and vascular structures mentioned above.

The *greater petrosal nerve* and filaments to the *lesser petrosal nerve* and the *tympanic plexus* are given off from the geniculate ganglion, while an inconstant *external petrosal branch* joins the middle meningeal arterial perivascular plexus.

*Stylomastoid Foramen and Beyond.* At or near its exit from the stylomastoid foramen, the facial nerve communicates with the auricular branch of the vagus nerve, the glossopharyngeal (IX) nerve (Plate 10), the internal carotid plexus and the great auricular and auriculotemporal nerves. On the face, there are many communications between branches of the facial and trigeminal nerves (Plate 7), and other communications exist between the posterior auricular branch of the facial nerve and the greater and lesser occipital nerves, and between the cervical branch of the facial nerve and the transverse cervical nerves.

On emerging from the stylomastoid foramen, the facial nerve runs anterolaterally between the bony styloid process and the stylohyoid muscle and posterior belly of the digastric muscle, and gives off the *posterior auricular nerve* and twigs to both these muscles. The nerve then curves upward behind the external acoustic meatus and splits into a smaller *auricular branch*, which supplies the often rudimentary intrinsic muscles on the cranial surface of the auricle and the posterior auricular muscle, and into a larger *occipital branch*, which runs along the superior nuchal line to supply the occipital belly of the occipitofrontalis muscle.

*Parotid Course.* Within 1.5 cm of leaving the stylomastoid foramen, the facial nerve passes over the external carotid artery and retromandibular vein to enter the posteromedial surface of the parotid gland, where it is grooved by the mastoid process and the posterosuperior border of the sternocleidomastoid muscle. Here, the nerve divides almost immediately into *temporofacial* and *cervicofacial divisions*; the former subdivides within the gland into *temporal* and *zygomatic branches*, and the latter, into *buccal, lingual, marginal mandibular* and *cervical branches*, all of which are interconnected by loops to constitute the *parotid plexus*.

The individual facial, scalp and cervical muscles innervated by the various branches are shown in the illustration; the only muscles not shown are the anterior and superior auricular muscles and the intrinsic muscles on the lateral surface of the auricle. These minuscule structures receive filaments from the temporal branches of the facial nerve. □

# Facial (VII) Nerve

| | |
|---|---|
| —— | **Motor fibers** |
| —— | **Sensory fibers** |
| ·····  | **Parasympathetic fibers** |
| - - - | **Sympathetic fibers** |

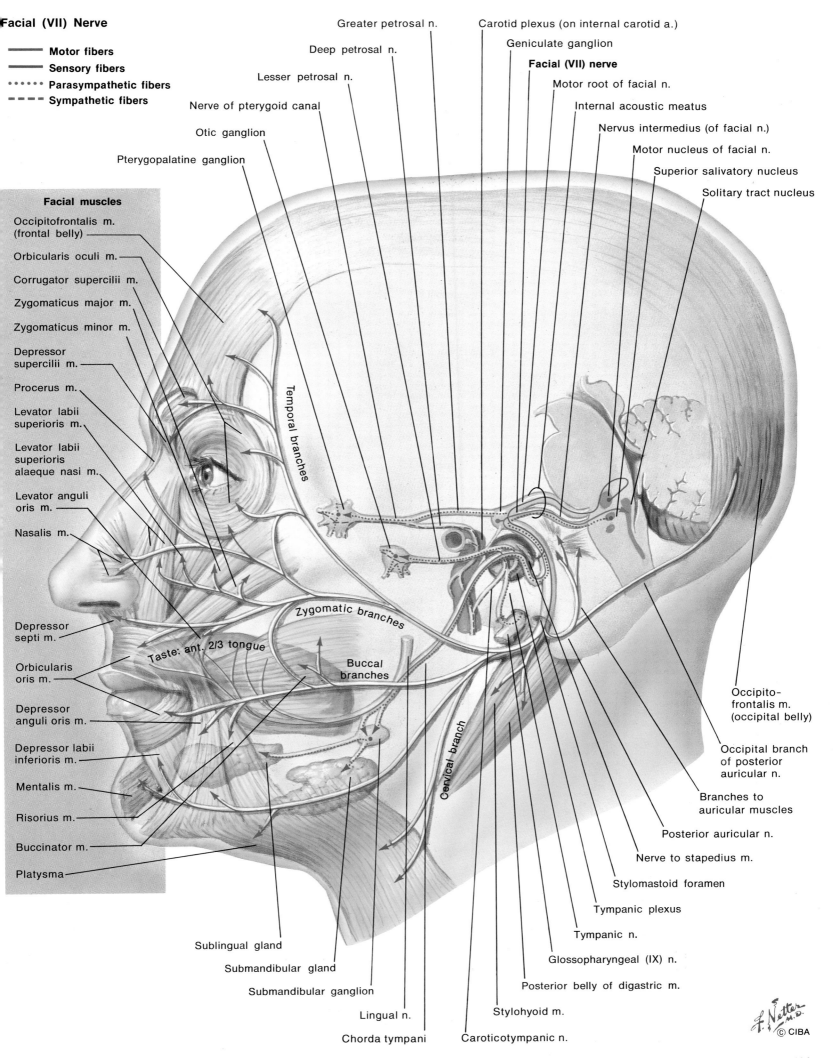

**Facial muscles**

Occipitofrontalis m. (frontal belly)
Orbicularis oculi m.
Corrugator supercilii m.
Zygomaticus major m.
Zygomaticus minor m.
Depressor supercilii m.
Procerus m.
Levator labii superioris m.
Levator labii superioris alaeque nasi m.
Levator anguli oris m.
Nasalis m.
Depressor septi m.
Orbicularis oris m.
Depressor anguli oris m.
Depressor labii inferioris m.
Mentalis m.
Risorius m.
Buccinator m.
Platysma

Greater petrosal n.
Deep petrosal n.
Lesser petrosal n.
Nerve of pterygoid canal
Otic ganglion
Pterygopalatine ganglion

Carotid plexus (on internal carotid a.)
Geniculate ganglion
**Facial (VII) nerve**
Motor root of facial n.
Internal acoustic meatus
Nervus intermedius (of facial n.)
Motor nucleus of facial n.
Superior salivatory nucleus
Solitary tract nucleus

Temporal branches

Zygomatic branches
Taste: ant. 2/3 tongue
Buccal branches
Cervical branch

Occipitofrontalis m. (occipital belly)
Occipital branch of posterior auricular n.
Branches to auricular muscles
Posterior auricular n.
Nerve to stapedius m.
Stylomastoid foramen
Tympanic plexus
Tympanic n.
Glossopharyngeal (IX) n.
Posterior belly of digastric m.
Stylohyoid m.
Caroticotympanic n.
Chorda tympani
Lingual n.
Submandibular ganglion
Submandibular gland
Sublingual gland

F. Netter M.D.
© CIBA

# Vestibulocochlear (VIII) Nerve

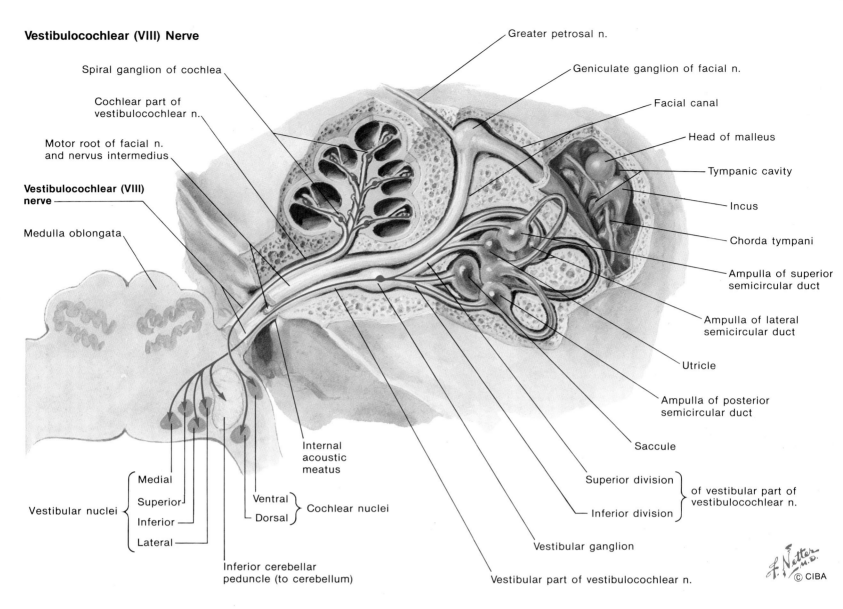

Spiral ganglion of cochlea

Cochlear part of vestibulocochlear n.

Motor root of facial n. and nervus intermedius

**Vestibulocochlear (VIII) nerve**

Medulla oblongata

Greater petrosal n.

Geniculate ganglion of facial n.

Facial canal

Head of malleus

Tympanic cavity

Incus

Chorda tympani

Ampulla of superior semicircular duct

Ampulla of lateral semicircular duct

Utricle

Ampulla of posterior semicircular duct

Saccule

Superior division / Inferior division } of vestibular part of vestibulocochlear n.

Vestibular ganglion

Vestibular part of vestibulocochlear n.

Internal acoustic meatus

Vestibular nuclei { Medial, Superior, Inferior, Lateral }

Ventral / Dorsal } Cochlear nuclei

Inferior cerebellar peduncle (to cerebellum)

## Vestibulocochlear (VIII) Nerve

The vestibulocochlear nerve consists of *vestibular* and *cochlear* parts. The former conveys afferent impulses concerned with equilibration, posture and muscle tone from the vestibular labyrinth of the internal ear, including the semicircular ducts (canals), utricle and saccule; the latter transmits auditory impulses from the spiral organ in the cochlea of the internal ear. The acoustic and vestibular pathways within the CNS are complex (see Section VIII, Plates 26, 27, 29 to 31, 38 and 39). The roots of the vestibular and cochlear nerves are attached to the brainstem, behind the facial (VII) nerve, in the triangular area bounded by the pons, cerebellar flocculus and medulla oblongata (see Section II, Plate 12); they enter the brainstem

separately and have different central connections (Plates 2 and 3). Sympathetic and parasympathetic fibers probably accompany both parts of the vestibulocochlear nerve. The vestibular and cochlear nerves usually unite over a variable distance and pass outward to enter the internal acoustic meatus, inferior to the motor root of the facial nerve and with the nervus intermedius interposed (see page 102; see also Section I, Plate 7 and Section III, Plate 13).

*Vestibular Nerve*. At the fundus of the internal acoustic meatus, the vestibular part of the vestibulocochlear nerve expands to form the *vestibular ganglion* and then splits into *superior* and *inferior divisions*. Both divisions contain peripheral processes of the vestibular bipolar cells, which penetrate tiny foramina in the superior and inferior vestibular areas of the fundus of the internal meatus. The peripheral processes then spread out and form contacts with hair cell receptors embedded in the neuroepithelium that lines the ampullae of the semicircular ducts (canals) and the maculae of the saccule and utricle (see Section VIII, Plate 28). The longer central processes of the bipolar cells transmit the impulses collected from these vestibular hair cells to the brainstem. Passing backward in the pontomedullary junctional area, the central processes divide into ascending and descending branches, which end predominantly in the *superior (cranial), inferior (caudal), medial* and *lateral vestibular nuclei* located

in the medulla oblongata and lower pons. However, other branches proceed directly through the homolateral inferior cerebellar peduncle to the flocculonodular cerebellar lobe (see Section VIII, Plates 29 and 37).

*Cochlear Nerve*. The fibers in the cochlear part of the vestibulocochlear nerve traverse many minute spirally arranged foramina in the fundus of the internal acoustic meatus and enter the modiolus, the central pillar of the cochlea. The fibers then run in tiny longitudinal and spiral canals in the modiolus and show numerous enlargements en route, which contain bipolar nerve cells and form the *spiral cochlear ganglion*. The short peripheral processes of these bipolar cells end in relation to special acoustic hair cells in the spiral organ of Corti in the cochlear duct (see Section VIII, Plate 25). The relatively long central processes of the bipolar cells of the cochlear nerve reach the brainstem lateral to the vestibular part and end in the *ventral* and *dorsal cochlear nuclei* located on the lateral aspect of the inferior cerebellar peduncle (see Section VIII, Plates 26 and 27).

*Clinical Factors*. Because of its anatomical relationships, the eighth cranial nerve is liable to be damaged by fractures involving the petrous part of the temporal bone, and by tumors affecting the brainstem or cerebellum. Together with its neighboring and associated structures, it is also predisposed to adverse reactions to some drugs and antibiotics. □

# Glossopharyngeal (IX) Nerve and Otic Ganglion

*The glossopharyngeal nerve* is closely related anatomically and functionally to the vagus (X) nerve. The two share common nuclei of origin and terminate in the *ambiguus* and *dorsal vagal* nuclei (Plate 11). However, the glossopharyngeal nerve also carries secretomotor fibers from the *inferior salivatory nuclei* scattered in the reticular formation (Plates 2 and 3).

As its name implies, the glossopharyngeal is a mixed nerve, distributed mainly to parts of the tongue and pharynx. Its rootlets appear at the dorsolateral sulcus of the medulla oblongata, above those of the vagus nerve (see Section II, Plate 12). The rootlets soon unite, and the nerve thus formed leaves the skull through the central part of the jugular foramen, between the inferior petrosal and sigmoid sinuses (see Section I, Plate 7 and Section III, Plate 13).

Two ganglia—a small *superior ganglion* and a larger *inferior ganglion*—are situated on the nerve in this part of its course. The pseudounipolar nerve cells contained in both ganglia transmit the following sensations: *special visceral sensation* (taste) from the posterior third of the tongue and part of the soft palate (see Section VIII, Plate 24); *general visceral sensation* (touch, pain, temperature) from the posterior third and adjacent areas of the tongue, fauces and pharynx; relatively few *general somatic afferent impulses* from small areas of postauricular skin and from the meninges in the posterior cranial fossa; and *visceral afferent impulses* from the carotid sinus and body (see Section VIII, Plate 28). The central cell processes concerned with taste end in the *solitary tract nucleus*; those concerned with visceral sensation end in the combined *dorsal glossopharyngeal-vagal nucleus*; and those concerned with general somatic sensibility end in the *spinal tract* and *nucleus of the trigeminal nerve*.

From the jugular foramen, the nerve arches forward between the internal jugular vein and internal carotid artery, passes deep to the styloid process, and curves behind the stylopharyngeus muscle to the side of the pharynx. It pierces the superior constrictor muscle (or passes between this muscle and the middle constrictor) to enter the base of the tongue, and finally divides into branches that supply the mucous membrane over the posterior third of the tongue, palatine tonsil, fauces and adjacent part of the pharynx and the vessels and glands in these parts.

The *lingual branches* convey special (taste) and general sensations from the vallate papillae and the tongue behind the sulcus terminalis. These branches are associated with small *lingual ganglia*, which serve as relay centers for the preganglionic and postganglionic vasomotor and secretomotor neurons.

Other glossopharyngeal branches include: the *tympanic nerve*, which arises from the inferior ganglion and ascends through the tympanic canaliculus to the middle ear (tympanic cavity), where it contributes to the *tympanic plexus* and gives off the *lesser petrosal nerve* (Plate 8); *communications* to the

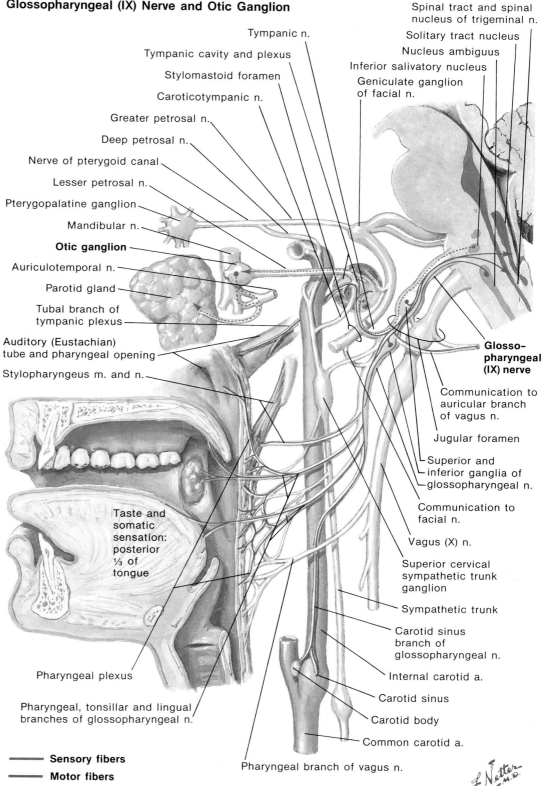

Spinal tract and spinal nucleus of trigeminal n.
Solitary tract nucleus
Nucleus ambiguus
Inferior salivatory nucleus
Geniculate ganglion of facial n.
Tympanic n.
Tympanic cavity and plexus
Stylomastoid foramen
Caroticotympanic n.
Greater petrosal n.
Deep petrosal n.
Nerve of pterygoid canal
Lesser petrosal n.
Pterygopalatine ganglion
Mandibular n.
**Otic ganglion**
Auriculotemporal n.
Parotid gland
Tubal branch of tympanic plexus
Auditory (Eustachian) tube and pharyngeal opening
Stylopharyngeus m. and n.
**Glosso-pharyngeal (IX) nerve**
Communication to auricular branch of vagus n.
Jugular foramen
Superior and inferior ganglia of glossopharyngeal n.
Communication to facial n.
Vagus (X) n.
Superior cervical sympathetic trunk ganglion
Sympathetic trunk
Carotid sinus branch of glossopharyngeal n.
Internal carotid a.
Carotid sinus
Carotid body
Common carotid a.
Pharyngeal branch of vagus n.
Taste and somatic sensation: posterior ⅓ of tongue
Pharyngeal plexus
Pharyngeal, tonsillar and lingual branches of glossopharyngeal n.

——— **Sensory fibers**
——— **Motor fibers**
•••••• **Parasympathetic fibers**

auricular vagal branch, the superior vagal ganglion, the superior cervical sympathetic trunk ganglion and the facial (VII) nerve; the *carotid sinus branch*; a branch to supply the *stylopharyngeus muscle*; and several *pharyngeal branches*, which unite with similar vagal branches and sympathetic filaments to form a plexus on the surface of the pharynx (see Section IV, Plates 5 and 6).

*The otic ganglion* lies immediately below the foramen ovale, between the mandibular nerve and the tensor veli palatini muscle, and anterior to the middle meningeal artery. Its main, parasympathetic, root is the *lesser petrosal nerve*, which contains the parotid secretomotor fibers. After

relaying in the ganglion, these fibers reach the gland through the parotid branches of the *auriculotemporal nerve*. The sympathetic root of the otic ganglion is a filament from the *middle meningeal plexus*. The ganglion may also communicate with the *chorda tympani*, the *nerve of the pterygoid canal* and the *medial pterygoid nerve*. Some taste fibers from the chorda tympani may pass through the communication with the ganglion and reach the facial nerve through its connection with the nerve of the pterygoid canal. The fibers from the medial pterygoid nerve traverse the ganglion without relaying, to supply the tensor veli palatini and tensor tympani muscles. □

# Vagus (X) Nerve

The vagus nerve contains both *afferent* and *efferent parasympathetic fibers*, which are widely distributed to visceral and vascular structures in the neck, thorax and abdomen. The nerve also conveys *somatic sensory fibers* in its auricular and meningeal branches, some *special sensory fibers* (taste) in its superior laryngeal branch, and *special visceral efferent fibers* that arise in the nucleus ambiguus and are distributed mainly to laryngeal and pharyngeal muscles.

The glossopharyngeal (IX), vagus and cranial parts of the accessory (XI) nerves may be regarded as a single nerve complex, because all are mainly parasympathetic in type and each has central connections with the *dorsal vagal nucleus*, the *solitary tract nucleus* and the *nucleus ambiguus* (Plates 10 and 12; see also Section II, Plates 12 and 13 and Section VIII, Plates 44 and 56).

## Vagal Nuclei

*The dorsal vagal nucleus* is mixed in type, since it represents fused visceral afferent and efferent columns of neurons. It consists of a longitudinal column of cells lying beneath the vagal trigone in the floor of the fourth ventricle, just lateral to the hypoglossal nucleus, and extending almost the entire length of the medulla oblongata (Plates 2 and 3; see also Section II, Plate 10). The *visceral afferent fibers* ending in the nucleus are the central processes of pseudounipolar sensory cells in the *inferior vagal ganglion*; the peripheral processes of the sensory cells convey impulses from the heart, aorta, trachea, bronchi, lungs, most of the alimentary tract (from the lower pharynx almost to the left colic flexure), liver, pancreas and possibly from the kidneys. *Preganglionic efferent fibers* carrying impulses for the same structures originate in the dorsal vagal nuclei and are distributed to these viscera through many *direct vagal branches* (see Section VIII, Plate 64), or through branches of the cardiac, celiac and other plexuses (see Section IV, Plates 6, 8, 9, 11 to 13 and 18).

The vagal preganglionic fibers end by forming synapses in ganglia situated near or within the viscera innervated. Because of this arrangement, the vagal parasympathetic postganglionic fibers are relatively short and more limited in their distribution than their sympathetic counterparts.

The *superior vagal ganglia* also contain pseudounipolar cells. They are concerned with sensory impulses conveyed in the auricular and meningeal vagal branches, although the fibers in the latter branches may be derived from interconnections between the ganglia and the upper cervical spinal nerves. The central processes of the superior vagal ganglion cells probably end in the *spinal nuclei of the trigeminal nerves*.

*The solitary tract nucleus* receives *afferent fibers*, which travel in the *superior laryngeal vagal branches*, from taste buds in the mucous membrane of the epiglottis and the epiglottic valleculae, although most of the gustatory fibers that end in this nucleus run in the *chorda tympani* and *glossopharyngeal nerves* (see Section VIII, Plate 24).

*The nucleus ambiguus* is developed from special visceral efferent columns and forms a row of discrete, multipolar neurons located deeply in the reticular formation of the medulla oblongata. Its axons emerge in the *glossopharyngeal* and *vagal nerves* and in the cranial parts of the *accessory nerves*, and are distributed mainly to the intrinsic laryngeal and pharyngeal muscles.

## Vagal Origin, Ganglia, Course and Branches

*Vagal Origin.* Each vagus nerve is attached to the medulla oblongata along the dorsolateral sulcus by 8 to 10 rootlets, above the radicles of the glossopharyngeal nerve and cranial parts of the accessory nerves (see Section II, Plate 12 and Section III, Plates 4, 5 and 10). The rootlets coalesce, and the nerve thus formed emerges from the skull through the *jugular foramen*, together with the glossopharyngeal nerve, the accessory nerve, the sigmoid sinus and several other blood vessels (see Section I, Plate 7 and Section III, Plate 13). Outside the skull, the vagus expands into *superior* and *inferior ganglia*.

*The superior vagal ganglion* communicates with the nearby superior cervical sympathetic trunk ganglion and with the facial, glossopharyngeal and accessory nerves. It gives off a *recurrent branch* to the meninges of the posterior cranial fossa and an *auricular branch*, which carries sensory impulses from parts of the tympanic membrane and the external acoustic meatus.

*The inferior vagal ganglion* (nodose ganglion) is connected with the cranial part of the accessory nerve. It communicates with the superior cervical sympathetic trunk ganglion, the hypoglossal nerve and the loop between the first and second cervical spinal nerves. It gives off *pharyngeal* and *superior laryngeal branches* and inconstant *carotid rami*, which assist the glossopharyngeal nerve in innervating the carotid sinus and body (see Section VIII, Plate 50).

*Cervical Vagal Course.* Below its inferior ganglion, each vagus nerve descends within the homolateral carotid sheath to the thoracic inlet, at first lying behind and between the internal jugular vein and internal carotid artery, and then between the former and the common carotid artery (see Section VI, Plate 2). Both vagi intercommunicate with filaments from the cervical sympathetic trunks or their branches, so that they are

really mixed parasympathetic-sympathetic nerves from the neck downward.

Apart from the meningeal, auricular, carotid, superior laryngeal and pharyngeal branches mentioned, the cervical parts of the vagi also supply *cardiac branches* (see Section III, Plate 9).

*The right vagus nerve* enters the thorax behind the internal jugular vein and in front of the first part of the subclavian artery. Here, it gives off the *right recurrent laryngeal nerve*, which hooks under the artery before ascending to the larynx. The main cord of the nerve now inclines posteromedially, behind the right brachiocephalic vein and the superior vena cava, and runs medial to the azygos vein to reach the root of the right lung. Here, it splits into smaller *anterior* and larger *posterior branches*, both of which contribute rami to the anterior and posterior pulmonary plexuses.

*The left vagus nerve* enters the thorax between the left common carotid and left subclavian arteries, behind the left brachiocephalic vein. It crosses the left side of the aortic arch, giving off the left recurrent laryngeal nerve; thereafter, as on the right side, it participates in the formation of the pulmonary and esophageal plexuses.

The *left recurrent laryngeal nerve* curves beneath the aorta on the outer side of the ligamentum arteriosum and then ascends to the larynx; like the corresponding right nerve, it runs in the groove between the esophagus and trachea, contributing motor, sensory, glandular and vascular fibers to both structures. The recurrent laryngeal nerves also supply all the laryngeal muscles except the cricothyroids, which are innervated by the superior laryngeal nerves.

*The vagal pulmonary branches*, along with filaments derived from the second to fifth or sixth thoracic sympathetic trunk ganglia, form smaller *anterior* and larger *posterior pulmonary plexuses* (see CIBA COLLECTION, Volume 7, page 22). The pulmonary plexuses become dispersed around the bronchial and vascular structures, and some of their terminal filaments reach the peripheral parts of the lungs. Small ganglia along the course of the larger bronchi provide relay stations for the preganglionic parasympathetic (vagal) fibers. The corresponding sympathetic fibers relay mostly in the sympathetic trunk ganglia. Sympathetic and parasympathetic pulmonary afferent fibers are also present. Microscopic plexuses, which can be traced as far as the smallest bronchioles, exist in the walls of the air passages.

*Esophageal Plexus.* Below the lung roots, the vagus nerves break up into two to four parts, which become closely apposed to the esophagus as it descends through the posterior mediastinum (see Section IV, Plates 8 and 12). Following the esophagus downward, they divide and reunite to form an open-meshed esophageal plexus containing small ganglia (see CIBA COLLECTION, Volume 3/I, pages 44 and 45). Most of the branches of the right vagus incline posteriorly, while most of those from the left vagus incline anteriorly. The esophageal plexus is reinforced by filaments from the thoracic parts of the sympathetic trunks and from the thoracic splanchnic nerves.

*Vagal Trunks.* At a variable distance above the esophageal hiatus in the diaphragm, the meshes of the esophageal plexus become reconstituted into two or more *vagal trunks*, which are situated anterior and posterior to the termination of the esophagus (see Section IV, Plates 13 to 15). □

# Vagus (X) Nerve

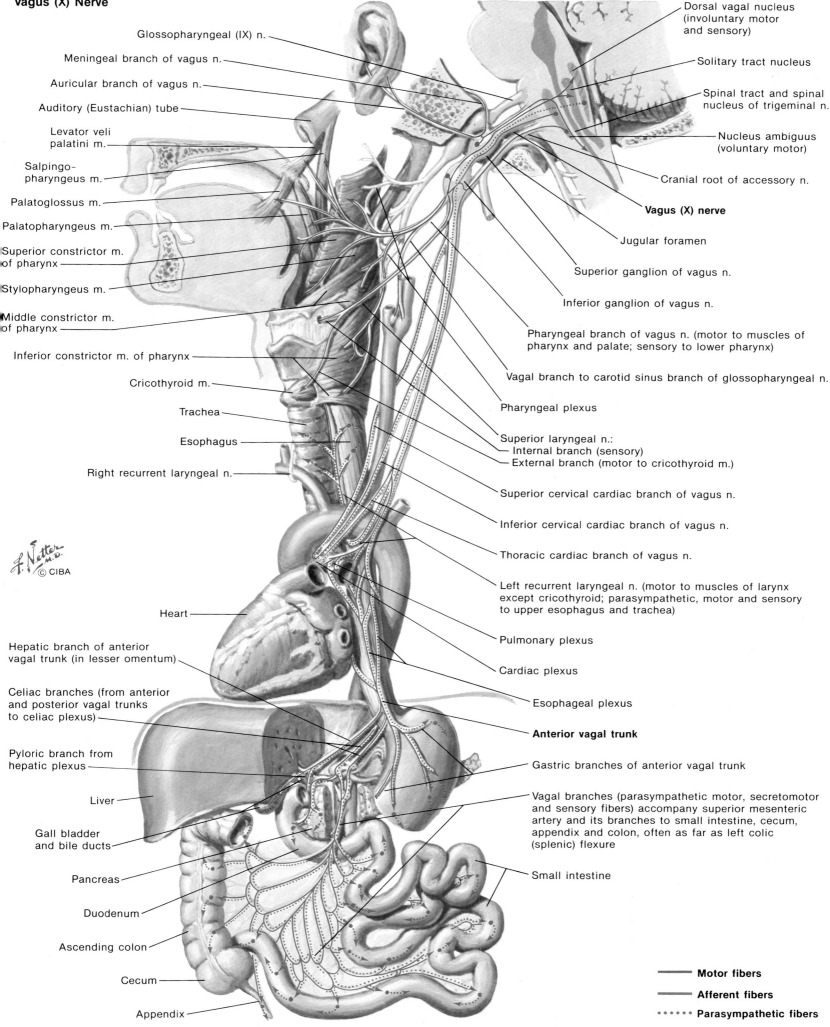

Glossopharyngeal (IX) n.

Meningeal branch of vagus n.

Auricular branch of vagus n.

Auditory (Eustachian) tube

Levator veli palatini m.

Salpingo-pharyngeus m.

Palatoglossus m.

Palatopharyngeus m.

Superior constrictor m. of pharynx

Stylopharyngeus m.

Middle constrictor m. of pharynx

Inferior constrictor m. of pharynx

Cricothyroid m.

Trachea

Esophagus

Right recurrent laryngeal n.

Heart

Hepatic branch of anterior vagal trunk (in lesser omentum)

Celiac branches (from anterior and posterior vagal trunks to celiac plexus)

Pyloric branch from hepatic plexus

Liver

Gall bladder and bile ducts

Pancreas

Duodenum

Ascending colon

Cecum

Appendix

Dorsal vagal nucleus (involuntary motor and sensory)

Solitary tract nucleus

Spinal tract and spinal nucleus of trigeminal n.

Nucleus ambiguus (voluntary motor)

Cranial root of accessory n.

Vagus (X) nerve

Jugular foramen

Superior ganglion of vagus n.

Inferior ganglion of vagus n.

Pharyngeal branch of vagus n. (motor to muscles of pharynx and palate; sensory to lower pharynx)

Vagal branch to carotid sinus branch of glossopharyngeal n.

Pharyngeal plexus

Superior laryngeal n.:
  Internal branch (sensory)
  External branch (motor to cricothyroid m.)

Superior cervical cardiac branch of vagus n.

Inferior cervical cardiac branch of vagus n.

Thoracic cardiac branch of vagus n.

Left recurrent laryngeal n. (motor to muscles of larynx except cricothyroid; parasympathetic, motor and sensory to upper esophagus and trachea)

Pulmonary plexus

Cardiac plexus

Esophageal plexus

**Anterior vagal trunk**

Gastric branches of anterior vagal trunk

Vagal branches (parasympathetic motor, secretomotor and sensory fibers) accompany superior mesenteric artery and its branches to small intestine, cecum, appendix and colon, often as far as left colic (splenic) flexure

Small intestine

Motor fibers
Afferent fibers
Parasympathetic fibers

# Accessory (XI) Nerve

The accessory nerve consists of cranial and spinal roots. The cranial root is associated in its central origins and peripheral distribution with the vagus (X) nerve.

*The cranial root* is the smallest component in this vital complex. Yet even this small element is important, because it conveys all or most of the fibers from the *recurrent laryngeal nerves* to the vagus nerve. Thus, the cranial root is an "accessory" part of the vagus nerve. Its fibers, which are classified as special visceral efferent, arise mainly from neurons in the caudal half of the *nucleus ambiguus*, with probable minor contributions from neurons in the *dorsal vagal nucleus* (Plates 2 and 3). These neurons are influenced, through internuncial neurons, by the corticonuclear (corticobulbar) subdivisions of both pyramidal tracts (see Section VIII, Plate 45), and their axons emerge as four to six rootlets from the dorsolateral sulcus, posterior to the olive of the medulla oblongata, in series with the rootlets of the glossopharyngeal (IX) and vagus nerves (see Section II, Plate 12 and Section III, Plates 4, 5 and 10). The accessory nerve rootlets coalesce to form the cranial root, which runs laterally and usually joins the larger spinal root before passing through the *jugular foramen* in the same dural and arachnoid sheaths as the vagus nerve (see Section I, Plate 7 and Section III, Plate 13). The cranial root communicates by one or two filaments with the superior vagal ganglion. However, most of its fibers continue onward as the *internal branch of the accessory nerve*, which joins the vagus nerve at or near its inferior ganglion and provides most of the motor fibers distributed in the pharyngeal and recurrent laryngeal branches of the vagus nerve (Plate 11). The *pharyngeal branches* supply the muscles of the soft palate (except the tensor veli palatini) and contribute motor fibers to the pharyngeal plexus. The fibers in the *recurrent laryngeal vagal branches* supply all the intrinsic laryngeal muscles except the cricothyroid. The theory that the internal accessory branch contains cardiac fibers has not been confirmed.

*The spinal root* fibers are the axons of an elongated strand of motor neurons—the *spinal nucleus of the accessory nerve*—reputedly developed from the special visceral efferent column that extends downward from the lower medulla oblongata into the dorsolateral part of the ventral gray column of the upper five or six cervical cord segments (see Section VII, Plate 3). The fibers emerge as a series of rootlets from the side of the spinal cord, about midway between the ventral and dorsal rootlets of the upper five or six cervical spinal nerves, and coalesce as they ascend behind the denticulate ligament to form the spinal root, which enters the skull through the *foramen magnum* behind the vertebral artery. Arching upward and outward, the spinal root usually unites over a short distance with the cranial root, and the two leave the skull through the *jugular foramen*, in the same dural sheath as the vagus nerve.

*Course of Accessory Nerve.* The cranial and spinal root fibers soon separate; the former constitute the *internal branch* of the accessory nerve,

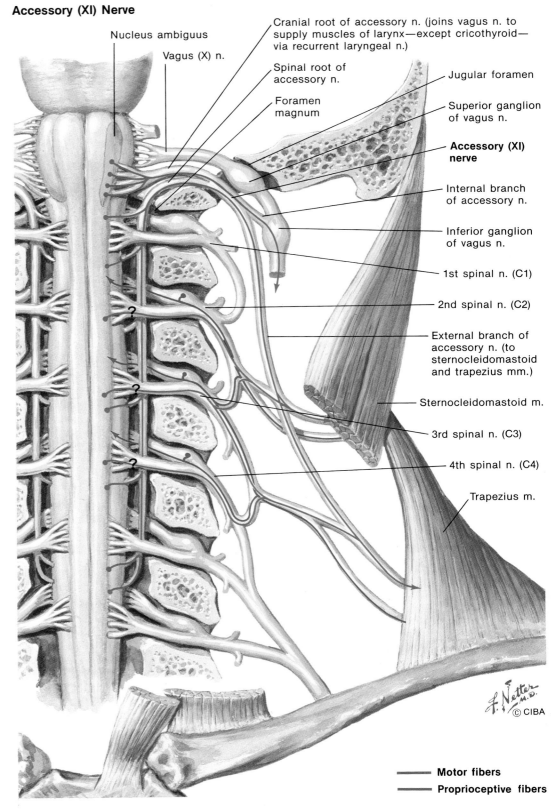

## Accessory (XI) Nerve

Nucleus ambiguus

Vagus (X) n.

Cranial root of accessory n. (joins vagus n. to supply muscles of larynx—except cricothyroid—via recurrent laryngeal n.)

Spinal root of accessory n.

Foramen magnum

Jugular foramen

Superior ganglion of vagus n.

**Accessory (XI) nerve**

Internal branch of accessory n.

Inferior ganglion of vagus n.

1st spinal n. (C1)

2nd spinal n. (C2)

External branch of accessory n. (to sternocleidomastoid and trapezius mm.)

Sternocleidomastoid m.

3rd spinal n. (C3)

4th spinal n. (C4)

Trapezius m.

—— **Motor fibers**
—— **Proprioceptive fibers**

which joins the vagus nerve, while the latter continue independently as the *external branch* of the accessory nerve. The external accessory branch is often mistakenly regarded as the entire accessory nerve, because it is the only part easily identified in routine dissections.

Below the jugular foramen, the external branch of the accessory nerve usually passes between the internal carotid artery and the internal jugular vein, and runs obliquely downward and backward over the transverse process of the atlas and deep to the styloid process, occipital artery and posterior belly of the digastric muscle before piercing the deep surface of the *sternocleidomastoid muscle*

(see Section VI, Plate 1). It passes through and supplies this muscle, and it is connected with branches of the *second* and, occasionally, the *third cervical spinal nerve*, which also end in the muscle. Emerging from about the midpoint of the posterior sternocleidomastoid border, the external branch then inclines downward across the posterior cervical triangle, crosses over the levator scapulae muscle and its covering of deep cervical fascia, and disappears under the trapezius muscle about 2 cm above the clavicle. Here, the nerve communicates with branches of the *third* and *fourth cervical spinal nerves* to form a pseudoplexus, which innervates the *trapezius muscle.* □

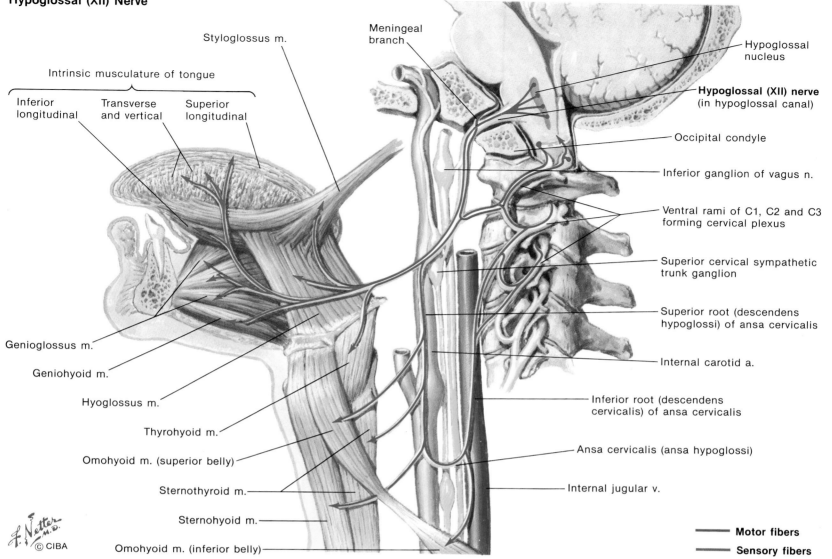

Meningeal branch

Styloglossus m.

Intrinsic musculature of tongue

Inferior longitudinal

Transverse and vertical

Superior longitudinal

Hypoglossal nucleus

**Hypoglossal (XII) nerve** (in hypoglossal canal)

Occipital condyle

Inferior ganglion of vagus n.

Ventral rami of C1, C2 and C3 forming cervical plexus

Superior cervical sympathetic trunk ganglion

Superior root (descendens hypoglossi) of ansa cervicalis

Internal carotid a.

Genioglossus m.

Geniohyoid m.

Hyoglossus m.

Thyrohyoid m.

Omohyoid m. (superior belly)

Sternothyroid m.

Sternohyoid m.

Omohyoid m. (inferior belly)

Inferior root (descendens cervicalis) of ansa cervicalis

Ansa cervicalis (ansa hypoglossi)

Internal jugular v.

**Motor fibers**

**Sensory fibers**

SECTION V    PLATE 13

# Hypoglossal (XII) Nerve

The hypoglossal nerve is the *motor nerve of the tongue*.

*The hypoglossal nucleus* is a column of cells 18 to 20 mm long and lies near the midline in the medulla oblongata (Plates 2 and 3). It extends from the level of the medullary striae of the fourth ventricle, almost to the lower end of the medulla, with its upper part subjacent to the hypoglossal trigone (see Section II, Plates 10 and 13). The main nucleus is composed of various subnuclei, which are probably associated with the individual muscles innervated.

The hypoglossal nucleus receives fibers through the corticonuclear (corticobulbar) tracts; most are from the heterolateral, but some are from the homolateral cerebral motor cortex (see Section VIII, Plate 45). The nucleus is also interconnected to the vagal, glossopharyngeal and trigeminal sensory nuclei, again probably through the reticular formation. Thus, it is presumably influenced

by visceral centers in the hypothalamus, through the impulses that reach the glossopharyngeal-vagal nuclei via the dorsal longitudinal fasciculus (Plates 7, 10 and 11; see also Section VIII, Plates 55 and 56). These numerous interconnections are implicated in controlling movements of the tongue in response to touch, pain, taste and thermal and proprioceptive stimuli from oral, lingual and pharyngeal sources.

***Course of Nerve.*** The axons of the hypoglossal nuclear cells emerge through the ventrolateral medullary sulcus as a series of rootlets (see Section II, Plate 12 and Section III, Plate 5). The rootlets coalesce to form two roots as they run outward behind the vertebral artery to leave the skull through the *hypoglossal canal* (see Section I, Plate 7 and Section III, Plate 13). At their exit into the upper neck, the two roots unite to form a single nerve, lying posteromedial to the internal carotid artery, internal jugular vein and the glossopharyngeal (IX), vagus (X) and accessory (XI) nerves. Inclining anteroinferiorly between the aforementioned artery and vein and communicating in passing with the nearby inferior vagal and superior cervical sympathetic trunk ganglia, the hypoglossal nerve continues forward, deep to the posterior belly of the digastric muscle and the occipital artery, before crossing over the external carotid artery, the lingual nerve and the middle pharyngeal constrictor muscle. It reaches the posterior border of the hyoglossus muscle above the

greater cornu of the hyoid bone, and then curves forward and upward over this muscle and the genioglossus muscle, lying deep to the central digastric tendon and the stylohyoid and mylohyoid muscles and inferior to the submandibular gland and its duct. Its terminal branches ascend into the tongue, where they communicate with branches of the lingual and glossopharyngeal nerves.

***Branches.*** The only true branches of the hypoglossal nerves are the *lingual*, and they convey general somatic efferent fibers to the muscles of the tongue. They supply all the *extrinsic muscles* (except the palatoglossi, which are innervated through the pharyngeal plexus)—the hyoglossus, styloglossus, chondroglossus and genioglossus muscles; and all the *intrinsic muscles*—the superior and inferior longitudinal, transverse and vertical lingual muscles.

The other apparent branches are actually offshoots from the cervical plexus (see Section VI, Plate 1), and are not connected with the hypoglossal nuclei. These include the *meningeal branch*, the *superior root* of the *ansa cervicalis* and the *nerves to the thyrohyoid* and *geniohyoid muscles*, which are derived from the ventral rami of the first and second cervical nerves. *Branches to the omohyoid, sternothyroid* and *sternohyoid muscles* from the *ansa cervicalis* itself are mainly derived from the ventral rami of the second and third cervical nerves via the *inferior root of the ansa.* □

Section VI

# Nerve Plexuses and Peripheral Nerves

Frank H. Netter, M.D.

*in collaboration with*

**G.A.G. Mitchell, Ch.M., D.Sc., F.R.C.S.** *Plates 1–16*

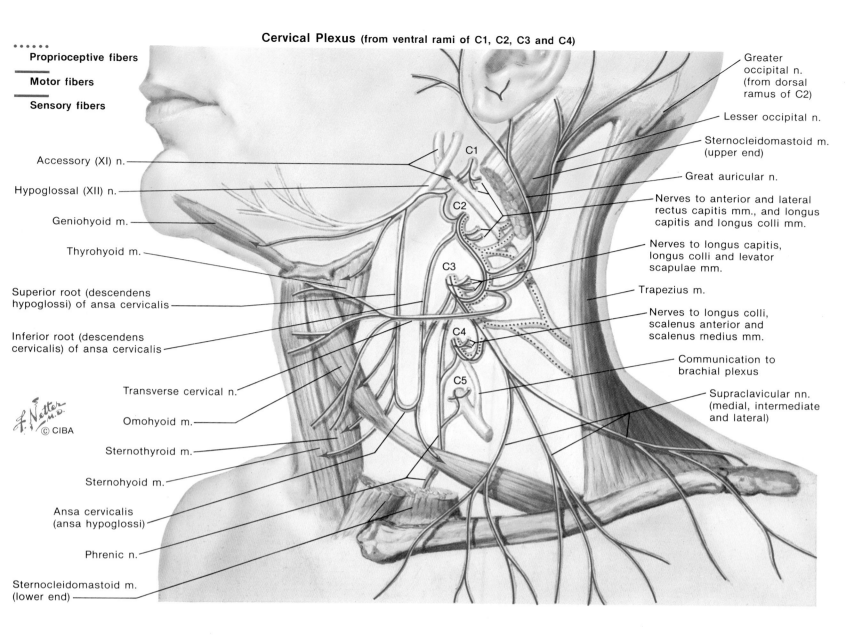

• • • • • Proprioceptive fibers

——— Motor fibers

——— Sensory fibers

Accessory (XI) n.

Hypoglossal (XII) n.

Geniohyoid m.

Thyrohyoid m.

Superior root (descendens hypoglossi) of ansa cervicalis

Inferior root (descendens cervicalis) of ansa cervicalis

Transverse cervical n.

Omohyoid m.

Sternothyroid m.

Sternohyoid m.

Ansa cervicalis (ansa hypoglossi)

Phrenic n.

Sternocleidomastoid m. (lower end)

Greater occipital n. (from dorsal ramus of C2)

Lesser occipital n.

Sternocleidomastoid m. (upper end)

Great auricular n.

Nerves to anterior and lateral rectus capitis mm., and longus capitis and longus colli mm.

Nerves to longus capitis, longus colli and levator scapulae mm.

Trapezius m.

Nerves to longus colli, scalenus anterior and scalenus medius mm.

Communication to brachial plexus

Supraclavicular nn. (medial, intermediate and lateral)

C1, C2, C3, C4, C5

SECTION VI PLATE 1

## Cervical Plexus

The cervical plexus lies deep to the sternocleidomastoid muscle. Its branches convey *motor fibers* to many cervical muscles and to the diaphragm; *sensory fibers* from parts of the scalp, neck and chest; *proprioceptive fibers*; and *autonomic vasomotor* and *sudomotor fibers* to vessels and glands. The superficial branches perforate the cervical fascia to supply cutaneous structures, while the deep branches supply mainly muscles and joints.

***The superficial branches*** are the lesser (minor) occipital, great auricular, transverse (cutaneous) cervical and supraclavicular nerves.

The *lesser occipital nerve* (C2, C3) curves around the accessory (XI) nerve, ascends near the posterior border of the sternocleidomastoid muscle, and divides into branches that supply the skin on the superolateral aspects of the neck, the upper part of the auricle and the adjacent area of the scalp.

The *great auricular nerve* (C2, C3) is larger than the lesser occipital and passes obliquely upward over the sternocleidomastoid muscle, lying near the external jugular vein before dividing into anterior and posterior branches. The former passes over or through the parotid gland to supply the skin of the posteroinferior part of the face. The latter supplies the skin over the mastoid process and over the medial and lateral surfaces of the lower part of the auricle.

The *transverse cervical nerve* (C2, C3) runs forward beneath the external jugular vein to divide into superior and inferior branches, which supply the skin over the anterolateral aspects of the neck from the mandible above to the sternum below.

The *supraclavicular nerves* (C3, C4) arise from a common trunk, which descends for a variable distance before dividing into medial, intermediate and lateral supraclavicular nerves. These supply the skin over the lower neck from near the midline to the acromioclavicular region and above the shoulder. They then pass in front of the clavicle to innervate the skin of the anterior chest wall to the level of the sternal angle and the second rib. The medial and lateral nerves, respectively, send twigs to the sternoclavicular and acromioclavicular joints.

***The deep branches*** are mainly motor, but they also carry proprioceptive, osseous, articular and autonomic fibers to and from muscles, bones, joints and vessels in their areas of distribution. Some motor branches pass *medially* to supply the rectus capitis anterior and rectus capitis lateralis (C1, C2), longus capitis (C1, C2, C3), longus colli and intertransverse (C2, C3, C4) muscles and the diaphragm through the phrenic nerve (Plate 2). Other muscular branches pass *laterally* to the sternocleidomastoid (C2, C3), trapezius (C3, C4), levator scapulae (C3, C4) and scalenus anterior and scalenus medius (C3, C4) muscles; the branches to the sternocleidomastoid and trapezius muscles are reputedly proprioceptive, but they nevertheless communicate with motor branches of the accessory nerve to these muscles.

A branch from the loop between C1 and C2 joins the hypoglossal (XII) nerve (see Section V, Plate 13). Some of these fibers continue onward along with the hypoglossal nerve to supply the thyrohyoid and geniohyoid muscles, while others leave it as a filament running downward, anterolateral to the carotid sheath, the *superior root (descendens hypoglossi)* of the *ansa cervicalis*, or *ansa hypoglossi*. The ansa ("loop") is completed by the *inferior root (descendens cervicalis)* derived from C2 and C3. Branches from the ansa supply the sternohyoid, sternothyroid and omohyoid muscles. □

**Phrenic Nerve** (C3, C4, C5)

## Phrenic Nerve

The phrenic nerve (C3, C4, C5) is the *motor nerve* of the *diaphragm*, although it also contains many sensory and sympathetic fibers. It is formed by a stout root from the fourth cervical ventral ramus, with smaller contributions from the third and fifth ventral rami, although the C3 fibers may join the phrenic nerve via a communication with the nerve to the sternohyoid muscle, and those from C5 may join it via the inconstant accessory phrenic nerve. The nerve receives gray rami communicantes from the superior and middle cervical sympathetic trunk ganglia and often from the vertebral ganglion and ansa subclavia.

The phrenic roots unite at the superolateral border of the scalenus anterior muscle, and the nerve thus formed descends almost vertically in front of this muscle to the thoracic inlet, lying behind the prevertebral fascia, the internal jugular vein and the transverse cervical and suprascapular arteries. It enters the thorax by passing between the subclavian vein and artery and inclining medially over the internal thoracic (internal mammary) artery. Thereafter, it runs downward alongside the pericardiacophrenic vessels and between the mediastinal pleura and fibrous pericardium to the diaphragm.

The *right phrenic nerve* runs almost vertically and is thus shorter than the left, which follows the leftward bulge of the heart. At the thoracic inlet, the right nerve is separated from the second part of the right subclavian artery by the scalenus anterior muscle, and lies lateral to the right brachiocephalic vein and superior vena cava. Continuing downward in front of the right lung root, it runs between the mediastinal pleura and the fibrous pericardium overlying the right atrium and thoracic portion of the inferior vena cava to reach the diaphragm.

At the thoracic inlet, the *left phrenic nerve* passes over the medial edge of the scalenus anterior muscle and the first part of the left subclavian artery, behind the termination of the thoracic duct. In the superior mediastinum, it runs between the left subclavian and left common carotid arteries, and slopes anteriorly over the left side of the aortic arch and left vagus nerve. It then continues onward, anterior to the left lung root and between the mediastinal pleura and fibrous pericardium covering the left surface of the heart to reach the diaphragm.

While passing through the thorax, both *phrenic nerves* supply sensory fascicles to the fibrous pericardium, to the mediastinal pleura and to the central areas of the diaphragmatic pleura. The sensory branches to the margins of the diaphragm and to the corresponding areas of overlying pleura and underlying peritoneum are provided by the lower intercostal nerves. The left phrenic nerve may send a twig to the left pulmonary plexus, and the right nerve supplies filaments to the inferior vena cava; both nerves communicate with the greater thoracic splanchnic nerves.

The right phrenic nerve pierces the central tendon of the diaphragm through or near the orifice for the inferior vena cava, and the left nerve penetrates the diaphragm close to the front edge of its central tendon, just lateral to the cardiac apex. Below the diaphragm, each nerve usually divides into three diverging *phrenicoabdominal branches*; these supply the diaphragm from its inferior surface and also supply sensory fibers to most of the peritoneum covering the diaphragm, except at the marginal areas; they also supply the coronary and falciform ligaments of the liver. The phrenico-abdominal branches communicate freely with the perivascular plexuses around the inferior phrenic arteries; on the right side (rarely, on the left), there is a *phrenic ganglion*. Offshoots from the inferior phrenic plexuses pass to the gastroesophageal junction, cardiac end of the stomach, porta hepatis and adrenal (suprarenal) plexuses. □

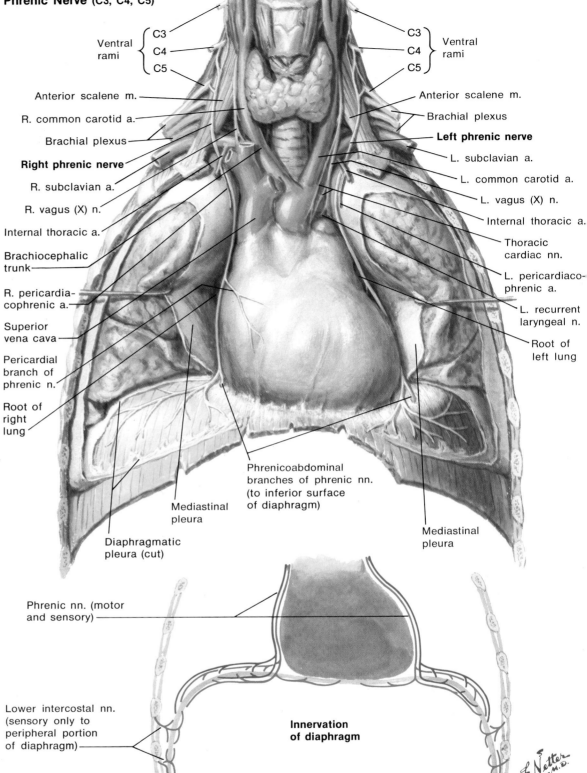

Ventral rami { C3 C4 C5 }

Ventral rami { C3 C4 C5 }

Anterior scalene m.

R. common carotid a.

Brachial plexus

**Right phrenic nerve**

R. subclavian a.

R. vagus (X) n.

Internal thoracic a.

Brachiocephalic trunk

R. pericardia-cophrenic a.

Superior vena cava

Pericardial branch of phrenic n.

Root of right lung

Anterior scalene m.

Brachial plexus

**Left phrenic nerve**

L. subclavian a.

L. common carotid a.

L. vagus (X) n.

Internal thoracic a.

Thoracic cardiac nn.

L. pericardiaco-phrenic a.

L. recurrent laryngeal n.

Root of left lung

Phrenicoabdominal branches of phrenic nn. (to inferior surface of diaphragm)

Mediastinal pleura

Diaphragmatic pleura (cut)

Mediastinal pleura

Phrenic nn. (motor and sensory)

Lower intercostal nn. (sensory only to peripheral portion of diaphragm)

**Innervation of diaphragm**

*f. Netter* © CIBA

# Course of Typical Thoracic Nerve

## Thoracic Nerves

The 12 pairs of thoracic nerves resemble other typical spinal nerves in their segmental attachments to the cord by *dorsal* and *ventral nerve roots*. These roots unite to form short *spinal nerve trunks*, which emerge through the corresponding intervertebral foramina, give off recurrent meningeal filaments, establish connections through white and gray rami communicantes with adjacent sympathetic trunk ganglia, and divide into larger *ventral* and smaller *dorsal rami*. (See Section II, Plates 15 and 16 for greater detail of these general arrangements.)

*The dorsal rami* of the thoracic nerves run backward near the zygapophyseal joints, which they supply, and divide into medial and lateral branches. Both sets of branches pass through the groups of muscles constituting the erector spinae and give off branches to them. The terminations of the upper six or seven *medial branches* innervate the skin adjacent to the corresponding spinous processes, but the lower five or six often fail to reach the skin. The terminations of all the *lateral branches* usually pierce the thoracolumbar fascia over the erector spinae muscles and divide into *medial* and *lateral cutaneous branches*, which innervate much of the skin of the posterior thoracic wall and upper lumbar regions.

*The ventral rami* of most of the thoracic nerves, unlike those in other regions, do not form plexuses. They retain their segmental character, and each pair runs separately in the corresponding intercostal spaces as the *intercostal nerves*. The first pair, however, divides into larger and smaller branches; the former, usually joined by twigs from the second pair, participate in the formation of the *brachial plexuses* (Plate 4), while the smaller branches are the first pair of intercostal nerves. The last (twelfth) pair of ventral rami course below the lowest ribs and are therefore termed the *subcostal nerves*.

*The intercostal nerves* are distributed mainly to structures in the thoracic and abdominal walls. The upper six pairs are limited to the thoracic parietes, while the lower five pairs extend from the thoracic into the abdominal walls and also contribute fibers to the diaphragm. The intercostal nerves give off *muscular, anterior* and *lateral cutaneous, mammary* and *collateral branches*, and supply filaments to adjacent vessels, periosteum, parietal pleura and peritoneum.

The upper six pairs supply *muscular branches* to the corresponding intercostal muscles and also to the subcostal, serratus posterior superior and

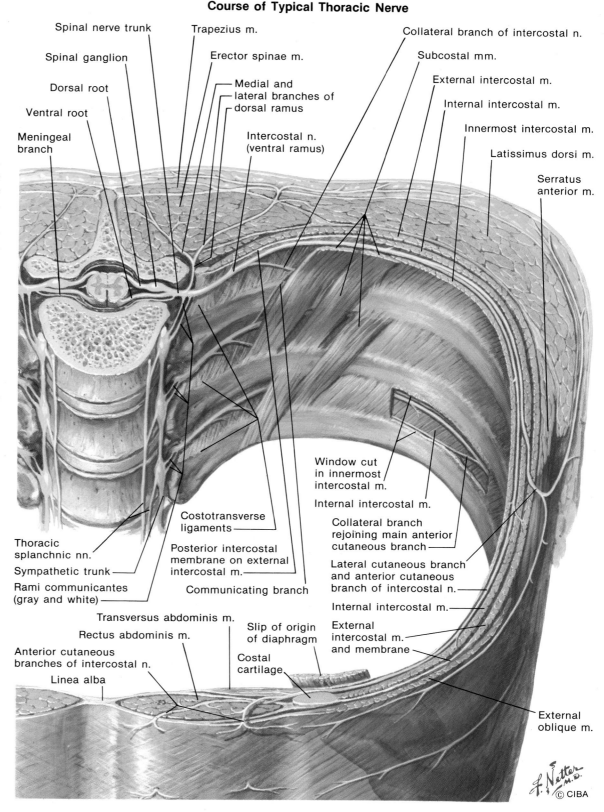

transverse thoracic muscles. The lower five pairs supply the lower intercostal muscles and the subcostal, serratus posterior inferior, transverse, oblique and rectus abdominal muscles. Fascicles from the lower intercostal nerves also enter the margins of the diaphragm, but they are sensory. The subcostal nerves supply the pyramidalis muscles.

The *anterior cutaneous branches* supply the front of the thorax. The *lateral cutaneous branches* pierce the internal and external intercostal muscles and end by dividing into branches that extend forward and backward to innervate the skin covering the lateral sides of the thorax and abdomen. The small

*lateral branch* of the *first intercostal nerve* supplies the skin of the axilla, and the lateral branch of the second is the *intercostobrachial nerve*, which is distributed to the skin on the medial side of the arm. The *lateral cutaneous branch* of the *subcostal nerve* pierces the internal and external oblique abdominal muscles and descends over the iliac crest to supply the skin of the anterior part of the gluteal region.

The *mammary glands* receive filaments from the lateral and anterior cutaneous branches of the fourth, fifth and sixth intercostal nerves, which convey autonomic and sensory fibers to and from the glands. □

## Right Brachial Plexus: Common Arrangement
**(from ventral rami of C5, C6, C7, C8 and T1 with contributions from C4 and T2)**

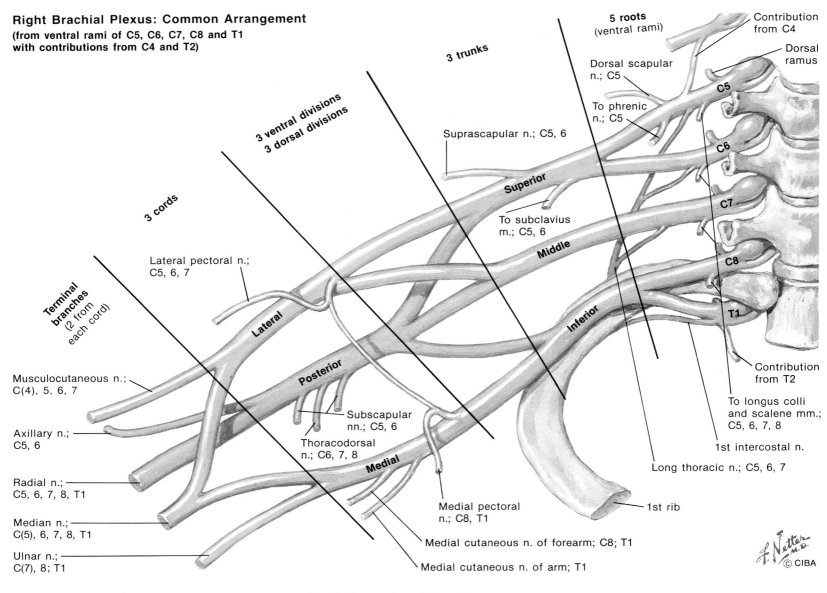

*f. Netter* ©CIBA

# Brachial Plexus

**Roots.** The brachial plexus is formed by the union of the ventral (anterior) rami of the *fifth, sixth, seventh* and *eighth cervical nerves* and the greater part of the *first thoracic nerve*—the roots of the plexus. Usually, a small branch from C4 joins the C5 root and one from T2 joins the T1 root; thus, C4 and T2 often provide minor contributions to the plexus. However, the contributions are variable in size, especially if so-called prefixation or postfixation exists. A "prefixed" plexus shows a cranial shift, and the C4 contribution is large, while the plexus from T1 is small, and that from T2 is often absent. In a "postfixed" plexus, the condition is reversed: the contribution from T2 is large, that from C5 is small, and that from C4 is often missing. The roots lie between the anterior and middle scalene muscles.

The plexus formation allows rearrangements of the efferent and afferent somatic and autonomic fibers (the latter reach the roots of the plexus through sympathetic rami communicantes), so that they are redirected through the various

trunks, divisions and cords into the most appropriate channels—the terminal branches—for distribution to the muscles, skin, vessels and glands in the upper limbs.

**Trunks.** The upper roots (C5, C6) unite to form the *superior trunk*, the C7 root continues alone as the *middle trunk*, and the lower roots (C8; T1) constitute the *inferior trunk* of the plexus. The trunks lie in the lower part of the posterior cervical triangle.

**Divisions and Cords.** Each trunk divides into three *ventral* (anterior) and three *dorsal* (posterior) *divisions*, which supply the ventral (flexor) and dorsal (extensor) structures in the upper limb. In the axilla, the divisions become regrouped as follows: the *ventral division* of the *inferior trunk* continues as the *medial cord* (C8; T1); the *ventral divisions* of the *superior* and *middle trunks* unite to form the *lateral cord* (C5, C6, C7); and all *three dorsal divisions* of the *trunks* join to produce the *posterior cord* (C5, C6, C7, C8; T1). (The terms "medial," "lateral" and "posterior" indicate the relationships of the cords to the second part of the axillary artery.)

**Branches.** Most of the branches of the plexus originate in the axilla from the *cords* located below the level of the clavicle—*infraclavicular branches*. However, several branches arise from the *roots* and *trunks* in the posterior cervical triangle above the clavicle—*supraclavicular branches*. Nerves derived from a cord do not necessarily contain fibers from

all its constituent roots; eg, the axillary nerve arising from the posterior cord (C5, C6, C7, C8; T1) contains fibers from only C5 and C6.

### Supraclavicular Branches

**From plexus roots**
To longus colli and scalene mm. . . . . . C5,6,7,8
Dorsal scapular . . . . . . . . . . . . . . . . . . . . C5
Branch to phrenic . . . . . . . . . . . . . . . . . . C5
Long thoracic . . . . . . . . . . . . . . . . . . . C5,6,7

**From superior trunk**
Suprascapular . . . . . . . . . . . . . . . . . . . . C5,6
To subclavius m. . . . . . . . . . . . . . . . . . . C5,6

### Infraclavicular Branches

**From lateral cord**
Lateral pectoral . . . . . . . . . . . . . . . . . . C5,6,7
Musculocutaneous . . . . . . . . . . . . . C(4),5,6,7
Lateral root of median . . . . . . . . . . . C(5),6,7

**From medial cord**
Medial pectoral . . . . . . . . . . . . . . . . . . C8; T1
Medial cutaneous n. of arm . . . . . . . . . . . T1
Medial cutaneous n. of forearm . . . . . . C8; T1
Ulnar . . . . . . . . . . . . . . . . . . . . . . C(7),8; T1
Medial root of median . . . . . . . . . . . . . C8; T1

**From posterior cord**
Upper subscapular . . . . . . . . . . . . . . . C5,6,(7)
Lower subscapular . . . . . . . . . . . . . . . . . C5,6
Axillary (circumflex humeral) . . . . . . . . C5,6
Thoracodorsal . . . . . . . . . . . . . . . . . . . C6,7,8
Radial . . . . . . . . . . . . . . . . . . . C5,6,7,8; T1

# Scapular, Axillary and Radial Nerves

*Scapular Nerves.* The *dorsal scapular nerve* (C5) arises from the uppermost root of the brachial plexus. It pierces the scalenus medius, runs deep to the levator scapulae, helping to supply it, and ends by supplying the minor and major rhomboid muscles. The *suprascapular nerve* (C5, C6) arises from the superior trunk of the brachial plexus. It runs outward, deep to the trapezius muscle, enters the supraspinous fossa through the scapular notch, and winds around the lateral border of the scapular spine to reach the infraspinous fossa. It supplies both the supraspinatus and infraspinatus muscles, and sends filaments to the shoulder and acromioclavicular joints and suprascapular vessels.

*The axillary (circumflex humeral) nerve* (C5, C6) arises from the posterior cord of the brachial plexus. Descending behind the axillary vessels, it curves posteriorly alongside the posterior circumflex humeral vessels and below the subscapularis muscle and the capsule of the shoulder joint, and gives a twig to the joint. It then passes through a quadrangular space, bounded above by the teres minor, below, by the teres major, medially, by the long head of the triceps brachii and laterally, by the humeral surgical neck to divide into *anterior* and *posterior branches*. The anterior branch passes between the humeral surgical neck and the deltoid muscle, which it supplies, and gives off small branches that pierce the muscle to supply the skin covering its lower half. The posterior branch also gives branches to the deltoid muscle, plus a branch to the teres minor, and terminates as the *upper lateral cutaneous nerve of the arm*.

*The radial nerve* (C5, C6, C7, C8; T1) is the largest branch of the brachial plexus and is the main continuation of its *posterior cord*. In the axilla, it lies behind the outer end of the axillary artery upon the subscapularis, latissimus dorsi and teres major muscles. Leaving the axilla, it enters the arm between the brachial artery and the long head of the triceps brachii muscle. Continuing downward and accompanied by the profunda brachii artery, it pursues a spiral course behind the humerus, lying close to the bone in the shallow radial nerve sulcus (hence its older name, the "musculospiral nerve"). It passes between the long and medial, and medial and lateral heads of the triceps brachii, and then lies deep to the lateral head of this muscle. On reaching the distal third of the arm at the lateral margin of the humerus, it pierces the lateral intermuscular septum to enter the anterior compartment of the arm. Then it descends anterior to the lateral humeral epicondyle and the articular capsule of the elbow joint, lying deep in the furrow between the brachialis muscle medially and the brachioradialis and extensor carpi radialis longus muscles laterally. At this point, it divides into its *superficial* and *deep terminal branches* (Plate 6).

*In the axilla,* the radial nerve gives off the small *posterior cutaneous nerve of the arm*. The muscular branch to the long head of triceps brachii usually arises near the boundary between the axilla and arm.

*In the arm,* the radial nerve supplies muscular, cutaneous, vascular, articular and osseous branches. The first muscular branch is long and slender, arising as the nerve enters the radial nerve sulcus; it accompanies the ulnar nerve to the lower arm to supply the distal part of the medial head of the triceps brachii and to furnish twigs to the elbow joint. A second, larger branch arises from the nerve as it lies in the radial nerve sulcus; it soon subdivides into smaller branches that enter the medial head of the triceps, with some filaments ending in the humeral periosteum and bone. A stouter subdivision supplies the lateral head of the triceps. It descends through the muscle, accompanied by the medial branch of the profunda brachii artery (which it supplies), then pierces and supplies the anconeus and sends filaments to the humerus and elbow joint.

Anterior to the lateral intermuscular septum, the radial nerve gives muscular branches to the lateral part of the brachialis, the brachioradialis, the extensor carpi radialis longus and, occasionally, to the extensor carpi radialis brevis. Vascular filaments are furnished to the arterial anastomoses around the elbow, and articular twigs are given off to the joint.

Three cutaneous branches arise from the radial nerve above the elbow: the *posterior cutaneous nerve of the arm*, the *lower lateral cutaneous nerve of the arm* and the *posterior cutaneous nerve of the forearm*.  □

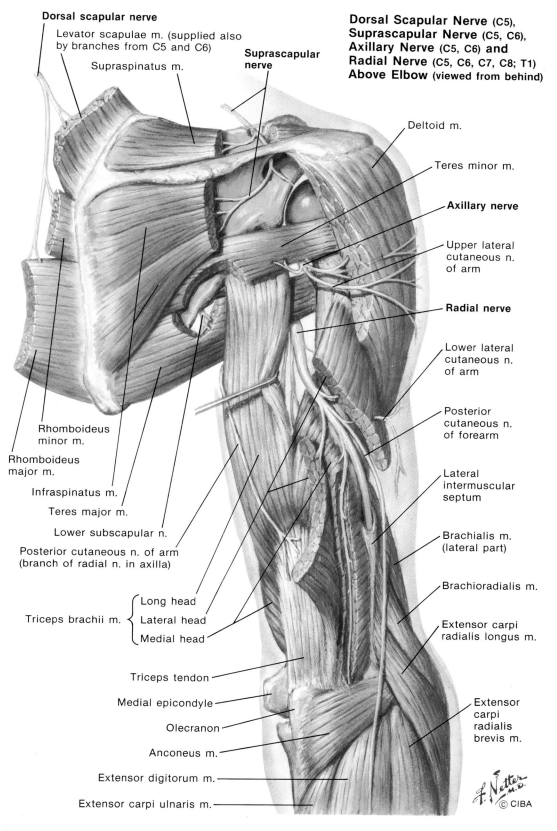

Dorsal scapular nerve

Levator scapulae m. (supplied also by branches from C5 and C6)

Supraspinatus m.

Suprascapular nerve

**Dorsal Scapular Nerve (C5),
Suprascapular Nerve (C5, C6),
Axillary Nerve (C5, C6) and
Radial Nerve (C5, C6, C7, C8; T1)
Above Elbow (viewed from behind)**

Deltoid m.

Teres minor m.

**Axillary nerve**

Upper lateral cutaneous n. of arm

**Radial nerve**

Lower lateral cutaneous n. of arm

Posterior cutaneous n. of forearm

Lateral intermuscular septum

Brachialis m. (lateral part)

Brachioradialis m.

Extensor carpi radialis longus m.

Extensor carpi radialis brevis m.

Rhomboideus minor m.

Rhomboideus major m.

Infraspinatus m.

Teres major m.

Lower subscapular n.

Posterior cutaneous n. of arm (branch of radial n. in axilla)

Triceps brachii m. { Long head / Lateral head / Medial head }

Triceps tendon

Medial epicondyle

Olecranon

Anconeus m.

Extensor digitorum m.

Extensor carpi ulnaris m.

# Radial Nerve in Forearm

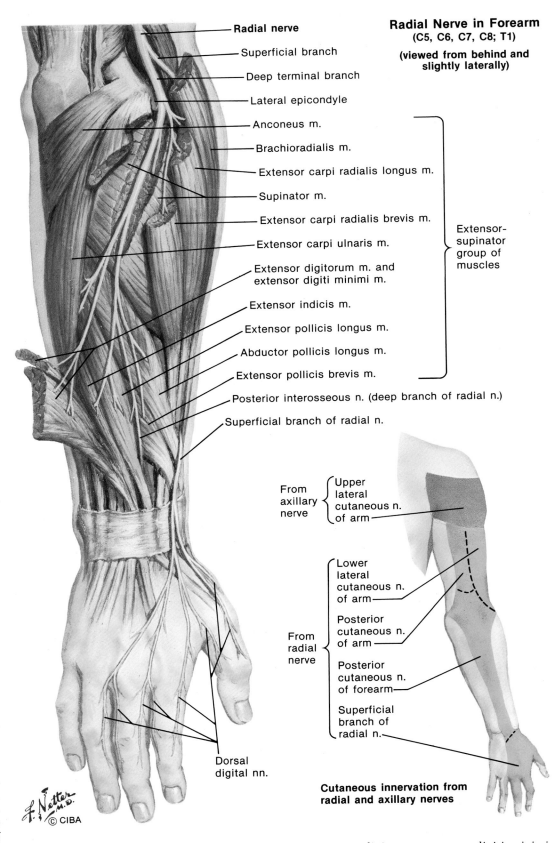

**Radial Nerve in Forearm**
(C5, C6, C7, C8; T1)
(viewed from behind and slightly laterally)

- Radial nerve
- Superficial branch
- Deep terminal branch
- Lateral epicondyle
- Anconeus m.
- Brachioradialis m.
- Extensor carpi radialis longus m.
- Supinator m.
- Extensor carpi radialis brevis m.
- Extensor carpi ulnaris m.
- Extensor digitorum m. and extensor digiti minimi m.
- Extensor indicis m.
- Extensor pollicis longus m.
- Abductor pollicis longus m.
- Extensor pollicis brevis m.
- Posterior interosseous n. (deep branch of radial n.)
- Superficial branch of radial n.

Extensor-supinator group of muscles

Dorsal digital nn.

From axillary nerve {
- Upper lateral cutaneous n. of arm

From radial nerve {
- Lower lateral cutaneous n. of arm
- Posterior cutaneous n. of arm
- Posterior cutaneous n. of forearm
- Superficial branch of radial n.

**Cutaneous innervation from radial and axillary nerves**

The radial nerve divides anterior to the lateral humeral epicondyle into superficial and deep terminal branches (Plate 5).

*The superficial terminal branch* descends along the anterolateral side of the forearm, deep to the brachioradialis and lying successively on the supinator, pronator teres, flexor digitorum superficialis and flexor digitorum longus muscles. In the upper third of the forearm, the superficial terminal branch and the radial artery converge; in the middle third, they are close together, with the nerve lying laterally; and in the lower third, they diverge as the nerve inclines posterolaterally, deep to the tendon of the brachioradialis. The nerve now pierces the deep fascia and commonly subdivides into two branches, which usually split into four or five *dorsal digital nerves.* The cutaneous area of supply is shown in the lower part of the illustration. The dorsal digital nerves also supply filaments to the adjacent vessels, joints and bones. (Note that the radial dorsal digital nerves extend only to the levels of the distal interphalangeal joints, and that the first dorsal digital nerve gives off a twig that curves around the radial side of the thumb to supply the skin over the lateral part of the thenar eminence.) The cutaneous areas on the hand supplied by the radial, median and ulnar nerves (Plates 8 and 9) show wide individual variations; communications exist between their branches, and considerable marginal overlaps are found in their zones of distribution.

*The deep terminal branch* winds posteroinferiorly around the lateral side of the radius and may supply additional twigs to the brachioradialis and extensor carpi radialis longus muscles, which supplement those given off the main stem of the radial nerve in the lower third of the arm. The deep terminal branch supplies branches to the extensor carpi radialis brevis and to the supinator

before passing between the humeral and radial heads of the supinator, or between this muscle and the upper end of the radial shaft, to reach the back of the forearm.

From this point onward, the nerve is generally called the *posterior (dorsal) interosseous nerve,* although this term is sometimes used as a synonym for the entire deep terminal branch. On emerging from or beneath the supinator muscle, the nerve becomes closely related to the posterior interosseous artery. The resulting neurovascular bundle lies at first between the superficial and deep extensor muscles in the forearm, where the nerve gives off short branches to the nearby muscular bellies of

the extensor digitorum, extensor digiti minimi and extensor carpi ulnaris muscles. Longer branches run distally to supply the extensor pollicis longus, extensor indicis, abductor pollicis longus and extensor pollicis brevis muscles. At the lower border of the extensor pollicis brevis, the nerve, now much reduced in size, passes deep to the extensor pollicis longus, and then descends posterior to the interosseous membrane to the back of the wrist. Here, it ends in a small nodule, a pseudoganglion, from which filaments are distributed to the distal radioulnar, radiocarpal and carpal bones, joints and ligaments, and the posterior interosseous and carpal vessels. □

# Musculocutaneous Nerve

**Musculocutaneous Nerve** (C5, C6, C7)

(only muscles innervated by musculocutaneous nerve are depicted)

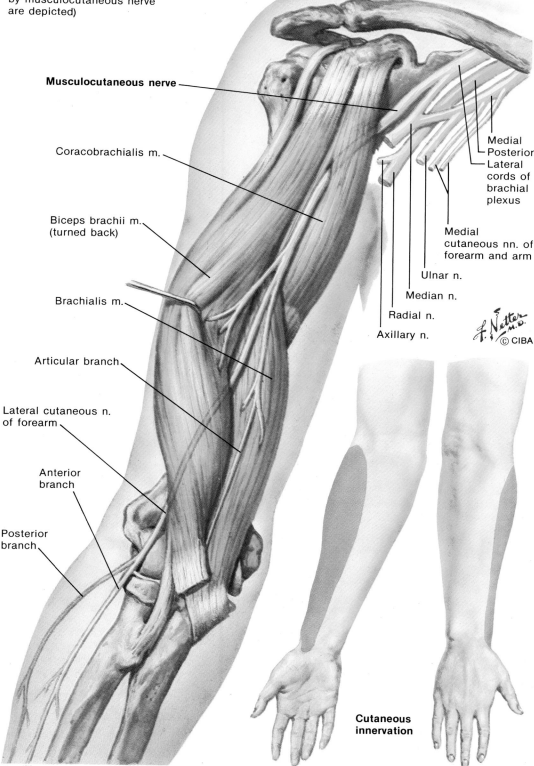

Musculocutaneous nerve

Coracobrachialis m.

Biceps brachii m. (turned back)

Brachialis m.

Articular branch

Lateral cutaneous n. of forearm

Anterior branch

Posterior branch

Medial
Posterior
Lateral
cords of
brachial
plexus

Medial cutaneous nn. of forearm and arm

Ulnar n.

Median n.

Radial n.

Axillary n.

**Cutaneous innervation**

The *musculocutaneous nerve* (C[4], C5, C6, C7), a branch of the *lateral cord* of the brachial plexus, arises opposite the lower border of the pectoralis minor muscle. It lies between the axillary artery and the coracobrachialis muscle, which it perforates and supplies. Continuing downward, it runs between the biceps and brachialis muscles, supplying branches to both heads of the biceps and most of the brachialis, and often communicating with the median nerve. In this part of its course, the musculocutaneous nerve inclines gradually toward the lateral side of the arm; at about the level of the elbow joint, it passes between the biceps and the brachioradialis to pierce the deep fascia and become the *lateral cutaneous nerve of the forearm*.

The branch to the coracobrachialis derives its fibers from C7 and usually arises from the main nerve before that nerve penetrates the muscle. Occasionally, the branch comes directly from the lateral cord of the brachial plexus. The branches to both heads of the biceps and to the brachialis arise from the nerve after it has emerged from the coracobrachialis. The branch supplying the brachialis gives off a filament that descends to help in the innervation of the elbow joint; other filaments supply the brachial artery and the profunda brachii artery and its nutrient humeral branch. Fibers innervating the periosteum on the distal anterior aspect of the humerus are reputedly conveyed with these vascular filaments.

*The lateral cutaneous nerve of the forearm* (lateral antebrachial cutaneous nerve) passes deep to the cephalic vein and soon divides into anterior and posterior branches. The *anterior branch* descends along the anterior aspect of the radial side of the forearm to the wrist and ends at the base of the thenar eminence. At the wrist, it lies in front of the radial artery and gives off filaments that penetrate the deep fascia to supply this part of the artery. The terminal filaments of the anterior branch communicate with corresponding filaments from the palmar cutaneous branch of the median nerve. The *posterior branch* is smaller. It curves around the radial border of the forearm and

breaks up into branches that supply a variable area of skin and fascia over the back of the forearm. The branches also communicate with those of the posterior cutaneous nerve of the forearm and with the superficial terminal branch of the radial nerve (Plate 6). The areas of skin and its appendages (sensory receptors, hairs, arrectores pilorum muscles, glands and vessels) supplied by the lateral cutaneous nerve of the forearm are shown in the lower right of the illustration, although, as is the case with the radial nerve of the forearm, these terminal cutaneous branches show considerable individual variation in the territories they supply. □

# Median Nerve

The *median nerve* (C[5], C6, C7, C8; T1) is formed by the union of *medial* and *lateral roots* arising from the corresponding cords of the brachial plexus.

*Course in Arm.* The median nerve runs from the axilla into the arm, at first lying lateral to the brachial artery. At about the level of the insertion of the coracobrachialis muscle, the nerve inclines medially over the brachial artery, and then descends along its medial side to the cubital fossa. Here, it lies behind the bicipital aponeurosis and intermediate (median) cubital vein, and in front of the insertion of the brachialis muscle and the elbow joint. (The close proximity of the vein, artery and nerve should be remembered when performing venipuncture in this area.) The only branches given off by the median nerve in the arm are filaments to the brachial vessels and an inconstant twig to the pronator teres muscle.

*Course in Upper Forearm.* The nerve passes into the forearm between the humeral and ulnar heads of the pronator teres, the latter separating it from the ulnar artery. It then runs deep to the aponeurotic arch between the humeroulnar and radial heads of the flexor digitorum superficialis, and continues downward between this muscle and the flexor digitorum profundus; it usually adheres to the deep surface of the superficial flexor. In the forearm, the nerve supplies branches to the pronator teres, flexor digitorum superficialis, flexor carpi radialis and palmaris longus muscles, and articular twigs to the elbow and proximal radio-ulnar joints. The longest branch is the *anterior interosseous nerve*, which, accompanied by the corresponding artery, runs downward on the interosseous membrane between the flexor pollicis longus and the flexor digitorum profundus; it supplies the former muscle and the lateral part of the latter (which provides the tendons for the index and middle fingers), and ends under the pronator quadratus, supplying this muscle and the distal radioulnar, radiocarpal and carpal joints. Vascular filaments help to innervate the ulnar and anterior interosseous vessels and the nutrient vessels of the radius and ulna. A *palmar cutaneous branch* arises about 3 to 4 cm above the flexor retinaculum, and descends over it to supply the skin of the median part of the palm and the thenar eminence. In the forearm, the median and ulnar nerves are occasionally interconnected by strand(s), and fibers passing through these communication(s) may explain certain anomalies in the nerve supplies of the hand muscles.

*In the lower forearm*, the median nerve becomes more superficial between the tendons of the palmaris longus and the flexor carpi radialis. It enters the palm together with the tendons of the digital flexor muscles, through the confined carpal tunnel that is bounded anteriorly by the tough flexor retinaculum, and posteriorly, by the carpal bones. Emerging from the tunnel, it splays out into its terminal muscular and palmar digital branches. The muscular branch arises close to, or is initially united with, the common palmar digital nerve to the thumb, and curves outward over

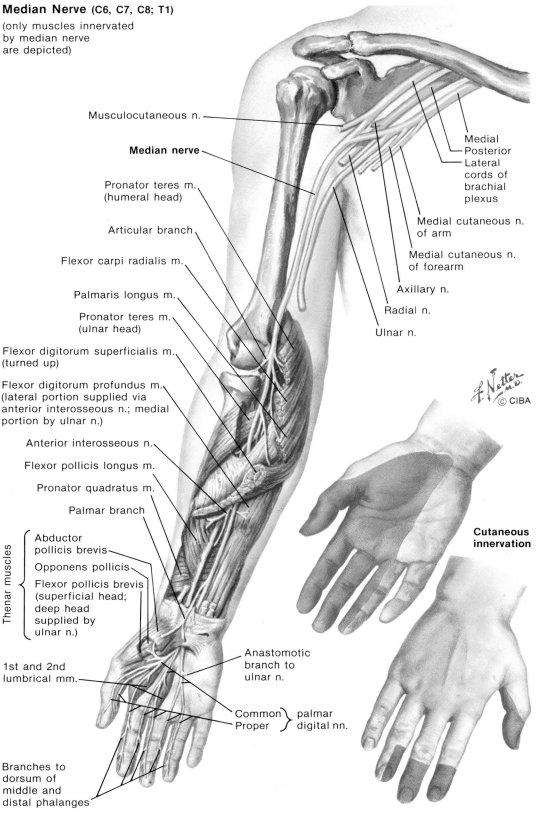

**Median Nerve** (C6, C7, C8; T1)
(only muscles innervated by median nerve are depicted)

Musculocutaneous n.

**Median nerve**

Pronator teres m. (humeral head)

Articular branch

Flexor carpi radialis m.

Palmaris longus m.

Pronator teres m. (ulnar head)

Flexor digitorum superficialis m. (turned up)

Flexor digitorum profundus m. (lateral portion supplied via anterior interosseus n.; medial portion by ulnar n.)

Anterior interosseous n.

Flexor pollicis longus m.

Pronator quadratus m.

Palmar branch

Thenar muscles { Abductor pollicis brevis
Opponens pollicis
Flexor pollicis brevis (superficial head; deep head supplied by ulnar n.)

1st and 2nd lumbrical mm.

Branches to dorsum of middle and distal phalanges

Medial
Posterior
Lateral
cords of brachial plexus

Medial cutaneous n. of arm

Medial cutaneous n. of forearm

Axillary n.

Radial n.

Ulnar n.

Anastomotic branch to ulnar n.

Common } palmar
Proper } digital nn.

**Cutaneous innervation**

or through the flexor pollicis brevis to supply its superficial head before dividing to supply the abductor pollicis brevis and opponens pollicis muscles. Sometimes, the muscular branch also supplies all or part of the first dorsal interosseus muscle. Rarely, it arises in the carpal tunnel and pierces the flexor retinaculum—an arrangement of potential clinical concern.

The *common* and *proper palmar digital nerves* vary in their origins and distributions, but the usual arrangement is that shown in Plates 8 and 9. The proper palmar digital nerves give off dorsal twigs, which innervate the skin (including the nail beds) over the distal, dorsal aspects of the lateral

3 1/2 digits. Occasionally, they supply only 2 1/2 digits. The proper palmar digital branches to the radial side of the index finger and to the contiguous sides of the index and middle fingers also carry motor fibers to supply, respectively, the first and second lumbrical muscles. Therefore, the digital nerves are not concerned solely with cutaneous sensibility. They contain an admixture of efferent and afferent somatic and autonomic fibers that transmit impulses to and from sensory endings, vessels, sweat glands and arrectores pilorum muscles, and between fascial, tendinous, osseous and articular structures in their areas of distribution. □

# Ulnar Nerve

The *ulnar nerve* is the main continuation of the *medial cord* of the brachial plexus. Its fibers are usually derived from C8 and T1, but it often receives additional fibers from C7.

*Course in Arm.* Initially, the ulnar nerve lies between the axillary artery and vein; as it enters the arm, it runs on the medial side of the brachial artery. At about the middle of the arm, it pierces the medial intermuscular septum and descends anterior to the medial head of the triceps brachii muscle, alongside the superior ulnar collateral artery. In the lower third of the arm, it inclines posteriorly to reach the interval between the medial humeral epicondyle and the olecranon. As it enters the forearm, it lies in the groove behind the medial epicondyle, between the humeral and ulnar heads of the flexor carpi ulnaris. Above the elbow, the nerve supplies no constant branches.

*Course in Forearm and Hand.* The ulnar nerve runs downward on the medial side of the forearm, lying first on the ulnar collateral ligament of the elbow joint and then on the flexor digitorum profundus, deep to the flexor carpi ulnaris. At elbow level, the ulnar nerve and artery are separated by a considerable gap, but they are closely apposed in the lower two thirds of the forearm. As the flexor carpi ulnaris narrows into its tendon, the nerve and artery emerge from under its lateral edge and are covered only by skin and fascia. They reach the hand by passing over the anterior surface of the flexor retinaculum, and the nerve splits almost immediately into its superficial and deep terminal branches.

*Branches.* In the forearm and hand, the ulnar nerve gives off articular, muscular, palmar cutaneous, dorsal, superficial and deep terminal, and vascular branches. Fine articular branches to the elbow arise from the main nerve as it runs posterior to the medial epicondyle; before splitting into its terminal branches, it supplies filaments to the wrist.

In the upper forearm, the ulnar nerve gives off branches to the flexor carpi ulnaris and the medial half of the flexor digitorum profundus. The *palmar cutaneous branch* arises to 7 cm above the wrist, descends near the ulnar artery, pierces the deep fascia, and supplies the skin over the hypothenar eminence; it communicates with the medial cutaneous nerve of the forearm and the palmar cutaneous branch of the median nerve. The *dorsal ulnar branch* arises 5 to 10 cm above the wrist, passes posteriorly, deep to the tendon of flexor carpi ulnaris, pierces the deep fascia, and continues distally along the dorsomedial side of the wrist. Here, it divides into branches that supply the areas of skin on the medial side of the back of the hand and fingers. There are usually two or three *dorsal digital nerves*, one supplying the medial side of the little finger, the other splitting into *proper dorsal digital nerves* to supply adjacent sides of the little and ring fingers, and the third (when present) supplying contiguous sides of the ring and middle fingers.

The *superficial terminal branch* supplies the palmaris brevis, innervates the skin on the medial

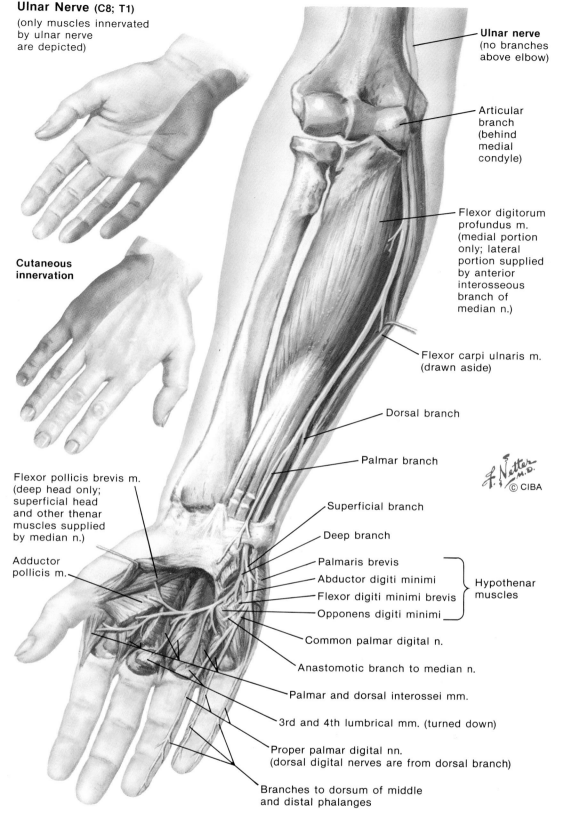

**Ulnar Nerve** (C8; T1)
(only muscles innervated by ulnar nerve are depicted)

Cutaneous innervation

Ulnar nerve (no branches above elbow)

Articular branch (behind medial condyle)

Flexor digitorum profundus m. (medial portion only; lateral portion supplied by anterior interosseous branch of median n.)

Flexor carpi ulnaris m. (drawn aside)

Dorsal branch

Palmar branch

Flexor pollicis brevis m. (deep head only; superficial head and other thenar muscles supplied by median n.)

Adductor pollicis m.

Superficial branch

Deep branch

Palmaris brevis
Abductor digiti minimi
Flexor digiti minimi brevis
Opponens digiti minimi
} Hypothenar muscles

Common palmar digital n.

Anastomotic branch to median n.

Palmar and dorsal interossei mm.

3rd and 4th lumbrical mm. (turned down)

Proper palmar digital nn. (dorsal digital nerves are from dorsal branch)

Branches to dorsum of middle and distal phalanges

side of the palm, and gives off two palmar digital nerves. One is the *proper palmar digital nerve* for the medial side of the little finger, and the other (a *common palmar digital nerve*) communicates with the adjoining common palmar digital branch of the median nerve before dividing into the two *proper palmar digital nerves* for the adjacent sides of the little and ring fingers. In a minority of individuals, the ulnar nerve supplies 2 1/2 rather than 1 1/2 digits, in which case the areas supplied by the median and radial nerves are reciprocally reduced.

The *deep terminal branch* runs between and supplies the abductor and flexor muscles of the little

finger, perforates and supplies the opponens digiti minimi, and then accompanies the deep palmar arterial arch behind the flexor digital tendons. In the palm, it gives branches to the third and fourth lumbricals and to the interossei, and usually ends by supplying the adductor pollicis and the flexor pollicis brevis.

Variations in the nerve supplies of the palmar muscles are as common as those in the cutaneous distribution; they are due to the variety of interconnections between the ulnar and median nerves, which allow interchanges of fibers from different nerve roots, and their clinical implications are important. □

# Lumbar, Sacral and Coccygeal Plexuses

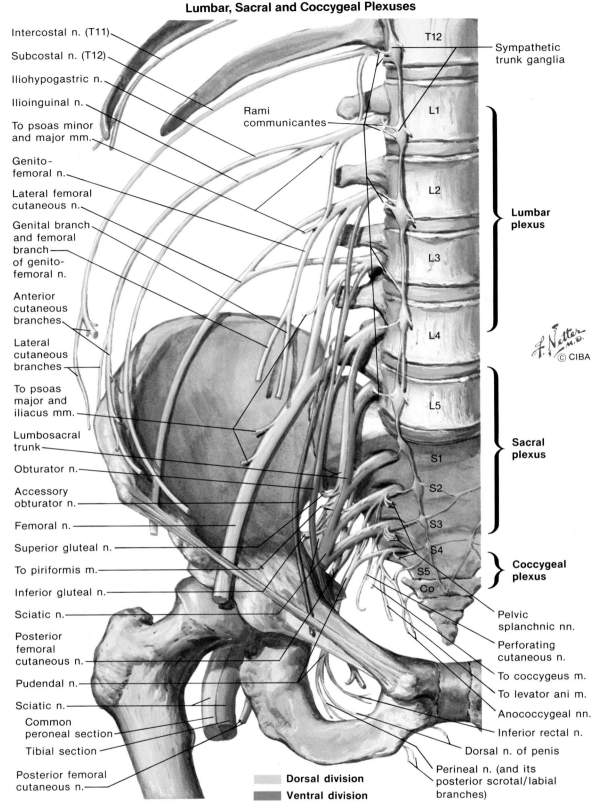

**Labels on illustration:**

Intercostal n. (T11)
Subcostal n. (T12)
Iliohypogastric n.
Ilioinguinal n.
To psoas minor and major mm.
Genito-femoral n.
Lateral femoral cutaneous n.
Genital branch and femoral branch of genito-femoral n.
Anterior cutaneous branches
Lateral cutaneous branches
To psoas major and iliacus mm.
Lumbosacral trunk
Obturator n.
Accessory obturator n.
Femoral n.
Superior gluteal n.
To piriformis m.
Inferior gluteal n.
Sciatic n.
Posterior femoral cutaneous n.
Pudendal n.
Sciatic n.
Common peroneal section
Tibial section
Posterior femoral cutaneous n.

Rami communicantes
T12
L1
L2
L3
L4
L5
S1
S2
S3
S4
S5
Co

Sympathetic trunk ganglia
Lumbar plexus
Sacral plexus
Coccygeal plexus
Pelvic splanchnic nn.
Perforating cutaneous n.
To coccygeus m.
To levator ani m.
Anococcygeal nn.
Inferior rectal n.
Dorsal n. of penis
Perineal n. (and its posterior scrotal/labial branches)

Dorsal division
Ventral division

The lumbar, sacral and coccygeal plexuses are interlinked and are formed from the ventral rami of the *lumbar, sacral* and *coccygeal nerves.* Variations in their makeup are common.

**The lumbar plexus** is produced by the union of the ventral rami of the first three lumbar nerves and the greater part of the fourth, with a contribution from the subcostal nerve. It lies anterior to the lumbar vertebral transverse processes, embedded in the posterior part of the psoas major muscle.

The first lumbar nerve receives a fascicle from the subcostal nerve and divides into upper and lower branches; the upper branch splits into the iliohypogastric and ilioinguinal nerves, while the lower branch joins a twig from the second lumbar nerve and becomes the genitofemoral nerve. Except near their terminations, all three nerves run parallel to the lower intercostal nerves and help to supply the transverse and oblique abdominal muscles. The *iliohypogastric nerve* gives off a lateral cutaneous branch to the skin on the anterolateral aspect of the buttock and ends as the anterior cutaneous branch to the skin above the pubis. The *ilioinguinal nerve* pierces the internal oblique muscle above the anterior part of the iliac crest and then runs above and parallel to the inguinal ligament to traverse the inguinal canal and supply the skin over the root of the penis, the adjoining part of the femoral triangle and the upper part of the scrotum (mons pubis and adjacent part of labium majus in the female). The *genitofemoral nerve* penetrates the psoas major muscle and divides into *genital* and *femoral branches.* The former passes through the inguinal canal and supplies the cremaster muscle and the skin of the scrotum; the latter supplies the skin over the upper part of the femoral triangle.

The larger part of the second lumbar nerve, the entire third lumbar nerve, and the offshoot from the fourth lumbar nerve to the lumbar plexus split into ventral (anterior) and dorsal (posterior) divisions, which unite to constitute, respectively, the *femoral* and *obturator nerves* (Plates 11 and 12). The *lateral femoral cutaneous nerve* (Plate 11) is formed by offshoots from the second and third posterior divisions.

The lower part of the ventral ramus of the fourth lumbar nerve joins the ventral ramus of the fifth to form the *lumbosacral trunk.* The trunk and the ventral rami of the first three sacral nerves and the upper part of the fourth sacral ramus constitute the *sacral plexus.*

**The sacral plexus,** by convergence and fusion of its roots, becomes a flattened band that gives rise to many branches before its largest part passes below the piriformis muscle and through the greater sciatic foramen as the *sciatic nerve* (Plate 13). The rami forming the sacral plexus divide into ventral (anterior) and dorsal (posterior) divisions, which subdivide and regroup to become branches of the plexus.

**Coccygeal Plexus.** The lower part of the ventral ramus of the fourth and fifth sacral nerves and the coccygeal nerves form the small coccygeal plexus. It consists of two loops on the pelvic surface of the coccygeus and levator ani muscles. Twigs are given off to these muscles, and fine *anococcygeal nerves* supply the skin between the anus and coccyx. □

# Femoral and Lateral Femoral Cutaneous Nerves

*The femoral nerve* (L2, L3, L4) is the largest branch of the lumbar plexus. It supplies the iliacus and anterior thigh muscles, twigs to the hip and knee joints and to adjacent vessels, and cutaneous branches to anteromedial aspects of the lower limb.

The femoral nerve originates from the dorsal divisions of the ventral rami of the second, third and fourth lumbar nerves (Plate 10), passes inferolaterally through the psoas major muscle, and then runs in a groove between this muscle and the iliacus, which it supplies. It enters the thigh behind the inguinal ligament to lie lateral to the femoral vascular sheath in the femoral triangle, where it divides into muscular and cutaneous branches.

*Muscular branches* supply the pectineus, sartorius and quadriceps femoris muscles. The nerve to the pectineus arises at the level of the inguinal ligament; the branches to the sartorius enter the upper two thirds of the muscle, several arising in common with the anterior femoral cutaneous nerves; the branches to the quadriceps femoris are arranged as illustrated; those to the rectus femoris and the vastus lateralis enter the deep surfaces of the muscles; that to the vastus intermedius enters its superficial surface and pierces the muscle to supply the underlying articularis genus; and the branch to the vastus medialis runs in the adductor canal for a variable distance, on the lateral side of the femoral vessels and saphenous nerve, giving off successive branches to this muscle, some of which end in the vastus intermedius and articularis genus muscles.

The *anterior femoral cutaneous nerves* arise in the femoral triangle. All these branches pierce the fascia lata 8 to 10 cm distal to the inguinal ligament and descend to knee level, supplying the skin and fascia over the front and medial sides of the thigh.

The *saphenous nerve* is the largest and longest of the femoral branches. It arises at the femoral triangle and descends through it on the lateral side of the femoral vessels to enter the adductor canal. Here, it crosses the vessels obliquely to lie on their medial side in front of the lower end of the adductor magnus. In the canal, the saphenous nerve communicates with branches of the anterior femoral cutaneous and obturator nerves to form the *subsartorial plexus.* At the lower end of the canal, it leaves the femoral vessels and gives off its *infrapatellar branch,* which curves around the posterior border of sartorius, pierces the fascia lata, and runs onward to supply the skin over the medial side and front of the knee and the patellar ligament. This branch assists offshoots from the anterior and lateral femoral cutaneous nerves in forming the *patellar plexus.*

The saphenous nerve continues its descent on the medial side of the knee, pierces the fascia lata between the tendons of the sartorius and gracilis muscles, courses downward on the medial side of the leg close to the great saphenous vein, and gives off its *medial crural cutaneous branches.* In the lower leg, it terminally subdivides: the *smaller branch* follows the medial tibial border to the level

## Femoral Nerve (L2, L3, L4) and Lateral Femoral Cutaneous Nerve (L2, L3)

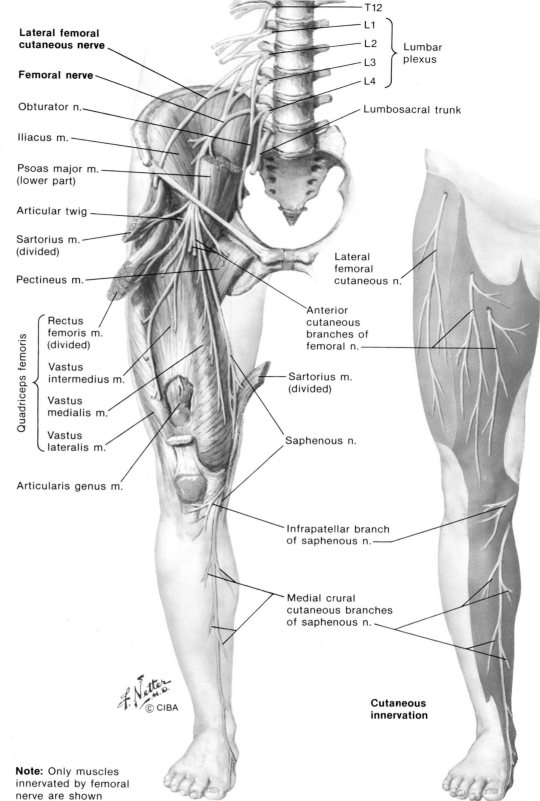

**Note:** Only muscles innervated by femoral nerve are shown

**Cutaneous innervation**

of the ankle, while the *larger branch* passes anterior to the medial malleolus to be distributed to the skin and fascia on the medial side and dorsum of the foot.

*Articular branches* arising from the nerve to the rectus femoris accompany the corresponding branches of the lateral circumflex femoral artery to the hip joint. Twigs from the branches to the vastus muscles and from the saphenous nerve supply the knee joint.

*The lateral femoral cutaneous nerve* (L2, L3) emerges from the lateral border of the psoas major muscle, passes obliquely over the iliacus behind

the parietal peritoneum and iliac fascia (which it supplies) toward the anterior superior iliac spine, and enters the thigh by passing over or through the lateral end of the inguinal ligament. The nerve then passes over or through the proximal part of the sartorius and descends deep to the fascia lata. It gives off a number of small branches to the overlying skin before piercing the fascia about 10 cm below the inguinal ligament. The terminal branches of the nerve supply the skin and fascia on the anterolateral surfaces of the thigh between the levels of the greater femoral trochanter and the knee. □

# Obturator Nerve

The *obturator nerve* (L2, L3, L4) supplies the obturator externus and the adductor muscles of the thigh, gives filaments to the hip and knee joints, and has a variable cutaneous distribution to the medial sides of the thigh and leg.

*Course.* The obturator nerve arises from the ventral divisions of the ventral rami of the second, third and fourth lumbar nerves (Plate 10). The contribution from the second lumbar nerve is commonly the smallest and is sometimes absent. These roots unite within the posterior part of the psoas major, forming a nerve that descends through the muscle to emerge from its medial border opposite the upper end of the sacroiliac joint. The obturator nerve runs outward and downward over the sacral ala and pelvic brim into the lesser pelvis, lying lateral to the ureter and internal iliac vessels, and then bends anteroinferiorly to follow the curvature of the lateral pelvic wall, anterior to the obturator vessels and lying on the obturator internus muscle, to reach the obturator groove at the upper part of the obturator foramen. The nerve passes through this groove to enter the thigh and divides into *anterior* and *posterior branches* at about this point.

*The anterior branch* runs in front of the obturator externus and adductor brevis muscles, and behind the pectineus and adductor longus muscles. Near its origin, it gives off an articular twig that enters the hip joint through the acetabular notch. It often supplies a branch to the pectineus and sends muscular branches to the adductor longus, adductor gracilis and adductor brevis muscles. The anterior branch finally divides into cutaneous, vascular and communicating branches.

The *cutaneous branch* is inconstant. When present, it unites with branches of the saphenous and anterior femoral cutaneous nerves in the adductor canal to form the *subsartorial plexus*, and assists in the innervation of the skin and fascia over the distal two thirds of the medial side of the thigh. Infrequently, this branch is larger and passes between the adductor longus and gracilis muscles to descend behind the sartorius to the medial side of the knee and the adjacent part of the leg, where it assists the saphenous nerve in the cutaneous supply of those areas.

The *vascular branches* end in the femoral artery. Other fine *communicating branches* may link the obturator nerve with the anterior and posterior femoral cutaneous nerves and the inconstant accessory obturator nerve.

*The posterior branch* pierces the anterior part of the obturator externus, and supplies this muscle. Thereafter, the nerve runs downward between

the adductor brevis and the adductor magnus and splits into branches that are distributed to the upper (adductor) part of the adductor magnus and sometimes to the adductor brevis, especially if the latter does not receive a supply from the anterior branch of the obturator nerve. A slender branch emerges from the lower part of the adductor magnus, passes through the hiatus of the adductor canal together with the femoral artery, and then continues to the knee joint. The posterior branch contributes filaments to the femoral and popliteal vessels, and ends by perforating the oblique popliteal ligament to supply the articular capsule, cruciate ligaments and synovial membrane of the

knee joint. The fibers to the capsule and ligaments are mostly of somatic origin, while those to the synovial membrane are mainly sympathetic.

*The accessory obturator nerve* (L3, L4) is inconstant. When present, it is small and is derived from the ventral divisions of the ventral rami of the third and fourth lumbar nerves. The accessory obturator nerve descends on the medial border of the psoas muscle and then crosses the superior pubic ramus to lie behind the pectineus. The nerve ends by helping to supply the pectineus, but may also supply a twig to the hip joint and another twig that joins the anterior branch of the obturator nerve. □

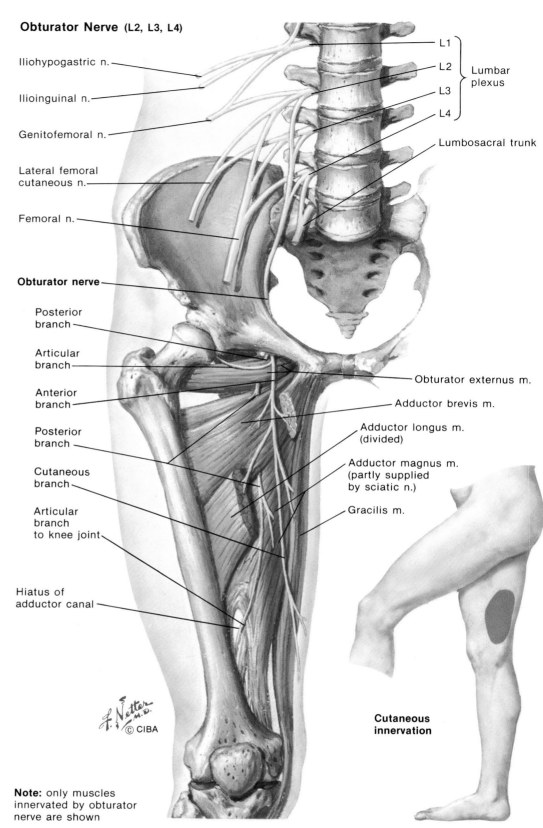

**Obturator Nerve (L2, L3, L4)**

Iliohypogastric n.

Ilioinguinal n.

Genitofemoral n.

Lateral femoral cutaneous n.

Femoral n.

L1
L2 } Lumbar plexus
L3
L4
Lumbosacral trunk

**Obturator nerve**

Posterior branch

Articular branch

Anterior branch

Posterior branch

Cutaneous branch

Articular branch to knee joint

Hiatus of adductor canal

Obturator externus m.

Adductor brevis m.

Adductor longus m. (divided)

Adductor magnus m. (partly supplied by sciatic n.)

Gracilis m.

*F. Netter M.D.* © CIBA

**Note:** only muscles innervated by obturator nerve are shown

**Cutaneous innervation**

# Sciatic, Tibial and Common Peroneal Nerves

## Sciatic Nerve

*Course*. The roots of the sciatic nerve arise from the ventral rami of the fourth lumbar to third sacral nerves (Plate 10) and unite to form a single trunk that is ovoid in cross section and 16 to 20 mm wide in adults (Plate 13). In the lesser pelvis, the nerve lies anterior to the piriformis, below which it enters the buttock through the greater sciatic foramen (in about 2% of individuals, the nerve pierces the piriformis). Next, the nerve inclines laterally beneath the gluteus maximus, where it rests on the posterior surface of the ischium and the nerve to quadratus femoris. On its medial side, it is accompanied by the posterior femoral cutaneous nerve and the inferior gluteal artery and its special branch to the nerve. On reaching a point about midway between the ischial tuberosity and the greater trochanter, the nerve turns downward over the gemelli, the obturator internus tendon and the quadratus femoris, which separate it from the hip joint, and leaves the buttock to enter the thigh beneath the lower border of the gluteus maximus.

The sciatic nerve then descends near the middle of the back of the thigh, lying on the adductor magnus and being crossed obliquely by the long head of the biceps femoris. Just above the apex of the popliteal fossa, it is overlapped by the contiguous margins of the biceps femoris and semimembranosus muscles. In about 90% of individuals, the sciatic nerve divides into its terminal *tibial* and *common peroneal branches* near the apex of the popliteal fossa, while in 10% of individuals the division occurs at higher levels. Rarely, the tibial and common peroneal nerves arise independently from the sacral plexus, but pursue closely related courses until they reach the apex of the popliteal fossa.

*Branches*. In the buttock, the sciatic nerve supplies an *articular branch* to the hip, which perforates the posterior part of the joint capsule. It may also supply *vascular filaments* to the inferior gluteal artery. Lower down, it supplies *muscular branches* to both heads of the biceps femoris, semimembranosus, semitendinosus and the ischial head of adductor magnus muscles. The branch to the short head of the biceps femoris comes from the common peroneal part of the nerve, while the branches for the other muscles are derived from the tibial division.

## Tibial Nerve

The tibial nerve is the larger, medial, terminal branch of the sciatic nerve (Plate 14). Its fibers are derived from the ventral divisions of the ventral rami of the fourth and fifth lumbar nerves and the first, second and third sacral nerves.

*Course*. The tibial nerve continues the line of the sciatic nerve through the popliteal fossa and into the leg. At its origin, the nerve is overlapped by the adjoining margins of the semimembranosus and biceps femoris muscles. In the popliteal fossa, the tibial nerve becomes more superficial, first lying lateral to the popliteal vessels and then crossing obliquely to their medial sides before disappearing into the leg between and beneath the

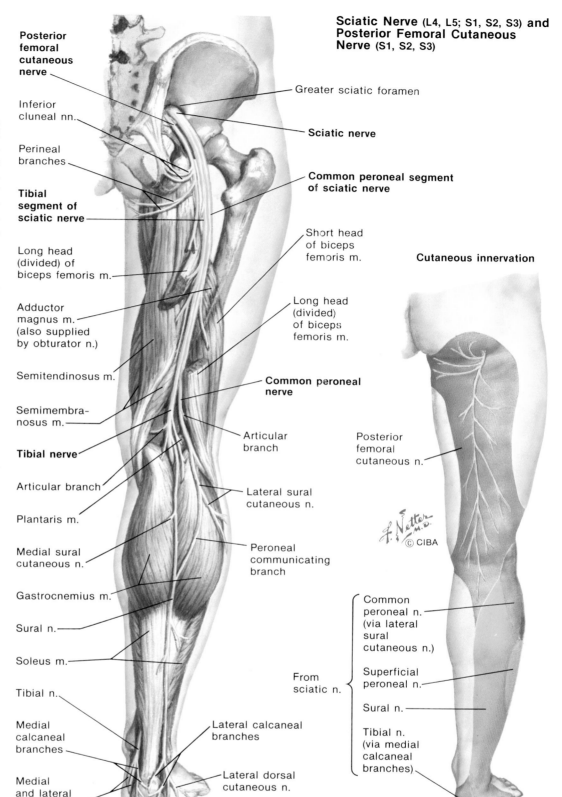

**Sciatic Nerve** (L4, L5; S1, S2, S3) **and Posterior Femoral Cutaneous Nerve** (S1, S2, S3)

Posterior femoral cutaneous nerve

Inferior cluneal nn.

Perineal branches

**Tibial segment of sciatic nerve**

Long head (divided) of biceps femoris m.

Adductor magnus m. (also supplied by obturator n.)

Semitendinosus m.

Semimembranosus m.

**Tibial nerve**

Articular branch

Plantaris m.

Medial sural cutaneous n.

Gastrocnemius m.

Sural n.

Soleus m.

Tibial n.

Medial calcaneal branches

Medial and lateral plantar nn.

Greater sciatic foramen

**Sciatic nerve**

**Common peroneal segment of sciatic nerve**

Short head of biceps femoris m.

Long head (divided) of biceps femoris m.

**Common peroneal nerve**

Articular branch

Lateral sural cutaneous n.

Peroneal communicating branch

Lateral calcaneal branches

Lateral dorsal cutaneous n.

**Cutaneous innervation**

Posterior femoral cutaneous n.

Common peroneal n. (via lateral sural cutaneous n.)

Superficial peroneal n.

Sural n.

Tibial n. (via medial calcaneal branches)

From sciatic n.

heads of the gastrocnemius and plantaris muscles. Passing over the popliteus and under the tendinous arch of the soleus on the medial side of the posterior tibial vessels, the tibial nerve next enters the space between the gastrocnemius and the soleus behind, and the upper part of the tibialis posterior, in front. Continuing downward, it crosses over the posterior tibial vessels to reach their lateral sides so as to lie between the contiguous margins of the flexor digitorum longus and flexor hallucis longus muscles. In the distal third of the leg, the nerve is covered only by skin and fascia as it descends toward the ankle region, where it curves anteroinferiorly into the sole of

the foot behind the medial malleolus, deep to the flexor retinaculum and between the tendons of the flexor hallucis longus and the flexor digitorum longus. The nerve ends at this level by dividing into the *medial* and *lateral plantar nerves*.

The tibial nerve consists of the following main branches: muscular, articular, sural, calcaneal and medial and lateral plantar; it also gives off smaller osseous (medullary) and vascular twigs.

*The muscular branches* supply both heads of the gastrocnemius, the plantaris, the popliteus, the soleus, the tibialis posterior, the flexor digitorum longus and the flexor hallucis longus. Branches to the gastrocnemius, the plantaris and

## Sciatic, Tibial and Common Peroneal Nerves
*(Continued)*

the popliteus, and a few that enter the posterior surface of the soleus arise in the popliteal fossa. The branch to the popliteus descends over the posterior surface of the muscle, hooks around its inferior border, and ascends to enter its anterior surface. Branches to the deep surface of the soleus and to the tibialis posterior, flexor digitorum longus and flexor hallucis longus muscles are given off in the upper third of the leg. Vasomotor filaments to the popliteal vessels arise from the main tibial nerve or its branches in the popliteal fossa.

*The articular branches* help to supply the knee, ankle and superior and inferior tibiofibular joints, and may arise in common with twigs supplying adjacent muscles, bones and vessels.

*The sural nerve*, a cutaneous branch, arises from the tibial nerve at about the middle or lower part of the popliteal fossa (Plate 13). Descending between the two heads of the gastrocnemius, the nerve pierces the deep fascia, gives off a small *medial sural cutaneous nerve* (it may be larger and arise directly from the tibial nerve), and is joined by the peroneal communicating branch of the lateral sural cutaneous nerve. As it continues downward near the small saphenous vein, passing over and then lateral to the Achilles tendon, the sural nerve contributes branches to the skin and fascia on the back and lateral sides of the lower leg. On reaching the space between the lateral malleolus and calcaneus muscles, it gives off *lateral calcaneal branches* to the skin and fascia of the lateral sides of the ankle and heel (the corresponding medial calcaneal branches come from the tibial nerve). The terminal part of the sural nerve runs forward as the *lateral dorsal cutaneous nerve*, along the lateral side of the foot and small toe.

*The medial plantar nerve* is larger than the lateral and is homologous with the median nerve in the hand (Plate 8). From its origin under the flexor retinaculum, the nerve runs first on the lateral side of the medial plantar vessels deep to the abductor hallucis, then onward between the abductor hallucis and the flexor digitorum brevis, and finally between the flexor hallucis brevis and flexor digitorum brevis muscles. At about the level of the tarsometatarsal joints, the nerve ends by dividing into a *proper plantar digital nerve* to the skin of the medial side of the great toe and three *common plantar digital nerves*. Before dividing, it supplies muscular twigs to the abductor hallucis, flexor digitorum brevis and flexor hallucis brevis muscles; cutaneous branches, which pierce the plantar aponeurosis to supply the posteromedial part of the sole of the foot; and articular and vascular filaments to the contiguous tarsal and tarsometatarsal joints and the medial plantar vessels. The *common plantar digital nerves* supply muscular twigs to the first and, occasionally, to the second lumbrical muscle; cutaneous branches to the medial two thirds of the anterior part of the sole; and articular and vascular filaments to adjacent joints and vessels. They finally divide into the *proper plantar digital nerves* that innervate the adjacent sides of the three medial interdigital

spaces and the plantar surfaces of the corresponding toes, and into upward-curving branches that supply the nail beds.

*The lateral plantar nerve* is homologous with the ulnar nerve in the hand (Plate 9). It arises deep to the flexor retinaculum and passes outward and forward in the sole of the foot on the medial side of the lateral plantar vessels. The nerve runs between the flexor digitorum brevis and the quadratus plantae, and then between the former and the abductor digiti minimi to end near the base of the fifth metatarsal bone by dividing into superficial and deep branches. Before dividing, it gives muscular branches to the quadratus plantae and

abductor digiti minimi muscles, and cutaneous branches that pierce the plantar aponeurosis to supply the lateral side of the sole.

The *superficial branch* splits into *proper* and *common plantar digital nerves*. The former supplies the skin and fascia on the plantar and lateral sides of the small toe, including the tip, muscular twigs to the flexor digiti minimi and the interossei of the fourth intermetatarsal space, and filaments to the fifth metatarsophalangeal and interphalangeal joints. The common plantar digital nerve divides into two *proper plantar digital nerves* supplying the skin and fascia of the plantar aspects, adjoining sides, and the nail beds of the fourth and fifth toes.

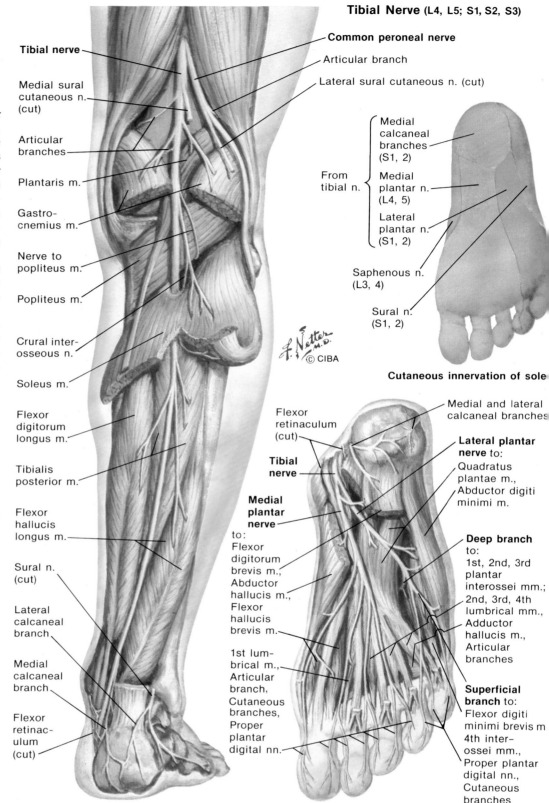

Cutaneous innervation of sole

## Sciatic, Tibial and Common Peroneal Nerves
*(Continued)*

The *deep branch* curves medially to accompany the plantar arterial arch on the deep surfaces of the digital flexor tendons and the oblique head of the adductor hallucis muscle. It supplies branches to the adductor hallucis, the second, third and fourth lumbricals and the interossei in the medial three metatarsal interspaces, and filaments to the plantar arch and to adjacent joints.

### Common Peroneal Nerve

*Course.* The common peroneal nerve (Plates 13 and 15) is the smaller, lateral, terminal branch of the sciatic nerve, and its fibers are derived from the dorsal divisions of the ventral rami of the fourth and fifth lumbar nerves and the first and second sacral nerves. From its origin, the nerve descends first along the lateral side of the popliteal fossa, overlapped by the medial margin of the biceps femoris, then passes between the biceps tendon and the lateral head of the gastrocnemius to reach the back of the fibular head, and finally winds around the back and outer side of the neck of the fibula between the two heads of the peroneus longus, where it divides into the *superficial* and *deep peroneal nerves*. At this point, the nerve can easily be compressed against the underlying bone.

*Branches.* Before dividing, the common peroneal nerve gives off three *articular filaments* to the knee, which accompany and help to supply the superior and inferior lateral genicular and anterior tibial recurrent arteries. It also gives off the *lateral sural cutaneous nerve*, which supplies the skin and fascia on the lateral and adjacent parts of the posterior and anterior surfaces of the upper part of the leg, and the *peroneal communicating branch*, which joins the sural branch of the tibial nerve and is distributed with it.

*The superficial peroneal nerve* descends between the extensor digitorum longus and peroneal muscles, and supplies the peroneus longus and the peroneus brevis, before piercing the deep fascia at about the junction of the middle and lower thirds of the leg. At this level, the nerve divides into medial and intermediate dorsal cutaneous nerves. The *medial dorsal cutaneous nerve* runs in front of the ankle and on to the dorsum of the foot, supplying twigs to the skin and fascia on the anterior surface of the distal third of the leg and the dorsum of the foot. Near the lower border of the inferior extensor retinaculum, it splits into two *dorsal digital nerves*, one of which supplies the medial and dorsal apsects of the dorsum of the foot and the great toe, and the other, the adjacent sides of the second and third toes. The *intermediate dorsal cutaneous nerve* runs along the lateral part of the dorsum of the foot, supplying the nearby skin and fascia and providing the *dorsal digital nerves* for the third and fourth, and fourth and fifth toes. It communicates with the lateral dorsal cutaneous nerve.

*The deep peroneal nerve* passes obliquely forward and downward around the fibular neck and between the peroneus longus and extensor digitorum longus muscles to the front of the crural interosseous membrane. The nerve descends

lateral to the tibialis anterior, and at first is medial to the extensor digitorum longus and then to the extensor hallucis longus, the tendon of which crosses the nerve obliquely above the ankle. In its downward course, the nerve lies first lateral to the anterior tibial vessels, then anterior to them, and finally lateral to them again in front of the lower end of the tibia and ankle, where the nerve divides into medial and lateral terminal branches. In the leg, the nerve sends branches to the tibialis anterior, extensor digitorum longus, extensor hallucis longus and peroneus tertius muscles, an articular branch to the ankle and filaments to the anterior tibial vessels. The *medial terminal branch*

gives rise to a *dorsal digital nerve*, which splits to supply the contiguous sides of the first and second toes. It also supplies filaments to the dorsalis pedis artery and nearby metatarsophalangeal and interphalangeal joints and, occasionally, a twig to the first dorsal interosseus muscle. The *lateral terminal branch* curves outward beneath the extensor digitorum brevis, becomes slightly expanded, and gives off several slender offshoots to supply the extensor digitorum brevis and its medial part (the extensor hallucis brevis), the adjacent tarsal and tarsometatarsal joints and, occasionally, the second and third dorsal interossei muscles. □

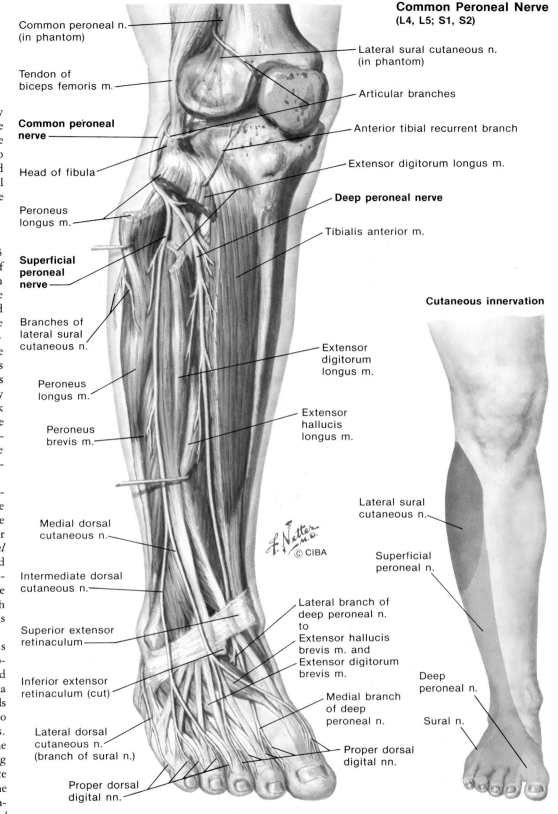

**Common Peroneal Nerve**
(L4, L5; S1, S2)

Common peroneal n. (in phantom)

Lateral sural cutaneous n. (in phantom)

Tendon of biceps femoris m.

Articular branches

**Common peroneal nerve**

Anterior tibial recurrent branch

Head of fibula

Extensor digitorum longus m.

**Deep peroneal nerve**

Peroneus longus m.

Tibialis anterior m.

**Superficial peroneal nerve**

Branches of lateral sural cutaneous n.

Extensor digitorum longus m.

Peroneus longus m.

Peroneus brevis m.

Extensor hallucis longus m.

Medial dorsal cutaneous n.

Intermediate dorsal cutaneous n.

Superior extensor retinaculum

Lateral branch of deep peroneal n. to Extensor hallucis brevis m. and Extensor digitorum brevis m.

Inferior extensor retinaculum (cut)

Medial branch of deep peroneal n.

Lateral dorsal cutaneous n. (branch of sural n.)

Proper dorsal digital nn.

Proper dorsal digital nn.

**Cutaneous innervation**

Lateral sural cutaneous n.

Superficial peroneal n.

Deep peroneal n.

Sural n.

F. Netter M.D. © CIBA

# Dermal Segmentation

The cutaneous area supplied by a single spinal nerve is called a *dermatome*. The cell bodies (cytons) of the afferent fibers involved are located in the dorsal spinal nerve root ganglia and in ganglia on cranial nerves V, VII, IX and X. One exception should be mentioned: the cell bodies of the trigeminal nerve proprioceptive fibers conveyed from the facial and masticatory muscles are located in the trigeminal mesencephalic nucleus and not in the trigeminal ganglion.

The spinal cord is segmental in character, and the spinal nerves are distributed to structures developed from the associated segments, or metameres (see Section VII, Plates 2 and 3). In the trunk, the correspondence between neural and bodily segments is clearly apparent, because they are arranged in consecutive encircling bands. In the limbs, however, due to plexus formation and interchange of nerve fibers in the nerves supplying them, the segmental distribution is obscured, although the arrangement is explicable embryologically. As the limb buds develop, they draw out parts of certain segments, together with their mesodermal cores, ectodermal coverings and corresponding segmental nerves and vessels. Thus, the more proximal dermatomes are elongated strips situated along the preaxial (outer) sides of the limbs, and the more distal ones are situated along their postaxial (medial sides). The oblique disposition in the lower limbs is due to the fact that during development, the limbs rotate medially around a longitudinal axis.

The fifth cervical to first thoracic metameres and the first lumbar to third sacral metameres contribute, respectively, to the formation of the upper and lower limbs. This is reflected in their nerve supplies, and explains why in the neck, trunk and upper limb the C5 and T1 dermatomes are in parts contiguous, and why in the trunk, perineum and lower limbs the L1 and L2 dermatomes are in places adjacent to those of S2 and S3: the intervening segments have migrated into the more distal parts of the limbs.

The nerves supplying neighboring dermatomes overlap, and thus division of one dorsal nerve root produces *hypoesthesia* rather than *anesthesia*. To effect complete cutaneous anesthesia in any area, at least three adjoining spinal nerves or their dorsal roots must be blocked or divided. The exception to this general rule is that section of the dorsal root of C2 produces an area of complete anesthesia in the occipital region of the scalp. The degree of nerve overlap varies for different sensations, being greater for touch than for pain and temperature. The segmental muscular supplies

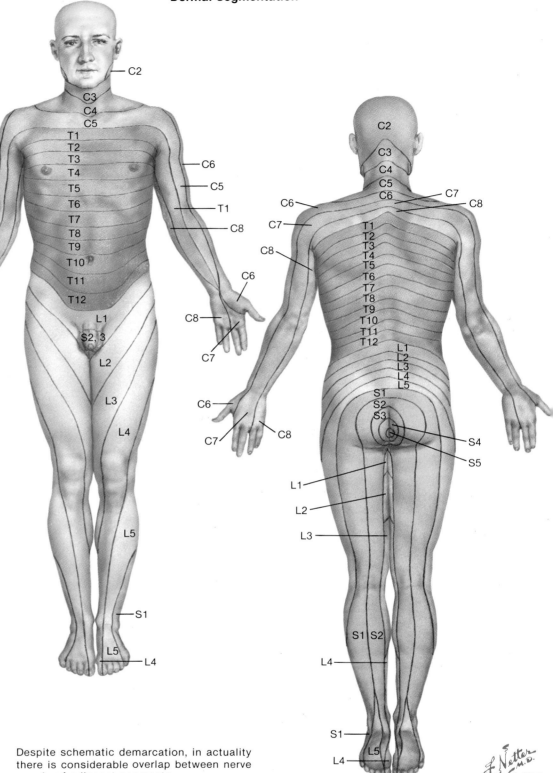

Despite schematic demarcation, in actuality there is considerable overlap between nerve supply of adjacent segments

also overlap, so that most of the larger muscles (especially those in the limbs) are innervated by fibers from several ventral nerve roots. Therefore, *paresis* occurs if only one or two roots are affected, but *paralysis* results if more roots are damaged or destroyed.

Knowledge of the dermatomes enables the clinician to locate lesions affecting the spinal cord or spinal nerves, and the dermatomes of the hand and foot deserve special attention.

### Levels of Principal Dermatomes

| | |
|---|---|
| C5 | clavicles |
| C5,6,7 | lateral parts of upper limbs |
| C8; T1 | medial sides of upper limbs |
| C6 | thumb |
| C6,7,8 | hand |
| C8 | ring and little fingers |
| T4 | level of nipples |
| T10 | level of umbilicus |
| T12 | inguinal or groin regions |
| L1,2,3,4 | inner and anterior surfaces of lower limbs |
| L4,5; S1 | foot |
| L4 | medial side of great toe |
| L5; S1,2 | outer and posterior sides of lower limbs |
| S1 | lateral margin of foot and little toe |
| S2,3,4,5 | perineum |

Section VII

# Embryology

Frank H. Netter, M.D.

*in collaboration with*

**Edmund S. Crelin, Ph.D., D.Sc.**  *Plates 1–15*

# Development of Nervous System

The development of the nervous system begins with the formation of the *embryonic disc*. The nervous system itself is derived from the *ectodermal* layer, and circumscribed parts of the disc ectoderm are predestined to contribute to the formation of specific parts of it (Plate 1).

*Eighteenth Day.* At the 18-day stage of embryonic development, the neural plate, tube and crest form. First, the midline notochordal tissue anterior to the blastopore induces the overlying head process to thicken and become the *neural plate*. A midsagittal *neural groove* then appears in the plate, on each side of which the ectodermal tissue predestined to contribute to the neural crest becomes elevated into the *neural folds* (Plate 2). These folds, in turn, fuse in the midline to form the *neural tube*. As the folds fuse, the tube coincidentally separates from its originating ectoderm. Certain cells at the margins of the folds are not included in the wall of the neural tube or in the superficial ectoderm as it closes above the newly formed tube, and these cells become the *neural crest*.

## Development of Brain

*Twenty-eighth Day.* During its early formative stage, the neural tube is a straight structure. However, even before the development of its caudal end is complete, the part anterior to the first cervical somite deviates from the shape of a simple tube. This area, the future brain, begins to form various bulges, flexures and cavities, each of which has significance in embryological development.

First, in the future brain region of the neural tube, three *primary bulges* appear—the *forebrain (prosencephalon)*, the *midbrain (mesencephalon)* and the *hindbrain (rhombencephalon)*. By the time the development of the caudal end of the tube is complete, *secondary bulges* called the *optic vesicles* extend from each side of the forebrain. At this time, a *cephalic flexure* and a *cervical flexure* of the future brain may be identified, and the *cavities* (which will become the ventricles) are visible. These cavities are the *prosocele* of the forebrain, the *mesocele* of the midbrain and the *rhombocele* of the hindbrain.

As each optic vesicle differentiates to form, first, an *optic cup* and *stalk* and, later, an *optic nerve* and a *part of the eyeball*, its original cavity is obliterated. Eventually, the original connection of each optic vesicle becomes located in the diencephalon.

*Thirty-sixth Day.* The forebrain has divided into two parts by the thirty-sixth day (Plate 3). The posterior (caudal) subdivision is the *diencephalon*; the anterior subdivision further differentiates into the two *telencephalic vesicles*, which eventually become the cerebral hemispheres. The telencephalic vesicles expand beyond the original anterior limit of the neural tube, which is called the *lamina terminalis*.

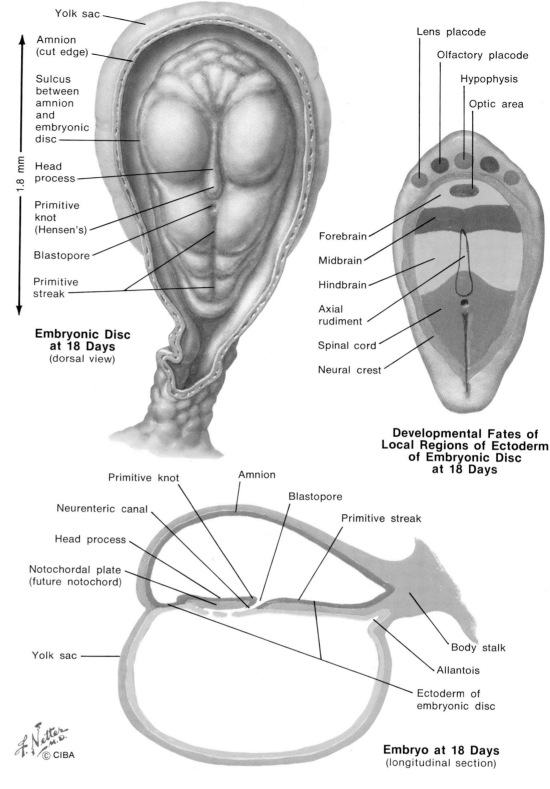

**Embryonic Disc at 18 Days** (dorsal view)

**Developmental Fates of Local Regions of Ectoderm of Embryonic Disc at 18 Days**

**Embryo at 18 Days** (longitudinal section)

Simultaneous with the subdivision of the forebrain, its original cavity undergoes related subdivisions. The two telencephalic vesicles, the *lateral teloceles*, are destined to become the lateral ventricles. The cavity between them, the *median telocele*, together with the *diocele* (the cavity of the diencephalon), will become the third ventricle. Similarly, the cavity of the mesencephalon, the *mesocele*, will become the cerebral aqueduct.

At the same time as the forebrain is dividing, the hindbrain is forming two structures: an anterior *metencephalon*, which is the future pons and cerebellum, and a posterior *myelencephalon*, which is the future medulla oblongata. Their cavities, the *metacele* and the *myocele*, become the fourth ventricle.

*Forty-ninth Day.* By seven weeks (Plates 4 and 7), not only has the telencephalon become the telencephalic vesicles, but a further subdivision has also appeared on each vesicle. These new structures are the two *olfactory lobes*, which are a part of the *rhinencephalon*. The more proximal area of the olfactory lobe, also known as the *paleopallium*, forms part of the wall of the cerebral hemisphere. These lobes originally have cavities that are later obliterated.

At the same time that the hindbrain (rhombencephalon) is dividing into the metencephalon and myelencephalon, a new, third flexure appears between these two structures—the *pontine flexure*. Simultaneously, the roof of the hindbrain starts to become thin.

## Development of Nervous System
(*Continued*)

*Three Months*. Growth and development continue, and, by three months, the two smooth-walled telencephalic vesicles, now easily identified as the cerebral hemispheres, have overgrown the diencephalon (Plates 4 and 7). By this time, the *spinal cord* has extended caudally to the coccygeal tip of the developing vertebral column. However, because of differential growth, this relationship between the tip of the cord and the vertebral column changes as development continues. By birth, the spinal cord ends at the level of the second lumbar vertebra (see page 36).

Also, as various parts of the brain change in shape with continued growth, the corresponding cavities adaptively change. As a result, the connections between the lateral ventricles (the former telocoeles) and the third ventricle (the former median telocoele and diocoele) are reduced in size, and may now be identified as the *interventricular foramina* (of Monro). During the third month, the *median aperture* (of Magendie) appears in the roof of the fourth ventricle, followed by the formation of the *lateral apertures* (of Luschka). (See Section II, Plates 8 and 9.)

### Development of Cerebral Hemispheres

As noted above, the telencephalic vesicles have overgrown the diencephalon by the third month and are recognizable as cerebral hemispheres (Plates 4 and 7). Each hemisphere has, by this time, divided into three parts that will differ functionally. The *first part* is the rhinencephalon, the *second part* is the thick basal or striatal area, ultimately the basal ganglia or basal nuclei, while the *third part* is the suprastriatal region, which will eventually be the cerebral cortex and its related underlying white matter.

*The rhinencephalon* began in part as outgrowths from the telencephalon, the olfactory lobes. (In fact, a translation of the word rhinencephalon is "nosebrain.") A second, significant part of the rhinencephalon, known as the *hippocampus* or *archipallium*, also forms a part of the wall of the cerebral hemisphere. This part began as a thickened bulging area on the medial wall of the lateral ventricles.

During evolution, the primitive olfactory sections of each cerebral hemisphere have acquired more complex and sophisticated structures and functions. Therefore, in man, the rhinencephalon includes, in addition to the bilaterally placed olfactory bulbs and hippocampi, such structures as the bilateral piriform lobes, the midline septum pellucidum, the midline fornix and its ramifications and the following bilaterally placed structures: the stria terminalis, amygdaloid body, medial and lateral olfactory gyri, parahippocampal gyrus and cingulate gyrus. In man, the rhinencephalon makes up that wall of the cerebral hemisphere which completely forms the border area where, during development, the superolateral surface of the diencephalon fuses with the inferomedial surfaces of the hemispheres. The rhinencephalon is therefore referred to as the *limbic*

*lobe*, because limbus means border (see Section II, Plates 5 and 6 and Section VIII, Plate 19).

The limbic lobe has profuse interconnections with the thalamus, the epithalamus and the hypothalamus, constituting the *limbic system*. The limbic system is intimately associated with emotional responses and the integration of olfactory information with visceral and somatic information (see Section VIII, Plates 62 to 64).

*Striatal Area*. The *basal ganglia*, or *basal nuclei*, form the second part of the telencephalon (Plates 6 and 7). They are located in the thick basal, or striatal, part of the telencephalic area, and are composed of groups of neuronal cell bodies. One of the more significant and larger of these ganglia is the *corpus striatum*, which becomes closely related, both developmentally and functionally, to the *thalamus* of the diencephalon. Until the end of the third month, the corpus striatum and the thalamus are separated by a deep groove. At about this time, the corpus striatum bulges into the lateral ventricle, while the thalamus protrudes into each side of the third ventricle. As the corpus striatum and the thalamus enlarge after the third month, the groove between them disappears, and they ultimately appear to be fused into one common mass.

*Suprastriatal Region*. In lower vertebrates, such as fish and amphibians, the older two parts of the telencephalon—the olfactory brain and basal ganglia—constitute the full extent of the cerebral hemispheres. In man, however, a third part of the telencephalon becomes predominant. This suprastriatal, nonolfactory part is known as the *neopallium*, which eventually constitutes almost all of the externally visible cerebral hemispheres.

*Cerebral Convolutions*. As the hemispheres increase in size so as to completely envelop the mesencephalon and the upper part of the cerebellum, their originally smooth surfaces become convoluted (Plates 4 and 5). The formation of the surface convolutions allows the outer layer of neurons, the *cerebral cortex* (1.5 to 4 mm thick), to increase greatly in area (to about $2,300 \text{ cm}^2$) without the overall size of the brain becoming prohibitively large.

The first conspicuous *depression*, or marking, to appear on the lateral aspect of each cerebral hemisphere is the *lateral (sylvian) sulcus*, which is evident during the third month. The slowly growing floor of the sulcus, lateral to the corpus striatum of the basal ganglia, is called the *insula*, which gradually becomes completely covered by adjacent areas of the hemisphere. Secondary and tertiary sulci, which are peculiar to the human brain, develop during the final months before birth.

*Continuing Development of Ventricles*. The ventricles continue to adapt to the changes occurring in various parts of the brain after the third month. In particular, the lateral ventricles each develop three *horns*, which protrude into the various lobes of the cerebral hemispheres: the *anterior* horn projects into the frontal lobe, the *inferior*, into the temporal lobe, and the *posterior*, into the occipital lobe (Plates 4 and 5; see also Section II, Plate 8 and Section III, Plate 15). Additionally, each lateral ventricle occupies a more lateral position relative to the third ventricle, and the originally wide interventricular foramen is transformed into a narrow *interventricular foramen* or *canal* (Plate 7). Simultaneously, the initially broad third ventricle reduces to a midline, slitlike cavity that

is quite narrow in its central part where the egg-shaped thalami bulge into the ventricle. Eventually, the two thalami usually bridge the ventricle to produce the *interthalamic adhesion* (Plate 6).

The *cerebral aqueduct*, which is also large in early developmental stages, becomes a long, slender tube connecting the third and fourth ventricles. The fourth ventricle also becomes proportionately smaller, while maintaining its basic rhomboid shape, and the relatively large, slitlike central canal of the spinal cord becomes a minute tube that is usually obliterated after age 40.

### Development of Choroid Plexuses

*The choroid plexuses* are formed in part from ependymal cells lining the ventricles of the brain (see page 135). Those areas of thin ependymal wall that form both the medial surfaces of each lateral ventricle and the roofs of the third and fourth ventricles become invaginated into the ventricles. As the ependymal cells invaginate, they are accompanied by blood vessels, now called the *choroidal vessels*, with adjacent pia mater. This mass is the *choroid plexus* (Plate 7; see also Section II, Plate 9).

A definite line of invagination, the *choroid fissure*, may be identified in each lateral ventricle. It first appears immediately behind the interventricular foramen, and then extends posteriorly in a curved line that ends along the medial wall of the inferior horn. Similarly, during the second month, the thin ependymal roofs of the third and fourth ventricles become invaginated along two parallel choroid fissures on each side of the midsagittal plane. The invaginations into the fourth ventricle extend laterally; ultimately, in the mature brain, the choroid plexuses traverse the full extent of the lateral recesses of the fourth ventricle to protrude through them into the subarachnoid space (Plate 8). In addition, the midline area of these plexuses may protrude through the median aperture of the fourth ventricle.

*Cerebrospinal Fluid*. The choroid plexuses are a source of cerebrospinal fluid (CSF), which fills the ventricles. The fluid escapes through the median and lateral apertures of the fourth ventricle into the subarachnoid space surrounding the brain and spinal cord. The lining of the plexuses forms a physiological "blood-CSF" barrier between the CSF and the blood supply to the brain.

### Development of Reticular Formation

One of the most ancient parts of the nervous system is the *reticular formation*. It is centrally located, and extends from the sacral part of the spinal cord to the thalamus. The reticular formation is a diffuse arrangement of neurons that forms a network, hence the term, "reticular." The brains of primitive vertebrates are made up chiefly of a reticular-type formation. During evolution, when the more organized parts of the nervous system appeared—consisting of circumscribed groups of neuron cell bodies known as *nuclei* and parallel bundles of their axonal extensions known as *tracts*—the reticular formation was retained as an important constituent of the mammalian nervous system.

The reticular formation receives input from both somatic and visceral sensory systems, including visual and olfactory, but is not concerned with discriminitive touch and proprioception. Neurons of the reticular formation transmit this sensory

# Development of Nervous System
*(Continued)*

information to thalamic nuclei which, in turn, transmit it (in general) to the cerebral cortex. This results in a pronounced effect on the waking state by sharpening attentiveness, and constitutes a part of what is known as the *reticular activating system.* Another part of this system is the *arousal-sleep cycle.* The reticular formation is organized to selectively filter all of the varied sensory input it receives. Only certain patterns of its modalities of sensory input trigger the reticular activating system to alert the cerebral cortex.

The *motor functions* of the reticular formation involve reticular neurons that synapse with motor neurons of both the pyramidal and extrapyramidal systems. Other groups of neurons in the reticular formation regulate visceral functions by synapsing with preganglionic autonomic motor neurons. Also, there are respiratory and cardiovascular centers in the reticular formation of the brainstem. Because these centers control such vital functions as respiratory rate, heart rate and blood pressure, injury to the brainstem can result in death.

The development of the more structurally organized parts of the nervous system will now be described.

## Alar and Basal Plates

While the neural tube is forming, a longitudinal groove, the *sulcus limitans,* appears on each side of its lumen, and divides the tube into a dorsal half (*alar plate*) and a ventral half (*basal plate*) (Plates 3 and 6). Because the basal plate does not participate in the formation of brain areas anterior to the midbrain, the diencephalon and telencephalic vesicles must arise from the alar plate. (Note that in the illustrations, the alar plate is colored yellow and the basal plate, brown.)

Within the alar plate, the cell bodies of *sensory* and *coordinating (internuncial) neurons* become located in a layer of gray matter called the *mantle layer* (see page 17). Similarly, in the basal plate, the cell bodies of *motor control (internuncial) neurons* also become situated in a mantle layer. This basal plate mantle layer is located in those areas of the developing brain that become the spinal cord, medulla oblongata and mesencephalon.

In the diencephalic area, a *hypothalamic sulcus,* comparable to, and contiguous with, the sulcus limitans, divides the alar plate into *dorsal* and *ventral* parts. The dorsal part becomes the *thalamus,* in which the cell bodies of sensory and coordinating neurons become located. The ventral part becomes the *hypothalamus,* in which the cell bodies of motor control neurons develop. Thus, the pattern established with the alar and basal plates—namely, that the *dorsal (alar) plate* is the site of *sensory* and *coordinating* neuronal cell bodies, while the *ventral (basal) plate* is the site of *motor control* neuronal cell bodies—is repeated, with the subsequent division of the alar plate of the diencephalon into dorsal and ventral segments. There is a difference, however, in that motor neurons whose axons pass out of the brainstem in cranial nerves *do not arise* from the cells of the ventral segment of the alar plate of the diencephalon, arising as they do from the basal plate of the remainder of the brainstem.

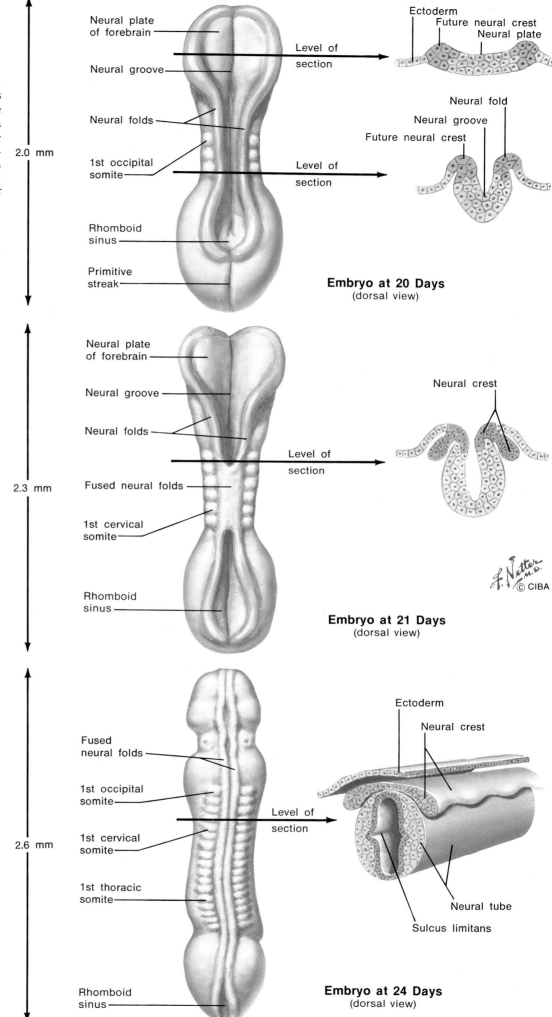

2.0 mm

2.3 mm

2.6 mm

**Embryo at 20 Days**
(dorsal view)

**Embryo at 21 Days**
(dorsal view)

**Embryo at 24 Days**
(dorsal view)

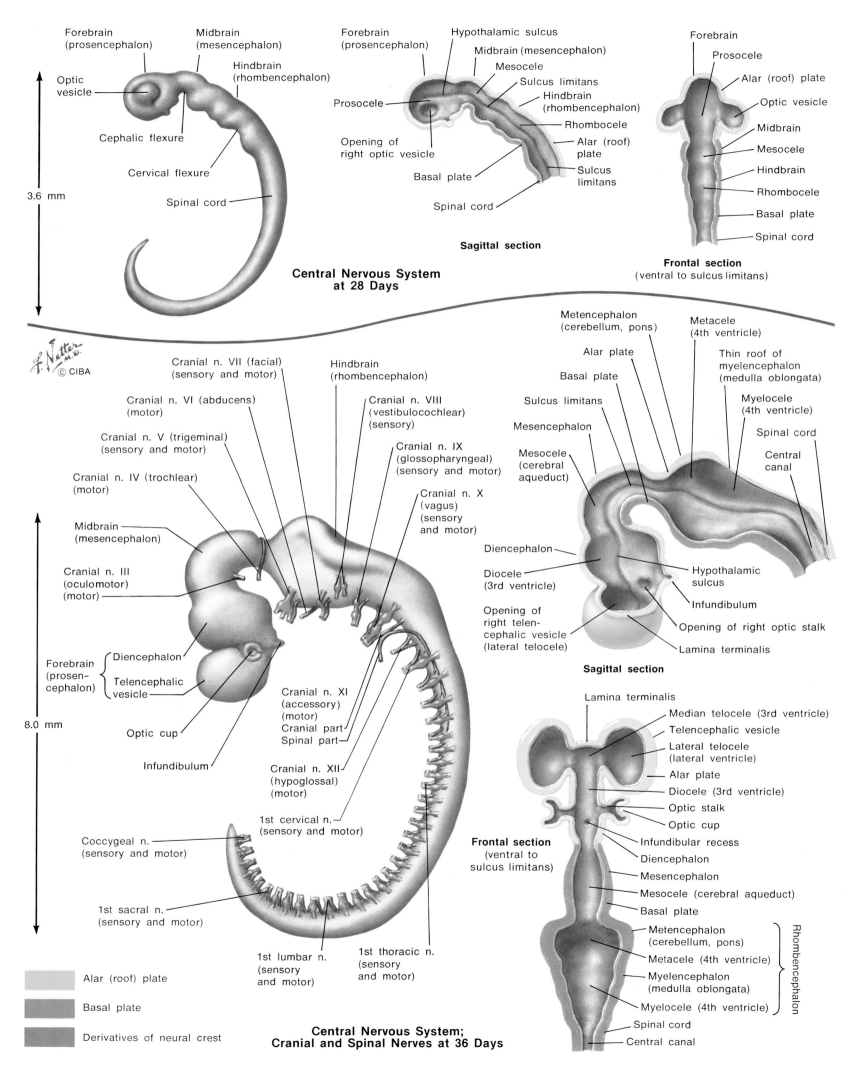

**Central Nervous System at 28 Days**

Forebrain (prosencephalon)
Midbrain (mesencephalon)
Hindbrain (rhombencephalon)
Optic vesicle
Cephalic flexure
Cervical flexure
Spinal cord
3.6 mm

Forebrain (prosencephalon)
Hypothalamic sulcus
Midbrain (mesencephalon)
Mesocele
Sulcus limitans
Hindbrain (rhombencephalon)
Prosocele
Rhombocele
Opening of right optic vesicle
Alar (roof) plate
Basal plate
Sulcus limitans
Spinal cord

**Sagittal section**

Forebrain
Prosocele
Alar (roof) plate
Optic vesicle
Midbrain
Mesocele
Hindbrain
Rhombocele
Basal plate
Spinal cord

**Frontal section**
(ventral to sulcus limitans)

F. Netter M.D.
© CIBA

Cranial n. VII (facial) (sensory and motor)
Cranial n. VI (abducens) (motor)
Cranial n. V (trigeminal) (sensory and motor)
Cranial n. IV (trochlear) (motor)
Midbrain (mesencephalon)
Cranial n. III (oculomotor) (motor)
Forebrain (prosencephalon) { Diencephalon / Telencephalic vesicle
Optic cup
Infundibulum
Coccygeal n. (sensory and motor)
1st sacral n. (sensory and motor)

Hindbrain (rhombencephalon)
Cranial n. VIII (vestibulocochlear) (sensory)
Cranial n. IX (glossopharyngeal) (sensory and motor)
Cranial n. X (vagus) (sensory and motor)
Cranial n. XI (accessory) (motor)
  Cranial part
  Spinal part
Cranial n. XII (hypoglossal) (motor)
1st cervical n. (sensory and motor)
1st lumbar n. (sensory and motor)
1st thoracic n. (sensory and motor)

8.0 mm

Alar (roof) plate
Basal plate
Derivatives of neural crest

**Central Nervous System;
Cranial and Spinal Nerves at 36 Days**

Metencephalon (cerebellum, pons)
Metacele (4th ventricle)
Alar plate
Basal plate
Thin roof of myelencephalon (medulla oblongata)
Sulcus limitans
Myelocele (4th ventricle)
Mesencephalon
Spinal cord
Mesocele (cerebral aqueduct)
Central canal
Diencephalon
Diocele (3rd ventricle)
Hypothalamic sulcus
Opening of right telencephalic vesicle (lateral telocele)
Infundibulum
Opening of right optic stalk
Lamina terminalis

**Sagittal section**

Lamina terminalis
Median telocele (3rd ventricle)
Telencephalic vesicle
Lateral telocele (lateral ventricle)
Alar plate
Diocele (3rd ventricle)
Optic stalk
Optic cup
Infundibular recess
Diencephalon
Mesencephalon
Mesocele (cerebral aqueduct)
Basal plate
Metencephalon (cerebellum, pons)
Metacele (4th ventricle)
Myelencephalon (medulla oblongata)
Myelocele (4th ventricle)
Rhombencephalon
Spinal cord
Central canal

**Frontal section**
(ventral to sulcus limitans)

## Development of Nervous System
*(Continued)*

*Functions of Diencephalon.* Phylogenetically, the *thalamus* is composed of ancient nuclei capable of acting independently of the cerebral cortex to control reflexes related to pleasant and unpleasant sensations. The thalamus exerts this control through its projectional (internuncial) neurons, which synapse with parts of the brain other than the cerebral hemispheres, especially with the hypothalamus. In addition to these ancient nuclei, in man, the larger part of the thalamus is formed by a new (dorsal) group of nuclei. These receive proprioceptive and general cutaneous, visceral, visual and acoustic impulses, which are then relayed to the cerebral cortex via other projectional (internuncial) neurons. However, so many modifications have occurred in the older parts of the thalamus during evolution that the structural and functional relationships of the older and newer parts are completely intermingled (see Section II, Plate 7 and Section VIII, Plate 41).

The *hypothalamus*, which is the ventral part of the alar-derived diencephalon, is a part of the *limbic system*. The hypothalamus controls the function of the *anterior lobe of the hypophysis* through the secretion of neurohormones (releasing factors), while the *infundibulum*, or *posterior lobe of the hypophysis*, is actually an extension of the hypothalamus. The hypothalamus may be considered the motor control headquarters of the autonomic system, which regulates emotional responses and such visceral functions as appetite, thirst, digestion, sleep, body temperature, sexual drive, heart rate and general smooth muscle action of the internal organs (see Section IV and Section VIII, Plates 51 to 64).

*Functions of Telencephalon.* The basal part of each cerebral hemisphere situated anterior and lateral to the hypothalamus is derived from the ventral part of the alar plate (ie, ventral to the hypothalamic sulcus). This basal area is made up of the *basal ganglia*, which contain the cell bodies of motor control neurons. The remainder of the cerebral hemispheres forms the bulk of the brain — the cerebral cortex and its related underlying white matter. The cell bodies of neurons, which are involved in analysis or thought, memory and voluntary and regulatory motor control over the entire nervous system, are located in the cortex (see Section VIII, Plates 43 to 47).

### Cellular Differentiation in Nervous System

As the neural tube takes form, three cell layers develop (Plate 9). Initially, the columnar epithelial cells lining the lumen of the neural tube differentiate into the *ependymal layer* of ciliated cells. (By birth, most, if not all, cilia will have been lost.) Some of the ependymal cells differentiate into *migrating neuroblasts*, which move peripherally to form the *mantle layer*. In turn, the processes of the cells of the mantle layer extend even more peripherally to form an outer region lacking nerve cell bodies, the *marginal layer*. As development continues, the layers form distinct *zones*.

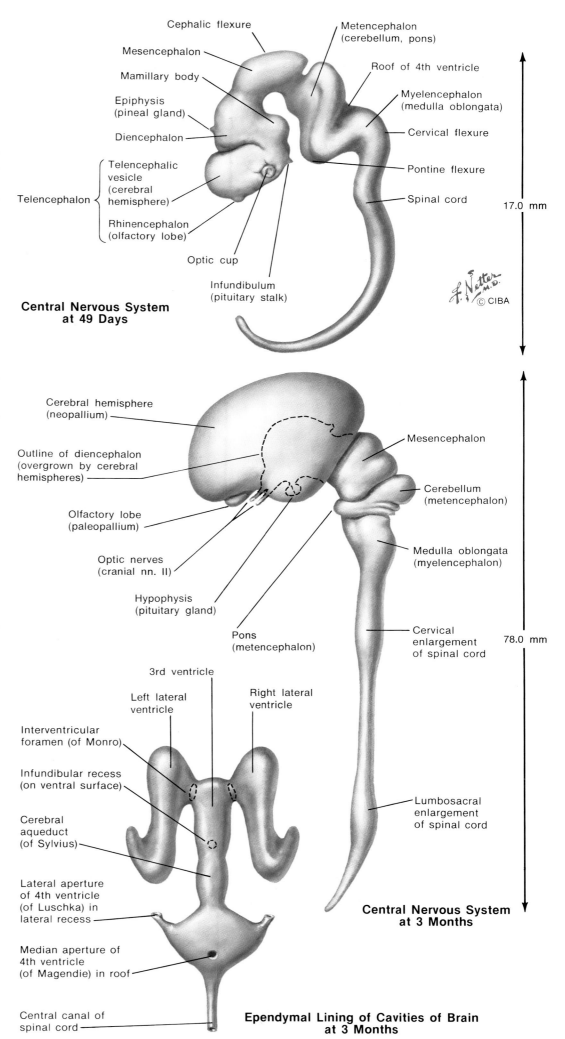

**Central Nervous System at 49 Days**

Cephalic flexure
Mesencephalon
Mamillary body
Epiphysis (pineal gland)
Diencephalon
Metencephalon (cerebellum, pons)
Roof of 4th ventricle
Myelencephalon (medulla oblongata)
Cervical flexure
Pontine flexure
Spinal cord
17.0 mm
Telencephalon { Telencephalic vesicle (cerebral hemisphere) / Rhinencephalon (olfactory lobe)
Optic cup
Infundibulum (pituitary stalk)

**Central Nervous System at 3 Months**

Cerebral hemisphere (neopallium)
Outline of diencephalon (overgrown by cerebral hemispheres)
Olfactory lobe (paleopallium)
Optic nerves (cranial nn. II)
Hypophysis (pituitary gland)
Pons (metencephalon)
Mesencephalon
Cerebellum (metencephalon)
Medulla oblongata (myelencephalon)
Cervical enlargement of spinal cord
Lumbosacral enlargement of spinal cord
78.0 mm

**Ependymal Lining of Cavities of Brain at 3 Months**

3rd ventricle
Left lateral ventricle
Right lateral ventricle
Interventricular foramen (of Monro)
Infundibular recess (on ventral surface)
Cerebral aqueduct (of Sylvius)
Lateral aperture of 4th ventricle (of Luschka) in lateral recess
Median aperture of 4th ventricle (of Magendie) in roof
Central canal of spinal cord

## Development of Nervous System
*(Continued)*

In Plate 6, the three layers are indicated by a distinct color scheme. The outer, marginal layer is colored yellow if it is derived from the alar plate and brown if from the basal plate, following the scheme used in Plate 3. Similarly, the mantle and ependymal layers are colored light blue if they are derived from the alar plate and dark blue, if from the basal plate. A thin black line separates the mantle layer from the ependymal layer. This color scheme is continued in subsequent illustrations to show the derivation of structures in the more developed states.

*Organizational Pattern in Spinal Cord.* In the spinal cord, the basic three-zone pattern is retained into maturity. The *ependymal zone* remains as columnar cells lining the lumen of the central canal. The cells of the *mantle zone* form the gray matter, and those of the *marginal zone* become the white matter.

Gradually, the *gray matter* assumes a roughly H-shaped mass, surrounded by the white matter (Plate 6). Following the pattern established with the division of the nervous system into alar and basal plates, the neuronal cells of the dorsal columns of gray matter (derived from the alar plate) are concerned with sensory and coordinating functions, whereas the neuronal cells in the lateral and ventral gray columns (derived from the basal plate) are motor in function. Similarly, the association and commissural (internuncial) neurons of the gray matter of the spinal cord are formed by other mantle zone neurons (Plate 11; see also Section VIII, Plate 49).

The *white matter*, for the most part, lacks neuronal cells, except for the scattered bodies of supporting neuroglia. Instead, bundles of axons, which arise from neurons located throughout all levels of the spinal cord and brain, form various tracts, or funiculi.

*Organizational Pattern in Brainstem.* The general plan of the spinal cord is continued into the brainstem, even though on casual inspection the two areas appear to have little in common. As in the spinal cord, the cell bodies of sensory and coordinating neurons within the brainstem are located dorsally, while those of motor neurons are positioned ventrally. However, because the brain undergoes a high degree of functional specialization, in the brainstem, the cell bodies of neurons in the mantle zone (gray matter), which have similar functions, become aggregated into masses known as *nuclei*, instead of forming the columns of gray matter as they do in the spinal cord. These nuclei are comparable to the autonomic ganglia of the peripheral nervous system, in which cell bodies of neurons with similar functions are also grouped together (see Section IV, Plates 2 and 3).

The increased specialization of the brain also leads to more complex arrangements of the axonal tracts that constitute the white matter of the brain. Thus, in the medulla oblongata, mesencephalon and diencephalon, the white matter of the marginal zone comes to surround the gray matter, here localized into nuclei.

As noted above, the mantle zone of the brainstem develops into several different kinds of

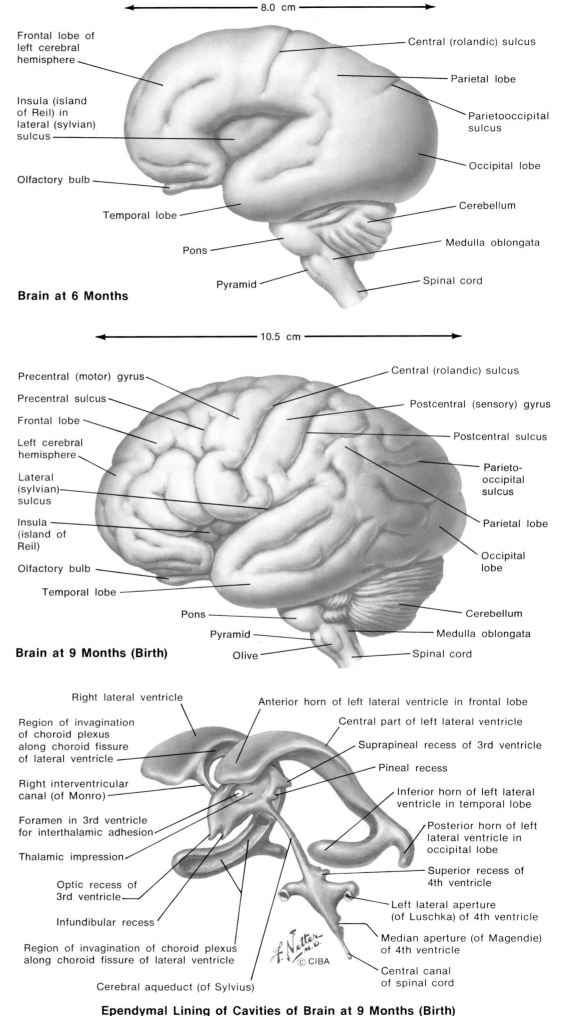

**Brain at 6 Months**

**Brain at 9 Months (Birth)**

**Ependymal Lining of Cavities of Brain at 9 Months (Birth)**

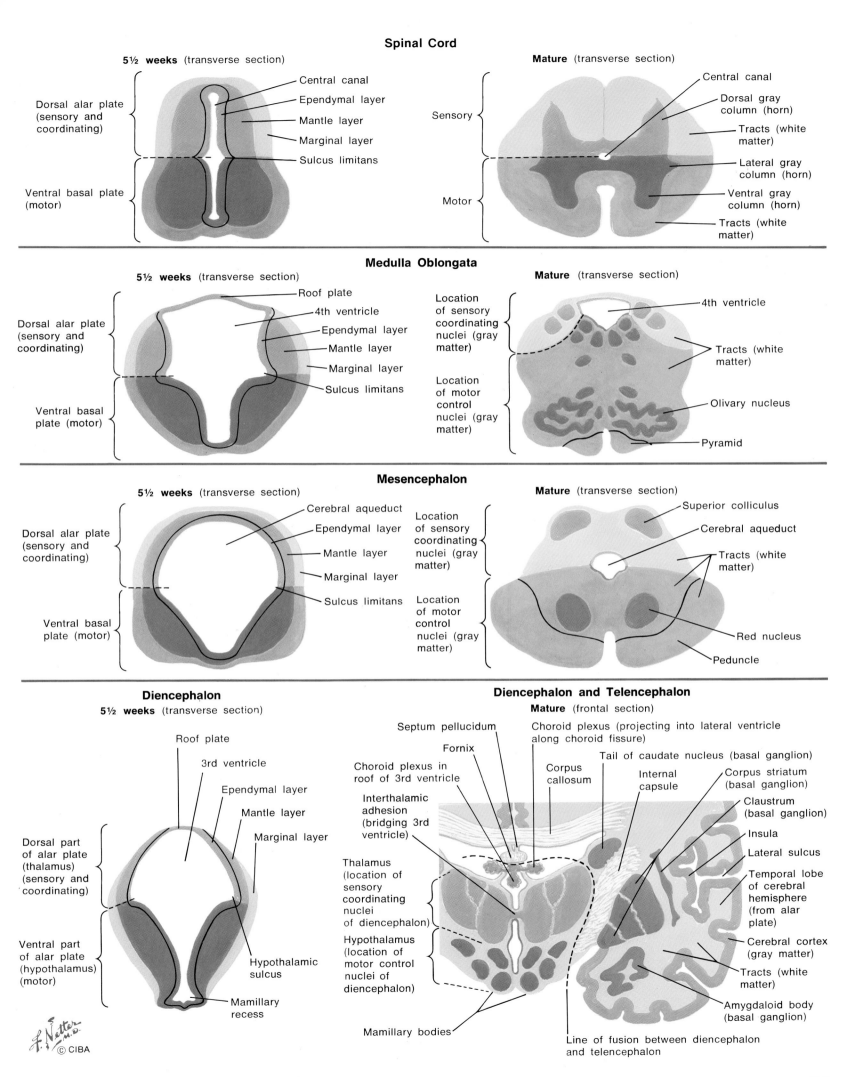

# Spinal Cord

**5½ weeks** (transverse section)

Dorsal alar plate (sensory and coordinating)

Ventral basal plate (motor)

- Central canal
- Ependymal layer
- Mantle layer
- Marginal layer
- Sulcus limitans

**Mature** (transverse section)

Sensory

Motor

- Central canal
- Dorsal gray column (horn)
- Tracts (white matter)
- Lateral gray column (horn)
- Ventral gray column (horn)
- Tracts (white matter)

# Medulla Oblongata

**5½ weeks** (transverse section)

Dorsal alar plate (sensory and coordinating)

Ventral basal plate (motor)

- Roof plate
- 4th ventricle
- Ependymal layer
- Mantle layer
- Marginal layer
- Sulcus limitans

**Mature** (transverse section)

Location of sensory coordinating nuclei (gray matter)

Location of motor control nuclei (gray matter)

- 4th ventricle
- Tracts (white matter)
- Olivary nucleus
- Pyramid

# Mesencephalon

**5½ weeks** (transverse section)

Dorsal alar plate (sensory and coordinating)

Ventral basal plate (motor)

- Cerebral aqueduct
- Ependymal layer
- Mantle layer
- Marginal layer
- Sulcus limitans

**Mature** (transverse section)

Location of sensory coordinating nuclei (gray matter)

Location of motor control nuclei (gray matter)

- Superior colliculus
- Cerebral aqueduct
- Tracts (white matter)
- Red nucleus
- Peduncle

# Diencephalon

**5½ weeks** (transverse section)

Dorsal part of alar plate (thalamus) (sensory and coordinating)

Ventral part of alar plate (hypothalamus) (motor)

- Roof plate
- 3rd ventricle
- Ependymal layer
- Mantle layer
- Marginal layer
- Hypothalamic sulcus
- Mamillary recess

# Diencephalon and Telencephalon

**Mature** (frontal section)

- Septum pellucidum
- Fornix
- Choroid plexus in roof of 3rd ventricle
- Interthalamic adhesion (bridging 3rd ventricle)
- Thalamus (location of sensory coordinating nuclei of diencephalon)
- Hypothalamus (location of motor control nuclei of diencephalon)
- Mamillary bodies
- Choroid plexus (projecting into lateral ventricle along choroid fissure)
- Corpus callosum
- Tail of caudate nucleus (basal ganglion)
- Internal capsule
- Corpus striatum (basal ganglion)
- Claustrum (basal ganglion)
- Insula
- Lateral sulcus
- Temporal lobe of cerebral hemisphere (from alar plate)
- Cerebral cortex (gray matter)
- Tracts (white matter)
- Amygdaloid body (basal ganglion)
- Line of fusion between diencephalon and telencephalon

*F. Netter M.D.*
© CIBA

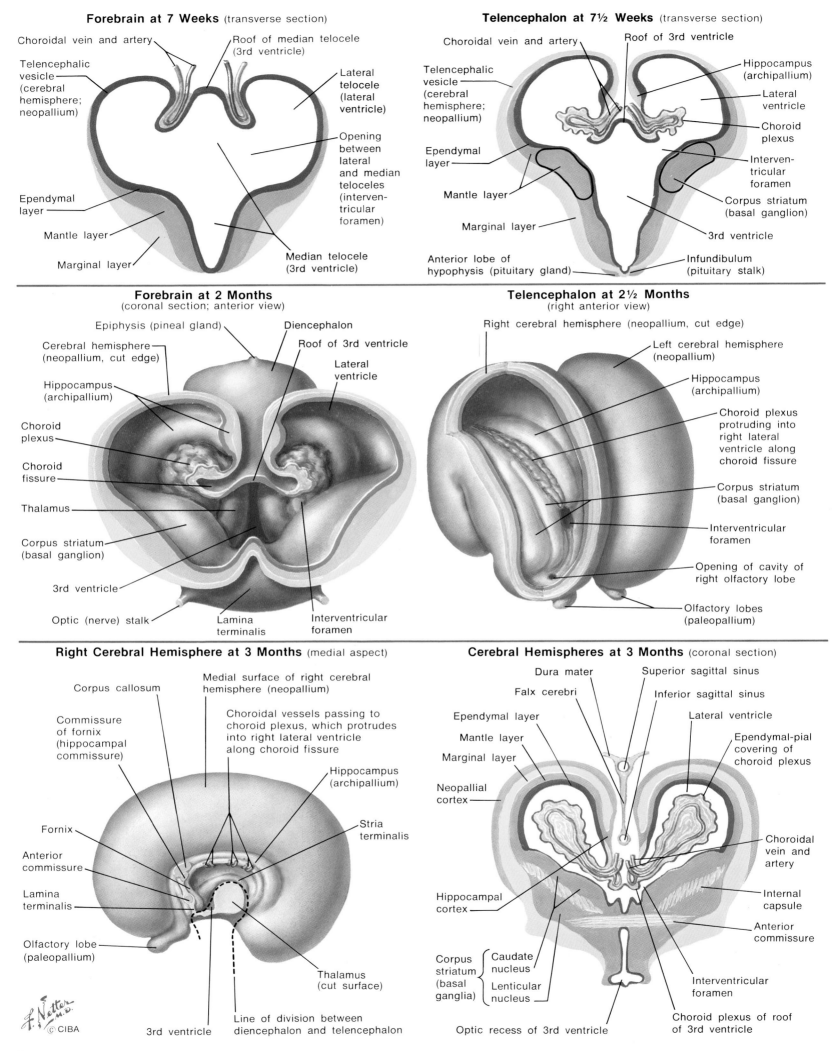

### Forebrain at 7 Weeks (transverse section)

Choroidal vein and artery

Roof of median telocele (3rd ventricle)

Telencephalic vesicle (cerebral hemisphere; neopallium)

Lateral telocele (lateral ventricle)

Opening between lateral and median teloceles (interventricular foramen)

Ependymal layer

Mantle layer

Marginal layer

Median telocele (3rd ventricle)

### Telencephalon at 7½ Weeks (transverse section)

Choroidal vein and artery

Roof of 3rd ventricle

Hippocampus (archipallium)

Telencephalic vesicle (cerebral hemisphere; neopallium)

Lateral ventricle

Choroid plexus

Ependymal layer

Interventricular foramen

Mantle layer

Corpus striatum (basal ganglion)

Marginal layer

3rd ventricle

Anterior lobe of hypophysis (pituitary gland)

Infundibulum (pituitary stalk)

### Forebrain at 2 Months (coronal section; anterior view)

Epiphysis (pineal gland)

Diencephalon

Roof of 3rd ventricle

Cerebral hemisphere (neopallium, cut edge)

Lateral ventricle

Hippocampus (archipallium)

Choroid plexus

Choroid fissure

Thalamus

Corpus striatum (basal ganglion)

3rd ventricle

Optic (nerve) stalk

Lamina terminalis

Interventricular foramen

### Telencephalon at 2½ Months (right anterior view)

Right cerebral hemisphere (neopallium, cut edge)

Left cerebral hemisphere (neopallium)

Hippocampus (archipallium)

Choroid plexus protruding into right lateral ventricle along choroid fissure

Corpus striatum (basal ganglion)

Interventricular foramen

Opening of cavity of right olfactory lobe

Olfactory lobes (paleopallium)

### Right Cerebral Hemisphere at 3 Months (medial aspect)

Corpus callosum

Medial surface of right cerebral hemisphere (neopallium)

Commissure of fornix (hippocampal commissure)

Choroidal vessels passing to choroid plexus, which protrudes into right lateral ventricle along choroid fissure

Hippocampus (archipallium)

Fornix

Stria terminalis

Anterior commissure

Lamina terminalis

Olfactory lobe (paleopallium)

Thalamus (cut surface)

3rd ventricle

Line of division between diencephalon and telencephalon

### Cerebral Hemispheres at 3 Months (coronal section)

Dura mater

Superior sagittal sinus

Falx cerebri

Inferior sagittal sinus

Ependymal layer

Lateral ventricle

Mantle layer

Ependymal-pial covering of choroid plexus

Marginal layer

Neopallial cortex

Hippocampal cortex

Choroidal vein and artery

Internal capsule

Anterior commissure

Corpus striatum (basal ganglia) { Caudate nucleus / Lenticular nucleus }

Interventricular foramen

Choroid plexus of roof of 3rd ventricle

Optic recess of 3rd ventricle

# Development of Nervous System
*(Continued)*

nuclei, generally following the same functional pattern as in the spinal cord. The sensory and coordinating nuclei of the cranial nerves develop from the dorsal (alar) part of the mantle layer, while the motor nuclei of the cranial nerves are derived from the ventral (basal) part. However, there are exceptions, and certain other motor control nuclei, such as the *red nucleus* in the mesencephalon, the *pontine nuclei* in the metencephalon and the *olivary nucleus* in the medulla oblongata, develop from neuroblasts of the dorsal (alar) part of the mantle layer that subsequently migrate into the ventral (basal) part. (In Plates 6 and 8, the olivary and red nuclei are shown in dark blue to indicate their *motor control function*, although their origins are from the dorsal (alar) plate, shown in light blue.) One possible explanation for the unique origin of these nuclei may be found in an understanding of their function. They all have interconnections, via the cerebellum and/or the basal ganglia, which enable them to monitor and coordinate muscle activity in relation to all types of sensory input (see Section VIII, Plates 37, 38 and 46).

Other important deviations from the basic structural pattern of the neural tube occur. Two such variations are the development of the ventricles, and the substantial thinning of the roof plates associated with the formation of the choroid plexuses in the medulla oblongata, diencephalon and telencephalon.

*Organizational Pattern in Cerebellum and Cerebral Hemispheres.* It is in the cerebellum and cerebrum that the greatest deviation from the basic structural pattern of the neural tube occurs. In these areas, migrating neuroblasts from the mantle zone invade the peripheral marginal zone to establish an outer gray cortex (Plate 9).

In the *cerebellum*, the original mantle zone gives rise to an inner level of gray matter composed of numerous nuclei, the largest of which is the *dentate nucleus*. Other migrating mantle zone neuroblasts form the outer *Purkinje cell layer* of the cortex. In turn, certain neuroblasts from the Purkinje cell layer migrate inward to give rise to the deeper *granular* and *Golgi cell layers* (see Section VIII, Plate 36).

Functionally, the cerebellum is the center for smooth coordination of muscular responses, especially those concerned with the subconscious maintenance of normal posture. With its feedback and dampening circuits, the cerebellum serves as a servomechanism to control complicated, integrated movements, such as talking and writing.

In the *telencephalon*, the mantle zone gives rise to the inner levels of gray matter made up of the basal ganglia. These ganglia consist of three parts, the *claustrum, amygdaloid body* and *corpus striatum.* The corpus striatum is, itself, made up of two sections, the *caudate* and *lenticular* nuclei. (Note that in Plate 7, the corpus striatum is shown in light blue to indicate the origin of this and all of the basal ganglia from the dorsal part of the alar plate. However, in Plate 6, which depicts the

mature state, the basal ganglia are shown in dark blue to indicate their motor control function.)

The neurons of the *corpus striatum* participate in the control, by initiation and inhibition, of gross intentional body movements that are normally performed unconsciously. Parts of the two nuclei of the corpus striatum provide background muscle tone while exact movements are being performed. The ancient part of the *amygdaloid body*, however, is closely related to the olfactory part of the cerebral hemisphere. The newer part is included in the limbic system, which interacts with the hypothalamus in the control of the visceral motor activity associated with emotional reactions.

In lower vertebrates lacking a cerebral cortex, the basal ganglia and the cerebellum serve as the

automatic brain regulators of muscle function related to posture and locomotion and to voluntary movements. Consequently, these areas of the brain are classified as part of the *extrapyramidal motor system*. By contrast, in man, voluntary control of muscle function is almost exclusively regulated through descending projectional tracts that arise from neurons in the cerebral motor cortex, constituting the *pyramidal motor system* (see Section VIII, Plates 45 and 46).

Initially, the basic neural tube structure of inner ependymal, intermediate mantle and outer marginal layers is also apparent in the wall of the neopallial section of the cerebral hemispheres. However, during the third month, migrating neuroblasts from the mantle zone pass into the

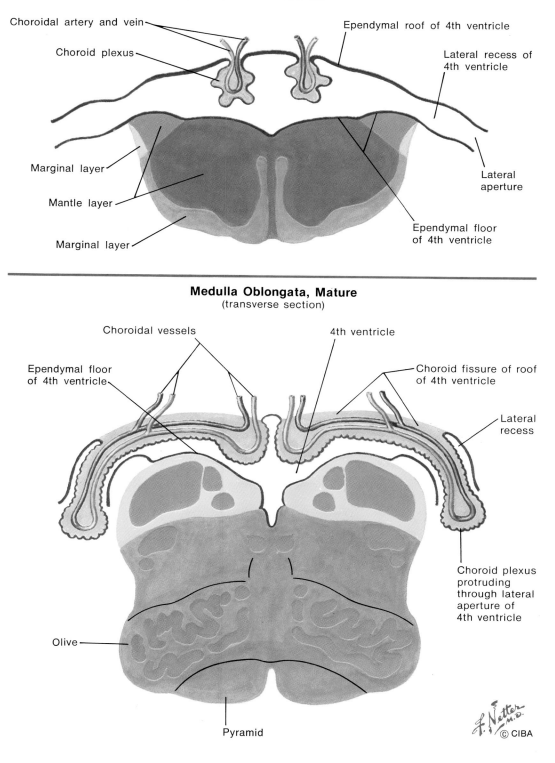

**Medulla Oblongata at 3½ Months**
(transverse section)

Choroidal artery and vein

Choroid plexus

Ependymal roof of 4th ventricle

Lateral recess of 4th ventricle

Marginal layer

Mantle layer

Marginal layer

Lateral aperture

Ependymal floor of 4th ventricle

**Medulla Oblongata, Mature**
(transverse section)

Choroidal vessels

4th ventricle

Ependymal floor of 4th ventricle

Choroid fissure of roof of 4th ventricle

Lateral recess

Choroid plexus protruding through lateral aperture of 4th ventricle

Olive

Pyramid

© CIBA

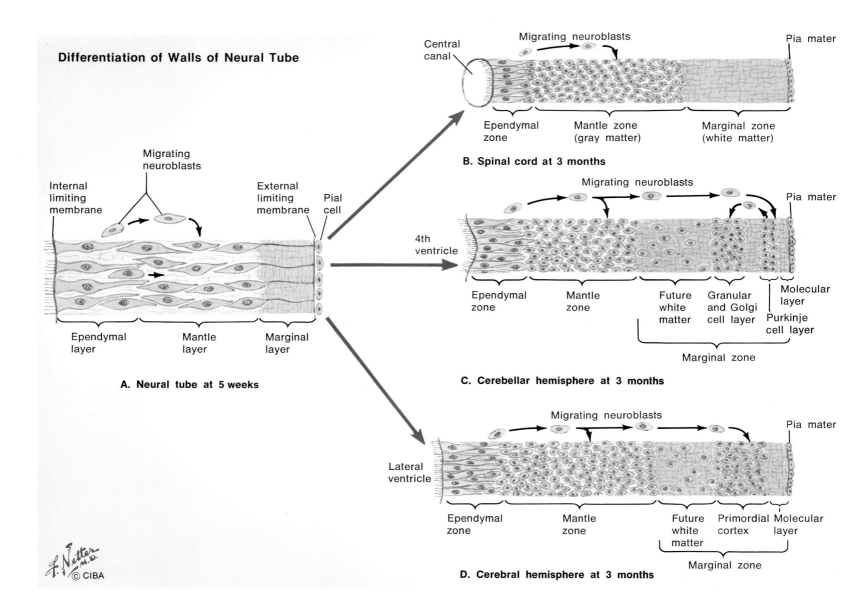

**Differentiation of Walls of Neural Tube**

Migrating neuroblasts

Central canal

Pia mater

Ependymal zone | Mantle zone (gray matter) | Marginal zone (white matter)

**B. Spinal cord at 3 months**

Internal limiting membrane

Migrating neuroblasts

External limiting membrane

Pial cell

Ependymal layer | Mantle layer | Marginal layer

**A. Neural tube at 5 weeks**

Migrating neuroblasts

4th ventricle

Pia mater

Ependymal zone | Mantle zone | Future white matter | Granular and Golgi cell layer | Purkinje cell layer | Molecular layer

Marginal zone

**C. Cerebellar hemisphere at 3 months**

Migrating neuroblasts

Lateral ventricle

Pia mater

Ependymal zone | Mantle zone | Future white matter | Primordial cortex | Molecular layer

Marginal zone

**D. Cerebral hemisphere at 3 months**

SECTION VII PLATES 9 AND 10

# Development of Nervous System
*(Continued)*

marginal zone to give rise to the neopallial *cerebral cortex*. Stratification within the cortex proceeds and, at six months, the six layers of cell bodies and their processes, which characterize the cerebral cortex, are demarcated. The final differentiation of the three outer layers is not complete, however, until middle childhood.

By the end of the sixth month of fetal development, nearly all of the neurons of the future nervous system are present, including the almost 10 billion cells of the cerebral cortex. (The 50 to 100 billion cells in the complete, mature cortex are chiefly glial cells, which are described below.) Extensions of the neuronal cells, the *dendrites* of the cortical neurons, begin to develop a few months before birth, although they are still quite rudimentary in the brain of a newborn infant (Plate 10). It is during the first year after birth that the processes of each cortical neuron develop to establish the single cell's ultimate 1,000 to 100,000 (average 10,000) connections with other neurons. In the young adult, the pattern of increasing interconnection is reversed, and the neurons of the brain begin to die in increasing numbers. In fact, by age 35, almost 100,000 cerebral cortical neurons are lost each day.

The unique pattern of neuron development is integral to the complex function of the cerebral cortex, which is primarily a vast information storage area. The cerebral cortex becomes the seat of intellectual reasoning, specialized memory banks and the capacity for symbolic communication. It is the storage site for many of the patterns of motor responses that can be called forth at will to control motor functions of the body. The cortex gives man voluntary control over how he will react to sensory stimuli.

### Development of Association, Commissural and Projectional Neurons

As described above, the thalamus receives all types of sensory input which are then relayed by projectional neurons either to the various nuclei of the brainstem or to the cerebral cortex.

Nearly all of the axons conveying such sensory input to each thalamus have crossed from the opposite side of the spinal cord or brainstem. Those fibers that have not crossed include half the optic nerve fibers, which enter the thalamus on the same side. *Projectional neurons* relay sensory impulses to the cerebral cortex from each thalamus, and there is a corresponding area of the thalamus for each area of the cerebral cortex (see Section VIII, Plate 41). Virtually all projectional neurons to the cerebral cortex, including those of visual and acoustic impulses but not those of olfaction, arise in the two thalami. Activation of a

minute part of the thalamus stimulates the corresponding and much larger area of the cerebral cortex via the axons of the thalamic projectional neurons. These axons pass to the cerebral hemispheres on the same side, and form part of the mass of projectional nerve fibers known as the *internal capsule*. The internal capsule is located between the thalamus and the corpus striatum of the basal ganglia. It is the inner part of the white matter encapsulating much of the basal ganglia. A thin *external capsule* of encapsulating white matter is located between the corpus striatum and the claustrum.

Above and anterior to the thalamus, the internal capsule partially divides the corpus striatum into two masses of gray matter, the *caudate* and *lenticular nuclei*. The striated appearance is the result of interconnecting strands of gray matter between the caudate and lenticular nuclei traversing the white matter of the internal capsule. Not shown in the illustrations are the further subdivisions of the lenticular nucleus into an internal (medial) *globus pallidus* and an external (lateral) *putamen*.

The cerebral cortex contains cell bodies of *association neurons*, which send their axons through the white matter of the hemisphere to end in another part of the cortex of the same side (see Section VIII, Plate 43). The cortex also contains the cell bodies of *commissural neurons*, which send their axons via the hemispheric white matter to

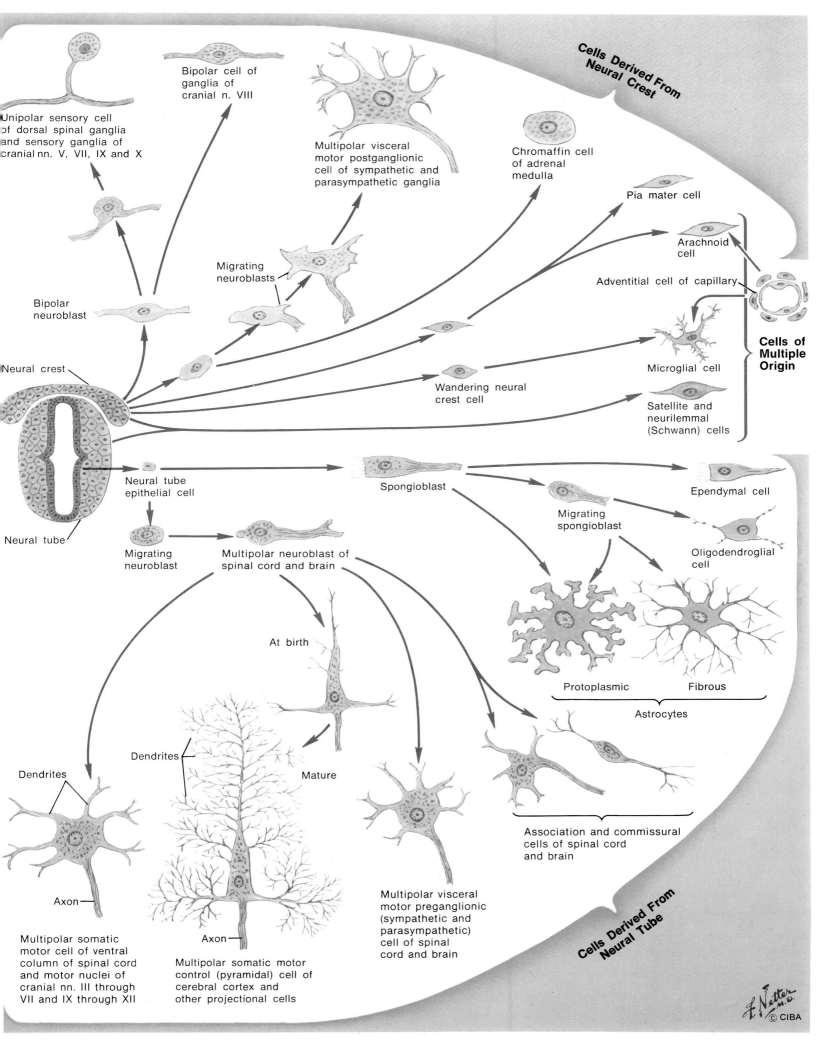

Unipolar sensory cell
of dorsal spinal ganglia
and sensory ganglia of
cranial nn. V, VII, IX and X

Bipolar cell of
ganglia of
cranial n. VIII

Multipolar visceral
motor postganglionic
cell of sympathetic and
parasympathetic ganglia

Chromaffin cell
of adrenal
medulla

Pia mater cell

Arachnoid
cell

Adventitial cell of capillary

**Cells of
Multiple
Origin**

Bipolar
neuroblast

Migrating
neuroblasts

Microglial cell

Neural crest

Wandering neural
crest cell

Satellite and
neurilemmal
(Schwann) cells

Neural tube
epithelial cell

Spongioblast

Migrating
spongioblast

Ependymal cell

Neural tube

Migrating
neuroblast

Multipolar neuroblast of
spinal cord and brain

Oligodendroglial
cell

At birth

Protoplasmic    Fibrous

Astrocytes

Dendrites

Dendrites

Mature

Dendrites

Axon

Axon

Association and commissural
cells of spinal cord
and brain

Multipolar somatic
motor cell of ventral
column of spinal cord
and motor nuclei of
cranial nn. III through
VII and IX through XII

Multipolar somatic motor
control (pyramidal) cell of
cerebral cortex and
other projectional cells

Multipolar visceral
motor preganglionic
(sympathetic and
parasympathetic)
cell of spinal
cord and brain

# Development of Nervous System
*(Continued)*

end in the opposite cerebral hemisphere. It is the commissural neurons that form bridges or *commissures* to allow functional interaction between the two sides of the brain (Plates 6 and 7; see also Section II, Plates 5 and 6).

The *anterior commissure* is the first to appear during development. It interconnects the olfactory amygdaloid nuclei and neopallial cortex parts of the cerebral hemispheres. The second commissure to appear is the *hippocampal commissure (commissure of the fornix)*, which unites the two hippocampal, olfactory parts of the hemispheres. The *habenular* and *posterior commissures*, interconnecting the diencephalon posteriorly in the region of the pineal body, are the next masses of commissural neurons to appear. The largest of the commissures, and the last to appear, is the great transverse bridge of the neopallial parts of the two hemispheres, the *corpus callosum*.

**Cortical Projectional Neurons.** The fibers from projectional neurons located in the cerebral cortex form tracts that pass from the cerebral cortex to other parts of the CNS. An example is the *corticospinal (pyramidal) tract*, which begins to form during the ninth week and reaches its caudal limits by the twenty-ninth week of development. Many of the cell bodies of the motor control neurons of the corticospinal tract are located in the cortex of the *precentral (motor) gyrus* (Plate 5). The pyramidal cells (Betz cells and smaller cells) of the motor cortex have been formed from neuroblasts that migrated from the mantle layer to a position peripheral to the marginal layer, thus establishing the cortex (Plates 9 and 10).

The axons of the pyramidal neurons pass down from each cerebral hemisphere to form the corticospinal tract section of each internal capsule. Farther distally, the two corticospinal tracts pass through the mesencephalon as part of the cerebral peduncles (Plate 6). As the tracts pass through the lower part of the medulla oblongata, they form elevations on the anterior or ventral surface known as the *pyramids*, from which the tracts derive their other name, the pyramidal tracts. At the level of the medulla oblongata, most of the fibers of the tracts decussate across the midline to pass down the opposite side of the spinal cord as the *lateral corticospinal* tract. The uncrossed fibers, which make up the *ventral corticospinal* tract, eventually cross to the opposite side at lower levels of the spinal cord.

The axons of the pyramidal motor control neurons of the cerebral cortex ultimately synapse with *ventral gray column motor neurons*. Thus, the cerebral hemisphere on one side exerts voluntary motor control over the opposite side of the body; as described above, it also receives sensory impulses from the opposite side of the body via fibers that have crossed to enter each thalamus.

## Development of Somatic and Autonomic Neurons

Neuroblasts from the neural tube (mantle layer) differentiate into somatic motor, preganglionic autonomic motor (sympathetic and parasympathetic) and internuncial neurons. Similarly, neuroblasts from the neural crest differentiate into

somatic sensory cells, visceral sensory cells, postganglionic autonomic motor (sympathetic and parasympathetic) neurons and the chromaffin cells of the suprarenal medulla (Plate 10).

The derivation of *internuncial (association, commissural* and *projectional) neurons* has been briefly described on page 140. The *chromaffin cells* of the adrenal medulla are primitive, modified, postganglionic sympathetic cells; their embryological development is discussed in the CIBA COLLECTION, Volume 4, page 77. There remain to be described three types of *motor neurons*—somatic motor, preganglionic autonomic motor and postganglionic autonomic motor—and two types of *sensory neurons*—somatic sensory and visceral sensory.

**Somatic Motor Neurons.** Near the end of the first month, the axons of motor neurons in the ventrolateral walls of the neural tube grow out from the tube (Plate 11). These axons will eventually innervate striated (voluntary) muscle, and will become part of the ventral motor root of a spinal nerve, or of the motor neuron contribution to the following cranial nerves: oculomotor (III), trochlear (IV), trigeminal (V), abducens (VI), facial (VII), glossopharyngeal (IX), vagus (X), accessory (XI) and hypoglossal (XII), (Plate 3; see also Section V). The peripheral somatic motor innervation of striated muscle is accomplished by a single neuron: ie, the axon passes from the cell body of a motor neuron directly to the neuromuscular junction (motor end plate) without synapsing (Plate 12).

**Autonomic Motor Neurons.** The autonomic motor neurons are more complicated than the somatic for three principal reasons. First, unlike the single fiber that carries peripheral somatic motor innervation, peripheral autonomic motor innervation requires two types of neurons—preganglionic and postganglionic (Plates 11 to 13). Secondly, autonomic motor neurons innervate glandular cells, smooth (involuntary) muscle and cardiac muscle, whereas somatic motor neurons only innervate striated (voluntary) muscle. Thirdly, autonomic motor neurons can be either sympathetic or parasympathetic, on a functional as well as an organizational basis (see Section IV).

Neuroblasts from the neural tube, which are destined to form *preganglionic* autonomic motor neurons (both *sympathetic* and *parasympathetic*), arise from the mantle layer of the ventral (basal) plate. These neuroblasts become located in the mantle layer of the neural tube immediately ventral to the sulcus limitans. The axon of each of these preganglionic neurons grows peripherally out of the brainstem or spinal cord to synapse with 100 or more postganglionic neurons.

As the axons of the *preganglionic sympathetic neurons* are growing peripherally, neuroblasts from the neural crest that are destined to become *postganglionic sympathetic neurons* are migrating and collecting into groups of cells, which will ultimately become *sympathetic ganglia*. Eventually, axons of the preganglionic sympathetic neurons synapse with the postganglionic sympathetic neurons in these ganglia. Such peripheral nerve ganglia are similar to the nuclei of the CNS.

The preganglionic sympathetic neurons are limited to the future lateral gray columns of the thoracic and upper lumbar segments of the spinal cord (Plate 6). Hence, the sympathetic system is also called the thoracolumbar outflow system. The ganglia of this system are located on each side

of the vertebral column (sympathetic trunk ganglia) or, in the abdominal region, anterior to the vertebral column (collateral ganglia).

The *preganglionic parasympathetic neurons*, which are derived from neuroblasts of the neural tube (mantle layer of the basal plate), are located in the mesencephalon, medulla oblongata and the second and third sacral segments of the spinal cord. Hence, the parasympathetic system is also called the craniosacral outflow system. Axons of these preganglionic parasympathetic neurons synapse with postganglionic parasympathetic neurons within the walls of the thoracic, abdominal and pelvic viscera.

Neuroblasts from the neural crest that give rise to *postganglionic parasympathetic neurons* also give rise to sensory neurons associated with the same general anatomical areas. Thus, the postganglionic parasympathetic neurons of the thoracic and abdominal viscera are derived from the same neural crest cells that ultimately form the neurons of the vagus nerve, which carries sensory fibers from the thoracic and abdominal viscera. Similarly, the postganglionic parasympathetic neurons of the pelvic viscera have a common origin from the neural crest with sensory neurons forming the sensory ganglia of the sacral nerves.

*In the head region*, the same general relationship holds true, except that the cell bodies of postganglionic parasympathetic neurons are grouped into ganglia that are external to, rather than in the walls of, the viscera they innervate (the *ciliary, pterygopalatine, submandibular* and *otic* ganglia). The postganglionic parasympathetic neurons are derived from the same neural crest cells that give rise to the sensory neurons of the sensory ganglia of the trigeminal, facial, vestibulocochlear, glossopharyngeal and vagus nerves.

As noted above, the cell bodies of the cranial *preganglionic parasympathetic motor neurons*, are located in the mesencephalon and medulla oblongata. The cell axons that synapse with the postganglionic neurons of the ciliary ganglion leave the mesencephalon with the oculomotor nerve. Similarly, the preganglionic parasympathetic cell axons that synapse with the cells of the pterygopalatine and submandibular ganglia leave the medulla oblongata with the facial nerve, while the preganglionic cell axons that synapse within the otic ganglion leave via the glossopharyngeal nerve.

**Somatic and Visceral Sensory Neurons.** The formation of somatic and visceral sensory neurons is closely related to the development of the spinal and cranial nerves, and will be discussed below.

## Development of Spinal and Cranial Nerves

All the sensory cells (both somatic and visceral) of the peripheral nervous system are derived from neural crest cells. With the exception of the bipolar cells of the spiral ganglion of the cochlea and the vestibular ganglion of the vestibulocochlear nerve, all the peripheral sensory cells ultimately become unipolar, although both classes of cell were originally bipolar (Plate 10).

**Spinal Cord.** The future sensory cells migrate from the neural crest and congregate alongside the spinal cord to form, on each side, a single ganglion for each segment of the spinal cord. As these cells transform into unipolar cells, their *central processes* grow into the neural tube to end on neuronal cell bodies of the dorsal gray column part of

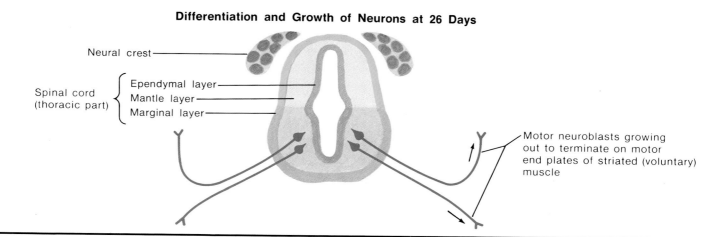

## Differentiation and Growth of Neurons at 26 Days

Neural crest

Spinal cord (thoracic part) { Ependymal layer / Mantle layer / Marginal layer

Motor neuroblasts growing out to terminate on motor end plates of striated (voluntary) muscle

## Differentiation and Growth of Neurons at 28 Days (right side of diagram shows newly acquired neurons only)

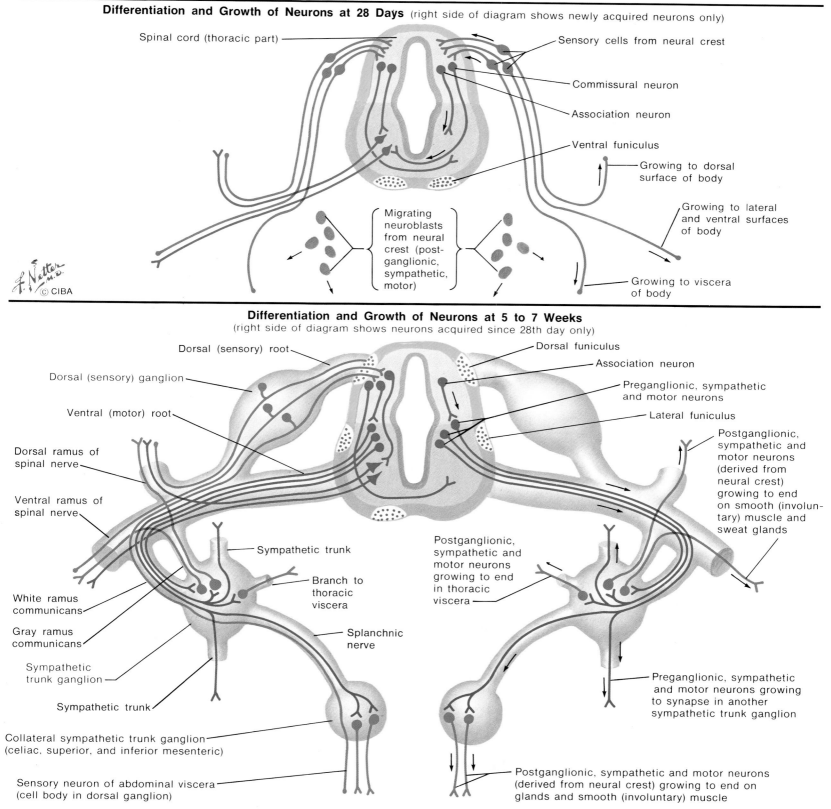

Spinal cord (thoracic part)

Sensory cells from neural crest

Commissural neuron

Association neuron

Ventral funiculus

Growing to dorsal surface of body

Growing to lateral and ventral surfaces of body

Migrating neuroblasts from neural crest (post-ganglionic, sympathetic, motor)

Growing to viscera of body

## Differentiation and Growth of Neurons at 5 to 7 Weeks
(right side of diagram shows neurons acquired since 28th day only)

Dorsal (sensory) root

Dorsal (sensory) ganglion

Ventral (motor) root

Dorsal ramus of spinal nerve

Ventral ramus of spinal nerve

White ramus communicans

Gray ramus communicans

Sympathetic trunk ganglion

Sympathetic trunk

Collateral sympathetic trunk ganglion (celiac, superior, and inferior mesenteric)

Sensory neuron of abdominal viscera (cell body in dorsal ganglion)

Dorsal funiculus

Association neuron

Preganglionic, sympathetic and motor neurons

Lateral funiculus

Postganglionic, sympathetic and motor neurons (derived from neural crest) growing to end on smooth (involuntary) muscle and sweat glands

Sympathetic trunk

Branch to thoracic viscera

Splanchnic nerve

Postganglionic, sympathetic and motor neurons growing to end in thoracic viscera

Preganglionic, sympathetic and motor neurons growing to synapse in another sympathetic trunk ganglion

Postganglionic, sympathetic and motor neurons (derived from neural crest) growing to end on glands and smooth (involuntary) muscle

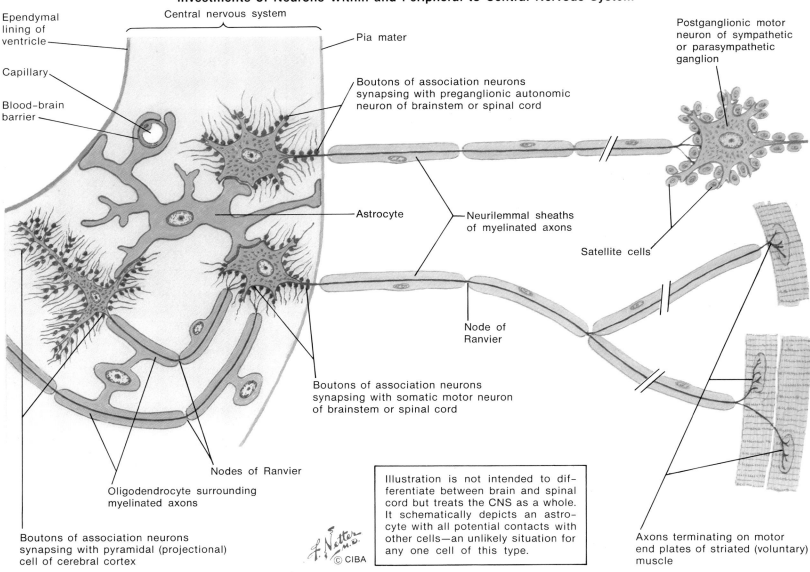

Ependymal lining of ventricle

Capillary

Blood-brain barrier

Central nervous system

Pia mater

Boutons of association neurons synapsing with preganglionic autonomic neuron of brainstem or spinal cord

Postganglionic motor neuron of sympathetic or parasympathetic ganglion

Astrocyte

Neurilemmal sheaths of myelinated axons

Satellite cells

Node of Ranvier

Boutons of association neurons synapsing with somatic motor neuron of brainstem or spinal cord

Nodes of Ranvier

Oligodendrocyte surrounding myelinated axons

Illustration is not intended to differentiate between brain and spinal cord but treats the CNS as a whole. It schematically depicts an astrocyte with all potential contacts with other cells—an unlikely situation for any one cell of this type.

Axons terminating on motor end plates of striated (voluntary) muscle

Boutons of association neurons synapsing with pyramidal (projectional) cell of cerebral cortex

SECTION VII PLATE 12

## Development of Nervous System
*(Continued)*

the mantle layer (Plates 11 and 13). Simultaneously, the *peripheral processes* grow distally to become enveloped in a sleeve of connective tissue along with the motor root fibers, or axons, of the same segment of the spinal cord; this combination constitutes a *spinal nerve*.

**Cranial Nerves.** In the brain region, the neural crest cells migrate to form sensory ganglia only in relation to the *trigeminal, facial, vestibulocochlear, glossopharyngeal* and *vagus* nerves (Plate 3). Of these, only the vestibulocochlear is purely sensory. (See Section V for details of all the nerves discussed.)

Although the *olfactory* (I) and *optic* (II) nerves are considered to be sensory nerves, they are, in fact, not typical nerves, because the olfactory bulbs and the eyeballs are extensions of the forebrain. Therefore, these "nerves" are actually tracts of the brain.

The remaining cranial nerves, namely, the *oculomotor, trochlear, abducens, accessory* and *hypoglossal*, are motor nerves. Of these, all except the accessory contain sensory fibers of proprioception. The cell bodies of the proprioceptive fibers, instead of clustering to form ganglia, are located

either among the axons of the motor neurons as they leave the brainstem, the trigeminal ganglion or the trigeminal sensory nucleus of the brainstem. Thus, only the trigeminal, facial, glossopharyngeal and vagus nerves have both a sensory ganglion and a motor root.

*The development of the accessory nerve* reveals that the cranial root, or bulbar accessory nerve, is actually an isolated root of the vagus that becomes sheathed in a common tube of connective tissue with the fibers of the so-called spinal root. The cranial root travels only a very short distance with the spinal root before it returns to the sheath of the vagus nerve, where it rightfully belongs.

The *cranial root* of the accessory nerve is composed chiefly of motor neuron fibers that innervate most of the striated laryngeal and pharyngeal muscles. The nerve fibers reach these muscles through the pharyngeal and laryngeal branches of the vagus nerve.

**Unmyelinated axons** are surrounded, or sheathed, by *parts* of either oligodendrocytes (within the CNS) or neurilemmal cells (peripheral nervous system). In either case, the oligodendrocyte or neurilemmal cell is rich in cytoplasm, and each oligodendrocyte or neurilemmal cell usually sheaths more than one axon of this type (Plate 14). Most axons of postganglionic autonomic (sympathetic and parasympathetic) neurons are unmyelinated (Plate 13). In unmyelinated

axons, the spaces between sheath cells, equivalent to the nodes of Ranvier, may be quite extensive.

*Myelinated axons*, by contrast, are those which are sheathed by *numerous layers* of the cell membrane of either oligodendrocytes (within the CNS) or neurilemmal cells (peripheral nervous system). There are differences between the myelin sheath formed by oligodendrocytes and that formed by neurilemmal cells. For instance, a single oligodendrocyte usually forms segments of myelin sheaths for a number of adjacent axons in the CNS, whereas a single neurilemmal cell typically forms a segment of myelin sheath for only one peripheral axon. In addition, the separation of the segments of the oligodendrocytes at the nodes of Ranvier (within the CNS) is greater than the separation of the segments between neurilemmal cells (peripheral nervous system).

### Myelin Sheath Formation

*Oligodendrocytes* and *neurilemmal cells* form myelin sheaths by similar processes (Plate 14). In an action similar to the continuous wrapping of a bolt of cloth, the sheath cell becomes wrapped around the axon many times, with the sheath cell or the axon or both causing the spiraling motion. As the wrapping occurs, the cytoplasm of the sheath cell retracts or is extruded, so that the two layers of the sheath cell's plasma membrane, which originally were separated by cytoplasm,

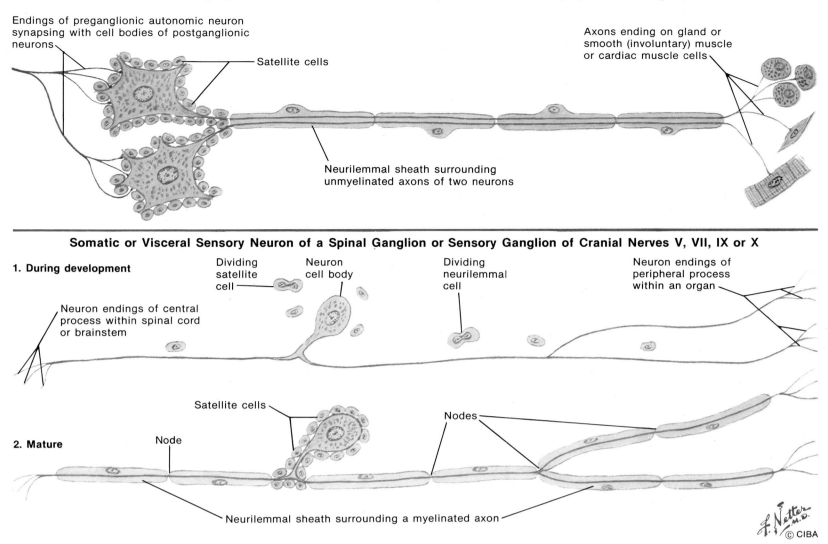

## Two Postganglionic Autonomic Neurons of a Sympathetic or Parasympathetic Ganglion

Endings of preganglionic autonomic neuron synapsing with cell bodies of postganglionic neurons

Satellite cells

Axons ending on gland or smooth (involuntary) muscle or cardiac muscle cells

Neurilemmal sheath surrounding unmyelinated axons of two neurons

## Somatic or Visceral Sensory Neuron of a Spinal Ganglion or Sensory Ganglion of Cranial Nerves V, VII, IX or X

**1. During development**

Dividing satellite cell

Neuron cell body

Dividing neurilemmal cell

Neuron endings of peripheral process within an organ

Neuron endings of central process within spinal cord or brainstem

Satellite cells

Nodes

**2. Mature**

Node

Neurilemmal sheath surrounding a myelinated axon

## Development of Nervous System
*(Continued)*

come together and fuse. Except for small islands of cytoplasm, which may be trapped between the fused membranes, the fusion is complete (Plate 15).

The cell membrane of the sheath cell, like cell membranes elsewhere, is composed of alternate layers of lipid and protein molecules. Thus, myelin is made up of numerous fused layers of lipo-protein membrane, and axons covered with fresh myelin assume a white, glistening appearance as a result of a lipid content of 60%. Tracts of white, glistening, myelinated axons make up the bulk of the white matter of the CNS. By contrast, the gray matter (a misnomer since it is actually pink in its fresh state) is composed chiefly of nerve cell bodies, dendrites and unmyelinated axons.

*Rami Communicantes*. The designation of the white and gray rami communicantes of the sympathetic nerves is based upon the axonal constituents of the rami at the invisible microscopic level. The majority of axons of a gray ramus communicans are postganglionic sympathetic and unmyelinated, whereas the majority of axons of a white ramus are myelinated preganglionic sympathetic and visceral sensory. However, when viewed with the naked eye, both the gray and white rami

appear white, because of their outer collagenous tissue sheaths (the epineurium and perineurium).

*Myelination and Function*. Myelination is closely associated with the development of the functional capacity of the neurons. Unmyelinated neurons have a low conduction velocity and show fatigue earlier, whereas myelinated neurons fire rapidly and have a long period of activity before fatigue occurs.

Neurons that ultimately are capable of rapid transmission of impulses become fully functional at about the time their axons become completely insulated with a myelin sheath. The formation of myelin in the spinal cord begins during the middle of fetal life, but is not completed until puberty. Myelin first appears in the cervical part of the spinal cord, and then extends progressively to lower levels. Similarly, during the fourth month of fetal development, the ventral motor root fibers are the first to acquire a myelin sheath, followed by the dorsal sensory roots. The last spinal tracts to be myelinated are the descending motor tracts, such as the corticospinal (pyramidal) and tectospinal tracts. These tracts become myelinated during the first and second years after birth.

In the brain, the process of myelination continues for years. It begins in the third and fourth months of fetal life, when the cranial nerves of the mesencephalon and medulla oblongata start to become myelinated. This sheathing is related to the well-developed abilities of the

newborn to suck and swallow, abilities which are vital to survival.

In general, the motor neurons of cranial nerves become myelinated before their sensory counterparts. Thus, it is not until the fifth and sixth months of development that the sensory neurons of the trigeminal nerve and the cochlear division of the vestibulocochlear nerve begin to acquire myelin. The optic nerve neurons begin to be sheathed at birth, and myelination is completed by the end of the second week after birth.

The *spinal root* of the accessory nerve is actually a unique cervical spinal motor nerve arising from the lateral surface of the upper five or six cervical segments of the spinal cord. The root passes up into the skull through the foramen magnum, and then leaves the skull through the jugular foramen to innervate the sternocleidomastoid and trapezius muscles in the neck.

### Development of Glial Cells

The non-neuronal elements of the CNS are important enough to warrant separate consideration.

The glial cells are the supporting structures of the CNS, and are composed of three types: *astrocytes, oligodendrocytes* and *microglia cells* (see Section VIII, Plate 2). The first two types of cell are derived from *spongioblasts* in the mantle layer, which, in turn, are derived from *neural tube epithelial cells* (Plate 10).

# Development of the Cellular Sheath of Axons

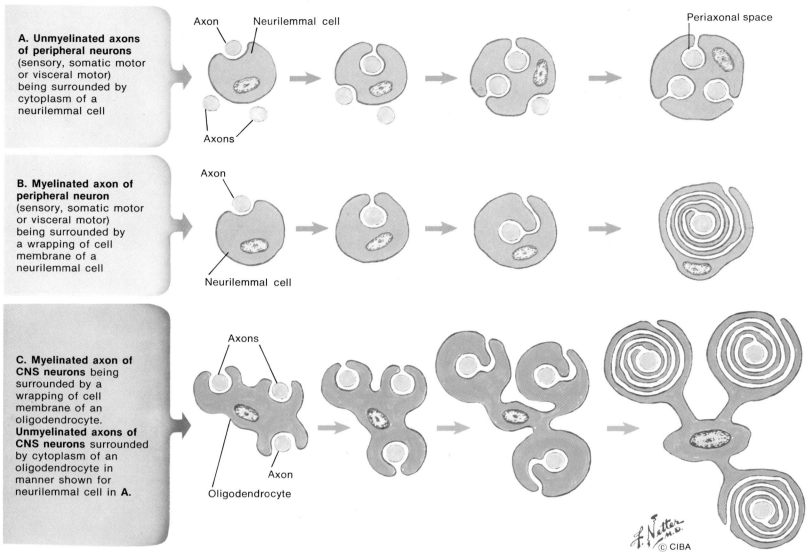

**A. Unmyelinated axons of peripheral neurons** (sensory, somatic motor or visceral motor) being surrounded by cytoplasm of a neurilemmal cell

Axon    Neurilemmal cell    Axons    Periaxonal space

**B. Myelinated axon of peripheral neuron** (sensory, somatic motor or visceral motor) being surrounded by a wrapping of cell membrane of a neurilemmal cell

Axon    Neurilemmal cell

**C. Myelinated axon of CNS neurons** being surrounded by a wrapping of cell membrane of an oligodendrocyte. **Unmyelinated axons of CNS neurons** surrounded by cytoplasm of an oligodendrocyte in manner shown for neurilemmal cell in **A.**

Axons    Axon    Oligodendrocyte

## Development of Nervous System
*(Continued)*

*The microglia* arise primarily from *mesenchyme*, the mesodermal embryonic connective tissue from which all layers of the blood vessels of the brain and spinal cord, including the adventitial layer, originate. Microglia also arise secondarily from the *neural crest cells* that enter the CNS along with the penetrating blood vessels. Microglia are the phagocytes of the nervous system.

*Astrocytes.* Two functionally different types of astrocyte exist. The *fibrous astrocytes* are abundant in the white matter, where they provide both support and binding for the tracts of nerve fibers by means of long, slender, smooth processes. The *protoplasmic astrocytes* are present in great numbers in the gray matter, where they fulfill the many different purposes depicted schematically in Plate 12. In the illustration, the single protoplasmic astrocyte represents a variety of such cells in the brain or spinal cord. As shown, the processes of protoplasmic astrocytes establish close contacts with neuronal cell bodies, blood capillaries and pia mater. Protoplasmic astrocytes occupy the spaces between axons and dendrites.

In addition, because these cells form "bridges" between neurons, capillaries and the CSF by means of boutons (end feet) terminating on the

ependyma and pia mater, they constitute water-ion compartments for the transport of metabolites. Furthermore, the perivascular boutons of protoplasmic astrocytes, in conjunction with the endothelial cells of capillaries, also form a highly selective blood-CSF barrier.

### Development of Sheath and Satellite Cells

As development continues, the nerve fibers (axons) of both the CNS and the peripheral nervous system eventually become sheathed or encapsulated. Within the CNS, association, commissural, projectional, somatic and autonomic motor neurons are—except for their boutons and at the nodes of Ranvier—eventually completely encapsulated by parts of other cells. The cell bodies become covered with the processes of *protoplasmic astrocytes* and the *boutons* of other neurons forming synapses; the axons, whether myelinated or unmyelinated, become surrounded by the glial cells known as *oligodendrocytes* (Plate 12).

In the peripheral nervous system, the neurons similarly become completely encapsulated by parts of other cells, except at their terminal endings and at the nodes of Ranvier. The *neurilemmal (Schwann) cell* is one such cell that sheathes both the myelinated and unmyelinated axons of somatic motor neurons and preganglionic autonomic motor neurons as they pass out of the CNS. These cells, derived from both the neural crest and the wall of the neural tube, also sheathe both

the central and peripheral processes of the somatic and visceral sensory neurons, as well as the axons of postganglionic autonomic (sympathetic and parasympathetic) motor neurons (Plate 13).

A second type of cell, which is derived from both the neural crest and the wall of the neural tube, and which participates in covering the neurons of the peripheral nervous system, is the *satellite cell*. Satellite cells completely encapsulate the cell bodies of sensory neurons in the sensory ganglia of both the cranial and spinal nerves, and also the postganglionic neurons of the sympathetic and parasympathetic ganglia.

Other cells of the neural crest, and, in some instances, mesenchymal cells as well, give rise to cells that form the coverings or meninges of the CNS (see Section III, Plates 11 and 12). In particular, the *arachnoid* develops from both neural crest and mesenchymal cells, whereas the *pia mater* arises only from neural crest cells. The outermost covering, the *dura mater*, is derived exclusively from mesenchyme.

### Myelinated and Unmyelinated Axons

Thus far, axons of neuronal cells of the nervous system have been characterized as either unmyelinated or myelinated, without further explanation.

At birth, the axons of the nerve cells of the brainstem (except the thalamic and projectional fibers to the cerebral cortex), together with the axons of the neuronal cells of the basal ganglia and

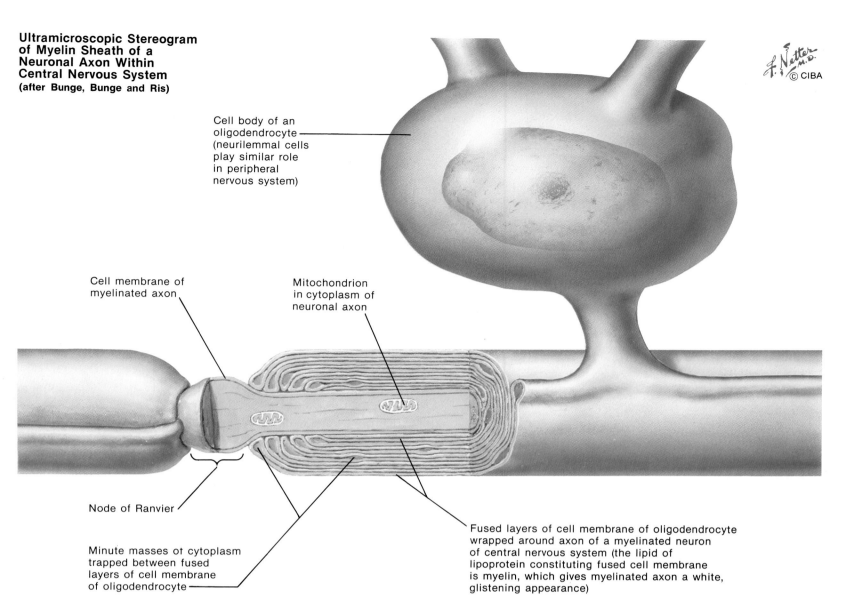

**Ultramicroscopic Stereogram of Myelin Sheath of a Neuronal Axon Within Central Nervous System**
(after Bunge, Bunge and Ris)

Cell body of an oligodendrocyte (neurilemmal cells play similar role in peripheral nervous system)

Cell membrane of myelinated axon

Mitochondrion in cytoplasm of neuronal axon

Node of Ranvier

Minute masses of cytoplasm trapped between fused layers of cell membrane of oligodendrocyte

Fused layers of cell membrane of oligodendrocyte wrapped around axon of a myelinated neuron of central nervous system (the lipid of lipoprotein constituting fused cell membrane is myelin, which gives myelinated axon a white, glistening appearance)

SECTION VII   PLATE 15

## Development of Nervous System
(*Continued*)

the connecting axons between the basal ganglia and the cerebellum, are all myelinated.

Axons of the neurons of the neopallial part of the cerebral hemispheres are among the last to become myelinated, the process beginning only at birth. First, axons of the cortical neurons of the olfactory, optic and acoustic areas become myelinated, followed by those arising from cell bodies in the somesthetic and motor cortices. The last fibers to be sheathed after birth are the projectional, commissural and association axons of the cerebral hemispheres. In fact, myelination of the axons of the association areas of the cerebral cortex continues throughout the adult years.

### Neurohormones

Phylogenetically, as small and uncomplicated organisms increased in size and complexity during evolution, it was essential that a central control system should be developed. Such a system required widespread extensions throughout the entire organism, so that sensory input and functional control over all body regions could be coordinated. The evolving neurons became grouped together to form a central nervous system, and the cell bodies of motor neurons in this

system developed extensions that passed out of the central system to accompany the peripheral processes of sensory neurons. Later, as the body greatly increased in size, some of the cell extensions (axons) became quite long, extending, in tall adults, for a distance of 1.5 m.

These many highly specialized neurons actually evolved from *glandular cells*, and some cells are structurally and functionally intermediate between typical endocrine cells and neurons. In this category are cells of the supraoptic and paraventricular hypothalamic nuclei, which possess axon terminations in the posterior lobe of the hypophysis (pituitary gland) that are rich in both cytoplasmic material and hormones (oxytocin and antidiuretic hormone). These hormones are produced by the neuron and pass along the axon to the hypophysis, where they are stored for release as needed. After being released, these posterior lobe hormones pass to the responsive (target) tissues of the body via the vascular system. Other similar hypothalamic cells secrete so-called releasing hormones that pass to the endocrine cells of the anterior lobe of the hypophysis through blood vessels, and regulate endocrine hormone secretion (see Section VIII, Plates 58 to 60).

The most primitive types of nerve cells in the human body are the *chromaffin cells* of the medulla of the adrenal gland (Plate 10). Although their morphology is typical of endocrine gland cells, these chromaffin cells, like the functionally

related postganglionic sympathetic motor neurons, secrete *epinephrine* and *norepinephrine*. These cells are both derived from the neural crest.

Although chromaffin cells and postganglionic sympathetic motor cells are functionally related because of their derivation and ability to secrete similar hormones, they have functional differences in respect to the extent and effect of their hormone secretions. Chromaffin cells, like endocrine cells, release their hormone (chiefly epinephrine) from a large part of the entire cell surface. After the hormone is released, it passes into adjacent capillaries and is distributed throughout the body via the vascular system. The epinephrine affects glands and both smooth and cardiac muscle to produce a total reaction, such as the "fight or flight" reaction of a threatened individual. By contrast, the postganglionic sympathetic motor cell, with its long, sheathed, axonal extension of cytoplasm, can only release its secretion (chiefly norepinephrine) at the unsheathed terminal endings (see Section IV, Plate 4). Consequently, the released norepinephrine exerts only a very limited and local effect in the particular effector organ.

Characteristically, all neurons secrete specific chemical substances (neurohumors or neurotransmitters) at the terminal endings of their axons, whether such an ending synapses on another neuron or terminates on a gland cell, a smooth muscle cell, a cardiac muscle cell or a striated voluntary muscle fiber (Plates 12 and 13). ☐

# Section VIII

# Physiology and Functional Neuroanatomy

Frank H. Netter, M.D.

*in collaboration with*

Jay B. Angevine, Jr., Ph.D.  *Plates 51–64*

Barry W. Peterson, Ph.D.  *Plates 1–2, 10, 13–39, 41–42, 44–50*

Barry W. Peterson, Ph.D. and Alexander Mauro, Ph.D.  *Plates 3–9, 11–12, 65–66*

Joe G. Wood, Ph.D.  *Plates 40, 43*

# Neuronal Structure and Synapses

*Neuronal Structure.* A typical neuron of the central nervous system consists of three parts: dendritic tree, cell body (soma) and axon.

The highly branched *dendritic tree* has a much greater surface area than the remainder of the neuron and is the receptive part of the cell. Incoming synaptic terminals make contact directly with the dendritic surface or with the small spines (gemmules) that protrude from it. The membrane potential induced in the dendrites spreads passively onto the cell soma, which allows all inputs acting on the neuron to summate in controlling the rate of neuronal discharge through the axon.

The *soma* contains the various organelles that control and maintain neuronal structure: nucleus, Golgi apparatus, lysosomes, ribosomes, mitochondria and smooth and rough endoplasmic reticula. The rough endoplasmic reticulum, studded with ribosomes, is called the *Nissl substance* because of its characteristic blue staining with Nissl stain. The *ribosomes* are the site of synthesis of neuronal proteins; as in other cells, the ribonucleic acid (RNA) templates that control protein structure are transcribed from patterns in the nuclear deoxyribonucleic acid (DNA). The soma membrane is also covered with synaptic endings separated by glial processes. Because of their proximity to the origin of the axon, these synaptic endings have an especially potent effect on the rate of discharge of the neuron.

In humans, the *axon* can extend for several feet. Such lengths pose supply problems, since the neuron must transport proteins and other synthesized substances as far as the axon terminals. Certain key substances are transported, at a rate as high as 400 mm/day, by rapid axonal transport, a process probably associated with the microtubules that originate in the soma and run the length of the axon. Other soluble and particulate substances, including mitochondria, move by *slow axonal transport* at a rate of 1 to 4 mm/day, aided partly by the peristalsislike motion of the axon.

The axon originates from a conical projection (axon hillock) on the soma (as shown in the illustration) or on one of the proximal dendrites. The axon membrane is specialized for the transmission of action potential (Plates 5 and 6). Because of its shape and high excitability, the initial segment of the axon is usually the site of action potential generation. The action potential then spreads down the axon and back to the soma and proximal dendrites. Because of the low excitability of the dendrites, the impulse usually does not spread very far into the dendritic tree.

At its distal end, the axon divides into numerous branches, which end in synapses.

*Types of Synapses.* The most common CNS synapses are those between axon terminals and dendrites (axodendritic) or between axon terminals and somata (axosomatic). *Axodendritic synapses* take several forms (A, B, C). Spine synapses are of particular interest, since they may be the site of morphological changes accompanying learning. *Axosomatic synapses* are of the simple type shown in A. Synaptic interconnections between a number

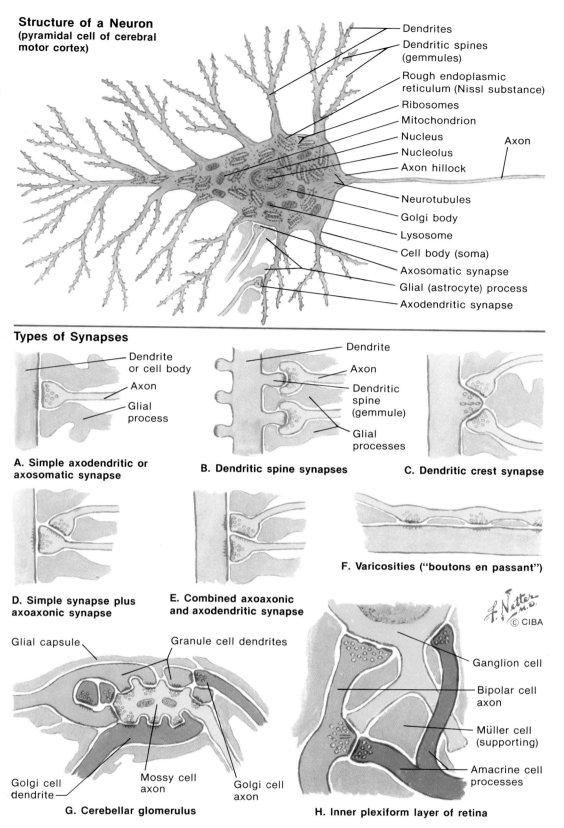

**Structure of a Neuron**
(pyramidal cell of cerebral motor cortex)

Dendrites
Dendritic spines (gemmules)
Rough endoplasmic reticulum (Nissl substance)
Ribosomes
Mitochondrion
Nucleus
Nucleolus
Axon hillock
Axon
Neurotubules
Golgi body
Lysosome
Cell body (soma)
Axosomatic synapse
Glial (astrocyte) process
Axodendritic synapse

**Types of Synapses**

Dendrite or cell body
Axon
Glial process

**A. Simple axodendritic or axosomatic synapse**

Dendrite
Axon
Dendritic spine (gemmule)
Glial processes

**B. Dendritic spine synapses**

**C. Dendritic crest synapse**

**D. Simple synapse plus axoaxonic synapse**

**E. Combined axoaxonic and axodendritic synapse**

**F. Varicosities ("boutons en passant")**

Glial capsule
Granule cell dendrites
Golgi cell dendrite
Mossy cell axon
Golgi cell axon

**G. Cerebellar glomerulus**

Ganglion cell
Bipolar cell axon
Müller cell (supporting)
Amacrine cell processes

**H. Inner plexiform layer of retina**

*F. Netter* © CIBA

of neurons occur within structures of a complex organization, such as the cerebellar glomerulus (G), although all synapses within the glomerulus are axodendritic.

Axons also form *axoaxonic synapses* with other axon terminals (D, E), and these are responsible for the phenomenon of presynaptic inhibition (Plate 9). Axoaxonic synapses are also seen in the efferent vestibular system (Plate 28) and in connection with motor neuron dendrites and other terminals ending on those dendrites.

The CNS also contains several less common types of synapses. *Dendrodendritic synapses* are found in the olfactory bulb (Plate 19). In the

internal plexiform layer of the retina, synaptic interactions involve *synaptic triads* of bipolar, amacrine and ganglion cell processes (H).

Other synapses are those formed between the peripheral axonal processses of sensory neurons and *sensory receptor cells*, as in the inner ear (Plates 25 and 28). Here, the axon terminal forms the postsynaptic element that is depolarized by the presynaptic sensory cell.

The specialized axosomatic synapses formed by efferent motor axons on muscle (motor end plates), and by autonomic axons on secretory cells (varicosities or "boutons en passant," F) are described in Plates 11 and 12. □

# Cell Types of Nervous System

**Sensory neurons** carry information from the periphery to the CNS in the form of sequences of action potentials (Plates 4 to 6). With the exception of olfactory, cochlear and vestibular sensory neurons, all sensory neurons are of the unipolar (modified bipolar) type. The *cell bodies* (somata) of these neurons lie in ganglia generally found outside the brain or spinal cord (Plate 48). The *proximal (central) processes* of these cells enter the CNS via the cranial nerves or the dorsal (posterior) spinal roots and terminate synaptically either on interneurons or, in the case of Group I muscle spindle afferents, on skeletal motor neurons. The *distal (peripheral) processes* of sensory neurons, which may be either myelinated or unmyelinated, terminate in one of three ways:

1. In the *free nerve ending*, the peripheral process branches widely and ends without obvious specialization or auxiliary structures (Plate 13). These endings respond primarily to intense stimuli, and are therefore thought to play a role in the perception of pain.

2. In the *encapsulated ending*, the terminal of the peripheral process is enveloped in an accessory structure that modifies the stimulus before it reaches the part of the nerve terminal membrane where the actual stimulus transduction occurs. Examples of encapsulated endings are Ruffini and Golgi endings, and Pacinian and Paciniform corpuscles (Plate 13). The muscle spindle and Golgi tendon organ are considered to be highly specialized forms of encapsulated endings, because stimulus transduction is also performed by the sensory nerve terminal in them (Plate 34).

3. In the *taste buds* and the *cochlear* and *vestibular systems*, sensory fibers end as synaptic terminals on the bodies of specialized receptor cells (Plates 23 and 25). These cells transduce chemical or mechanical stimulation into a shift in membrane potential, which is then synaptically transmitted to the peripheral process terminal. Action potential initiation occurs in the terminal at a rate governed by the strength of the synaptic influence of the receptor cell on the terminal.

*Olfactory* and *optic afferent neurons* do not fit into any of the three types of endings described above (Plates 18 to 21). Olfactory stimuli are detected by specialized receptor cells, which have axons that project directly to the interneurons of the olfactory bulb. The retina, which is formed by an outgrowth of the brain, differs from other sensory receptor structures in that it contains both receptor cells and several types of interneurons. The optic nerve, therefore, corresponds more to a central sensory tract than to a sensory nerve.

*Interneurons* may be defined as neurons that do not project beyond the CNS; they are by far the most numerous of all neurons, numbering some 20 billion in man. Interneurons may act on other neurons via postsynaptic excitation or inhibition, presynaptic inhibition, or mechanisms that increase or decrease the sensitivity of the target neuron to other synaptic inputs received (Plates 9 and 10). The last-mentioned mechanisms are often elicited by interneurons that employ catecholamines as neurotransmitters and appear to involve cyclic AMP as a mediator in the target cell. Typically, a given interneuron will produce the same response in all the neurons with which it synapses.

Neurons of the CNS are organized in several hierarchical levels, each more complex than the preceeding one. The most basic level of organization is the path of a *spinal reflex* (Plate 33), through which the sensory information that reaches the spinal cord is relayed to motor neurons by a small number of spinal interneurons. *Brainstem neurons* occupy a second level of complexity: they receive sensory input relayed from the body via spinal interneurons and directly from special sensory systems, and then project directly or indirectly back to the spinal cord, where they influence the activity of motor neurons or spinal interneurons. *Cerebellar* and *cerebral cortical neurons* are more complex (Plates 1, 36 and 42). On receipt of sensory input, they act to modulate the activity of brainstem and spinal interneurons or, in the case of pyramidal cells in the precruciate cortex, to modulate the activity of motor neurons. The pathways in the *hypothalamus* and *association areas* of the *cerebral cortex* are indirect and exceedingly complicated (Plates 43 and 56).

Also commonly encountered is the *recurrent feedback loop*. In many instances, the final neuron in the loop is inhibitory, so that the loop functions as a negative feedback circuit (eg, the Renshaw cell, which is excited by motor neuron collaterals and acts to inhibit motor neurons). Instances of positive feedback also exist.

**Motor Neurons.** All neurons that send efferent axons to the periphery can be broadly described as effector, or motor, neurons, which are typically medium-to-large, multipolar cells with long myelinated axons. There are three classes of motor neurons:

1. *Motor neurons supplying skeletal muscles* are located in the anterior horn of the spinal cord, and they project to the periphery via the anterior (ventral) spinal roots (see Section II, Plates 15 and 16). Motor neurons supplying muscles of the face and some muscles of the neck and throat are located in the various brainstem motor nuclei; they project to their target muscles via the fifth, seventh and ninth to twelfth cranial nerves (see Section V). Motor neurons supplying skeletal muscles are of two kinds: *alpha motor neurons*, which supply the main extrafusal muscle fibers and *fusimotor (gamma motor) neurons*, which supply the intrafusal fibers of muscle spindles (Plate 6). The alpha motor neurons have conduction velocities ranging from 50 to 100 m/sec; fusimotor axons have velocities in the range of 20 to 40 m/sec.

Skeletal motor neurons are often referred to as the "final common path," because they integrate all CNS activity controlling a given muscle—from spindle afferent fibers, spinal interneurons involved in spinal reflexes, brainstem nuclei and cortical pyramidal cells.

2. *Extraocular motor neurons* are located in the nuclei of the third, fourth and sixth cranial nerves (Plate 30). Since human extraocular muscles lack muscle spindles, these neurons are all of the alpha motor type. The contractions of these muscles in various combinations direct the eyes during slow (pursuit, vestibuloocular) and rapid (saccadic) eye movements (Plate 31).

3. *The motor innervation of the autonomic nervous system* differs from the innervation of skeletal and extraocular muscles in that two neurons are involved. The first, called the *preganglionic neuron*, is located in the intermediate horn of the spinal cord or in the brainstem and sends a thin myelinated axon to one of the various sympathetic or parasympathetic ganglia. The sympathetic ganglia are located near the spinal cord, whereas parasympathetic ganglia are located close to or within the organ being innervated. Within the ganglion, the preganglionic fiber forms an excitatory (cholinergic) synapse with a ganglionic neuron. The ganglionic neuron then sends an unmyelinated *postganglionic axon* to innervate the target structure (see Section IV).

*Glia.* More than half the volume of the CNS consists of glial cells, which are believed to be important in maintaining the functioning of neurons. There are three basic classes of glial cells:

1. *Astrocytes* occupy much of the space between neural processes in the gray matter. Their processes serve to wall off and separate synaptic endings from each other. Astrocytes also have processes that form end feet, which adhere closely to the walls of capillaries in the CNS. Because of this close relationship, it is thought that astrocytes may play a role in the transport of substances between capillaries and neurons. They may also play an active, symbiotic role in neural metabolism.

2. Another class of glial cells forms the coverings that envelop axons in both the central and peripheral nervous systems and surround the neurons of the sensory and autonomic ganglia. Axonal sheaths of either the myelinated or the unmyelinated type are formed by *oligodendrocytes* in the CNS, and by *Schwann cells* in the peripheral nervous system. The glial cells surrounding sensory ganglion neurons are called *satellite cells.* An analogous type of glial cell is found in autonomic ganglia.

3. *Microglia* comprise the remaining class of glial cells. They are small cells that enter the nervous system from blood vessels and function there as macrophages. Because of their mesodermal origin, microglia are not considered to be true neuroglia.

Although the electrical properties of glial cells have not been shown to play a role in neural functioning, these properties are of interest to physiologists because they influence records of CNS electrical activity. Glial cells are not electrically excitable and therefore do not produce action potentials. Like in many other cells, however, their resting potentials depend on the internal and external concentration of potassium ions. In the presence of extracellular potassium ions freed from neighboring neurons during activity, glial cells can become highly depolarized from their normal resting potential of 90 mV. Astrocytes have also been found to be linked by electrical synaptic junctions. Because of this coupling, the depolarization of glia in one area may spread quite widely and cause current flows that can influence EEG and evoked potential recordings. □

## Some Cell Types of the Nervous System

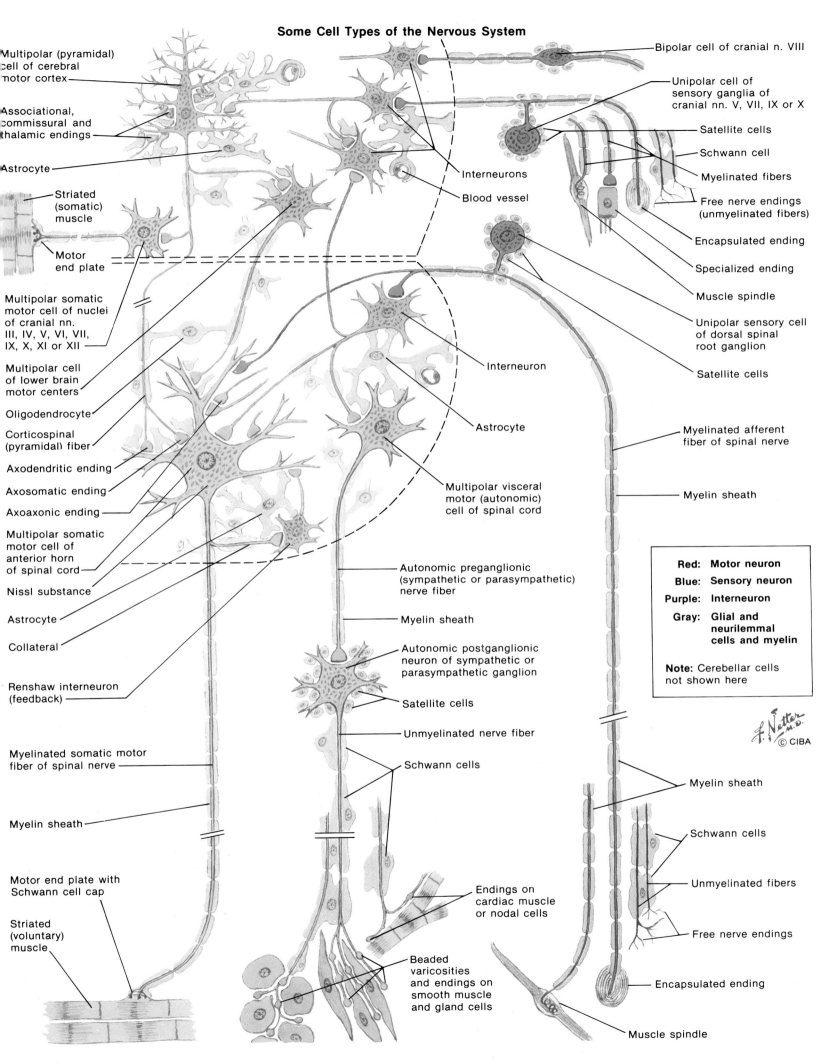

Multipolar (pyramidal) cell of cerebral motor cortex

Associational, commissural and thalamic endings

Astrocyte

Striated (somatic) muscle

Motor end plate

Multipolar somatic motor cell of nuclei of cranial nn. III, IV, V, VI, VII, IX, X, XI or XII

Multipolar cell of lower brain motor centers

Oligodendrocyte

Corticospinal (pyramidal) fiber

Axodendritic ending

Axosomatic ending

Axoaxonic ending

Multipolar somatic motor cell of anterior horn of spinal cord

Nissl substance

Astrocyte

Collateral

Renshaw interneuron (feedback)

Myelinated somatic motor fiber of spinal nerve

Myelin sheath

Motor end plate with Schwann cell cap

Striated (voluntary) muscle

Interneurons

Blood vessel

Interneuron

Astrocyte

Multipolar visceral motor (autonomic) cell of spinal cord

Autonomic preganglionic (sympathetic or parasympathetic) nerve fiber

Myelin sheath

Autonomic postganglionic neuron of sympathetic or parasympathetic ganglion

Satellite cells

Unmyelinated nerve fiber

Schwann cells

Endings on cardiac muscle or nodal cells

Beaded varicosities and endings on smooth muscle and gland cells

Bipolar cell of cranial n. VIII

Unipolar cell of sensory ganglia of cranial nn. V, VII, IX or X

Satellite cells

Schwann cell

Myelinated fibers

Free nerve endings (unmyelinated fibers)

Encapsulated ending

Specialized ending

Muscle spindle

Unipolar sensory cell of dorsal spinal root ganglion

Satellite cells

Myelinated afferent fiber of spinal nerve

Myelin sheath

Myelin sheath

Schwann cells

Unmyelinated fibers

Free nerve endings

Encapsulated ending

Muscle spindle

Red: **Motor neuron**
Blue: **Sensory neuron**
Purple: **Interneuron**
Gray: **Glial and neurilemmal cells and myelin**

**Note:** Cerebellar cells not shown here

F. Netter M.D.
© CIBA

# Resting Membrane Potential

At the resting state of a neuron, the electrical potential of its protoplasm is more negative than the electrical potential of extracellular fluid by approximately 70 mV. This difference across the neuronal membrane is referred to as the *resting membrane potential* (RMP).

Experiments with neurons in both vertebrates and invertebrates (the giant axons and neurons of squids and mollusks are particularly favorable for such experiments) have shown that the RMP is dependent on the intracellular and extracellular concentrations of sodium ions ($Na^+$), potassium ions ($K^+$) and chloride ions ($Cl^-$), concentrations which are normally markedly different. As expressed by the comparative sizes of the rectangles in the illustration, extracellular fluid contains mostly $Na^+$ and $Cl^-$, with only a small amount of $K^+$. Protoplasm contains less $Cl^-$ than does extracellular fluid, a high concentration of $K^+$ and only a small amount of $Na^+$. Also protoplasm contains organic anions (mostly negatively charged proteins and amino acids), too large to diffuse through the neuronal membrane.

Two major factors are responsible for the differences between intracellular and extracellular ion concentrations. The first is that the negative charge of organic anions in the protoplasm must be balanced by a reduced concentration of $Cl^-$ and/or by increased concentrations of $K^+$ or $Na^+$. The second is the presence of an active transport mechanism, the *sodium-potassium ion pump*. This mechanism uses metabolic energy (in the form of ATP) to remove $Na^+$ from the inside of a neuron and replace it with $K^+$.* In the resting state, the rate of transport of $Na^+$ and $K^+$ by the pump is equal and opposite to the rate at which these ions diffuse across the membrane down their concentration gradients. The large differences between external and internal concentrations of $Na^+$ and $K^+$ contribute to the RMP and play a vital part in the production of action potentials.

Studies have indicated that the RMP can best be explained in terms of potentials that result from the tendency of $Cl^-$, $K^+$ and $Na^+$ ions to move down their concentration gradients. By means of the Nernst equation, the equilibrium potential (E) for each ion can be calculated from the concentration of that ion on the inside and outside of the neuron. E represents the transmembrane potential necessary to counter the tendency of the ion to move into or out of the neuron. For $K^+$ at body temperature the equation becomes:

$$E_{K^+} = +61 \log \left[ \frac{[K^+] \text{ outside}}{[K^+] \text{ inside}} \right]$$

$$= +61 \log \left[ \frac{.005 \text{ molar}}{.150 \text{ molar}} \right] = -90 \text{ mV}$$

Similar calculations yield values of $+50$ mV for $E_{Na^+}$ and of $+70$ mV for $E_{Cl^-}$. Were the

*In some neurons, the amount of $Na^+$ extrusion by the pump exceeds the amount of $K^+$ intake by a ratio of approximately 3:2. A pump with these properties is called "electrogenic," because it produces a net transfer of positive ions from the neuron. The net extrusion of positive ions makes the membrane potential more negative and gives rise to passive flows of other ions that preserve electroneutrality.

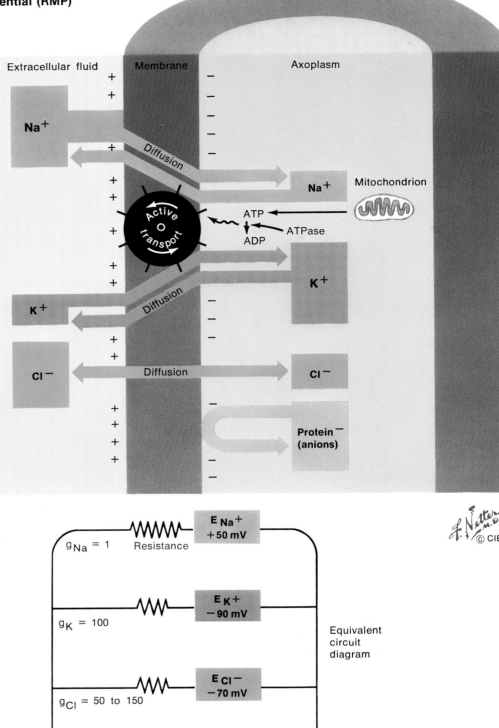

**Resting Membrane Potential (RMP)**

Extracellular fluid — Membrane — Axoplasm

Na+ — Diffusion — Na+ — Mitochondrion

Active transport — ATP — ATPase — ADP

K+ — Diffusion — K+

Cl⁻ — Diffusion — Cl⁻

Protein⁻ (anions)

$g_{Na} = 1$ — Resistance — E Na⁺ +50 mV

$g_K = 100$ — E K⁺ −90 mV

Equivalent circuit diagram

$g_{Cl} = 50$ to $150$ — E Cl⁻ −70 mV

RMP −70 mV

membrane permeable to only one ion, the RMP would be equal to E for that ion. Because the membrane is permeable to several ions, the RMP is calculated by combining E values for those ions weighted according to the permeability of the membrane for each ion. Thus $K^+$ and $Cl^-$, for which the membrane has higher permeability, contribute more strongly to the RMP than $Na^+$, for which the membrane has only 1% of the permeability for $K^-$.

The theory of the RMP is represented by the equivalent circuit diagram. The individual equilibrium potentials produced by differences in ionic concentration act as batteries (each battery is shown as a rectangle) connected in series to a resistor, the magnitude of which is inversely related to the conductance (permeability) of the membrane to the ion in question. A large resistance represents the low permeability of the membrane to $Na^+$; smaller resistances represent its higher permeability to $K^+$ and $Cl^-$. The net potential that results from connecting the three battery-resistance combinations in parallel appears across the neuronal membrane. Because of its thinness and relatively high electrical resistance compared to that of the surrounding cytoplasm and extracellular fluid, the membrane behaves like a capacitor charged to $-70$ mV. □

## Action Potential

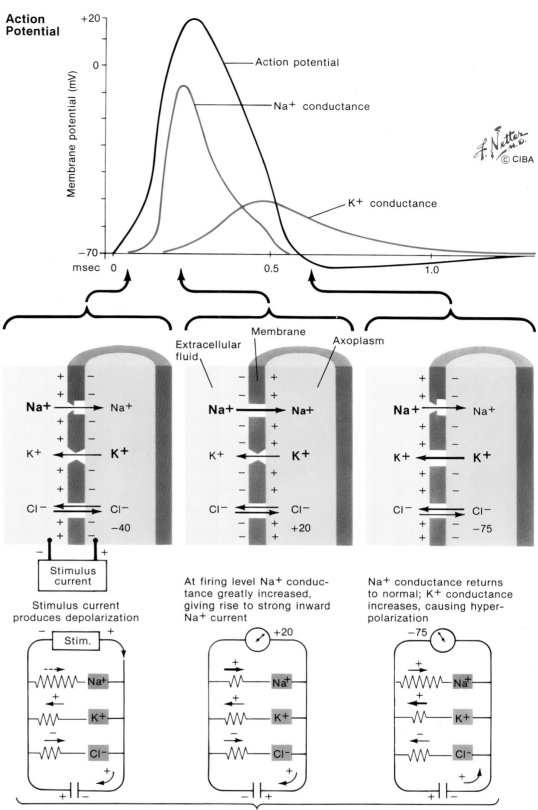

**Action Potential**

If the membrane of a neuron is depolarized from −70 mV to approximately −40 mV, the neuron responds with a brief, impulsive flow of ionic current that shifts the membrane potential to +20 mV and then back to −75 mV, below resting level. This response, the *action potential*, is the basic mechanism that allows the axons of neurons to carry information over long distances.

*Sodium Ion (Na⁺) Permeability.* The principal factor underlying the action potential is that depolarization causes the membrane to become more permeable to Na⁺. This increase in permeability and the resulting increase in Na⁺ influx cause the membrane potential to move in a depolarizing direction—toward the Na⁺ equilibrium potential. If the initial depolarization is greater than a certain *threshold* value (typically, a depolarization of 20 to 30 mV), the membrane achieves an unstable, positive-feedback state in which a further increase in Na⁺ permeability produces further membrane depolarization; this gives rise to yet greater Na⁺ permeability, which in turn causes more depolarization, etc. The overall result is a rapid rise in Na⁺ permeability and a reversal of the membrane potential from its normal −70 mV back to +20 mV. If the initial depolarization does not reach the threshold level, the membrane potential returns to its resting level, and no action potential takes place.

If Na⁺ permeability remained at the maximum level attained during the action potential, the neuron would remain in a depolarized state. However, within 0.5 msec after the initial depolarization, a mechanism known as *sodium ion inactivation* causes the Na⁺ permeability to decrease rapidly to resting levels. At the same time, potassium ion (K⁺) permeability, which increases with membrane depolarization but at a slower rate than Na⁺ permeability, reaches its peak. Because $E_{K^+}$ is −90 mV, this permeability change acts in concert with Na⁺ inactivation to bring the membrane potential back to the RMP.

*Potassium ion (K⁺) permeability*, which is not inactivated, declines slowly with repolarization of the neuron and causes a period of slight hyperpolarization at the end of the action potential. The residual K⁺ permeability also combines with continuing Na⁺ inactivation to make the neuron nonexcitable during a brief *refractory period*.

Three pairs of diagrams show the ionic currents and permeability changes that occur during the action potential. Different membrane pores, or channels, are shown for Na⁺, K⁺ and chloride ions (Cl⁻, based on pharmacological evidence that the voltage-dependent Na⁺ and K⁺ permeability changes can be independently blocked by different drugs (see page 218).

*In the left pair* of diagrams, a depolarizing stimulus current is being applied across the membrane. It causes an inward flow of Cl⁻, enhances the outward flow of K⁺, and reduces the inward flow of Na⁺. Positive current flows into the membrane capacitor and causes depolarization.

*In the center pair* of diagrams, the applied depolarization has caused the Na⁺ channels to open, which has resulted in a strong inward flow of Na⁺ down its concentration gradient. Part of the inward current carried by Na⁺ is balanced by an outward flow of K⁺ and an inward flow of Cl⁻. The remaining current charges the membrane capacitance to +20 mV.

*In the right pair* of diagrams, Na⁺ inactivation has closed the Na⁺ channel and the K⁺ channel has opened, causing an outward flow of K⁺. Part of the current carried by K⁺ is balanced by an outward flow of Cl⁻. The remaining current charges the membrane capacitance to −75 mV. □

# Impulse Propagation

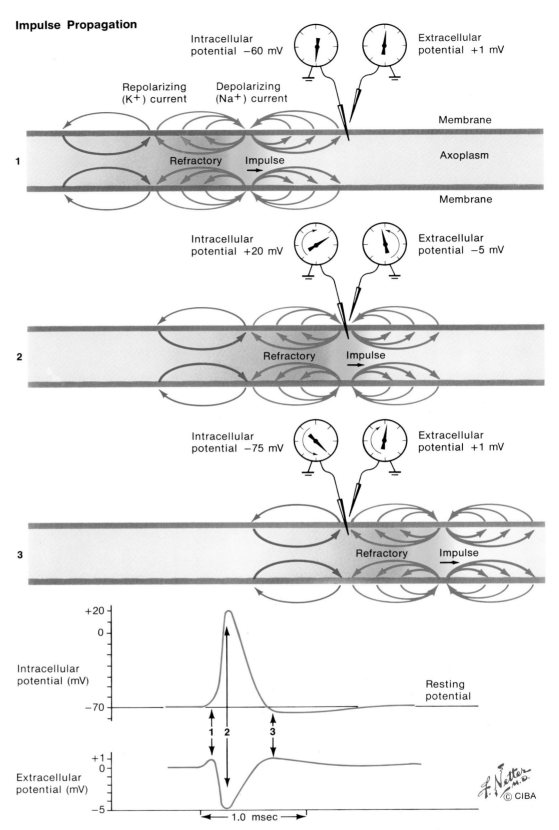

**Impulse Propagation**

The description of the nerve action potential on page 155 applies to a situation in which a long length of axonal membrane becomes active simultaneously. In the case of a normal propagating action potential, only a small section of the membrane is active at one time. As a result, part of the current associated with the action potential in the active region passes through adjacent, inactive parts of the axonal membrane. According to the theory of impulse propagation, this spread of current is the factor responsible for the propagation of nerve impulses.

*Action Potential Propagation.* Three stages illustrate the propagation of an action potential past a point on an axon at which microelectrodes have been positioned to record intracellular and extracellular potentials, each with respect to "ground" (the bath fluid). The intracellular electrode records the transmembrane potential, while the extracellular electrode records the much smaller voltage changes produced by the flow of current through the extracellular fluid.

*Stage 1.* The nerve impulse is approaching the recording point from the left. Inward current flow at the active region gives rise to compensatory outward current flow through a section of axonal membrane on either side of the active region. (The inward flow of sodium ion [$Na^+$] current in excess of that required to charge the membrane capacitance must be balanced by the outward flow of other ionic currents.) The outward current flow is passive in that it is not initiated by a change in membrane permeability, as is the inward $Na^+$ current. According to Ohm's law, such a passive flow of outward current through the membrane resistance causes a voltage drop that depolarizes the axonal membrane at the recording point. The intracellular electrode, therefore, records depolarization of the membrane, and the extracellular electrode records a positive voltage shift caused by the outward flow of current away from the recording point.

*Stage 2.* As the activity approaches, the transmembrane depolarization at the recording point becomes greater, until it reaches the threshold for action potential initiation. At this point, the membrane becomes active. The passive outward current flow shifts to an active inward flow of $Na^+$ current. In accordance with this reversal in the direction of current flow, the voltage recorded by the extracellular electrode shifts from positive to negative. Rather than changing sign, however,

the intracellular potential moves farther in the depolarizing direction. This happens because the inward current flow is caused by a change in membrane permeability to $Na^+$, which shifts the membrane potential toward $E_{Na^+}$($+50$ mV).

The strong flow of inward current at the recording point gives rise to a passive flow of outward current through the axonal membrane to the right and to the left. Depolarization caused by this current triggers an action potential in the axon to the right. Re-excitation of the axon to the left does not occur immediately, because the membrane is temporarily refractory as a result of the passage of the nerve impulse.

*Stage 3.* The axon to the right has become active, while the potential at the recording point has fallen to $-75$ mV. This takes place because $Na^+$ inactivation has returned $Na^+$ permeability to a low level and potassium ion ($K^+$) permeability has increased, thus moving the potential toward $E_{K^+}$ ($-90$ mV). The increase in $K^+$ permeability and the active zone to the right give rise to an outward current flow, which is revealed by a final positive extracellular voltage. Because of the altered permeability of the membrane to $K^+$ and $Na^+$ inactivation during the refractory period, this outward current cannot give rise to another action potential. □

# Conduction Velocity

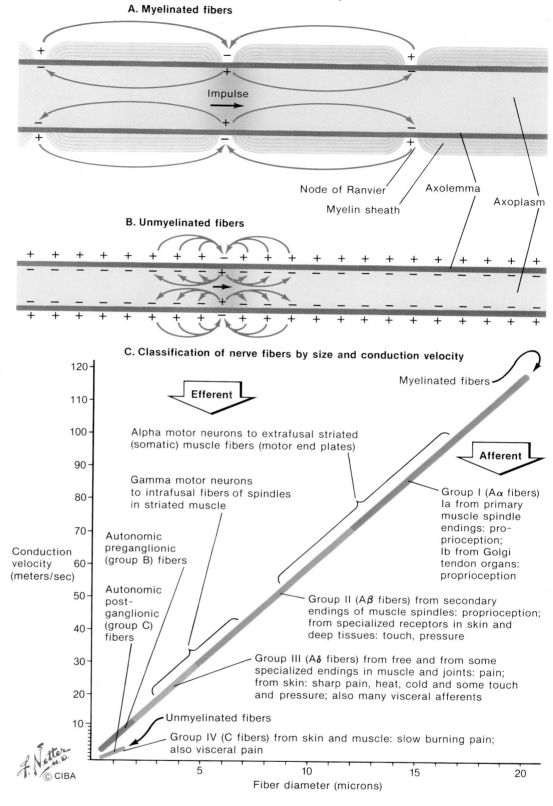

**Conduction Velocity**

**A. Myelinated fibers**

Impulse

Node of Ranvier    Axolemma

Myelin sheath    Axoplasm

**B. Unmyelinated fibers**

**C. Classification of nerve fibers by size and conduction velocity**

Myelinated fibers

Efferent

Afferent

Alpha motor neurons to extrafusal striated (somatic) muscle fibers (motor end plates)

Gamma motor neurons to intrafusal fibers of spindles in striated muscle

Autonomic preganglionic (group B) fibers

Autonomic post-ganglionic (group C) fibers

Conduction velocity (meters/sec)

Group I (Aα fibers) Ia from primary muscle spindle endings: proprioception; Ib from Golgi tendon organs: proprioception

Group II (Aβ fibers) from secondary endings of muscle spindles: proprioception; from specialized receptors in skin and deep tissues: touch, pressure

Group III (Aδ fibers) from free and from some specialized endings in muscle and joints: pain; from skin: sharp pain, heat, cold and some touch and pressure; also many visceral afferents

Unmyelinated fibers

Group IV (C fibers) from skin and muscle: slow burning pain; also visceral pain

Fiber diameter (microns)

The velocity of action potential propagation along an axon depends on the distance that sra-threshold depolarization spreads in front of the active zone. This distance can be increased either by increasing the axonal diameter (which decreases the longitudinal resistance of the axoplasm) or by increasing the transverse resistance of the outer covering of the axon. Increasing the axonal diameter alone (as would be needed in unmyelinated fibers) would require excessively large diameters in order to attain the high action potential conduction velocities observed in the human nervous system. In myelinated fibers, where the transverse resistance is increased by the addition of the myelin sheath, conduction velocities in excess of 100 m/sec are achieved with axonal diameters of less than 20 $\mu$m.

In a myelinated nerve fiber, successive 1- to 2-mm segments of axon, called *internodes*, are enveloped by multiple layers of Schwann cell membrane (Plate 2). Between these segments are short lengths of axon with little or no covering, called *nodes of Ranvier*. According to the saltatory conduction theory, myelin increases the transverse resistance of the internodes, while the resistance at the nodes remains normal. As a result, when the axonal membrane at a node becomes active (A), the passive outward currents produced by this activity are prevented from flowing through the membrane of the adjacent internode; instead, they flow through the membrane of the next node.

The resulting depolarization triggers an action potential at this node. Thus, unlike impulse propagation in an unmyelinated axon (B), which proceeds continuously in very small steps, the impulse in a myelinated axon jumps from node to node and results in a much greater conduction velocity.

As shown in C, mammalian peripheral nerves contain myelinated fibers with diameters of 0.5 to 20 $\mu$m and conduction velocities of 3 to 120 m/sec, and unmyelinated fibers with diameters of less than 2 $\mu$m and conduction velocities of 0.5 to 2.0 m/sec. In 1930, Erlanger and Gasser published a classification of peripheral nerve fibers, based on conduction velocity. Three groups of fibers were defined according to descending conduction velocity, designated A (with subgroups α, β and γ), B and C. A further subgroup, Aδ, was added later. This classification refers to both afferent (sensory) and efferent (motor) fibers, whereas a more recent classification of nerve fibers into groups I, II, III and IV refers only to afferent fibers. This second classification is based on

Lloyd's studies of reflex physiology and is preferred when dealing with muscle afferent fibers (Plate 34).

The properties and functions of the different classes of nerve fibers are summarized in C. In the somatic efferent system, fibers supplying skeletal muscle fibers (alpha motor axons) have conduction velocities ranging from 50 to 100 m/sec (Aα and Aβ ranges), and fibers supplying the intrafusal muscle fibers of muscle spindles (gamma motor axons) have conduction velocities ranging from 10 to 40 m/sec Aγ and Aδ ranges). Autonomic efferent fibers fall either into group B (preganglionic fibers) or group C (postganglionic fibers).

In the afferent system, the larger myelinated fibers carry information from specialized receptors that respond to only one type of stimulus, whereas many smaller myelinated fibers carry information about noxious stimuli that give rise to the sensation of prickling pain (Plates 13 and 14). The function of unmyelinated sensory fibers (group IV, or C, fibers) is not entirely clear. Stimulation of these fibers as a group evokes only the sensation of burning pain, but experiments have shown that many of these fibers carry information about a specific type of stimulus (touch, pressure, temperature), and only a restricted group is specifically sensitive to noxious stimuli. □

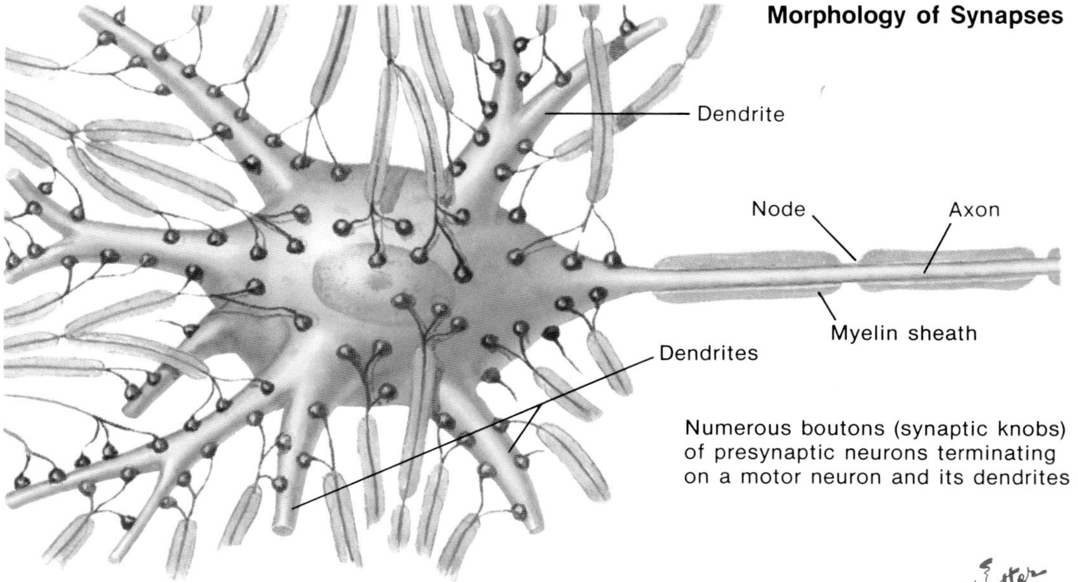

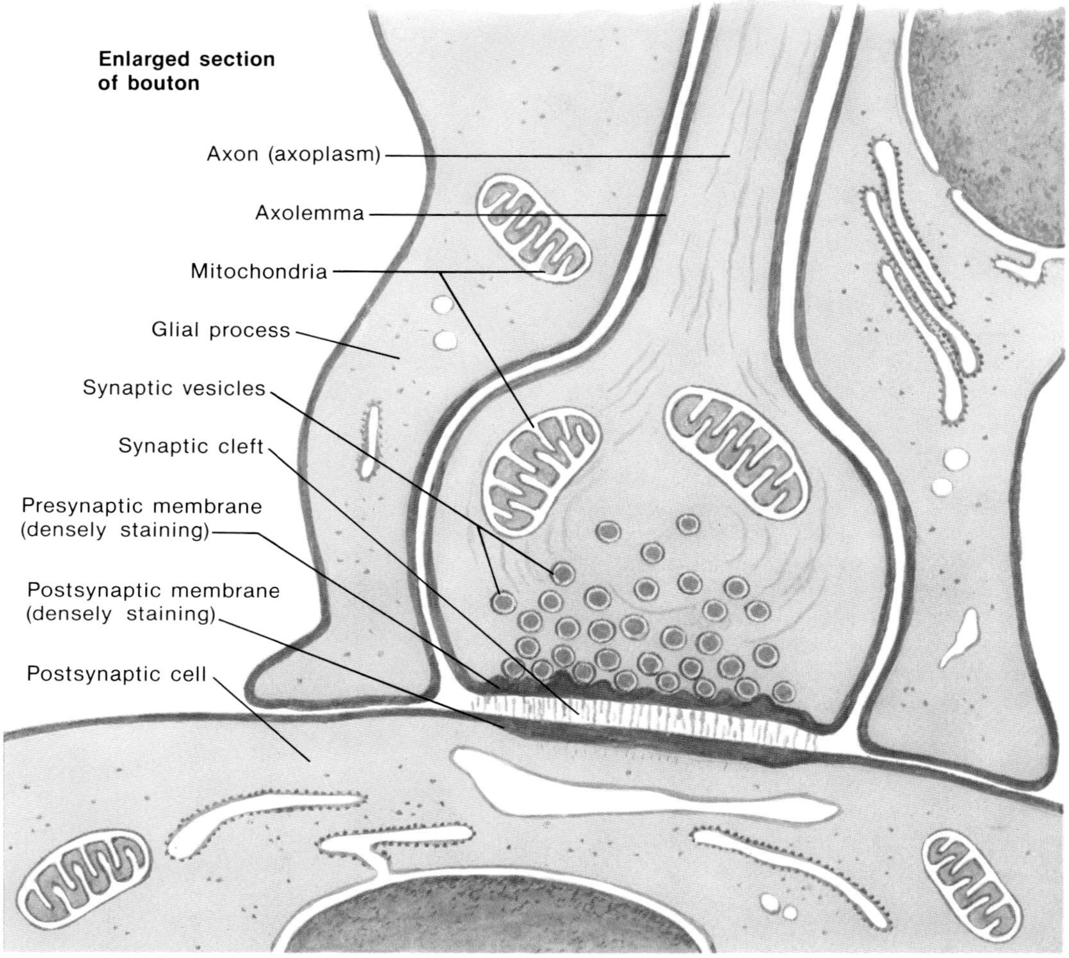

# Morphology of Synapses

Dendrite

Node

Axon

Myelin sheath

Dendrites

Numerous boutons (synaptic knobs)
of presynaptic neurons terminating
on a motor neuron and its dendrites

**Enlarged section
of bouton**

Axon (axoplasm)

Axolemma

Mitochondria

Glial process

Synaptic vesicles

Synaptic cleft

Presynaptic membrane
(densely staining)

Postsynaptic membrane
(densely staining)

Postsynaptic cell

Information is transferred from one neuron to another, or between neurons and receptor or effector cells, at specialized regions of cellular contact called *synapses*. The illustration shows the morphology of typical synapses between neurons in the mammalian CNS.

As shown in the upper half of the illustration, the neuronal axons about to terminate on a motor neuron lose their myelin sheaths and sprout numerous preterminal branches. At the point of termination on the soma or on the dendrites of the motor neuron, the final part of each branch swells to produce a synaptic *bouton*, or knob, which increases the effective area of contact. These boutons cover a large part of the somatic and dendritic membranes, but do not impinge on the motor axon itself, which is covered by a myelin sheath. Areas of somatic and dendritic membrane not contacted by synaptic boutons are covered by glial cell processes.

The lower part of the illustration shows the structure of a typical synapse and the surrounding glial processes as revealed by scanning electron microscopy; this is a chemically transmitting synapse (Plate 8), the only type known to exist in the human nervous system (electrically transmitting synapses are found in invertebrates and lower vertebrates). In the chemically transmitting synapse, the membranes of both the bouton (presynaptic membrane) and the motor neuron (postsynaptic membrane) are intact and are separated by a *synaptic cleft* 200Å to 300Å wide. This distance is greater than the space that separates neurons from the surrounding glial cells, which is 150Å to 200Å wide. Under scanning electron microscopy, both the presynaptic and postsynaptic membranes generally stain more intensely with heavy metal than do nonsynaptic membranes, and this staining often reveals striated or filamentous structures within the synaptic cleft itself. The functional significance of these staining features is unknown.

Boutons contain a unique cellular organelle, the *synaptic vesicle*. These vesicles are round or oval structures, approximately 500Å in diameter, which are bounded by a lipoprotein membrane. They are found within the cytoplasm of the terminal, typically clustered close to the presynaptic membrane. A variety of biochemical and cytological evidence indicates that these vesicles contain the chemical transmitter substance by means of which the synaptic ending produces excitation or inhibition of the postsynaptic neuron. Recent evidence suggests that the shape of synaptic vesicles as seen on electron microscopy may provide an indication of the specialized function of the synapse;

thus, vesicles of excitatory synapses usually have round profiles, whereas those of inhibitory synapses have oval, or flattened, profiles. Synapses with dense-staining cores appear to contain monoamines such as norepinephrine or serotonin. In addition to synaptic vesicles, boutons also contain neurotubules, neurofilaments and numerous mitochondria.

The cytoplasm of the postsynaptic cell contains all of the organelles of typical neurons (Plate 1), and in some cases, shows specialized saclike structures that lie just beneath the postsynaptic membrane. The functional significance of these structures is unknown. □

# Chemical Synaptic Transmission

Chemical synaptic transmission proceeds in three steps: (1) the release of the transmitter substance from the bouton in response to the arrival of an action potential; (2) the change in the ionic permeabilities of the postsynaptic membrane caused by the transmitter; and (3) the removal of the transmitter from the synaptic cleft. Depending on the type of permeability changes produced in the second step, synaptic activation may have either an excitatory or an inhibitory effect on the postsynaptic cell.

As described on page 158, synaptic transmitter substances are concentrated in *synaptic vesicles* within the bouton. Although the exact mechanism of its release is unknown, it appears that the transmitter substance is released in packets, or quanta, of 1,000 to 10,000 molecules at a time, and that the probability of release of these quanta increases with the degree of depolarization of the terminal membrane. Thus, the intense depolarization caused by an action potential actuates the nearly simultaneous release of a large number of quanta. A reasonable hypothesis to account for the quantal nature of transmitter release is that the contents of an entire vesicle are discharged at once into the synaptic cleft, perhaps by the process of *exocytosis*.

Following their release, transmitter molecules diffuse across the synaptic cleft and combine with specific receptor molecules in the postsynaptic membrane. This combination gives rise to a change in the ionic permeability of the postsynaptic membrane and results in a flow of ions down their electrochemical potential gradients. This ionic flow is not synchronous with the arrival of the action potential in the terminal, but begins after a *synaptic delay* of 0.3 to 0.5 msec, which is the time required for transmitter release and diffusion and for the completion of reactions within the postsynaptic membrane, which alter membrane permeability.

The direction of current flow produced by transmitter action depends upon which ionic permeabilities are altered. In an *excitatory synapse*, the transmitter causes an increase in the permeability of the postsynaptic membrane to sodium ions ($Na^+$) and potassium ions ($K^+$). Because of their respective concentration gradients across the neuronal membrane (Plate 3), $Na^+$ tends to move into the postsynaptic cell, and $K^+$, out of it. The negative potential of the neuronal cytoplasm, however, assists the inward flow of positive ions and retards their outward flow, so that the combined electrochemical force for $Na^+$ influx greatly exceeds that for $K^+$ efflux. Thus, the predominant ionic movement across the postsynaptic membrane is an *inward flow of $Na^+$*. As shown, the resulting current flow causes a shift of the postsynaptic cell membrane potential in the depolarizing direction. This depolarizing potential change, which is called an *excitatory postsynaptic potential (EPSP)*, brings the postsynaptic cell closer to its threshold for action potential initiation.

In an *inhibitory synapse*, transmitter action causes an increase of the postsynaptic membrane's permeability to $K^+$ and chloride ions ($Cl^-$) but

## Chemical Synaptic Transmission

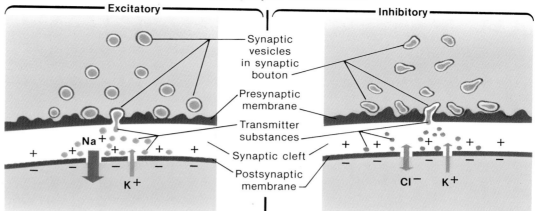

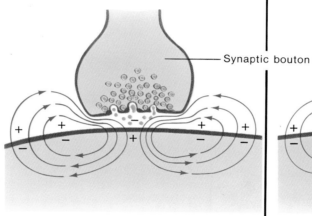

When impulse reaches excitatory synaptic bouton, it causes release of a transmitter substance into synaptic cleft. This increases permeability of postsynaptic membrane to $Na^+$ and $K^+$. More $Na^+$ moves into postsynaptic cell than $K^+$ moves out, due to greater electrochemical gradient

Resultant net ionic current flow is in a direction which tends to depolarize postsynaptic cell. If depolarization reaches firing threshold, an impulse is generated in postsynaptic cell

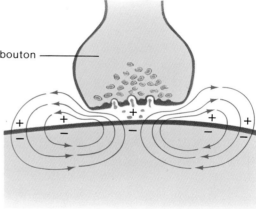

At inhibitory synapse, transmitter substance released by an impulse increases permeability of postsynaptic membrane to $K^+$ and $Cl^-$ but not to $Na^+$. $K^+$ moves out of postsynaptic cell but no net flow of $Cl^-$ occurs at resting membrane potential

Resultant ionic current flow is in direction which tends to hyperpolarize postsynaptic cell. This makes depolarization by excitatory synapses more difficult—more depolarization is required to reach threshold

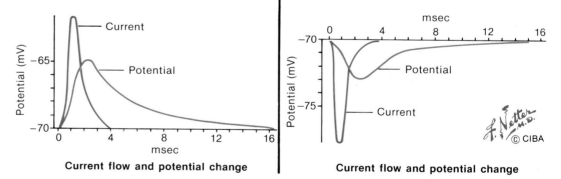

**Current flow and potential change**

**Current flow and potential change**

not to $Na^+$. Since $Cl^-$ is approximately at electrochemical equilibrium across the neuronal membrane, the major ionic movement is an *outward flow of $K^+$*. The resulting current flow is in the opposite direction to that of the current flow in an excitatory synapse, and gives rise to a shift of the postsynaptic cell membrane potential in the hyperpolarizing direction. This hyperpolarizing potential change, which is called an *inhibitory postsynaptic potential (IPSP)*, moves the membrane potential away from the threshold for action potential initiation. The increased ionic permeability of the postsynaptic membrane also contributes to the inhibitory effect by tending to "short

out" any membrane depolarization occurring simultaneously.

As shown, the ionic current and the resulting membrane potential change have different time courses because the synaptic current charges the membrane capacitance, which then discharges passively over a period of 10 to 15 msec. The short duration of the synaptic current is the consequence of the removal of transmitter from the synaptic cleft. This removal is accomplished in part by passive diffusion, and in part, by specific mechanisms that lead to transmitter uptake by surrounding cells or transmitter breakdown by enzymatic degradation. □

# Synaptic Inhibitory Mechanisms

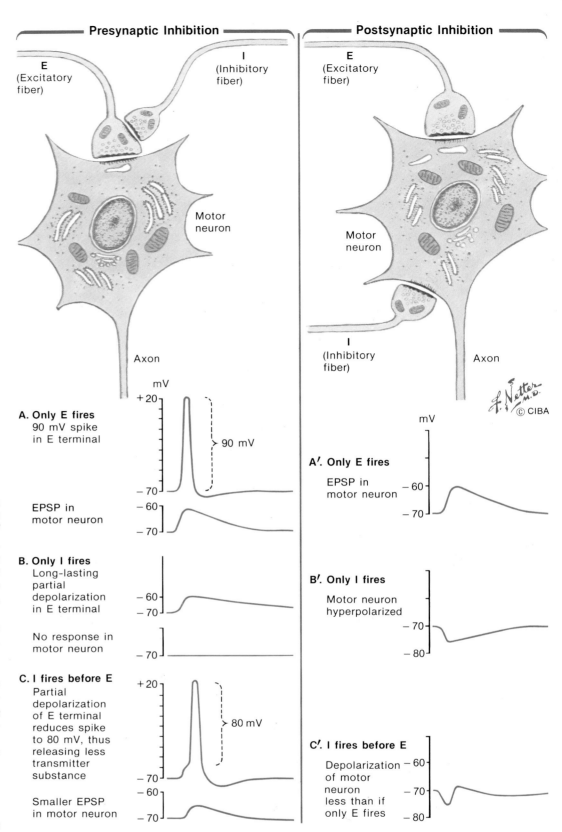

**Presynaptic Inhibition**

E (Excitatory fiber)

I (Inhibitory fiber)

Motor neuron

Axon

mV

**A. Only E fires**
90 mV spike in E terminal

+20

−70

90 mV

EPSP in motor neuron

−60
−70

**B. Only I fires**
Long-lasting partial depolarization in E terminal

−60
−70

No response in motor neuron

−70

**C. I fires before E**
Partial depolarization of E terminal reduces spike to 80 mV, thus releasing less transmitter substance

+20

−70

80 mV

Smaller EPSP in motor neuron

−60
−70

**Postsynaptic Inhibition**

E (Excitatory fiber)

Motor neuron

I (Inhibitory fiber)

Axon

mV

**A′. Only E fires**
EPSP in motor neuron

−60

−70

**B′. Only I fires**
Motor neuron hyperpolarized

−70

−80

**C′. I fires before E**
Depolarization of motor neuron less than if only E fires

−60

−70

−80

The discharge of neuronal action potentials in response to an excitatory synaptic input may be prevented or decreased by two distinct kinds of inhibitory mechanism. One mechanism, known as *postsynaptic inhibition*, acts directly on the target neuron to decrease its excitability. The other mechanism, known as *presynaptic inhibition*, acts on the terminals of incoming excitatory fibers to decrease their power to excite the target neuron. Anatomical and physiological evidence suggests that both forms of inhibition are found throughout the CNS.

*Postsynaptic inhibition* is produced by inhibitory axosomatic or axodendritic synapses, whose activation increases the permeability of the target neuron's membrane to potassium and chloride ions (see page 159). When such synapses are activated alone, they cause a hyperpolarizing inhibitory postsynaptic potential (IPSP) in the target neuron. If activation of inhibitory synapses precedes activation of excitatory synapses, the excitatory depolarization is diminished in two ways. First, the excitatory postsynaptic potential (EPSP) evoked by excitatory transmitter release starts from an already hyperpolarized membrane, as a result of the IPSP. Secondly, the increase of membrane conductance caused by inhibitory transmitter action lowers the net transmembrane resistance, so that a larger proportion of the excitatory synaptic current can flow through the membrane. Thus, less current is available to charge the membrane capacitance, and the size of the EPSP is therefore decreased. The combination of a smaller EPSP riding on an initially hyperpolarized membrane potential results in a diminution of the excitation produced by excitatory synaptic input.

*Presynaptic inhibition* is mediated by axoaxonic synapses that end upon the terminals of excitatory fibers. Activation of these synapses has

no direct effect on the target neuron, but causes a decrease in the ability of the excitatory synapses to depolarize that neuron. Although the mechanism responsible for this decrease in excitatory synaptic efficacy has not definitely been established, experiments have shown that it is associated with a relatively long-lasting depolarization of the excitatory terminals. One reasonable theory suggests that depolarization of the excitatory presynaptic terminal diminishes the membrane potential change that is caused by an action potential in the terminal, and that this decrease in action potential amplitude results in a decrease in the amount of transmitter release.

*Pharmacology.* In addition to their physiological differences, the two forms of inhibition differ pharmacologically. Studies of inhibition in the spinal cord have shown that postsynaptic inhibition is blocked by strychnine, whereas presynaptic inhibition is resistant to strychnine but is blocked by picrotoxin. The chemical transmitter substance at strychnine-sensitive inhibitory synapses is thought to be the amino acid glycine, whereas the transmitter substance for presynaptic inhibition is unknown. Gamma-aminobutyric acid (GABA) has been implicated as a postsynaptic inhibitory transmitter in the brain. Its action is specifically blocked by the drug bicuculline. ☐

# Summation of Excitation and Inhibition

Summation of excitation and inhibition is the vital principle on which the functioning of the CNS is based. The illustration shows the various intracellular potential changes observed during temporal and spatial summation of excitation and inhibition, as voltage-versus-time tracings similar to those produced by an oscilloscope.

The principle of summation relates to the fact that a neuron typically has a large number of synaptic terminals (boutons) ending upon it (A); alone, each bouton is capable of producing only a small synaptic potential. As shown in B, the small excitatory postsynaptic potential (EPSP) produced by a single excitatory terminal is not sufficient to depolarize the motor neuron to its threshold point. For suprathreshold depolarization to be produced, either temporal or spatial summation of excitation must take place.

*Temporal summation* occurs when a burst of action potentials reaches a nerve fiber terminal. If the terminal is excitatory, the first action potential in the burst produces a depolarizing EPSP in the motor neuron that begins to decay toward the resting potential (C). Before the decay is complete, another action potential arrives in the terminal and evokes a second EPSP. The depolarization caused by this EPSP adds to the residual depolarization remaining from the first EPSP and moves the membrane potential closer to the threshold level. Finally, the EPSP evoked by a third action potential adds its depolarization to that produced by the first two to drive the membrane potential past the threshold level and to trigger an action potential in the motor neuron. Thus, because of temporal summation, a burst of action potentials in an excitatory fiber is able to evoke the firing of a target neuron, even though the individual EPSPs evoked by single action potentials are too small to produce a suprathreshold depolarization. In a similar manner, the inhibitory postsynaptic potentials (IPSPs) produced by a burst of action potentials in an inhibitory fiber can summate to produce a large hyperpolarizing potential.

*Spatial summation* involves the activation of two or more terminals at approximately the same time. When such synchronous activation occurs, the inward and outward currents evoked by excitatory and inhibitory terminals summate to produce a net shift in the membrane potential of the target cell. If two excitatory terminals are activated (D), the net membrane potential shift will be a depolarization approximately equal to the sum of the EPSPs that would be evoked by each terminal acting alone; this combined depolarization exceeds the threshold level and triggers an action potential. If, in addition to the two excitatory terminals an inhibitory terminal is also activated (E), the net depolarization will be reduced by an outward flow of current at the inhibitory synapse. Under these conditions, additional excitation is required to produce a suprathreshold depolarization.

Spatial summation plays a vital role in the interaction of patterns of activity originating in

various neuronal pathways. For example, in the case of the effect of central motor tone on the reflex evoked by muscle stretch, the stretch produces a volley of action potentials in the group Ia fibers from the stretched muscle (Plate 33). The synaptic action of the Ia fiber terminals evokes medium-to-large EPSPs in motor neurons supplying the stretched muscle, and small EPSPs in motor neurons supplying synergistic muscles. If the body is in a relaxed state, only the motor neurons receiving large EPSPs will discharge action potentials, causing a small twitch of the stretched muscle; the remaining motor neurons, which receive EPSPs too small to evoke firing, constitute

the *subliminal fringe* of the stretch reflex. If the body is in an active state, central nervous pathways will produce a steady excitatory input to the motor neurons involved in the stretch reflex. Thus, many of the neurons in the subliminal fringe will receive sufficient additional excitation to cause them to fire, and muscle stretch may result in a vigorous contraction of that muscle and its synergists. In a similar way, motor neurons that fall within the subliminal fringe of two different reflexes may be fired when both reflexes occur together. This kind of reflex interaction by spatial summation helps to adapt reflex patterns to meet the demands of different external conditions. □

## Temporal and Spatial Summation of Excitation and Inhibition

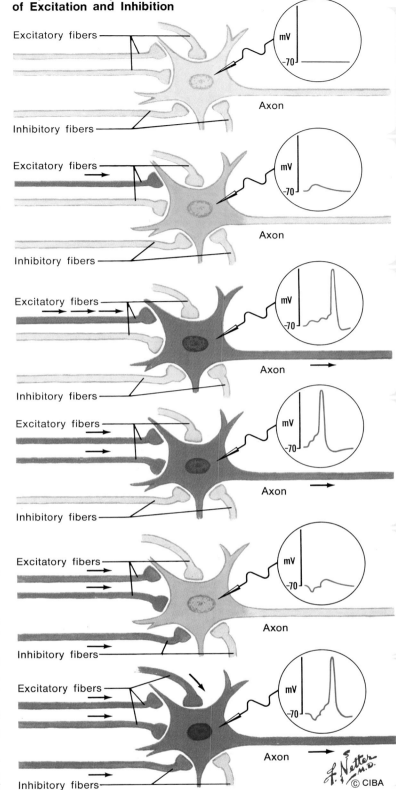

**A. Resting state:** motor nerve cell shown with synaptic boutons of excitatory and inhibitory nerve fibers ending close to it

**B. Partial depolarization:** impulse from one excitatory fiber has caused partial (below firing threshold) depolarization of motor neuron

**C. Temporal excitatory summation:** a series of impulses in one excitatory fiber together produce a suprathreshold depolarization that triggers an action potential

**D. Spatial excitatory summation:** impulses in two excitatory fibers cause two synaptic depolarizations that together reach firing threshold triggering an action potential

**E. Spatial excitatory summation with inhibition:** impulses from two excitatory fibers reach motor neuron but impulses from inhibitory fiber prevent depolarization from reaching threshold

**E. (continued):** motor neuron now receives additional excitatory impulses and reaches firing threshold despite a simultaneous inhibitory impulse; additional inhibitory impulses might still prevent firing

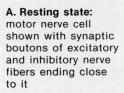

# Somatic Neuromuscular Transmission

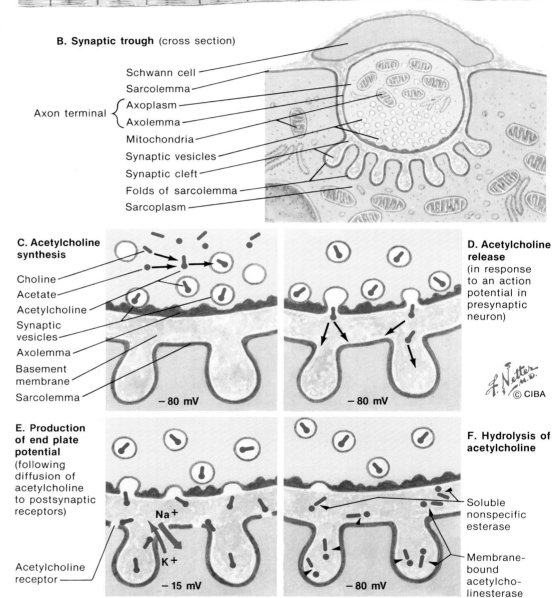

**A. Neuromuscular junction (motor end plate)** (longitudinal section)

Schwann cell

Axon terminal in synaptic trough

Axoplasm
Myelin sheath
Sarcolemma
Sarcoplasm
Muscle cell nucleus
Myofibrils

**B. Synaptic trough** (cross section)

Axon terminal {
Schwann cell
Sarcolemma
Axoplasm
Axolemma
Mitochondria
Synaptic vesicles
Synaptic cleft
Folds of sarcolemma
Sarcoplasm

**C. Acetylcholine synthesis**

Choline
Acetate
Acetylcholine
Synaptic vesicles
Axolemma
Basement membrane
Sarcolemma

−80 mV

**D. Acetylcholine release** (in response to an action potential in presynaptic neuron)

−80 mV

**E. Production of end plate potential** (following diffusion of acetylcholine to postsynaptic receptors)

Na+

K+

Acetylcholine receptor

−15 mV

**F. Hydrolysis of acetylcholine**

Soluble nonspecific esterase

Membrane-bound acetylcholinesterase

−80 mV

## Somatic Neuromuscular Transmission

The *neuromuscular junction* (motor end plate) is a specialized synapse between the axon of a motor neuron and a somatic muscle fiber. The structure of this synapse is adapted in such a way that a single action potential in the motor axon will produce sufficient synaptic depolarization of the muscle fiber to trigger a muscle action potential.

As shown in A, the motor axon gives rise to branches that lie in troughs within the muscle fiber membrane (sarcolemma). The exposed branches of the motor axon and the outer surface of the synaptic trough are covered by Schwann cells (B). Extensive folding of the sarcolemma within the synaptic trough greatly increases the surface area of the postjunctional membrane, thereby increasing the depolarizing power of the synapse. The axon terminal contains numerous mitochondria and a large number of globular synaptic vesicles (round on microscopic section) containing the synaptic transmitter *acetylcholine*.

C, D, E and F illustrate four phases of the activity of the neuromuscular junction. C shows the synthesis of acetylcholine from choline and an activated form of acetate. This synthesis, which takes place continuously within the axon terminal, is catalyzed by the enzyme choline acetyltransferase. This enzyme has been found both in the terminal cytoplasm and within the synaptic vesicles themselves, raising the possibility that acetylcholine synthesis may occur within the vesicles.

Following the arrival of an action potential in the axon terminal, acetylcholine is released from the vesicles into the synaptic cleft, presumably by the mechanism of exocytosis (D). The acetylcholine then diffuses across the synaptic cleft and combines with specific receptor sites on the surface of the postjunctional membrane. This combination triggers an increase in postjunctional membrane permeability to sodium ions ($Na^+$) and potassium ions ($K^+$), (E). Because of the large amounts of acetylcholine released from the numerous axon terminal branches and the extensive area of the postjunctional membrane, the flow of $Na^+$ and $K^+$ produced by these permeability changes drives the muscle fiber membrane toward the sodium-potassium ion equilibrium potential, which is −15 mV. However, before this level of muscle fiber membrane potential is reached, the depolarization triggers a muscle action potential that leads to a contraction of the myofibrils. Because it is large, the *neuromuscular*

*synaptic potential* (often referred to as the end plate potential, or EPP) is usually studied in the presence of blocking agents such as curare, which reduce its maximum depolarization to levels below the action potential threshold. Under these conditions, the EPP has properties similar to those of a typical EPSP, described on page 159.

Acetylcholine is removed from the synaptic cleft by diffusion and by hydrolysis, which is catalyzed by enzymes known as esterases (F). Most of the hydrolysis is catalyzed by a specific *acetylcholinesterase* that is bound to the basement membrane lining the sarcolemma. A small quantity of acetylcholine that diffuses away from the junction

is hydrolyzed by soluble, nonspecific esterases found in interstitial fluids. In the resting state, the axon terminal releases packets of approximately 10,000 acetylcholine molecules at irregular intervals. These packets, which are thought to represent the contents of one synaptic vesicle, produce small postjunctional depolarizations (termed miniature EPPs), about one hundredth the size of an EPP. Continuous release of acetylcholine may play some role in maintaining the localized sensitivity of the postjunctional membrane to acetylcholine. When the axon terminal degenerates following nerve section, this sensitivity spreads over the entire sarcolemma (see page 219). □

## Visceral Efferent Endings

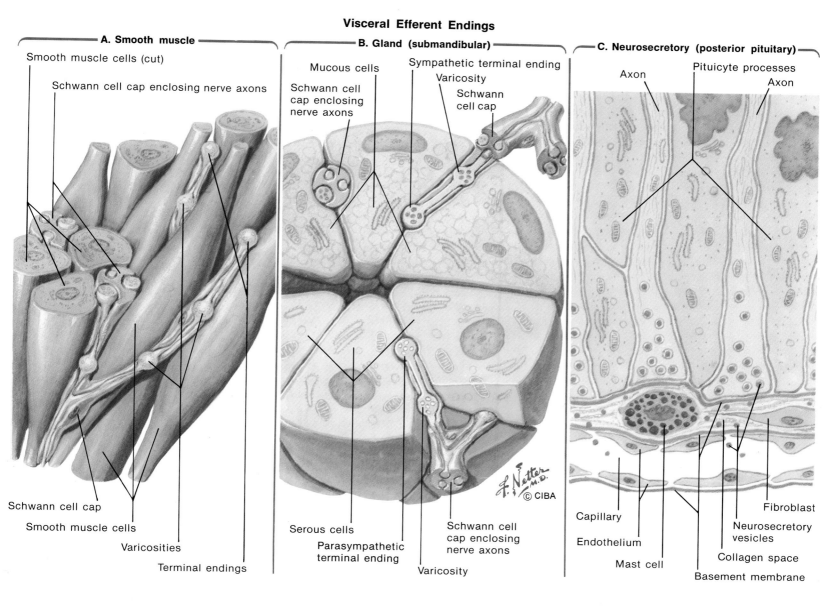

**A. Smooth muscle**

Smooth muscle cells (cut)

Schwann cell cap enclosing nerve axons

Schwann cell cap

Smooth muscle cells

Varicosities

Terminal endings

**B. Gland (submandibular)**

Mucous cells

Schwann cell cap enclosing nerve axons

Sympathetic terminal ending

Varicosity

Schwann cell cap

Serous cells

Parasympathetic terminal ending

Varicosity

Schwann cell cap enclosing nerve axons

**C. Neurosecretory (posterior pituitary)**

Axon

Pituicyte processes

Axon

Capillary

Endothelium

Mast cell

Fibroblast

Neurosecretory vesicles

Collagen space

Basement membrane

SECTION VIII PLATE 12

# Visceral Efferent Endings

Efferent endings involved in the control of smooth muscle and glandular activity and in neurosecretion do not exhibit the discrete one-to-one type of relationship between presynaptic endings and postsynaptic cells characteristic of neuromuscular junction or central synapses (Plates 7 and 11). Instead, neural transmitter substances released by such efferent endings are discharged into the interstitial space or into the bloodstream, where they can influence the activity of numerous effector cells. In agreement with this functional difference, ultrastructural studies of visceral efferent endings have failed to demonstrate the type of close apposition of specialized presynaptic and postsynaptic membranes that characterizes other chemical synaptic junctions. A functional visceral efferent junction can be as wide as 2,000 Å.

Autonomic neuromuscular endings control such diverse functions as heart rate, intestinal and urogenital activity, pupillary size and blood pressure (see Section IV). The morphological features of this type of ending are shown in A, which illustrates a three-dimensional reconstruction of the smooth muscle lining the colon. Bundles of the unmyelinated postganglionic fibers that innervate intestinal muscle are enveloped by individual Schwann cells. As these bundles run between smooth muscle cells, each axon exhibits beadlike swellings filled with synaptic vesicles at various points along its length. At these *varicosities* (boutons en passant), the surrounding Schwann cell membranes are drawn back so that the released transmitter substance can diffuse into the interstitial space and act on nearby smooth muscle cells. After forming numerous varicosities, an individual axon loses its Schwann cell sheath; after a short distance, it forms a final terminal ending similar in structure to the earlier varicosities.

Autonomic nerve endings in exocrine glands are structurally similar to autonomic neuromuscular endings. In the case of the mandibular gland (B), bundles of unmyelinated postganglionic fibers in Schwann cell sheaths form varicosities and terminal endings in the spaces between secretory cells. In this gland, as in many structures innervated by autonomic fibers, two types of endings are seen. *Sympathetic endings*, which in this gland excite mucous cells to produce mucous saliva, are filled with densely staining vesicles indicating the presence of the transmitter norepinephrine. *Parasympathetic endings*, which act on serous cells to produce watery saliva, are filled with clear vesicles that contain acetylcholine.

The neurosecretory endings of the posterior pituitary gland (C) and adrenal medulla are adapted to allow the transmitter substance released by the arrival of an action potential in the nerve terminal to enter the bloodstream and be carried to target cells in other parts of the body. In the posterior pituitary, axons of neurons in the supraoptic and paraventricular nuclei of the hypothalamus run between supporting cells called pituicytes to terminate directly on the basement membrane that delimits the collagen space around a capillary (Plates 59 and 60). Vesicles within the terminals contain one of the two posterior pituitary hormones, oxytocin and vasopressin (antidiuretic hormone). The morphology of the endings suggests that a hormone released by the arrival of action potentials in the terminals is able to diffuse through the collagen space and enter the capillary via pores between the endothelial cells. This diffusion process may be aided by mast cells, which are known to play a role in capillary permeability. □

# Cutaneous Receptors

Glabrous and hairy skin both contain a wide variety of receptors for the purpose of detecting mechanical, thermal or painful stimuli applied to the body surface. Because of the difficulty in visualizing these receptors and in stimulating an individual receptor in isolation, the identification of the function of different receptor types is still tentative in many cases. The situation is further complicated in that a receptor specialized to respond to one stimulus may also respond (usually more weakly) to another stimulus. How "crosstalk" of this kind is resolved by the CNS is still unknown.

Three types of receptors are common to glabrous and hairy skin: Pacinian (lamellated) corpuscles, Merkel's discs and free nerve endings. The *Pacinian corpuscle* has been identified as a quickly adapting mechanoreceptor, and its mechanical transduction process has been extensively studied (Plate 14). The primary role of Pacinian corpuscles appears to be the sensing of brief touch or vibration.

*Merkel's discs* are slowly adapting mechanoreceptors structured to respond to maintained deformation of the skin surface. Typically, one afferent fiber of a large-to-medium diameter branches to form a cluster of Merkel's discs, situated at the base of a thickened region of epidermis. Each nerve terminal branch ends in a disc enclosed by a specialized accessory cell (Merkel cell). The distal surface of the Merkel cell is held to nearby epidermal cells by cytoplasmic protrusions and desmosomes, while the base of the cell is embedded in the underlying dermis. Thus, movement of the epidermis relative to the dermis will exert a shearing force on the Merkel cell. The Merkel cell also contains numerous granulated vesicles, which suggests that some form of chemical synaptic transmission may occur, although attempts to demonstrate this have failed. Direct mechanical transduction by the nerve ending has not been ruled out as a possibility. However, whatever the transduction mechanism, the Merkel-cell/Merkel-disc ending appears to play a role in the sensing of both touch and pressure.

The so-called *free nerve ending* is made up of a branching nerve axon, which is entirely or

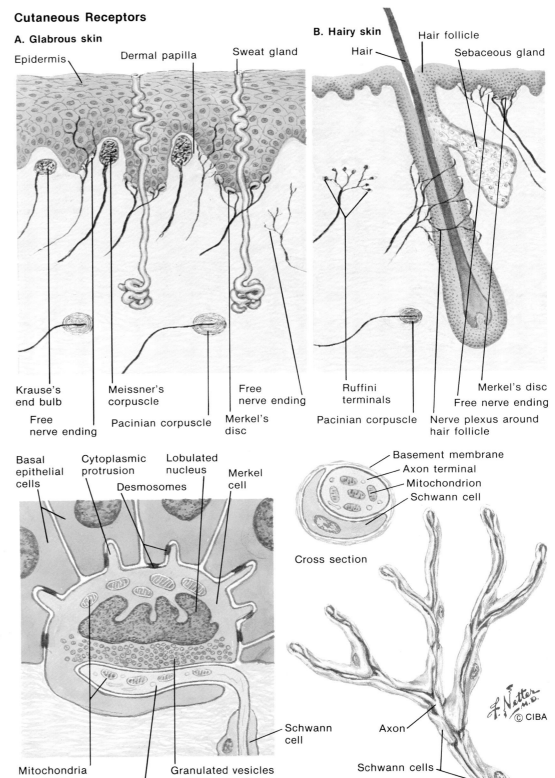

## Cutaneous Receptors

### A. Glabrous skin

Epidermis
Dermal papilla
Sweat gland

Krause's end bulb
Meissner's corpuscle
Free nerve ending

Free nerve ending
Pacinian corpuscle
Merkel's disc

### B. Hairy skin

Hair follicle
Hair
Sebaceous gland

Ruffini terminals
Merkel's disc
Free nerve ending

Pacinian corpuscle
Nerve plexus around hair follicle

Basal epithelial cells
Cytoplasmic protrusion
Lobulated nucleus
Merkel cell
Desmosomes

Basement membrane
Axon terminal
Mitochondrion
Schwann cell

Cross section

Mitochondria
Expanded axon terminal
Granulated vesicles
Schwann cell

Axon
Schwann cells

**C. Detail of Merkel's disc**

**D. Detail of free nerve ending**

partially surrounded by Schwann cells. The axon/Schwann-cell complex is further surrounded by a basement membrane. Free nerve endings originate from fine myelinated or unmyelinated fibers that branch extensively in the dermis and may penetrate into the epidermis. These endings respond to strong mechanical and thermal stimuli, and they are particularly activated by painful stimuli.

The other receptors found in glabrous skin are *Meissner's corpuscles* (tactile corpuscles), in which the terminal branches of a myelinated axon intertwine in a basketlike array of accessory cells, and *Krause's end bulbs*, in which a fine myelinated fiber

forms a club-shaped ending. Meissner's corpuscles have been tentatively identified as quickly adapting mechanoreceptors subserving the sense of touch, whereas Krause's end bulbs may be thermoreceptors.

The most important receptors in hairy skin are the *hair follicle endings*, in which axon terminals of sensory nerve fibers wrap themselves around a hair follicle. These endings are quickly adapting mechanoreceptors that provide information about any force applied to the hair and, thus, to the skin. Hairy skin also contains the spraylike *Ruffini terminals*, which may be involved in the sensing of steady pressure applied to hairy skin. □

# Pacinian Corpuscle

**Pacinian Corpuscle
as Pressure Transducer**

To amplifier

Pressure

Generator potential

Action potential

1st node
Myelin sheath
Lamellated capsule
Central core
Unmyelinated axon terminal

**A.** Sharp "on and off" changes in pressure at start and end of pulse applied to lamellated capsule are transmitted to central axon and provoke generator potentials which in turn may trigger action potentials; there is no response to a slow change in pressure gradient. Pressure at central core and, accordingly, generator potentials are rapidly dissipated by viscoelastic properties of capsule. (Action potentials may be blocked by pressure at a node or by drugs)

To amplifier

Pressure

Generator potential

Action potential

**B.** In absence of capsule, axon responds to slow as well as to rapid changes in pressure. Generator potential dissipates slowly, and there is no "off" response

The Pacinian corpuscle is one of a group of receptors, known as mechanoreceptors, which transform mechanical force, or displacement, into action potentials (Plate 13). In a simple mechanoreceptor such as the Pacinian corpuscle, transduction of the mechanical stimulus into action potentials occurs in three stages. First, the mechanical stimulus is modified by the viscoelastic properties of the receptor and the accessory cells surrounding it. Then, the modified mechanical stimulus acts on the mechanically sensitive membrane of the receptor cell to produce a change —a generator potential— in the transmembrane potential of the receptor cell. Finally, the generator potential acts to produce action potentials in the afferent nerve fiber linked to the mechanoreceptor.

The Pacinian corpuscle consists of the unmyelinated terminal part of an afferent nerve fiber that is surrounded by concentric lamellae formed by the membranes of numerous supporting cells. The axon terminal membrane is adapted in such a way that its ionic permeability increases when it is deformed by applied pressure. Although the permeability change appears to be nonspecific, the principal ion flux that occurs is an inflow of sodium ions ($Na^+$), because of the great difference in the electrochemical potential of this ion on the two sides of the membrane. The $Na^+$ influx causes a depolarizing current to flow through the axon terminal and the nearby nodes of Ranvier of the afferent fiber. The depolarization caused by this current comprises the generator potential. If the depolarization is great enough, it will produce an action potential at the point of lowest threshold—in this case, at the first node. This action potential then propagates along the afferent fiber to the CNS.

Pressure   **Na+**

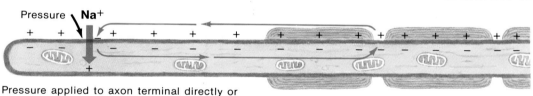

Pressure applied to axon terminal directly or via capsule causes increased permeability of membrane to Na+, thus setting up ionic generator current through 1st node

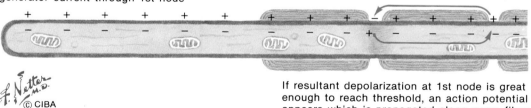

If resultant depolarization at 1st node is great enough to reach threshold, an action potential appears which is propagated along nerve fiber

The Pacinian corpuscle is specifically adapted to respond to rapidly changing mechanical stimulation. Experiments on isolated Pacinian corpuscles have shown that this adaptation involves both the physical structure of the receptor and the properties of the action-potential generating mechanism.

When pressure is applied to an intact Pacinian corpuscle, single action potentials are evoked at the beginning and end of the pressure pulse. If action potentials are blocked by a drug such as tetrodotoxin, the generator potentials evoked by the pressure pulse can be recorded. In the intact Pacinian corpuscle, these potentials consist of rapidly decaying depolarizations that occur at the beginning and end of the pulse.

If all the lamellae of the sheath except the innermost are dissected away, the response of the Pacinian corpuscle to the pressure pulse is modified. The generator potential now decays slowly throughout the period of applied pressure, and no additional depolarization appears at the termination of the pulse. This finding indicates that the viscoelastic properties of the intact capsule dissipate applied pressure, which means that only sudden pressure changes can reach the membrane of the nerve terminal and produce a generator potential. □

## Somesthetic System of Body

Neural pathways conveying somatosensory information to the cerebral cortex can be divided into two major systems: *posterior* (dorsal) and *anterolateral* (ventral). Studies of posterior system interruptions suggest that the posterior pathways are involved in mediating fine tactile and kinesthetic sensations and that the anterolateral pathways conduct impulses for pain and temperature, and for touch and deep pressure (Plate 48).

*The posterior funiculus*, made up of the *fasciculus gracilis* and the *fasciculus cuneatus*, carries fibers that signal discriminative touch or pressure, muscle length and tension, and joint position (Plate 37). Some afferent fibers, principally those from quickly adapting cutaneous receptors, ascend the entire length of the spinal cord to synapse directly with neurons in the *gracile* and *cuneate nuclei*, which relate to the lower and upper parts of the body. Other fibers leave the posterior columns and either activate spinal neurons for reflex purposes or project upward in the dorsolateral funiculus. In man, most of these secondary ascending fibers also end in the gracile or cuneate nuclei, although a small number of axons— the *spinocervical tract*—apparently terminate in the upper cervical segments, in the *lateral cervical nucleus*. The *nucleus Z* (not shown), also involved in somesthetic pathways, acts as a relay for muscle spindle afferents from the lower part of the body. All of the above nuclei send their axons via the *medial lemniscus* to the contralateral *ventral posterolateral (VPL) nucleus* of the thalamus (Plate 41), which projects to the *somatosensory regions* of the cerebral cortex (Plate 43).

The relay neurons in the gracile, cuneate and VPL nuclei and the neurons of the primary somatosensory cortex are activated by a single sensory modality over a restricted receptive field. The receptive fields of neurons within each nucleus are arranged in an orderly fashion and give rise to a somatotopic representation of the body surface. Thus, a high degree of specificity and order is maintained throughout the pathway.

*Anterolateral Funiculus.* Two somatosensory pathways ascend in the anterolateral spinal white matter: the conjoined lateral and ventral (anterior) spinothalamic tracts and the smaller spinoreticulothalamic pathway. The *spinothalamic tracts* arise from neurons in the regions of the posterior horn of the spinal cord that correspond to laminae I, IV, V and VI of Rexed (Plate 49). Most axons cross in the anterior white commissure at about the level of their cell somata and ascend in the contralateral lateral and anterior funiculi, although a few fibers ascend ipsilaterally. The spinothalamic axons end principally in the *VPL nucleus* (neospinothalamic projection) and in the *posterior nuclear group* and *intralaminar nuclei* (paleospinothalamic projection). Some spinothalamic neurons (especially those in lamina I) respond only to strong, noxious stimuli, but most of these neurons are excited by the activity of a wide variety of afferent fibers related to touch, pressure, vibration and temperature sense. All spinothalamic neurons have large, unilateral receptive fields and transmit information about a wide variety of peripheral

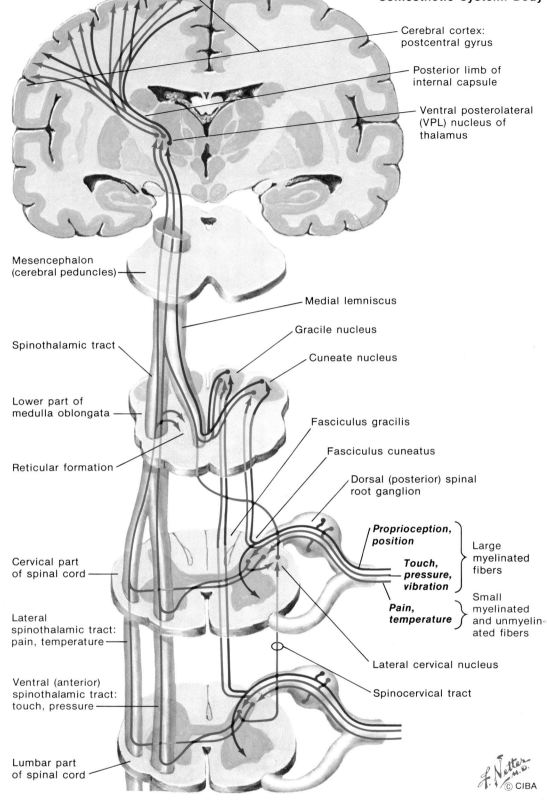

Cerebral cortex: postcentral gyrus

Posterior limb of internal capsule

Ventral posterolateral (VPL) nucleus of thalamus

Mesencephalon (cerebral peduncles)

Medial lemniscus

Gracile nucleus

Spinothalamic tract

Cuneate nucleus

Lower part of medulla oblongata

Fasciculus gracilis

Fasciculus cuneatus

Reticular formation

Dorsal (posterior) spinal root ganglion

*Proprioception, position*

Large myelinated fibers

*Touch, pressure, vibration*

Cervical part of spinal cord

*Pain, temperature*

Small myelinated and unmyelinated fibers

Lateral spinothalamic tract: pain, temperature

Lateral cervical nucleus

Ventral (anterior) spinothalamic tract: touch, pressure

Spinocervical tract

Lumbar part of spinal cord

stimuli, but with less specificity than is shown by neurons in the posterior spinal pathways.

*The spinoreticulothalamic pathway* (not shown) begins with neurons in the regions corresponding to laminae V to VIII, which ascend in the lateral and anterior funiculi to activate neurons in the *brainstem reticular formation*, which in turn project to the *intralaminar nuclei* of the thalamus. The spinoreticulothalamic neurons respond to the same stimuli as spinothalamic neurons, but tend to have very large, bilateral receptive fields. This fact, together with the nonspecific nature of the intralaminar nuclei, suggests that this pathway may be more important in generalized arousal

reactions than in discriminative processing of sensation.

*Lesions.* Since the principal pathways of the posterior and anterolateral columns cross in the medulla and in the spinal cord, and since each pathway transmits specific modalities, damage from spinal cord lesions presents specific and characteristic deficits. *Posterior column destruction* results in ipsilateral loss of discriminatory touch and vibration sense, as well as loss of position sense below the level of the lesion. *Anterolateral column interruption* produces contralateral loss of pain and temperature sense accompanied by diminished touch and vibratory sense below the lesion. □

# Somesthetic System of Head

Most of the nerve cell bodies for somesthetic information from the head are located in the trigeminal (semilunar) ganglion. The primary relay nuclei are the principal sensory trigeminal nucleus and the spinal (descending) trigeminal nucleus, the upward continuation of the substantia gelatinosa (Plate 49). In addition, the mesencephalic trigeminal nucleus contains cell bodies of neurons responsible for proprioception in the head. The somesthetic pathways from the head, like those from the body (Plate 15), can be divided into two major systems.

*The first somesthetic system* is functionally similar to the posterior spinal pathways, mediating fine tactile and kinesthetic sensations. It includes relay neurons in the *principal sensory nucleus* and the *rostral (oral) part* of the *spinal trigeminal nucleus*. These neurons receive input from large myelinated fibers signaling touch, pressure, muscle length or tension and joint position. Most of these relay neurons project to the *contralateral ventral posteromedial (VPM) nucleus* of the thalamus via the *ventral trigeminal lemniscus*, which is contiguous with the medial lemniscus. A smaller number of relay neurons project to the *ipsilateral VPM nucleus* via the *dorsal trigeminal lemniscus*, the projection responsible for ipsilateral face representation in the primary somatosensory cortex. Throughout this system, neurons have the small receptive fields, modality specificity and somatotopic arrangement that are consistent with their participation in fine sensory discrimination.

*The second somesthetic system* is functionally related to the anterolateral spinal pathways. It mediates the sensations of temperature and pain, as well as tactile sensation, which is less refined. The second system involves relay neurons in the *caudal part* of the *spinal trigeminal nucleus*, which receives input from both myelinated and unmyelinated afferent fibers. The fibers enter via the trigeminal (V), facial (VII) and vagus (X) nerves and descend in the *spinal trigeminal tract* before entering the nucleus; They carry information about touch, pressure and thermal and noxious stimuli. Because of the alternative pathways available for touch and pressure sensation in the first somesthetic system, sectioning of the spinal trigeminal tract leads primarily to a loss of pain and temperature sensitivity on the ipsilateral side of the head. Relay neurons more *rostrally placed* in the caudal part of the spinal nucleus project principally to the *contralateral posterior* and *intralaminar thalamic nuclei*, a projection analogous to that of the paleospinothalamic fibers. Neurons in the *more caudal* parts of the nucleus project to both the *ipsilateral* and *contralateral intralaminar nuclei* via relay neurons in the *brainstem reticular formation*. This projection resembles that of the spinoreticulothalamic pathway. Neurons in the caudal part of the spinal nucleus exhibit a wide variety of responses to peripheral stimulation, which range from discrete responses, such as those seen in the main sensory nucleus, to the mixed-modality and nociceptive responses observed in spinothalamic neurons. Proprioceptive cell bodies

located in the *mesencephalic trigeminal nucleus* send bilateral projections to the *thalamus*. They also have monosynaptic connections to the motor trigeminal nucleus. The latter connection is responsible for the "jaw jerk" reflex.

*Modulation of Somesthetic Pathways.* The somesthetic pathways are under continuous dynamic control by local and descending pathways, which may inhibit transmission at various relays within each pathway. The inhibition is typically mediated by *presynaptic* or *postsynaptic inhibitory interneurons* located either within or close to the sensory relay nuclei being controlled. Examples of descending control systems are those

originating in the brainstem reticular formation or within the somatosensory cortex itself, the activation of which can lead to the suppression of pain (Plates 44 and 17).

*Trigeminal Disorders.* In some cases of *skull fracture*, peripheral branches of the trigeminal nerve are damaged at their exits through the respective foramina, resulting in a distributive sensory loss. The major disorder is *trigeminal neuralgia*, which is characterized by sensory loss, with paroxysms of severe pain in one (or more) of the divisions, often triggered by a local irritation. The etiology of this usually unilateral disorder is unclear. □

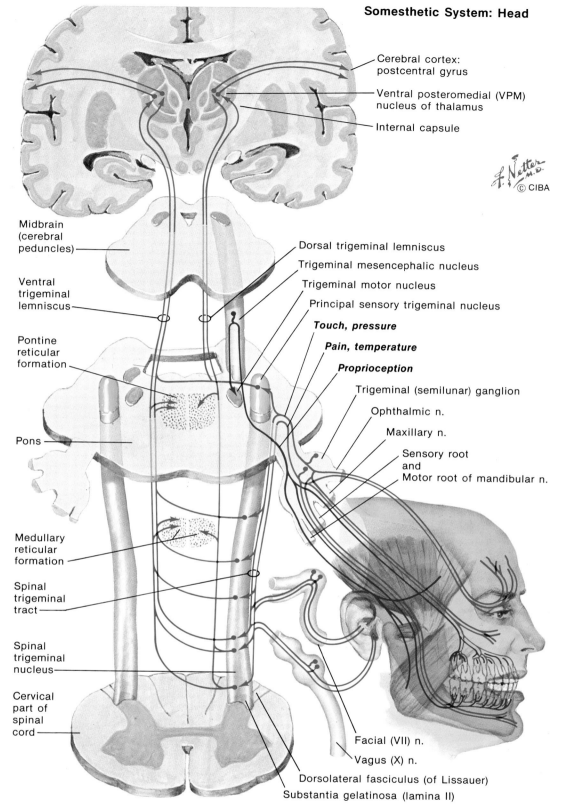

**Somesthetic System: Head**

Cerebral cortex: postcentral gyrus

Ventral posteromedial (VPM) nucleus of thalamus

Internal capsule

Dorsal trigeminal lemniscus

Trigeminal mesencephalic nucleus

Trigeminal motor nucleus

Principal sensory trigeminal nucleus

*Touch, pressure*

*Pain, temperature*

*Proprioception*

Trigeminal (semilunar) ganglion

Ophthalmic n.

Maxillary n.

Sensory root and Motor root of mandibular n.

Midbrain (cerebral peduncles)

Ventral trigeminal lemniscus

Pontine reticular formation

Pons

Medullary reticular formation

Spinal trigeminal tract

Spinal trigeminal nucleus

Cervical part of spinal cord

Facial (VII) n.

Vagus (X) n.

Dorsolateral fasciculus (of Lissauer)

Substantia gelatinosa (lamina II)

# Endorphin System

**Endorphin System**

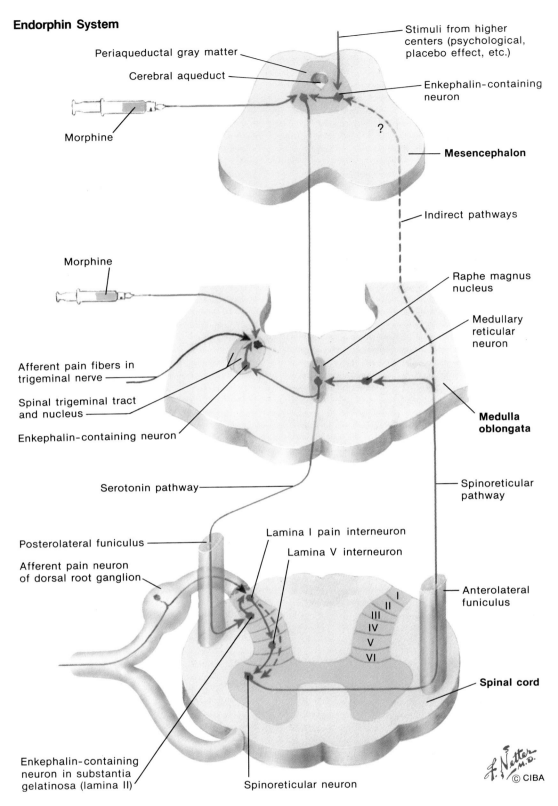

Stimuli from higher centers (psychological, placebo effect, etc.)

Periaqueductal gray matter

Cerebral aqueduct

Enkephalin-containing neuron

Morphine

Mesencephalon

?

Indirect pathways

Morphine

Raphe magnus nucleus

Medullary reticular neuron

Afferent pain fibers in trigeminal nerve

Spinal trigeminal tract and nucleus

Enkephalin-containing neuron

Medulla oblongata

Serotonin pathway

Spinoreticular pathway

Posterolateral funiculus

Lamina I pain interneuron

Lamina V interneuron

Afferent pain neuron of dorsal root ganglion

Anterolateral funiculus

Enkephalin-containing neuron in substantia gelatinosa (lamina II)

Spinoreticular neuron

Spinal cord

*Endorphins.* Neurons in the CNS of lower mammals have specific receptor sites that bind the drug morphine and related compounds. It has recently been determined that these sites act as receptors for a class of endogenously produced chemical transmitter substances, the endorphins, examples of which are the two related pentapeptides—*methionine* and leucine *enkephalin*. Neurons containing endorphins or having endorphin receptors on their surfaces are found in many sensory relay nuclei in the midbrain, pons and medulla oblongata and in structures such as the periaqueductal gray matter. These areas are involved in the analgesia that can be produced by electrical stimulation of the brainstem. Endorphin-containing neurons apparently function as key links in the theoretical pain control system shown in the illustration—possibly in man, as well as in the rat and the cat. The system mediates analgesia produced by the placebo effect, by painful stimuli (as in acupuncture), by opiate drugs and by electrical brain stimulation, all of which can be antagonized by naloxone, a drug that blocks endorphin receptor sites.

*Pathways.* Beginning at the level of the *periaqueductal gray matter*, enkephalin-containing neurons are excited by painful stimuli reaching them over convergent *reticular pathways*, or by central signals originating in the *cerebral cortex*. Stimulation of these neurons leads to activation of *projection neurons*, which in turn excite the neurons of the *raphe magnus nucleus* in the medulla oblongata. Raphe magnus neurons may also be directly activated by some of the same painful or central stimuli that activate the periaqueductal gray matter, and there is some evidence that the raphe magnus nucleus may contain endorphin neurons of its own.

Raphe neurons, which are thought to use serotonin as their transmitter substance, project to a number of *sensory relay nuclei*, including the spinal trigeminal nucleus and the substantia gelatinosa of the posterior horn of the spinal cord, where their action reduces the level of excitation of the

sensory relay neurons by painful stimuli, thus causing analgesia. This effect can be mimicked by the injection of serotonin into sensory nuclei, and blocked by drugs that antagonize the effect of serotonin.

The exact way in which raphe neurons act at the level of the sensory nuclei is uncertain, but several lines of evidence suggest the scheme shown in the illustration. Painful sensations are carried by thin afferent fibers that use the peptide, substance P, as a transmitter to excite relay neurons, such as those in spinal lamina I, that inform the brain about painful stimuli. The release of substance P by these fibers is reduced by enkephalin, perhaps in a manner analagous to the presynaptic inhibition described in Plate 9. It is

therefore possible that raphe neurons act by activating local enkephalin neurons in the spinal cord or in the trigeminal nucleus, which produce analgesia by presynaptic inhibition of afferent fibers carrying pain signals. Inhibition may also occur at later stages in the nociceptive pathway.

*Morphine* injected systemically can cause analgesia by acting either at the level of the periaqueductal gray matter or directly within the sensory relay nuclei. The former site appears to be more sensitive, since analgesia produced by low doses of morphine can be blocked by lesions that destroy the raphe magnus nucleus or its projection; these lesions do not prevent analgesia produced by larger doses of morphine, which apparently act directly on the sensory nuclei. □

# Olfactory Receptors

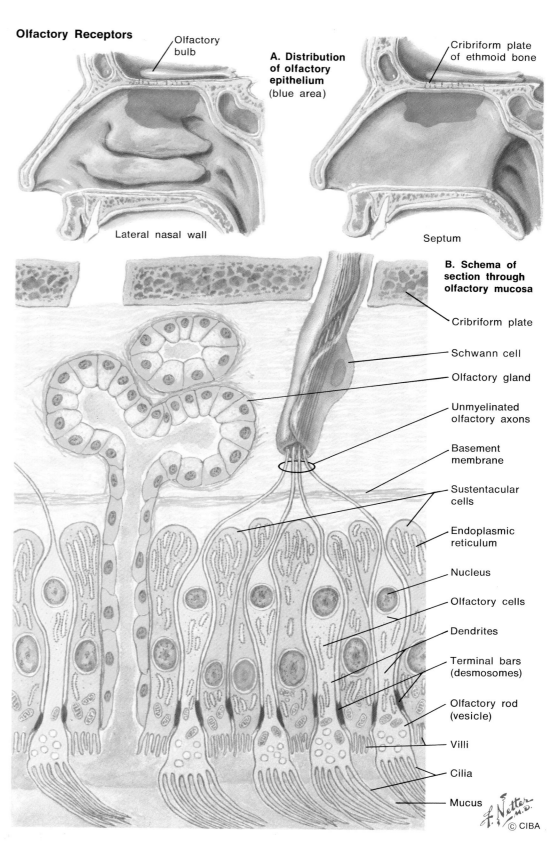

**Olfactory Receptors**

Olfactory bulb

**A. Distribution of olfactory epithelium** (blue area)

Lateral nasal wall

Cribriform plate of ethmoid bone

Septum

**B. Schema of section through olfactory mucosa**

- Cribriform plate
- Schwann cell
- Olfactory gland
- Unmyelinated olfactory axons
- Basement membrane
- Sustentacular cells
- Endoplasmic reticulum
- Nucleus
- Olfactory cells
- Dendrites
- Terminal bars (desmosomes)
- Olfactory rod (vesicle)
- Villi
- Cilia
- Mucus

Receptors responsible for the sense of smell are found in the patch of olfactory epithelium that lines the medial and lateral walls of the roof of the nasal cavity (see Section V, Plate 4). In addition to the receptor cells, this epithelium contains olfactory (Bowman's) glands and sustentacular cells, both of which contribute to the mucous secretion that coats the epithelial surface. The sustentacular cells also act as supporting cells for the slender olfactory receptors.

*Olfactory receptor cells* may be considered specialized, primitive-type, bipolar neurons. Their nuclei are located at the base of the epithelial layer. From the nuclear region, a dendritic process extends toward the surface of the epithelium. At its apical end, this process widens into an olfactory rod, or vesicle, which gives rise to the 10 to 15 motile cilia that project into the mucous layer covering the epithelium. Desmosomes at the base of the olfactory vesicle provide a tight seal between the membranes of olfactory and sustentacular cells, thus barring external substances from entering the intercellular spaces. At its base, the olfactory receptor cell narrows and gives rise to a fine (0.2 to 0.3 $\mu$m) unmyelinated axon. Large numbers of these axons converge to run together within a single Schwann cell sheath, eventually penetrating the cribriform plate to collectively form the olfactory (I) nerve (Plate 19). In humans, this nerve contains on the order of 100 million axons.

*Odorant Transduction.* Because of the small size and inaccessibility of first-order olfactory cells, the mechanisms of olfactory transduction have not been investigated as thoroughly as other sensory mechanisms. However, it is known that odorous substances enter the mucous layer coating the olfactory epithelium and act on the apical ends (including the cilia) of olfactory cells to cause a depolarization of those cells. The mechanism of interaction of the odorant and the cell membrane is not completely clear. It may be a binding of the odorant to specific receptor sites, as in the taste system (Plate 23), or the odorant may directly penetrate the lipid membrane and thus open channels. Also, there is evidence that the molecular size, shape and configuration of the odorant are important elements in olfactory discrimination. Whatever the form of interaction, indirect measurements suggest that an increase in the ionic conductance of the membrane accompanies

the depolarization of olfactory receptors. This depolarization acts directly at the site of action potential initiation, which is located at the point of origin of the axon of the sensory cell, to produce a train of action potentials.

*Sense of Smell.* As in the case of taste fibers, which may respond to a variety of taste stimuli, individual olfactory nerve fibers respond to a number of different odors. Man differentiates the odors of thousands of chemicals; nevertheless, it has not been possible to identify a set of primary odor qualities analogous to the four primary tastes. Investigation of this mechanism is proceeding through studies of specific hereditary

defects in the sense of smell (anosmias) that make it impossible to detect certain odors. Despite our present lack of knowledge about olfaction, it seems likely that, as with the gustatory system, the neural message for olfactory perceptions consists of activity across large populations of olfactory fibers.

Skull fractures involving the cribriform plate of the ethmoid bone can damage the mucosa and the tiny olfactory nerve fibers, and thus cause unilateral or bilateral anosmia. The common cold, which causes irritation and swelling of the nasal mucous membranes, frequently provokes transient bilateral anosmia. □

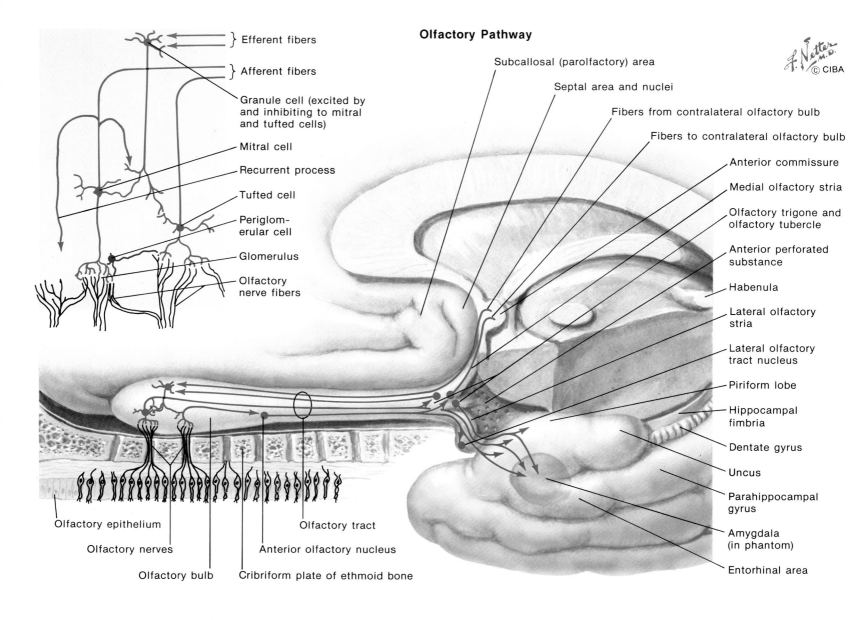

**Olfactory Pathway**

*Efferent fibers*

*Afferent fibers*

Granule cell (excited by and inhibiting to mitral and tufted cells)

Mitral cell

Recurrent process

Tufted cell

Periglom-erular cell

Glomerulus

Olfactory nerve fibers

Subcallosal (parolfactory) area

Septal area and nuclei

Fibers from contralateral olfactory bulb

Fibers to contralateral olfactory bulb

Anterior commissure

Medial olfactory stria

Olfactory trigone and olfactory tubercle

Anterior perforated substance

Habenula

Lateral olfactory stria

Lateral olfactory tract nucleus

Piriform lobe

Hippocampal fimbria

Dentate gyrus

Uncus

Parahippocampal gyrus

Amygdala (in phantom)

Entorhinal area

Olfactory epithelium

Olfactory nerves

Olfactory bulb

Anterior olfactory nucleus

Olfactory tract

Cribriform plate of ethmoid bone

# Olfactory Pathway

*Olfactory Bulb.* In the first stage of the olfactory pathway, about 100 million olfactory afferent fibers (Plate 18) enter the *olfactory bulb*, a flattened, oval mass lying near the lateral margin of the cribriform plate of the ethmoid bone. As explained in Section VII, Plates 4 and 5, the olfactory lobes originally have cavities that are obliterated during embryological development. Hence, the olfactory bulb has a radial organization consisting of a number of superimposed layers. The incoming olfactory fibers join together in the outermost layer to form presynaptic nets called glomeruli. Each *glomerulus* is composed of the terminals of about 25,000 axons of receptor cells. Within the glomeruli, the afferent terminals synapse with and excite the dendrites of *mitral* and *tufted cells*. These cells make up the second order of neurons in the olfactory bulb. Each of

the estimated 50,000 mitral cells sends its dendrite to only a single glomerulus, while each of the 150,000 tufted cells sends dendrites to several glomeruli. Olfactory afferents within the glomeruli also activate *periglomerular cells*, which in turn inhibit mitral and tufted cells. Further inhibition arises at the dendrodendritic contacts between mitral and tufted cells and the processes of *granule cells*, which lie deeper still within the olfactory bulb. These contacts are an example of two-way, synaptic feedback connections: the granule cells are excited by mitral and tufted cells and, in turn, inhibit them. Integration of olfactory information occurs when excitation is spread throughout the multiple-branched granule cell processes, and also when granule cells are excited by the centrifugal efferent fibers that reach the olfactory bulb from higher centers. Another factor in this highly complex integrative process are the recurrent collaterals of mitral cells that appear to excite mitral, tufted and granule cells.

These synaptic arrangements result in a series of local circuits, which forms the basis for integrative processes within the olfactory bulb, so that there is a striking transformation in the response to odors from the glomeruli to the mitral cells. The glomeruli have response profiles for different substances, which are directly related to the physiochemical properties of the odorant molecules concerned (and unrelated to human, subjective

response profiles for these substances), whereas mitral cells tend to respond similarly to groups of substances that evoke similar subjective sensations.

*Olfactory Tract and Central Connections.* The axons of mitral and tufted cells form the *olfactory tract*, through which they project to the *olfactory trigone* and into the *lateral* and *medial olfactory striae*, where they establish a complex pattern of central connections. Some mitral and tufted cell axons terminate in the *anterior olfactory nucleus* (a continuation of the granule cell layer throughout the olfactory tract) and *olfactory tubercle*, which are the sites of origin of the efferent fibers projecting to both the ipsilateral and contralateral olfactory bulbs. Other axons reach the prepiriform cortex and the amygdala (amygdaloid body), as well as the septal nuclei and the hypothalamus; some, after relaying in the *lateral olfactory tract nucleus*. Relatively little is known about the properties of neurons in the areas that receive lateral olfactory tract projections, but it is interesting to note that both the prepiriform cortex and the amygdala are closely linked to the hypothalamus (Plate 56). This close linkage may explain the powerful effect of olfactory stimuli upon feeding, sexual and other affective behaviors (Plate 62). In addition, olfactory "hallucinations" are known to occur in temporal lobe disease involving the central olfactory areas, such as the uncus and other related regions. ☐

# Visual Receptors

*The human eye* is a highly developed sense organ containing numerous accessory structures that modify visual stimuli before they reach the photoreceptors. The *extraocular muscles* pivot the eyeball, thus causing the image of the object viewed to fall on the *fovea*, the retinal area of highest visual acuity (Plate 30). The shape of the eyeball, its surfaces and the refractive properties of the *cornea, lens* and *aqueous* and *vitreous humors* assist in focusing the image on the retina. To allow viewing of near and far objects, this focus can be adjusted by the action of the *ciliary muscle*, which changes the shape of the lens. The intensity of the light reaching the retina is controlled by the muscles of the *iris*, which vary the size of the *pupillary aperture* (see Section V, Plate 6). Incident light must traverse most of the retinal layers before it reaches the *photoreceptor cells* lying in the outer part of the retina. Beyond the photoreceptors is a layer of *pigment cells*, which eliminates back reflections by absorbing any light passing through the photoreceptor layer.

*The photoreceptor cells* are called rods and cones because of the shapes of their outer segments. *Rods* function as receptors in a highly sensitive, monochromatic visual system, whereas *cones* serve as receptors in the color vision system, which is less sensitive but more acute. Both receptors, however, are activated in a similar manner—they are hyperpolarized by photons of light falling directly upon them.

For example, the detection of light in the rod begins with the absorption of photons by the visual pigment, *rhodopsin*. Rhodopsin is a combination of the protein, opsin and the *cis* isomer of retinine, a compound derived from vitamin A. It is located within the membranous lamellae of the rod's outer segment, a highly modified cilium associated with a typical basal body. Upon the absorption of a photon, rhodopsin is converted to *lumirhodopsin*, which is unstable and changes spontaneously to *metarhodopsin*, which is then degraded by a chemical reaction known as bleaching. Rhodopsin lost by this bleaching process is restored to its active form by enzymatic reactions that require metabolic energy and vitamin A.

After a brief time lag, the absorption of a photon leads to changes in the ionic permeability of the membrane of the outer segment. Although the mechanism of this chain of events is unknown, the time lag suggests that the permeability change is not directly related to the photochemical reaction of rhodopsin with light (which occurs instantaneously), but is instead triggered by one of the intermediaries in the bleaching breakdown of rhodopsin.

The change in the receptor membrane triggered in the rod by light absorption is not the typical increase in ion permeability most sensory receptors undergo when activated; rather, there is a *decrease* in the permeability of the outer segment membrane to sodium ions ($Na^+$). In the absence of light, this permeability is relatively high, and there is a steady inward flow of $Na^+$ (the current

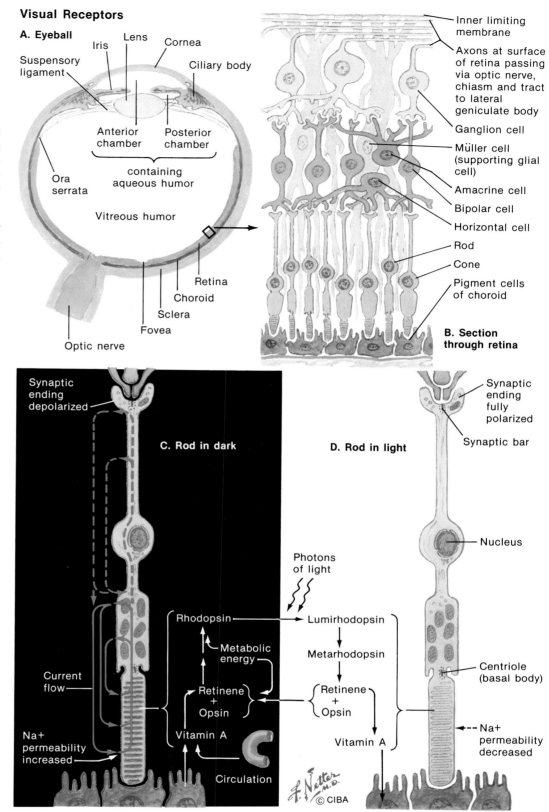

## Visual Receptors

### A. Eyeball

Iris — Lens — Cornea
Suspensory ligament
Ciliary body
Anterior chamber — Posterior chamber
containing aqueous humor
Ora serrata
Vitreous humor
Retina
Choroid
Sclera
Fovea
Optic nerve

Inner limiting membrane
Axons at surface of retina passing via optic nerve, chiasm and tract to lateral geniculate body
Ganglion cell
Müller cell (supporting glial cell)
Amacrine cell
Bipolar cell
Horizontal cell
Rod
Cone
Pigment cells of choroid

### B. Section through retina

### C. Rod in dark
Synaptic ending depolarized
Current flow
Na+ permeability increased
Rhodopsin
Metabolic energy
Retinene + Opsin
Vitamin A
Circulation

### D. Rod in light
Synaptic ending fully polarized
Synaptic bar
Photons of light
Lumirhodopsin
Metarhodopsin
Retinene + Opsin
Vitamin A
Nucleus
Centriole (basal body)
Na+ permeability decreased

flow resulting from this ionic movement, known as the "dark current," keeps the entire rod in a depolarized state). When light absorption provokes a decrease in $Na^+$ permeability, the dark current is cut off and the rod becomes more hyperpolarized. This hyperpolarization influences the synaptic action of the rod on horizontal and bipolar cells (Plate 21) in a way that is not clearly understood. Polarization changes in one rod may also spread to neighboring receptors via electrical synapses. Any photon that is successfully absorbed by photopigment produces the same electrochemical result, regardless of the wavelength of that photon. However, the probability

that a photon will be absorbed by photopigment varies considerably with the wavelength of the incident light; and rhodopsin has a maximal absorbency for light with a wavelength of 500 nm.

Cones may contain one of three different photopigments, with a maximum absorbency at 445 nm (blue), 535 nm (green) and 570 nm (red). Cone pigments all contain *cis* retinine, but have different forms of opsin that modify the light absorption pattern. By analyzing the relative activity produced by the three types of cones, the CNS is able to determine the wavelength of the incident light, and a sensation of color vision results. □

# Retinogeniculostriate Visual Pathway

*The retina* has several distinct layers. *Rods* (R) and *cones* (C), (Plate 20) form synaptic connections with bipolar (B) and horizontal (H) cells. *Bipolar cells* are relay neurons that transmit visual signals from the inner to the outer plexiform layer of the retina; *horizontal cells* are interneurons activated by rods and cones in one area and sending their axons laterally to act on neighboring bipolar cells. As a result of the actions of horizontal cells, bipolar cells have concentric receptive fields; ie, their membrane potentials are shifted in one direction by light reaching the center of their receptive field, and in the opposite direction, by light reaching the surrounding area. Neither bipolar nor horizontal cells generate action potentials; all information is transferred by changes in membrane potential, which spread passively through the cell bodies and axons.

The processes of bipolar cells that reach the inner plexiform layer form synapses with ganglion cells (G) and amacrine cells (A). *Ganglion cells* are output neurons whose axons comprise the optic nerves and optic tracts; *amacrine cells* are interneurons that contribute to the perception of motion and change. Unlike other retinal neurons, both amacrine and ganglion cells generate action potentials.

*Visual Pathways.* In mammals, most retinal ganglion cells send excitatory or inhibitory impulses via the *optic nerves* and *tracts* to the *dorsal lateral geniculate nucleus* of the lateral geniculate body of the thalamus, from where retinal information is relayed to the primary visual cortex via the *geniculostriate projection*, or *optic radiation*. In man, this cortical area covers both walls of the posterior calcarine fissure and adjacent parts of the occipital pole (Brodmann's area 17), (Plates 30 and 43).

The transmission of information from retina to visual cortex is *topographically organized*. Stimuli in the right half of the visual field activate neurons in the left half of each retina. Ganglion cells from these areas project to the left lateral geniculate body, which then projects to the left visual cortex. Input from both eyes is relayed by neurons in different layers of the lateral geniculate body. Similarly, stimuli in the left half of the visual field are relayed to the right visual cortex.

The upper and lower visual fields are also topographically mapped onto the lateral geniculate body and visual cortex. The upper field is represented in the lateral parts of the lateral geniculate

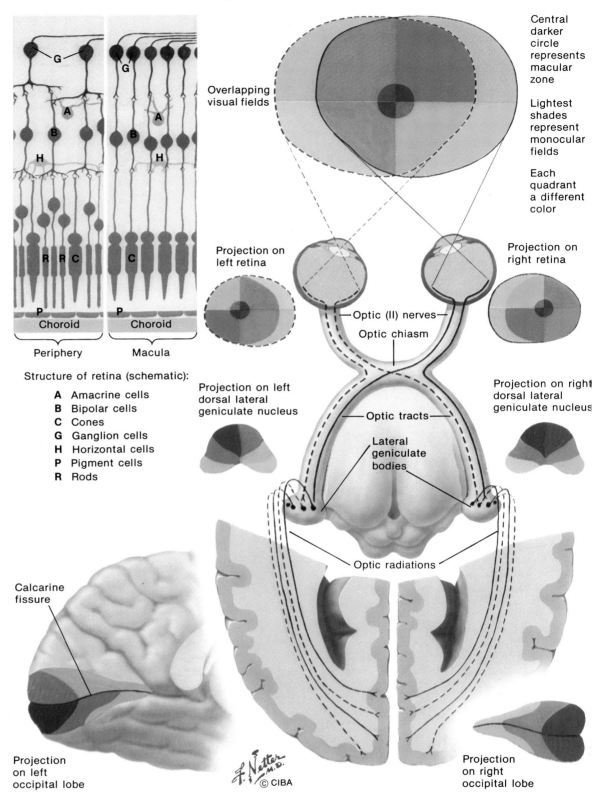

Structure of retina (schematic):

A Amacrine cells
B Bipolar cells
C Cones
G Ganglion cells
H Horizontal cells
P Pigment cells
R Rods

Central darker circle represents macular zone

Lightest shades represent monocular fields

Each quadrant a different color

Overlapping visual fields

Projection on left retina

Projection on right retina

Optic (II) nerves
Optic chiasm

Projection on left dorsal lateral geniculate nucleus

Projection on right dorsal lateral geniculate nucleus

Optic tracts

Lateral geniculate bodies

Optic radiations

Calcarine fissure

Projection on left occipital lobe

Projection on right occipital lobe

nuclei and the inferior portions of the visual cortex, and the lower visual field is represented in the corresponding medial and superior regions. The *macula* (central visual field) is represented in the central parts of the lateral geniculate nuclei and the posterior visual cortex, and the *peripheral retina*, in the peripheral parts of the lateral geniculate nuclei and the anterior visual cortex. The fovea, the central spot of the macula, is represented by a proportionally larger cortical area than the periphery of the retina.

*Neurological deficits* in the visual system caused by tumors, hemorrhage, vascular occlusion, infectious disease or trauma can be localized by determining the type and extent of the resultant visual field deficit. Retinal damage produces localized signs at the level of the primary receptor, whereas optic nerve disease causes partial or total blindness in the affected eye. Pressure at the optic chiasm will result in bitemporal hemianopsia, caused by a compression of the fibers from the nasal segment of both retinas. Interruption of the visual tract between the chiasm and lateral geniculate body results in a homonymous hemianopsia, and a similar deficit occurs if the striate cortex is lost unilaterally. Incomplete field deficits (scotomas) occur from partial damage to the geniculostriate radiations. ☐

**Retinal Projections to Thalamus, Midbrain and Brainstem**

## Visual System: Retinal Projections

As illustrated in Plate 21, the main retinal projection is to the *dorsal lateral geniculate nucleus*, which then projects to the visual cortex and receives projections from it. The retinogeniculostriate system thus formed is the basis for essentially the entire visual consciousness in man.

Other optic nerve fibers terminate within the *superior colliculus*. This multilayered structure plays an important role in orienting the reactions that shift the head and eyes in order to bring an object of interest into the center of the visual field (Plate 30). In addition to direct optic nerve input, the superior colliculus receives indirect visual input via the visual cortex. As is the case throughout the visual system, this input is topographically organized so that each point within the colliculus corresponds to a particular region within the visual field. Collicular neurons tend to respond best to interesting or moving stimuli, and the discharge of neurons in the deeper layers of the colliculus is closely related to the orienting movements of the eyes evoked by such stimuli.

The deeper collicular layers are the source of several efferent projections, shown in the lower part of the illustration. One group of fibers crosses the midline and runs caudally, sending terminals to the brainstem reticular formation and then continuing on to cervical and thoracic levels as the *tectospinal tract*; these fibers are probably involved in the orienting movements of the head and body. A second group of fibers projects to the posterior thalamus (pulvinar), which then projects to the cortical association areas (Plate 42). Fiber projections responsible for eye movements relay in the mesencephalic reticular formation below the superior colliculus (vertical eye movements), and in the medial pontine reticular formation (horizontal eye movements).

The *pretectum*, like the superior colliculus, receives visual information from optic nerve fibers and from the visual cortex. This area appears to be involved in visual reflexes, such as the light reflex (which regulates the size of the pupil) and the accommodation reflex (which controls the degree of curvature of the lens). The former is a subcortical reflex and relays in the accessory oculomotor (Edinger-Westphal) nucleus (see Section V, Plate 6), whereas the latter involves pathways through the cerebral cortex.

The *ventral lateral geniculate nucleus* receives visual input from optic nerve fibers, the visual cortex and the superior colliculus. It projects to other visual structures and also sends fibers to the pontine nuclei, which then project to the cerebellum (Plate 37). The deep nuclei of the cerebellum, in turn, project back to the ventral lateral geniculate nucleus. The precise function of these connections is unknown, but they are thought to be significant in visually evoked motor behavior.

The *nucleus of the accessory optic tract* is a small group of neurons located on the lateral aspect of the mesencephalon. This nucleus receives input from the optic nerve and projects to the inferior olive, the nucleus reticularis tegmenti pontis and

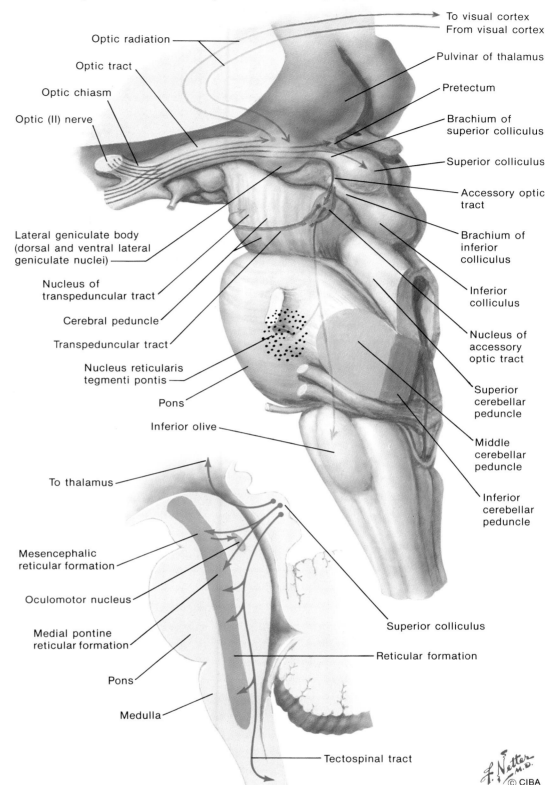

the nucleus of the transpeduncular tract. The connections to the inferior olive (the source of the climbing fibers that project to the cerebellum) and to the nucleus reticularis tegmenti pontis (the source of mossy fibers projecting to the cerebellum [Plate 37]) provide signals about the movement of images on the retina, which modulate visual tracking reflexes mediated by the vestibulocerebellum (Plates 38 and 39). The role of the transpeduncular projection is unknown.

***Neurological Disorders***. The two regions of this system most susceptible to specific clinical deficits are the superior colliculi and the pretectal region. Since the *superior colliculi* are responsible

for visuomotor coordination, including skeletal movements to assist eye fixation and eye movements for vertical and horizontal gaze, damage to this area results in the loss of fixation and tracking ability. Tumors of the pineal gland may produce pressure on the superior colliculi, initially resulting in an inability to gaze upward. Further damage causes other gaze changes, as well as a loss of ability to orient the eyes, head and body to external signals. The *pretectal area* may be affected by diseases such as CNS syphilis, alcoholism or encephalitis. When this occurs, there is a loss of the pupillary reflex to light but not to accommodation (Argyll-Robertson pupil). □

# Taste Receptors

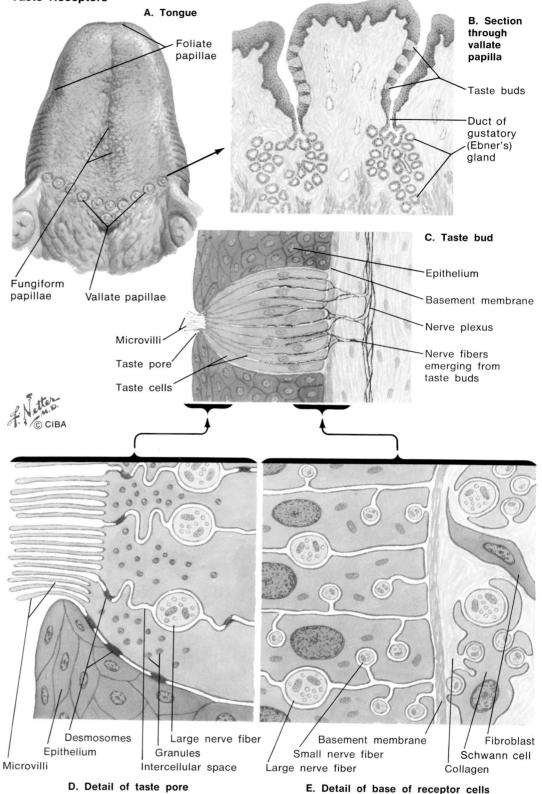

**Taste Receptors**

**A. Tongue**

Foliate papillae

Fungiform papillae

Vallate papillae

**B. Section through vallate papilla**

Taste buds

Duct of gustatory (Ebner's) gland

**C. Taste bud**

Epithelium

Basement membrane

Nerve plexus

Nerve fibers emerging from taste buds

Microvilli

Taste pore

Taste cells

**D. Detail of taste pore**

Microvilli

Epithelium

Desmosomes

Granules

Large nerve fiber

Intercellular space

**E. Detail of base of receptor cells**

Basement membrane

Small nerve fiber

Large nerve fiber

Fibroblast

Schwann cell

Collagen

***Taste Buds***. Gustatory caliculi contain the receptors responsible for the sensation of taste. They are located in the epithelium of the tongue, mouth and throat. The greatest concentration of taste buds is on the sides of the *vallate papillae* at the base of the tongue, with lesser numbers located on the walls surrounding these papillae. Taste buds are also numerous on the *foliate papillae* found on the sides and tip of the tongue, but are sparingly distributed on the *fungiform papillae, soft palate, epiglottis* and *pharynx.*

Each *taste bud* consists of a bundle of columnar cells, which lies within the epithelium and penetrates its surface at an opening called a *taste pore.* Although the cells making up the taste bud can be subdivided into four types on the basis of detailed morphological criteria, they are actually rather similar and may all function as chemoreceptors. At their apical ends, the taste cells give rise to microvilli, which project from the taste pore. Just below their apical ends, the cells are joined by desmosomes, which seal off the intracellular spaces from the taste pore.

Taste buds are innervated by both *large* and *small fibers*, which emerge from a subepithelial nerve plexus and enter the bud at its base. The larger fibers run in clefts between taste cells, while the smaller fibers (possibly terminal branches derived from large fibers) tend to run in invaginations found in the basal parts of taste cells. The central course of these fibers in the various cranial nerves involved in taste is shown in Plate 24.

***The sensation of taste*** can be divided into four primary qualities, each of which can be elicited by a specific test compound. These are: *sweet* (sucrose), *sour* (hydrochloric acid), *salty* (sodium chloride) and *bitter* (quinine). The tip of the tongue is sensitive to all four stimuli, but especially to sweet and salty substances; the sides of the tongue, to sour substances; and the base of the tongue, to bitter substances.

Compounds evoking taste sensations are thought to act by *binding to specific receptor sites* on the apical parts (microvilli) of the taste cells. By a mechanism that is not yet understood, this binding causes an increase in the ionic conductance of the taste cell membrane, which then gives rise to a depolarization of the taste cell; this depolarization, in turn, leads to an increase in the rate of discharge of the taste fibers. Recent observations of synapticlike structures involving taste cells and

nerve fibers suggest that the transmission of excitation from taste cells to gustatory fibers may be mediated by *chemical synaptic transmission.*

A single taste cell often responds to more than one of the four primary taste stimuli, but not equally to each sensation. Similar multiple responses are observed in taste fibers, each of which synapses with several taste cells. However, the patterns of responses to the four taste stimuli by single fibers are not entirely random, because experimental studies of large groups of fibers have revealed a tendency for certain fiber groups to respond specifically to certain sets of stimuli. For instance, a considerable number of fibers have

been observed to respond well to both salt and acid stimuli, whereas fibers responding strongly to both salt and sweet stimuli are rare. Even within a given responding group, the relative sensitivity to different stimuli varies widely.

There are no hard-and-fast rules by which the gustatory system operates to produce a single taste sensation from a single stimulus. Instead, the neural message for gustatory quality is a pattern composed of the relative amounts of activity across a population of many fibers. A major challenge facing neurophysiologists is to discover how these patterns are analyzed and interpreted by the CNS. □

# Taste Pathways

The chemosensitive cells found in the taste buds of the tongue, epiglottis and larynx (Plate 23) are innervated by three groups of sensory neurons (see Section V, Plates 8, 10 and 11).

*Sensory Neurons.* The cell bodies of the first group of neurons are located in the *geniculate ganglion.* They project to the brain via the *nervus intermedius* of the facial (VII) nerve, and their distal axonal processes project to the tongue via the *facial nerve* and *chorda tympani* or the *greater (superficial) petrosal nerve* and *otic ganglion.* Both groups of fibers eventually join the *lingual nerve,* which innervates the tip of the tongue. Since the fungiform and foliate papillae found in this part of the tongue are especially sensitive to sweet, salty and sour substances, the sensory cells of the geniculate ganglion are especially important for sensing these three taste qualities.

A second group of sensory taste neurons is found in the *petrosal (inferior) ganglion* of the glossopharyngeal (IX) nerve. Their central connections are with the nucleus of the solitary tract, while their peripheral branches connect with the taste buds at the base of the tongue via the *glossopharyngeal nerve.* The third group of neurons is located in the *nodose (inferior) ganglion* of the vagus (X) nerve. They project to the brainstem nuclei via the roots of the vagus nerve and to the epiglottis and larynx via the *superior laryngeal nerve.* Since taste cells in the vallate papillae at the base of the tongue and in the epiglottis and larynx are especially sensitive to bitter substances, the petrosal and nodose ganglia play an important role in producing the sensation of bitterness.

*Central Connections.* Within the brain, all three groups of taste fibers project to the *rostral part of the nucleus of the solitary tract,* where they activate second order taste relay neurons. These neurons then project to neurons in the *pontine taste area,* which in turn project to the thalamus, lateral hypothalamic area and amygdala. The projection to the *thalamus* originates bilaterally and terminates in the *ventral posteromedial* (VPM) nucleus (Plate 42). The VPM nucleus is the specific thalamic relay nucleus that sends fibers to the taste region of the *sensory cortex,* located just below the face. Thus, the taste connections of the thalamus appear to be involved in the conscious perception of taste. The bilaterality of taste projections provides for an overall appreciation of taste qualities, although this diffusion results in the relative inability to localize taste perception to a specific side of the tongue. The *hypothalamic* and *amygdalar* taste connections, on the other hand, appear to be primarily involved in reflex and motivational responses to taste stimuli, and thus control food intake (Plate 62).

The reflex-type brainstem connections of the taste pathway nuclei with the autonomic nuclei for salivation (superior and inferior salivatory nuclei) form the anatomical basis for the salivation reflexes that accompany taste responses to food stimuli on the tongue. Other autonomic brainstem connections are responsible for "gustation

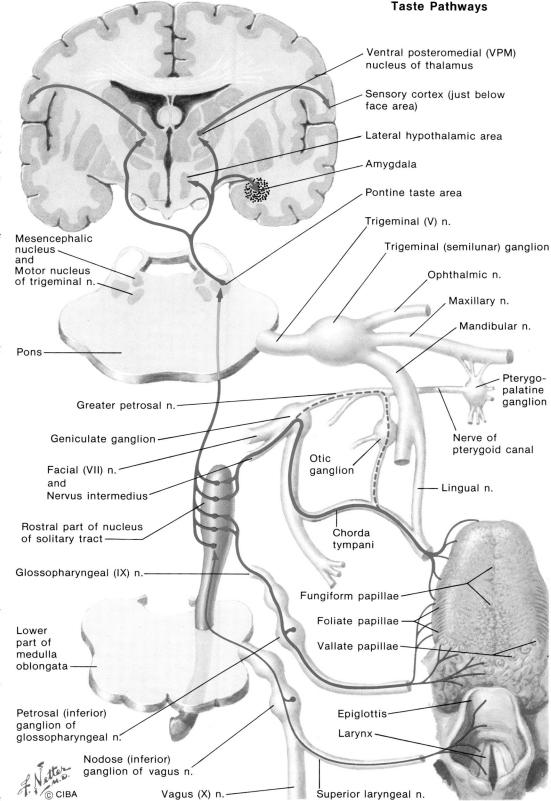

Ventral posteromedial (VPM) nucleus of thalamus

Sensory cortex (just below face area)

Lateral hypothalamic area

Amygdala

Pontine taste area

Trigeminal (V) n.

Trigeminal (semilunar) ganglion

Ophthalmic n.

Maxillary n.

Mandibular n.

Pterygopalatine ganglion

Nerve of pterygoid canal

Lingual n.

Ventral posteromedial (VPM) nucleus of thalamus

Mesencephalic nucleus and Motor nucleus of trigeminal n.

Pons

Greater petrosal n.

Geniculate ganglion

Facial (VII) n. and Nervus intermedius

Rostral part of nucleus of solitary tract

Glossopharyngeal (IX) n.

Lower part of medulla oblongata

Petrosal (inferior) ganglion of glossopharyngeal n.

Nodose (inferior) ganglion of vagus n.

Vagus (X) n.

Otic ganglion

Chorda tympani

Fungiform papillae

Foliate papillae

Vallate papillae

Epiglottis

Larynx

Superior laryngeal n.

sweating," which is characterized by localized facial and forehead sweating in response to eating spicy or peppery foods. Although this is a normal response, it can be pathological if sweating is profuse.

As explained on page 174, individual taste fibers respond to all four taste qualities in a weighted fashion, rather than to a single taste stimulus. This diversity of response appears to arise from the complex connnections of each fiber with multiple sensory cells. The same weighted multiple-taste responses happen in neurons at all stages of the taste pathway shown in the illustration. In addition, taste-sensitive neurons in the

VPM thalamic nucleus have been found to respond to thermal, although not to mechanical, stimulation of the tongue. The mechanism by which individual taste qualities are derived from the mixed sensory signals transmitted by the taste pathways has not yet been determined.

*Lesions* of the facial nerve, proximal to the emergence of the chorda tympani nerve but distal to the geniculate ganglion, result in an ipsilateral loss of taste, but not in a loss of general sensation on the anterior two thirds of the tongue. Glossopharyngeal nerve lesions cause a loss of general sensation, as well as of taste, on the posterior part of the tongue. □

# Cochlear Receptors

*The human cochlea* is a spiral channel located within the petrous portion of the temporal bone at the base of the skull. It is divided into three spaces by the *vestibular (Reissner's) membrane* and the *basilar membrane*. Between these membranes is the *cochlear duct (scala media)*, filled with potassium-rich endolymph and continuous with the vestibular labyrinth (Plate 28). The two remaining spaces, the *scala vestibuli* and the *scala tympani*, are external to the membranous labyrinth and are filled with perilymph. At the basal end of the scala vestibuli is the *oval window*, which is connected to the auditory ossicles that transmit vibration from the eardrum. At the basal end of the scala tympani is the membrane-covered *round window*, whose movements provide a compensatory release of the vibratory pressures at the oval window.

The cochlea receives dual innervation: afferent fibers, which originate from cell bodies in the *spiral ganglion* adjacent to the cochlear duct (Plate 26), and efferent fibers, which originate in the *brainstem* (Plate 27). Both types of fibers form synapses with sensory hair cells in the *spiral organ of Corti* (experimental studies have shown that activity in the efferent fibers can inhibit the discharge of cochlear afferent fibers). At the center of the organ of Corti is the *tunnel of Corti*, flanked by two sets of supporting *rods of Corti* (pillar cells).

*Hearing.* Vibrations applied to the oval window spread through the cochlea and induce vibrations in the basilar membrane, which are then transduced into afferent nerve excitation by the hair cells. The *hair cells* are arranged in inner and outer groups, and each cell is capped with 50 to 100 hairlike *stereocilia*. The inner hair cells, about 3,500 in number, are arranged in a single row on the inner side of the inner rods of Corti; the 12,000 outer hair cells are longer, and are arranged in three rows in the basal coil of the cochlea, and in four or five rows in the apical coil. Physiological studies suggest that cochlear hair cells behave like their vestibular counterparts: by an unknown mechanism, bending of stereocilia in one direction leads to a depolarization of hair cells and an accelerated rate of nerve discharge, while bending in the opposite direction produces hyperpolarization and a slowing of discharge.

In the illustration, C shows how the spiral organ of Corti transforms vibrations of the basilar membrane into a force bending the sensory hairs. The cells themselves are held in a fixed relationship to the basilar membrane by supporting cells and the rods of Corti. The stereocilia of both groups of hair cells are embedded in the overlying *tectorial membrane*, which is suspended in such a way that the up-and-down movement of the basilar membrane causes the tectorial membrane to slide back and forth across the surface of the hair cells, thereby producing a shearing force on the stereocilia. When the basilar membrane moves in response to incident sound vibrations, the afferent fibers are excited and tend to fire during that part of the vibratory cycle which corresponds to the maximum outward bending of the stereocilia. This "phase-locked firing" helps the CNS to analyze sound frequencies.

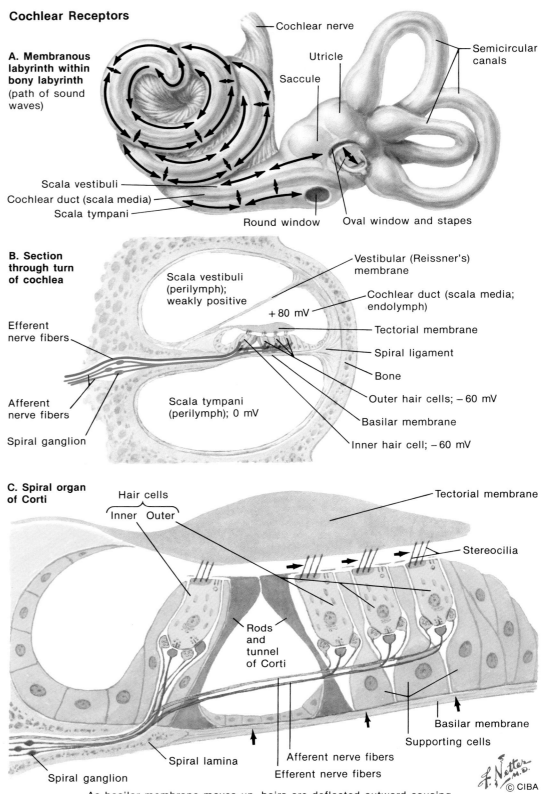

## Cochlear Receptors

**A. Membranous labyrinth within bony labyrinth** (path of sound waves)

Cochlear nerve
Semicircular canals
Utricle
Saccule
Scala vestibuli
Cochlear duct (scala media)
Scala tympani
Round window
Oval window and stapes

**B. Section through turn of cochlea**

Scala vestibuli (perilymph); weakly positive
Vestibular (Reissner's) membrane
+ 80 mV
Cochlear duct (scala media; endolymph)
Tectorial membrane
Spiral ligament
Bone
Outer hair cells; – 60 mV
Basilar membrane
Inner hair cell; – 60 mV
Efferent nerve fibers
Afferent nerve fibers
Spiral ganglion
Scala tympani (perilymph); 0 mV

**C. Spiral organ of Corti**

Hair cells
Inner   Outer
Tectorial membrane
Stereocilia
Rods and tunnel of Corti
Basilar membrane
Supporting cells
Spiral lamina
Afferent nerve fibers
Efferent nerve fibers
Spiral ganglion

As basilar membrane moves up, hairs are deflected outward causing depolarization of hair cells and increased firing of afferent nerve fibers

Another type of frequency analysis is based on the differences in the shape and stiffness of the basilar membrane located between the base and the apex of the cochlea. Because of these variations, the basilar membrane at the base of the cochlea resonates most readily at high frequencies, whereas at the apex it resonates best at low frequencies. The dimensions of the basilar membrane alter gradually, so that for each vibration frequency between the two extremes, a region of the membrane, and hence a group of afferent fibers, responds most vigorously. The cochlea is therefore said to be *tonotopically organized*: each afferent fiber will respond to some extent to a range of frequencies, while within the range is one frequency to which it will respond most readily.

*Deafness.* The cochlea is often the source of deafness, either to a specific pitch or to a broad range of frequencies. Head trauma can produce transient deafness, but severe injury involving a fracture of the petrous part of the temporal bone can cause permanent spiral ganglion or cochlear damage. Intense noise can cause temporary deafness; if it is sustained, permanent cochlear damage will result. The most common cause of deafness in adult life is *otosclerosis*, a non-neural process that results in the fixation of the stapes to the oval window. □

# Afferent Auditory Pathways

Auditory afferent fibers, upon entering the brainstem in the vestibulocochlear (VIII) nerve (Plate 25; see also Section V, Plate 9), branch to innervate two primary receiving areas within the medulla oblongata—the *dorsal* and *ventral cochlear nuclei*. Neurons in these nuclei have similar properties: each is excited by a relatively narrow range of sound frequencies and may be inhibited by tones outside that range. Within each nucleus, neurons sensitive to different frequencies are arranged in an orderly manner, which gives rise to a *tonotopic* distribution within the nucleus.

Beyond the cochlear nuclei, the auditory pathway consists of a series of nuclei—the *superior olivary complex*, the *nucleus of the lateral lemniscus*, the *inferior colliculus* and the *medial geniculate body*. Within these nuclei, signals from both ears interact on their way toward the cerebral cortex (some of the complex interconnections between these nuclei are shown). As the signals ascend the pathway, they do not necessarily relay at each nucleus along the line. Thus, fibers from the cochlear nuclei project directly to the nucleus of the lateral lemniscus, and fibers from the superior olive pass without interruption to the inferior colliculus.

Eventually, auditory signals reach the *medial geniculate body*, the lateral portion (pars principalis) of which projects to the primary auditory cortex (Plate 43). In man, Brodmann's area 41 in the temporal lobe has been identified as the *primary auditory area*; it is not known whether secondary auditory areas also exist, as in lower mammals. Despite the extensive intermixing among afferent fibers, the bulk of the neural activity reaching the auditory cortex originates in the contralateral ear. Tonotopic ordering is preserved throughout the ascending pathway, so that individual cortical regions are sensitive to specific frequencies. The width of the band of frequencies to which an individual neuron responds is approximately the same in area 41 as at the level of the cochlear nuclei.

In the analysis of acoustic information, relatively little is known about the function of the various stages within the auditory pathway. Recently, it has been shown that neurons within the *superior olivary complex* are specifically adapted for analyzing the location of a sound in space. Olivary neurons receive excitatory input from the contralateral cochlear nuclei and inhibitory input from the ipsilateral cochlear nuclei. In the medial portion of the complex, where neurons are sensitive to sounds of low frequency, these opposing inputs result in individual neurons becoming attuned to a fixed time delay between the arrival of sound at each ear. In the lateral portion of the complex, where neurons are sensitive to higher frequencies, the opposing inputs result in neurons becoming sensitive to differences in the intensity of sound reaching each ear. Psychophysical studies have shown that interaural time delays and intensity differences are the key features responsible for localizing a sound. However, even though the

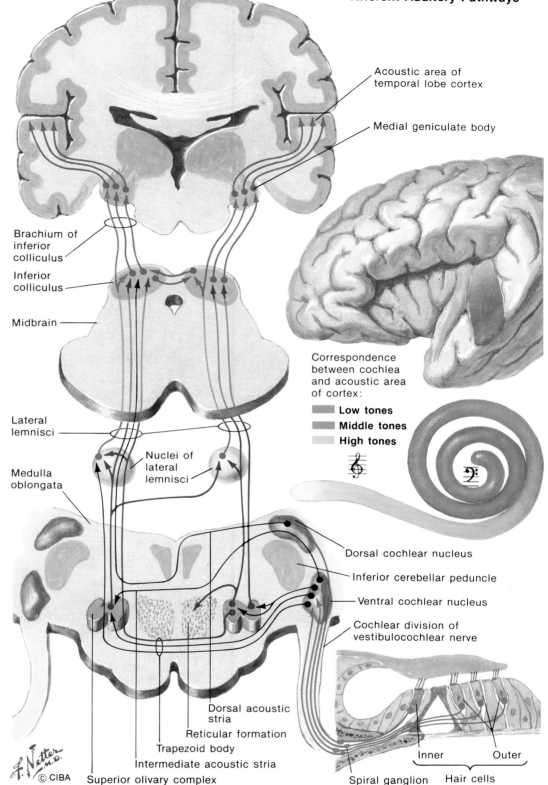

Acoustic area of temporal lobe cortex

Medial geniculate body

Brachium of inferior colliculus

Inferior colliculus

Midbrain

Lateral lemnisci

Nuclei of lateral lemnisci

Medulla oblongata

Correspondence between cochlea and acoustic area of cortex:

Low tones
Middle tones
High tones

Dorsal cochlear nucleus

Inferior cerebellar peduncle

Ventral cochlear nucleus

Cochlear division of vestibulocochlear nerve

Dorsal acoustic stria

Reticular formation

Trapezoid body

Intermediate acoustic stria

Superior olivary complex

Spiral ganglion

Inner / Outer — Hair cells

analysis of these features is carried out by neurons in the superior olivary complex, studies involving CNS lesions have shown that the entire auditory pathway, including the auditory cortex, must be intact for sound localization to take place. Similarly, auditory structures as far as the level of the *inferior colliculus* are required for frequency discrimination, even though neurons at all levels of the auditory pathway are frequency selective. Intensity discriminations, on the other hand, can be made following the destruction of the inferior colliculus and higher centers. Such discrimination may involve the collateral pathways that relay auditory signals to the *brainstem reticular formation*.

These pathways are probably also involved in the reflex reaction to a sudden sound.

*Disorders.* A common auditory pathway deficit is acoustic neuroma. The patient suffers loss of sound localization, diminished speech discrimination and diminution of the stapedius reflex. Nerve-type deafness can be caused by toxins (eg, arsenic, lead, quinine) and by antibiotics such as streptomycin, which can also damage the cochlea directly. Because of the multisynaptic and highly complex system of crossed pathways, damage to auditory brainstem tracts and nuclei by trauma, tumors or vascular disorders results in only a slight hearing impairment. ☐

# Centrifugal Auditory Pathways

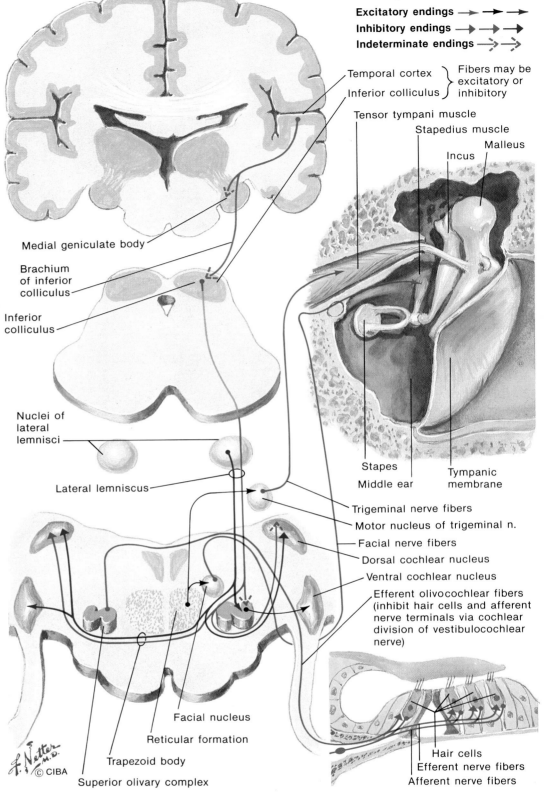

**Centrifugal Auditory Pathways**

Excitatory endings →→→

Inhibitory endings →→→

Indeterminate endings ⇢⇢

Temporal cortex ⎫ Fibers may be
Inferior colliculus ⎬ excitatory or
 ⎭ inhibitory

Tensor tympani muscle

Stapedius muscle

Malleus

Incus

Medial geniculate body

Brachium of inferior colliculus

Inferior colliculus

Nuclei of lateral lemnisci

Lateral lemniscus

Stapes
Middle ear

Tympanic membrane

Trigeminal nerve fibers

Motor nucleus of trigeminal n.

Facial nerve fibers

Dorsal cochlear nucleus

Ventral cochlear nucleus

Efferent olivocochlear fibers (inhibit hair cells and afferent nerve terminals via cochlear division of vestibulocochlear nerve)

Facial nucleus

Reticular formation

Trapezoid body

Superior olivary complex

Hair cells
Efferent nerve fibers
Afferent nerve fibers

Centrifugal connections are a prominent feature of the auditory system. Within the brain, such connections arise from each of the areas involved in the auditory system, including the primary auditory cortex, and project to nuclei one or two levels below their point of origin. Individual connections may be either excitatory or inhibitory, but the centrifugal pathways appear to be activated by the inhibition of transmission of auditory signals through the ascending auditory pathways (Plate 26).

Centrifugal auditory pathways also include efferent projections to the sensory hair cells of the cochlea (Plate 25) and to the muscles of the middle ear. The cochlear efferent fibers originate from a group of neurons on the medial side of the contralateral superior olive (retroolivary group), and pass to the cochlea via the crossed olivocochlear bundle and the cochlear division of the vestibulocochlear (VIII) nerve. They are joined by a smaller number of fibers, which originate in the ipsilateral superior olive (not shown in the illustration). The efferent fibers produce hyperpolarization in the cochlear hair cells and afferent nerve terminals, thereby decreasing the afferent response produced when sound reaches the cochlea. Fibers innervating the muscles of the middle ear originate in the trigeminal motor nucleus and the facial nucleus (the tensor tympani muscle and the stapedius muscle). By contracting, these muscles decrease the transmission of sound vibrations from the eardrum to the oval window by the ossicles (incus, malleus and stapes).

Several functions have been proposed for the centrifugal auditory pathways. One possibility is that efferent impulses can dampen the sensitivity of the auditory system, thus preventing damage to it from too strong a stimulus. The middle ear muscles contract during loud noises and self-initiated vocalization, thereby helping to prevent saturation or damage of the cochlear receptors. Sound-activated efferent fibers in the olivocochlear bundle may additionally contribute to the suppression of sensory input that could saturate the central nervous pathways. A related mechanism, possibly also mediated by olivocochlear fibers, is one whereby auditory discrimination is improved by the attenuation of the response of the auditory system to loud background noise, although it is not known to what extent centrifugal connections within the CNS may contribute to this suppression of strong sounds.

The phenomenon of selective attention to auditory signals may also be an effect of the centrifugal auditory pathways. Changes in the activity of the ear muscle have been observed during attentive behavior. Evidence also shows that the inhibition occurring within the cochlear nuclei may be related to the habituation that occurs when an auditory stimulus is presented repeatedly.

Finally, centrifugal connections may play a role in the shaping of neural signals underlying auditory discrimination. Neurons at higher levels of the auditory pathway tend to respond to transient changes in auditory input rather than to steady signals. Centrifugal inhibition may be a factor in eliminating responses to steady signals, thus accentuating sensitivity to transient ones. Together with the inhibition that takes place within each level of the auditory system, it may also contribute to the processes that sharpen neuronal responses by restricting the ranges of the frequencies to which each neuron responds.

Evidence to support the roles proposed for the centrifugal auditory system is fragmentary; rather, these theories should be regarded as hypotheses requiring verification. The wide extent of centrifugal auditory connections, however, indicates that they are important in controlling man's responses to auditory stimuli. □

# Vestibular Receptors

*The membrane labyrinth*, filled with potassium-rich endolymph, is a system of thin-walled intercommunicating tubes and ducts situated within the petrous part of the temporal bone at the base of the skull. In addition to the *cochlear duct* (Plate 25), it consists of five vestibular structures, each containing a specialized mechanoreceptor. The saclike *utricle* and *saccule* contain areas called *maculae*, which specifically respond to linear acceleration, such as the pull of gravity. Connected to the utricle are the three *semicircular canals*. Within swellings of the canals, called *ampullae*, are the specialized detectors of angular acceleration, the *cristae*.

The vestibular labyrinth receives a dual innervation, which consists of the distal axonal processes of bipolar vestibular afferent neurons (whose cell bodies are in the *vestibular ganglion*) and the vestibular efferent fibers that originate in the *brainstem*. The afferent axons terminate on the mechanoreceptive vestibular *hair cells* that are the basic sensory transducers of the labyrinth.

*Hair Cells*. On some hair cells (type I), the afferent terminal takes the form of a large, goblet-shaped nerve calyx; on others (type II), only small, budlike, terminal synaptic boutons are found. Type I hair cells are thought to be more sensitive than those of type II. Efferent fibers form typical chemical synapses with hair cells or with afferent terminals, which act to increase the discharge rate of afferent fibers and to modulate their response to mechanical stimuli.

The apical ends of both types of hair cells bear a tuft of 40 or more sensory hairs, or *stereocilia*, whose bases are embedded in a stiff cuticle, and a single, lower *kinocilium*, which originates from a basal body and has a structure similar to that of a motile cilium. The entire group of hairs is joined together at its free end. The effective stimulus for a hair cell is a shearing force that bends its sensory hairs; when the stereocilia are bent toward the kinocilium, the cell becomes depolarized, thus increasing the discharge frequency of the afferent nerve. Bending in the opposite direction leads to hyperpolarization and a decrease in discharge frequency. The mechanism that transduces hair bending into changes in hair cell membrane potential is not known, but the structure of the hair tuft suggests that these changes may be related to a deformation of the region around the basal body, which is more compliant than the cuticle.

*The cristae and maculae* are especially sensitive to angular and linear acceleration, because of accessory structures that convert head movements to bending forces on the sensory hairs. The sensory hairs of the mechanoreceptors in the *cristae* are embedded in the gelatinous *cupula* that extends to the opposite wall of the ampulla. Angular acceleration in the plane of the semicircular canal causes the fluid within the canal, the inertia of which tends to resist movement, to press against the cupula. This pressure causes the cupula to flex into a concave or a convex shape, thus bending the sensory hairs. Since all hair cells in the crista are oriented in the same direction as their kinocilia, this bending either increases or

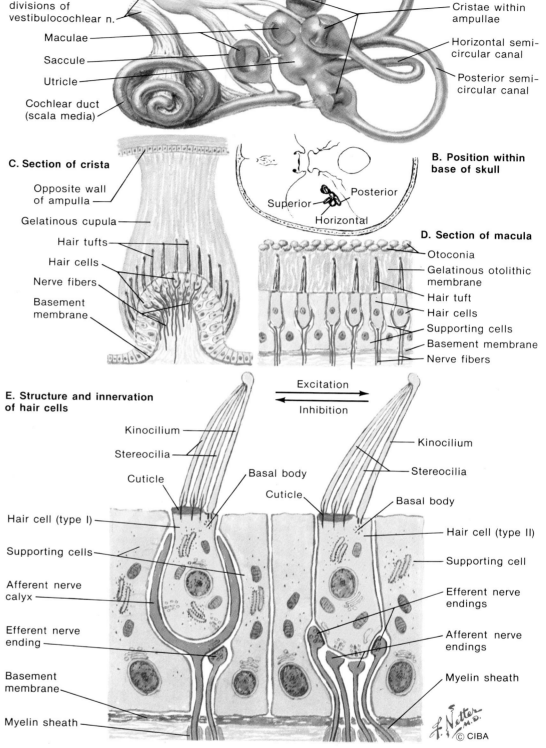

### Vestibular Receptors

**A. Membranous labyrinth**

Vestibular ganglion
Vestibular and cochlear divisions of vestibulocochlear n.
Maculae
Saccule
Utricle
Cochlear duct (scala media)
Superior semicircular canal
Cristae within ampullae
Horizontal semicircular canal
Posterior semicircular canal

**C. Section of crista**

Opposite wall of ampulla
Gelatinous cupula
Hair tufts
Hair cells
Nerve fibers
Basement membrane

**B. Position within base of skull**

Superior
Posterior
Horizontal

**D. Section of macula**

Otoconia
Gelatinous otolithic membrane
Hair tuft
Hair cells
Supporting cells
Basement membrane
Nerve fibers

**E. Structure and innervation of hair cells**

Excitation
Inhibition

Kinocilium
Stereocilia
Cuticle
Hair cell (type I)
Supporting cells
Afferent nerve calyx
Efferent nerve ending
Basement membrane
Myelin sheath

Basal body
Cuticle

Kinocilium
Stereocilia
Basal body
Hair cell (type II)
Supporting cell
Efferent nerve endings
Afferent nerve endings
Myelin sheath

decreases the discharge rate of all the afferent fibers.

The hairs of the sensory cells found in the *maculae* are embedded in a gelatinous otolithic membrane covered with crystals of calcium carbonate, called *otoconia*. Because the otoconia are denser than the surrounding fluid, the otolithic membrane tends to move under the influence of linear acceleration. For instance, when the normally horizontal utricular macula is tilted, the pull of gravity tends to make the otolithic membrane slide downward, thus bending the sensory hairs. Since the macula contains hair cells that have two different orientations, this bending

increases the discharge rate of some utricular afferent fibers and slows the discharge rate of others. These signals are analyzed by the CNS for information on the position of the head. The macula of the *saccule* is in a vertical position and is therefore sensitive to vertical acceleration. The saccule may also contribute to the sensing of head position when the head is oriented with one ear down.

*Vestibular dysfunction* is often accompanied by such autonomic events as sweating, nausea, vomiting, tachycardia and decreased blood pressure, probably because of reflex connections between the vestibular input and the autonomic visceral motor centers in the brainstem. □

# Vestibulospinal Tracts

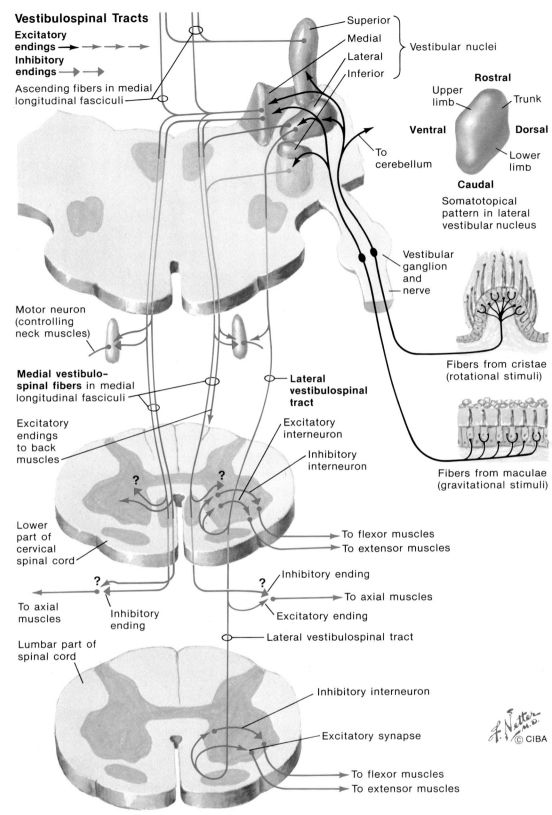

**Vestibulospinal Tracts**

Excitatory endings →
Inhibitory endings →
Ascending fibers in medial longitudinal fasciculi

Superior
Medial
Lateral — Vestibular nuclei
Inferior

Rostral
Upper limb
Trunk
Ventral
Dorsal
Lower limb
Caudal
Somatotopical pattern in lateral vestibular nucleus

To cerebellum

Vestibular ganglion and nerve

Fibers from cristae (rotational stimuli)

Fibers from maculae (gravitational stimuli)

Motor neuron (controlling neck muscles)

Medial vestibulospinal fibers in medial longitudinal fasciculi

Excitatory endings to back muscles

Lower part of cervical spinal cord

Lateral vestibulospinal tract

Excitatory interneuron

Inhibitory interneuron

To flexor muscles
To extensor muscles

To axial muscles
Inhibitory ending

Inhibitory ending
To axial muscles
Excitatory ending
Lateral vestibulospinal tract

To axial muscles
Lumbar part of spinal cord

Inhibitory interneuron

Excitatory synapse

To flexor muscles
To extensor muscles

*The vestibular nuclei* consist of four major groups of neurons—the *superior, medial, lateral* and *inferior vestibular nuclei*—situated in the dorsolateral part of the pons and medulla oblongata (see Section V, Plate 9). Three of these neuronal groups—the medial, lateral (Deiters') and inferior (descending) vestibular nuclei—comprise the major central termination of the vestibular afferent fibers that supply the otolithic organs (utricle and saccule) of the labyrinth (Plate 28). Vestibular afferent fibers supplying the semicircular canals end primarily in the superior, medial and lateral vestibular nuclei, but many fibers also terminate in the vestibulocerebellum (Plate 39). In addition to these vestibular afferent impulses, the vestibular nuclei also receive input from the spinal cord, cerebellum, reticular formation and higher centers.

The known output pathways from the vestibular nuclei include projections to the spinal cord, oculomotor nuclei, cerebellum and reticular formation. Vestibular activity also reaches the thalamus, superior colliculus and other higher centers, but the exact pathways are not known.

*Vestibulospinal Tracts.* The illustration shows the projections of vestibular neurons to the spinal cord via the *lateral vestibulospinal tract (LVST)* and *medial vestibulospinal tract (MVST)*. These two tracts, which lie in the anterior and anteromedial funiculi (Plate 48), act primarily on the motor apparatus that controls the proximal muscles, and therefore are important in the regulation of postural equilibrium.

The *LVST* originates primarily from the *lateral vestibular nucleus.* Some of the neurons of this nucleus extend for the entire length of the spinal cord, while others reach only part of the distance; they may also branch to innervate several regions along their path of descent. The lateral nucleus is *somatotopically organized*—neurons projecting to the lower (hindlimb) levels of the spinal cord are located in the dorsocaudal portion of the nucleus, and neurons ending at higher levels are situated in the ventrorostral portion. The former region receives a heavy projection from the cerebellar vermis (Plate 38), whereas the latter region receives a heavy input of vestibular afferent fibers.

The predominant action of the LVST is to produce the contraction of extensor (antigravity)

muscles and the relaxation of flexor muscles. In the case of neck, trunk and some lower limb extensor muscles, contraction is produced in part by direct (monosynaptic) excitation of motor neurons. The excitation of other limb extensor muscles and the inhibition of flexor muscles are mediated by pathways that include spinal interneurons.

The *MVST* extends only as far as the thoracic spinal segments. It contains fibers that originate in the *medial vestibular nucleus* and produce direct inhibition of motor neurons controlling neck and axial muscles. In addition, the tract contains fibers originating in the medial, lateral and inferior

vestibular nuclei, which excite motor neurons in the neck and back, and probably other neurons as well. Anatomical data indicate that MVST fibers also terminate within the cervical enlargement of the spinal cord, chiefly on interneurons.

The two vestibulospinal tracts are important factors in *vestibular reflex reactions* that are triggered by the movement of the head in space. Particularly significant in this regard is the strong vestibular action on the neck muscles, which helps to stabilize the position of the head. However, these tracts and the reticulospinal tracts (Plate 47) also appear to play a much wider role in the control of the proximal musculature. □

# Control of Eye Movements

The extraocular muscles responsible for eye movements are controlled by motor neurons located in various nuclei. Thus, the lateral rectus is controlled by the abducens nucleus; the superior oblique, by the trochlear nucleus; and the superior, inferior and medial recti and the inferior oblique muscles, by the oculomotor nucleus. Both smooth (pursuit) and rapid (saccadic) eye movements depend on patterns of activity produced in these muscles by direct projections from the vestibular nuclei and the reticular formation (Plate 31), and by indirect activation from the superior colliculus and the cerebral cortex.

*The vestibular projection* is important for the maintaining of visual fixation during head movements. To effect smooth movement, tracking and proper visualization, the contraction of one eye muscle must be accompanied by the relaxation of its antagonist. The action of turning the head excites *vestibular afferent fibers* from semicircular canal receptors. Fibers from an individual semicircular canal excite two specific groups of relay neurons in the *vestibular nuclei*. One group excites the extraocular motor neurons that cause the eyes to move in the direction opposite to the head movement, and the other group inhibits motor neurons that activate movement of the eyes in the same direction as the head. (For example, turning the head to the right will excite fibers from the right horizontal semicircular canal, which in turn will activate neurons in the right medial and lateral vestibular nuclei. Some of these vestibular neurons will then excite motor neurons controlling the right medial and left lateral rectus muscles. Other vestibular neurons will inhibit motor neurons controlling the right lateral rectus and internuclear neurons controlling the left medial rectus. The result will be a compensatory movement of both eyes to the left.) The vestibulocerebellum modulates the vestibulo-extraocular reflex in such a way that the resulting eye movement precisely compensates for the head movement and thus keeps the gaze fixed on the same point (see page 191).

The connections of the right vestibular nuclei to the *abducens, trochlear* and *oculomotor nuclei* can be divided into two sections. The first section comprises vestibular projections to motor neurons supplying the superior and inferior rectus and superior and inferior oblique muscles. These motor neurons all receive excitatory input from the contralateral medial nucleus, and inhibitory input from the ipsilateral superior nucleus. The innervation of medial and lateral rectus motor neurons, which mediate horizontal eye movements, is organized differently. The medial vestibular nucleus sends excitatory fibers to the contralateral abducens nucleus and inhibitory fibers to the ipsilateral abducens nucleus. These fibers excite or inhibit the lateral rectus motor neurons and another group of neurons within the abducens nucleus, the internuclear neurons, which project to the opposite oculomotor nucleus to excite the medial rectus motor neurons. The latter neurons are also excited by fibers that originate in the lateral vestibular nucleus and pass upward in the ascending tract of Deiters. If the

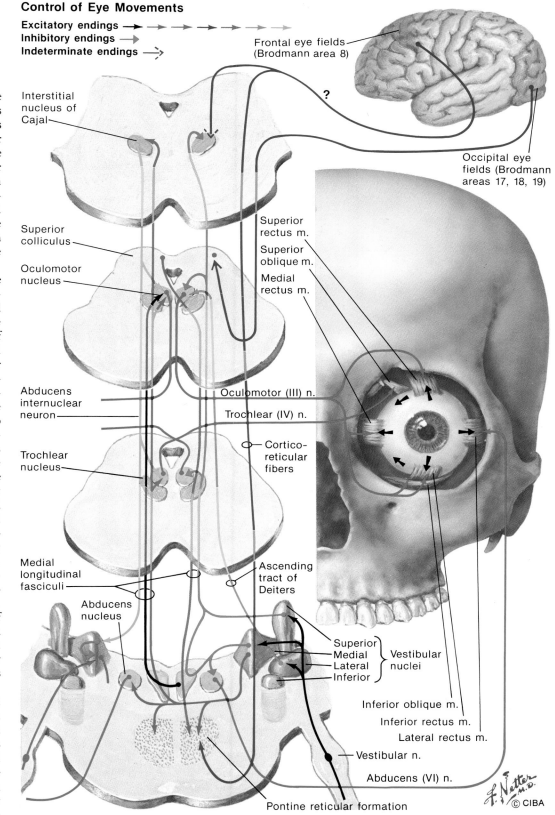

## Control of Eye Movements

Excitatory endings →  →  →  →  →  →
Inhibitory endings →
Indeterminate endings ⇢

Frontal eye fields (Brodmann area 8)

Occipital eye fields (Brodmann areas 17, 18, 19)

Interstitial nucleus of Cajal

Superior colliculus

Oculomotor nucleus

Abducens internuclear neuron

Trochlear nucleus

Medial longitudinal fasciculi

Abducens nucleus

Superior rectus m.
Superior oblique m.
Medial rectus m.

Oculomotor (III) n.
Trochlear (IV) n.
Cortico-reticular fibers

Ascending tract of Deiters

Superior
Medial
Lateral
Inferior
} Vestibular nuclei

Inferior oblique m.
Inferior rectus m.
Lateral rectus m.

Vestibular n.
Abducens (VI) n.

Pontine reticular formation

axons of internuclear neurons are interrupted by lesions of the medial longitudinal fasciculus, this results in the paresis of the medial rectus, seen in internuclear ophthalmoplegia.

*Other Pathways.* In addition to the relatively direct pathways described above, each nucleus also receives input via more complex pathways involving the reticular formation. These pathways are also modulated by semicircular canal activity and can produce compensatory movements similar to those mediated by the disynaptic pathways. The *reticular formation*, however, appears to be especially important in organizing fast, saccadic eye movements, which may be initiated by signals

from the frontal cortical eye fields or the superior colliculus (Plate 31).

Two other structures are related to gaze control. The *interstitial nucleus of Cajal* receives input from the frontal cortex and vestibular nuclei and excites the motor neurons in the oculomotor and trochlear nuclei that produce vertical and oblique eye movements. It also activates inhibitory interneurons in the vestibular nuclei, thereby diminishing the activity of vestibulo-extraocular relay neurons. The *superior colliculus* receives input from the retina and visual cortex and sends excitatory fibers to neurons in the pontine reticular formation that produce saccadic eye movements (Plate 22). □

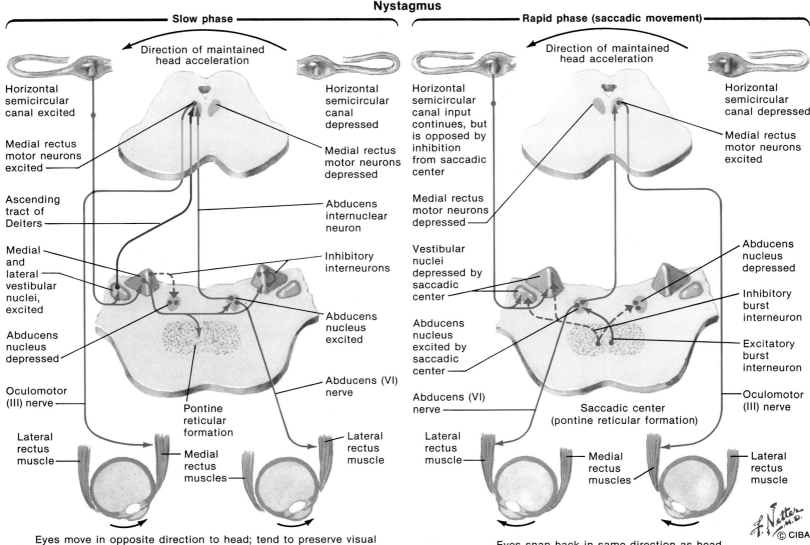

**Nystagmus**

## Slow phase

Direction of maintained head acceleration

Horizontal semicircular canal excited

Medial rectus motor neurons excited

Ascending tract of Deiters

Medial and lateral vestibular nuclei, excited

Abducens nucleus depressed

Oculomotor (III) nerve

Lateral rectus muscle

Pontine reticular formation

Medial rectus muscles

Abducens internuclear neuron

Inhibitory interneurons

Abducens nucleus excited

Abducens (VI) nerve

Lateral rectus muscle

Horizontal semicircular canal depressed

Medial rectus motor neurons depressed

Eyes move in opposite direction to head; tend to preserve visual fixation: rate determined by degree of horizontal canal excitation

## Rapid phase (saccadic movement)

Direction of maintained head acceleration

Horizontal semicircular canal input continues, but is opposed by inhibition from saccadic center

Medial rectus motor neurons depressed

Vestibular nuclei depressed by saccadic center

Abducens nucleus excited by saccadic center

Abducens (VI) nerve

Lateral rectus muscle

Saccadic center (pontine reticular formation)

Medial rectus muscles

Horizontal semicircular canal depressed

Medial rectus motor neurons excited

Abducens nucleus depressed

Inhibitory burst interneuron

Excitatory burst interneuron

Oculomotor (III) nerve

Lateral rectus muscle

Eyes snap back in same direction as head

CIBA

# Nystagmus

Nystagmus consists of alternating back-and-forth movements of the eyes. The movement in one direction resembles the slow eye movement seen during the *tracking of an object* (pursuit), whereas the return movement in the opposite direction consists of a *saccadic* (quick) "beat." By convention, the direction of the quick eye movement is used to specify the direction of the nystagmus. In most cases, nystagmus can be classified into two categories.

*Optokinetic nystagmus* is produced by prolonged, recurrent activation of the visual pathways sensitive to image motion (Plates 21 and 22). This form of nystagmus can be clinically induced by having the patient view a rotating drum marked with alternating dark and light stripes.

*Vestibular nystagmus* arises from a prolonged asymmetrical input from semicircular canal receptors of the vestibular labyrinth or from neurological disorders that induce asymmetrical activity in the vestibular nuclei or in the vestibulocerebellum on the two sides of the brain (Plates 38 and 39). Vestibular nystagmus can also be clinically induced, and is then known as "caloric" nystagmus. Warm or cold water is syringed into one ear, and, depending on the orientation of the patient's head, the heating or cooling produces a prolonged excitation of one or more of the semicircular canal receptors, thus causing nystagmus.

The illustration shows the neuronal mechanisms responsible for the slow and quick phases of vestibular nystagmus. Asymmetrical labyrinthine input is produced by a maintained horizontal angular acceleration of the head. (A similar effect could be produced by a sudden stopping of horizontal rotation.) Only the connections of neurons whose activity exceeds their resting level are illustrated. Thus, during the slow phase, the input of the left horizontal semicircular canal excites neurons in the lateral and medial vestibular nuclei on the left side, whereas the right vestibular nuclei receive less than their usual input from the right horizontal semicircular canal. As described on page 181, neurons in the left vestibular nuclei act to excite motor neurons controlling the left medial and right lateral rectus muscles

and to activate the abducens internuclear neurons that add to the excitation of the left medial rectus. Simultaneously, motor neurons controlling the antagonists of these muscles are inhibited by vestibular inhibition of the left abducens motor neurons and internuclear neurons. As the steady semicircular canal input continues, the circuitry in the vestibular nuclei and reticular formation acts as an integrator to produce a steady increase in the excitatory and inhibitory signals that reach the extraocular motor neurons. The eyes, therefore, move steadily to the right.

When the vestibulo-extraocular activity responsible for the slow phase of nystagmus reaches a certain level, it is abruptly terminated by the quick-phase mechanism. This mechanism depends on a separate group of neurons that suddenly becomes active when the oculomotor drive reaches a high level. Many lines of evidence suggest that neurons in the *pontine reticular formation* (saccadic center) participate in the quick-phase mechanism. Since this region receives signals from the vestibular nuclei, it may contain neurons that become active when those signals exceed a certain threshold. Neurons *within* the vestibular nuclei are probably also involved in the quick-phase mechanism, which appears to reverse the slow-phase eye movement both by direct excitation or inhibition of extraocular motor neurons and by influencing vestibular relay neurons. □

# Spinal Effector Mechanism

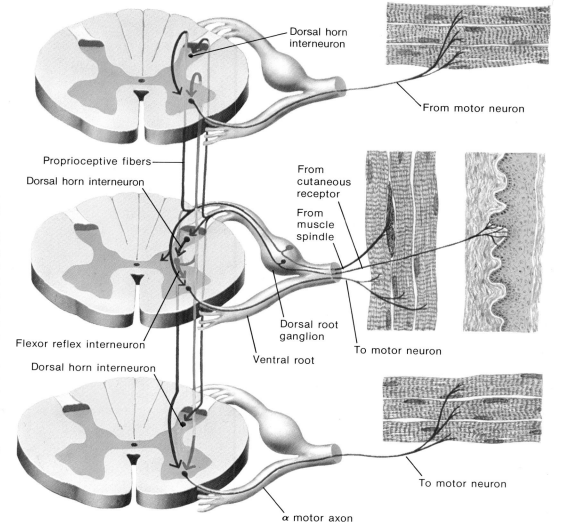

Dorsal horn interneuron

From motor neuron

Proprioceptive fibers

Dorsal horn interneuron

From cutaneous receptor

From muscle spindle

Flexor reflex interneuron

Dorsal root ganglion

To motor neuron

Dorsal horn interneuron

Ventral root

To motor neuron

α motor axon

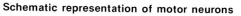

## Schematic representation of motor neurons

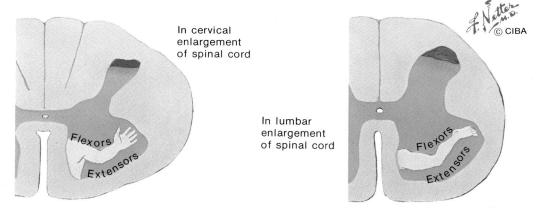

In cervical enlargement of spinal cord

In lumbar enlargement of spinal cord

Flexors

Extensors

Flexors

Extensors

The illustration shows a schematic representation of the structure of the spinal motor nuclei and their segmental connections.

*Motor Neurons.* Except for muscles innervated by the cranial nerves, each somatic muscle receives its motor supply from a column of motor neurons arranged longitudinally in the anterior horn of the spinal cord. Motor neurons fall into three classes (Plates 22 and 34). The large *alpha motor neurons* supply the extrafusal fibers of the muscle, and each motor neuron may innervate several to more than one thousand fibers distributed throughout the muscle. The fibers innervated by a single motor neuron are called a *motor unit*. The small *gamma motor neurons* (fusimotor neurons) innervate the intrafusal muscles of the spindles, thus regulating proprioceptive feedback of information about muscle length. The intermediate-sized *beta motor neurons* project to both extrafusal and intrafusal muscles; their activity causes contraction and also adjusts length feedback to compensate for that contraction.

*Motor nuclei* may extend longitudinally over several segments of the spinal cord. Despite this, the nuclei supplying different muscles tend to be arranged in an orderly, somatotopic pattern (Plate 49). In the upper cervical and thoracic segments, which innervate only axial muscles, the anteromedial group is the only group of somatomotor neurons present; in the cervical and lumbar enlargements of the spinal cord (lower part of illustration), additional motor columns supplying limb muscles appear more laterally in the anterior horn. Moving from the rostral to the caudal end of the two enlargements, the motor nuclei supplying the proximal limb muscles appear first, lying adjacent to the anteromedial column. They are followed by the nuclei supplying the more distal muscles, which tend to lie more posteriorly and laterally. Nuclei supplying the extensor muscles also tend to lie anteriorly and laterally to those supplying the flexor muscles. Even the small movement of an extremity involves activity in the medial and lateral cell columns extending over several spinal cord segments.

*Proprioceptive and Exteroceptive Fibers.* Motor neurons can be influenced by both the proprioceptive and the exteroceptive fibers that enter the spinal cord. Upon entering the spinal cord (upper part of illustration), these fibers may give off ascending and descending branches that send terminal branches into the posterior or anterior horn over a distance of several segments, which approximately matches the extent of the corresponding motor nucleus. Further afferent fiber branches may continue rostrally to various sensory relay nuclei (Plates 15 and 37).

The most numerous *proprioceptive fibers* are those carrying information from muscle spindles (Group Ia and II fibers), and from Golgi tendon organs (Group Ib fibers), (Plates 34 and 35). The Ia fibers are unique in that they enter the anterior horn motor nuclei and establish direct connections with motor neurons. These connections form the basis of the *stretch reflex* (Plate 33). One Ia afferent fiber from a spindle in a given muscle produces direct excitation in virtually every motor neuron supplying that muscle and in a smaller proportion of motor neurons supplying closely related synergistic muscles. This selectivity may be explained by the fact that the terminal field of the Ia fiber is approximately coextensive with the motor nucleus of its muscle and overlaps slightly with synergist motor nuclei located nearby.

The principal reflex elicited by *exteroceptive fibers* is the *flexor withdrawal reflex* (Plate 33). The distribution of motor effects in this reflex is much broader than that of the stretch reflex, comprising most of the flexor muscles of the limb, as well as crossed activation of the contralateral extensor muscles. This distribution does not derive from the projection pattern of the afferent fibers, however, but rather from the divergent projection of chains of interneurons in the posterior and anterior horns that subserve the withdrawal reflex. □

# Spinal Reflex Pathways

The illustration shows some of the intrinsic circuitry within the spinal cord that influences the reflex activity of motor neurons. It is important to emphasize that these circuits are ordinarily under the control of higher centers (Plates 45 to 47). Nevertheless, despite the complexities introduced by a higher control, a knowledge of the basic spinal circuits is an important step toward understanding motor behavior.

*Stretch Reflex.* A and B show some of the connections made by Group Ia and II (not shown) afferent fibers from muscle spindle receptors (Plates 34 and 35). These afferent fibers are responsible for the stretch reflex, in which the stretching of a muscle elicits a contraction of that muscle and its close synergists and a relaxation of its antagonists (Plate 32). When the muscle is stretched, its spindle receptors are activated, thus causing increased firing of the spindle afferent fibers. The direct monosynaptic excitation of the motor neurons by these spindle afferent fibers contributes to the contraction of the stretched muscle and its synergists (B). Relaxation of the antagonist muscles is produced by a disynaptic inhibitory pathway involving an interneuron. The stretching of an extensor muscle leads to a reflex contraction of the extensors acting at that particular joint, and to a simultaneous relaxation of the antagonistic flexor muscles.

Excitation and inhibition of motor neurons (B) are mediated by axosomatic or axodendritic synapses (Plate 1). Muscle spindle afferents, as well as other afferents, may also activate the circuits that modulate the action of afferent fibers by means of *presynaptic afferent inhibition* (A). Here, Ia fibers from either the flexors or the extensors activate an inhibitory neuron, which forms an axoaxonic synapse with a muscle spindle afferent fiber that terminates on an extensor motor neuron. As described on page 160, the action of these synapses blocks or decreases the excitation of a motor neuron by muscle spindle afferents.

*Recurrent inhibition* is another type of neural interaction that controls the activity of motor neurons (C). It is produced by the collaterals of motor neurons that excite inhibitory interneurons known as Renshaw cells (Plate 2). When the motor neurons discharge, the Renshaw cells are activated by the motor neuron collaterals and fire a train of action potentials. The firing of the Renshaw cells causes the inhibition of motor neurons of the same muscle and of other related, synergistic muscles. In addition to limiting the firing rate of motor neurons, this inhibition is also thought to restrict motor activity to the most intensely excited motor neurons.

*Tendon Organ Reflex.* Reflex actions evoked by Ib afferent fibers from Golgi tendon organs are shown in D. As described on page 185, these fibers are activated by active (strong) tension in a muscle. When thus activated, the Ib fibers excite spinal interneurons, which inhibit the motor neurons that supply the particular muscle from which

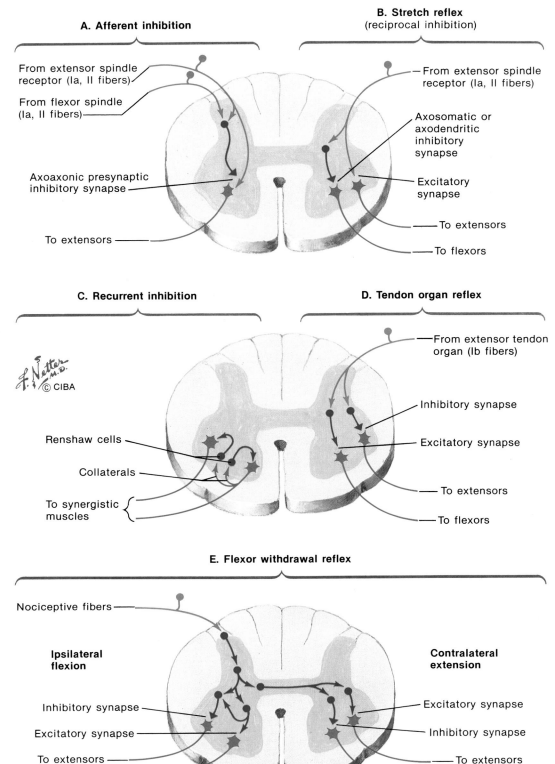

**Spinal Reflex Pathways**

**A. Afferent inhibition**

From extensor spindle receptor (Ia, II fibers)

From flexor spindle (Ia, II fibers)

Axoaxonic presynaptic inhibitory synapse

To extensors

**B. Stretch reflex** (reciprocal inhibition)

From extensor spindle receptor (Ia, II fibers)

Axosomatic or axodendritic inhibitory synapse

Excitatory synapse

To extensors

To flexors

**C. Recurrent inhibition**

Renshaw cells

Collaterals

To synergistic muscles

**D. Tendon organ reflex**

From extensor tendon organ (Ib fibers)

Inhibitory synapse

Excitatory synapse

To extensors

To flexors

**E. Flexor withdrawal reflex**

Nociceptive fibers

Ipsilateral flexion

Inhibitory synapse

Excitatory synapse

To extensors

To flexors

Contralateral extension

Excitatory synapse

Inhibitory synapse

To extensors

To flexors

the Ib fibers originate, and simultaneously excite the motor neurons that supply antagonist muscles. Thus, the tendon organ reflex action is opposite to that produced by muscle spindle afferent fibers. The tendon organ reflex was once thought to play a role in protecting the muscles from excessive tension. Instead, it now appears that tendon organ discharge provides a "force feedback" signal whose inhibitory action opposes the excitatory "length feedback" signal provided by muscle spindle afferents during periods when the muscle is actively generating tension.

*Flexor Withdrawal Reflex.* Complex pathways are involved in the familiar flexor withdrawal reflex evoked by a painful stimulus (E). Such a stimulus activates nociceptive afferent fibers, which produce the firing of chains of neurons in the posterior horn of the spinal cord. These neurons, in turn, activate the interneurons in the anterior horn that excite flexor motor neurons and inhibit extensor motor neurons on the side of the painful stimulus. At the same time, commissural neurons activate circuits that excite extensor motor neurons and inhibit flexor motor neurons on the opposite side. The resulting reflex response is flexion or withdrawal of the stimulated limb, and extension of the opposite limb (see page 183). □

## Muscle and Joint Receptors

Several types of mechanoreceptors located in the joints and muscles provide the CNS with vital proprioceptive information about the position of the parts of the body and the length and tension of various muscles.

*Joint Receptors.* Four types of receptors have been described in the joint capsule and ligaments. *Golgi-type* endings are located in ligaments but not in the capsule, and are innervated by large diameter (Aα) fibers (Plate 6); they are slowly adapting receptors that respond to joint position with changes in their tonic discharge rates. *Ruffini terminals* and *Paciniform corpuscles*, which resemble Pacinian corpuscles but are smaller (Plate 13), are found in the joint capsule and are innervated by medium-diameter (Aβ) fibers. Ruffini terminals respond to both movement and position, whereas Paciniform corpuscles respond only to movement. *Free nerve endings*, supplied by small group III (Aδ) fibers and unmyelinated C fibers, are found in both ligaments and joint capsules; they are thought to respond to extreme, painful movement of the joint. The part played by these four receptor types in signaling joint position is not well understood. A particular difficulty arises from the fact that the majority of receptors respond only at maximum joint extension or flexion, whereas position sense is realized throughout the entire range of a movement.

*Muscle Receptors.* Muscles also contain four types of receptors, two of which—Golgi tendon organs and muscle spindles—are specific to muscle and contribute to the proprioceptive control of reflexes (Plates 32, 33 and 35).

*Golgi tendon organs* are encapsulated receptors located in a tendon, close to the junction of the tendon and the corresponding muscle. The tendon organ capsule surrounds a bundle of tendon fascicles, which are connected to between 3 and 25 muscle fibers. Each tendon organ is innervated by a single group Ib (Aα) fiber that enters the capsule and forms spraylike endings in contact with the tendon fascicles. Because it is connected in series with the muscle fibers, the tendon organ is stretched and thereby excited when muscle tension increases. Tension produced by active muscle contraction has been shown to be more effective in exciting tendon organs than tension produced by passive muscle stretch.

The *muscle spindle* is a complex receptor consisting of *intrafusal fibers*, a bundle of small muscle fibers encased in a sheath. The fibers typically do not run the entire length of the muscle; instead, they insert into one or both ends of the sheath of a large extrafusal muscle fiber. The intrafusal fibers are of two types: smaller *nuclear chain fibers*, in which the cell nuclei lie in a line along the middle portion of the fiber, and larger *nuclear bag fibers*, in which the nuclei are more clustered. Both nuclear bag and nuclear chain fibers are innervated by small-diameter gamma motor fibers, which

### Muscle and Joint Receptors

Alpha motor neurons to extrafusal striated muscle end plates

Gamma motor neurons to intrafusal striated muscle end plates

Ia (Aα) fibers from annulospiral endings (proprioception)

II (Aβ) fibers from flower spray endings (proprioception); from paciniform corpuscles (pressure) and pacinian corpuscles (pressure)

III (Aδ) fibers from free nerve endings and from some specialized endings (pain and some pressure)

IV (unmyelinated) fibers from free nerve endings (pain)

Ib (Aα) fibers from Golgi tendon organs (proprioception)

Aα fibers from Golgi-type endings

Aβ fibers from paciniform corpuscles and Ruffini terminals

Aδ and C fibers from free nerve endings

Alpha motor neuron to extrafusal muscle fiber end plates

Gamma motor neuron to intrafusal muscle fiber end plates

II (Aβ) fiber from flower spray endings

Ia (Aα) fiber from annulospiral endings

Extrafusal muscle fiber

Intrafusal muscle fibers

Sheath

Lymph space

Nuclear bag fiber

Nuclear chain fiber

**Detail of muscle spindle**

Efferent fibers

Afferent fibers

increase the sensitivity of the spindle by causing a contraction of the intrafusal muscle fibers. Each spindle receives afferent innervation from a single, large group Ia (Aα) fiber, which forms large *annulospiral* (primary) endings around both nuclear chain and nuclear bag fibers, and from one to five medium group II (Aα) fibers, which form *flower spray* (secondary) endings chiefly on nuclear chain fibers. Because these spindles lie parallel to the extrafusal muscle fibers, they are stretched when the muscle lengthens. The range of muscle stretch encountered during normal movement excites both kinds of afferent fibers, but in somewhat different fashions. The group II fibers respond to lengthening with an increase in their tonic discharge rate, which remains constant as long as the muscle is stretched, whereas the group Ia fibers respond especially vigorously to the dynamic phase of muscle lengthening, and more weakly, to maintained stretch.

The remaining two classes of muscle receptors include *Pacinian* or *Paciniform corpuscles*, which are innervated by group II (Aβ) fibers and respond to vibratory stimuli, and *free nerve endings*, which are innervated by group III (Aδ) or IV (C) fibers and respond to strong, noxious stimuli. Thus, they resemble corresponding types of receptors found in other tissues (Plates 2 and 13). □

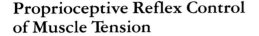

# Proprioceptive Reflex Control of Muscle Tension

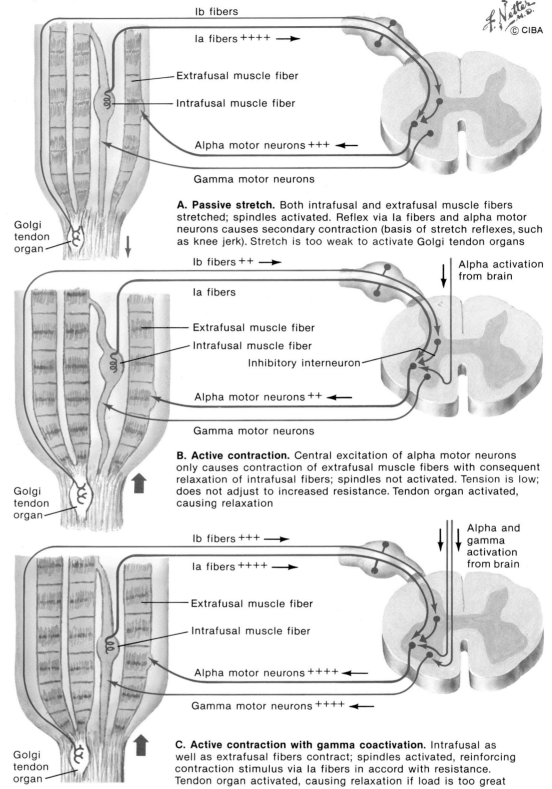

**Proprioceptive Reflex Control of Muscle Tension**

Ib fibers

Ia fibers ++++ →

Extrafusal muscle fiber

Intrafusal muscle fiber

Alpha motor neurons +++ ←

Gamma motor neurons

Golgi tendon organ

**A. Passive stretch.** Both intrafusal and extrafusal muscle fibers stretched; spindles activated. Reflex via Ia fibers and alpha motor neurons causes secondary contraction (basis of stretch reflexes, such as knee jerk). Stretch is too weak to activate Golgi tendon organs

Ib fibers ++ →

Ia fibers

Extrafusal muscle fiber

Intrafusal muscle fiber

Inhibitory interneuron

Alpha motor neurons ++ ←

Gamma motor neurons

Golgi tendon organ

Alpha activation from brain

**B. Active contraction.** Central excitation of alpha motor neurons only causes contraction of extrafusal muscle fibers with consequent relaxation of intrafusal fibers; spindles not activated. Tension is low; does not adjust to increased resistance. Tendon organ activated, causing relaxation

Ib fibers +++ →

Ia fibers ++++ →

Extrafusal muscle fiber

Intrafusal muscle fiber

Alpha motor neurons ++++ ←

Gamma motor neurons ++++ ←

Golgi tendon organ

Alpha and gamma activation from brain

**C. Active contraction with gamma coactivation.** Intrafusal as well as extrafusal fibers contract; spindles activated, reinforcing contraction stimulus via Ia fibers in accord with resistance. Tendon organ activated, causing relaxation if load is too great

The higher motor control centers of the brain receive information from *muscle spindles* and *Golgi tendon organs* (Plate 34) primarily via the group I fibers of the posterior spinal roots. The central processing of this proprioceptive information leads to the smoothness of normal muscle activity and coordinated movement. Even without the higher processing, however, muscle spindle and tendon organ activity can work directly at the spinal level via group I and II collateral fibers and result in the reflexes that occur when there is a need to compensate for rapid changes in body position and orientation (Plate 33). This segmental processing in the sensorimotor system operates effectively even when there is a loss of connection with the brain centers, such as after spinal cord transection or in certain disease states.

When muscle spindles respond to stretching or to a change in the length of a given muscle, there is increased activity in the Ia afferent fibers, which then directly stimulates the alpha motor neurons supplying that particular muscle. (The same Ia fibers inhibit antagonist muscles through interneuron connections.) By contrast, activity in Ib afferent fibers caused by Golgi tendon organs, which respond to muscle tension, stimulates spinal interneurons to inhibit the alpha motor neurons supplying a particular muscle.

***Passive Stretch.*** When the muscle is passively lengthened, both extrafusal and intrafusal fibers are stretched (A). The *muscle spindles* are activated, causing a volley of activity in group Ia and group II (not shown) fibers; this provokes reflex excitation of alpha motor neurons, thus stimulating the extrafusal fibers to contract and oppose the applied force. Golgi tendon organs, which respond poorly to passive stretch, do not discharge under these circumstances. The more rapid or intense the stretching and the change in length, the more rapid or intense the contraction, an example of which is the knee jerk. Thus, the spinal stretch reflex enables the muscle to perform like a spring; if either the afferent or the efferent limb of the nerve supply is damaged, such action is not possible.

***Active Contraction.*** The role of spinal reflexes during active contraction of a muscle is shown in

B and C. A situation in which there is *higher stimulation of alpha motor neurons only* (B), brings about the contraction of the extrafusal fibers, which leads to a shortening of the muscle overall and a slackening of the intrafusal fibers. This results in a termination of activity in the muscle spindles and Ia fibers. The increase in muscle tension, however, is sufficient to activate the *Golgi tendon organs* and the Ib afferent fibers that attempt to inhibit the alpha motor neurons via interneurons. Sufficient Ib inhibition will lead to relaxation or cessation of muscle contraction.

In a *normal situation during voluntary contraction of a muscle* (C), commands from the brain excite

both alpha and gamma motor neurons, resulting in the stimulation and shortening of both extrafusal and intrafusal fibers. The *muscle spindles* are activated and produce a discharge of Ia fibers, which thus reinforce the higher stimulation of the alpha motor neurons. This reinforced motor neuron activity increases the springlike tension of the contracting muscle and helps it adjust to changes in the load. The activated Ib afferent fibers from the *Golgi tendon organs* oppose the alpha motor neurons through a feedback mechanism that reduces tension and causes relaxation if the load becomes too great. The role of this "force feedback" mechanism is not well understood. □

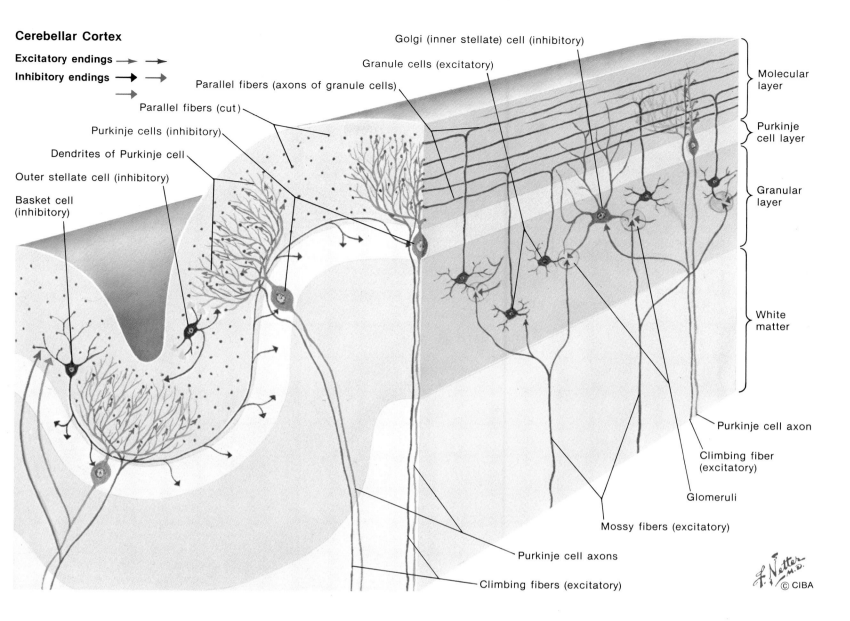

## Cerebellar Cortex

**Excitatory endings** →  →

**Inhibitory endings** ■→  ▬→
  ■→

Golgi (inner stellate) cell (inhibitory)

Granule cells (excitatory)

Parallel fibers (axons of granule cells)

Parallel fibers (cut)

Purkinje cells (inhibitory)

Dendrites of Purkinje cell

Outer stellate cell (inhibitory)

Basket cell (inhibitory)

Molecular layer

Purkinje cell layer

Granular layer

White matter

Purkinje cell axon

Climbing fiber (excitatory)

Glomeruli

Mossy fibers (excitatory)

Purkinje cell axons

Climbing fibers (excitatory)

# Cerebellar Cortex

The cerebellar cortex is a highly folded sheet of neural tissue composed of five types of neurons arranged in three distinct layers. The outermost *molecular layer* contains the functionally similar outer stellate and basket cells; the intermediate *Purkinje cell layer* contains the Purkinje cell bodies; the innermost *granular layer* contains the granule and Golgi (inner stellate) cell bodies. Beneath the three cortical layers lies the cerebellar white matter, through which run afferent and efferent fibers (Plates 37 and 38).

*Afferent fibers* are of two types, mossy fibers and climbing fibers. The majority of cerebellar afferent pathways terminate as *mossy fibers*. These fibers branch in the white matter and then terminate within the granular layer in glial-encased structures called *glomeruli* (Plate 39). Within each glomerulus, the mossy fiber forms excitatory synapses with dendrites of both *granule* and *Golgi cells*. Impulses generated in the granule cells are conducted upward along the cell's axon to the molecular layer, where it bifurcates to form longitudinally running parallel fibers. These parallel fibers form excitatory synapses with *Purkinje, basket* and *outer stellate cells* along a narrow longitudinal segment of cortex; the basket and outer stellate cells are inhibitory interneurons and produce long-lasting inhibition of Purkinje cells, locally and for a considerable distance lateral to the longitudinal strip of active parallel fibers. Therefore, Purkinje cell activity produced by a localized mossy fiber input consists of a brief burst of action along the course of active parallel fibers, surrounded by a band of inhibited cells.

The excitation of Purkinje cells by mossy fibers is further controlled and restricted by the *Golgi cells*. These cells are excited both by mossy fibers, with which they synapse within the glomeruli, and by parallel fiber synapses on their apical dendrites. When Golgi cells discharge in response to this excitation, inhibitory impulses are conducted back to the glomeruli, where they decrease the excitability of granule cells to subsequently arriving impulses from mossy fibers. Because of the wide spread within the cortex of Golgi cell dendrites and axons, their action further restricts the focus of excitation produced by mossy fiber action and reinforces the surrounding zone of inhibition.

The action of *climbing fibers*, the second type of afferent fiber, is quite different from that of mossy fibers. As far as is known, each climbing fiber originates in the inferior olive, branches deep in the cerebellar white matter, and then innervates several widely separated cortical regions situated in the same parasagittal plane. Within the cortex, the climbing fiber forms so dense a network of excitatory synapses on the soma and dendrites of a single *Purkinje cell* that a single arriving impulse produces a massive depolarization in the Purkinje cell. In addition, climbing fibers excite *Golgi* and *basket cells*, which then depress the activity of many nearby Purkinje cells. This particular depressive effect appears to have a greater influence on overall cortical output than does the restricted intense activation of the small number of Purkinje cells receiving direct excitation from each climbing fiber. The significance of the abnormally intense synaptic action of climbing fibers on Purkinje cells is still obscure, but it may be related to motor learning in the cerebellum.

*Efferent Fibers*. All cerebellar cortical output is conducted centrally in *Purkinje cell* axons. Under normal circumstances, Purkinje cells discharge rhythmically, so that both excitatory and inhibitory modulation of their baseline activity can vary the amount of inhibition produced in their target neurons in the deep cerebellar or vestibular nuclei (Plate 39). □

# Cerebellum: Subdivisions and Afferent Pathways

The cerebellar cortex can be divided into three subregions on both phylogenetic and functional criteria, although some differences exist between the subdivisions (see Section II, Plates 10 and 11). In phylogenetic terms, the oldest subdivision is the *archicerebellum*. It includes part of the uvula, the nodulus and the flocculus, which together make up the flocculonodular lobe and the lingula. These cerebellar regions are closely related to the vestibular system (Plate 39), and in the functional classification, therefore, they are termed the *vestibulocerebellum*. The second subdivision is the *paleocerebellum*. It includes most of the vermis (midline portion) and uvula, and the pyramids. These regions primarily control movements of the trunk and girdle muscles. Because of their close relationship to the spinal cord, these regions, as well as the adjacent gracile lobules and intermediate regions of the cerebellar hemispheres, are functionally classified as the *spinocerebellum*. The most recent subdivision is the *neocerebellum*. It includes the middle part (lobule VI) of the vermis and the cerebellar hemispheres. As mentioned above, part of this cerebellar subdivision consists of regions (the intermediate parts of the hemispheres in the anterior lobe and the gracile lobules in the middle [posterior] lobe) that receive extensive spinal input and are functionally classified as the spinocerebellum. The remaining regions are functionally classified as the *pontocerebellum*, because of their close relationship to the pontine nuclei, which relay information from the cerebral cortex.

As explained on page 187, there are two types of cerebellar afferent fibers: *mossy fibers* and *climbing fibers*. Each type is the termination of afferent pathways.

## Mossy Fiber Pathways

*Vestibulocerebellar Pathways.* Vestibular input reaches the vestibulocerebellum by direct projections of vestibular afferent fibers and by projections of neurons in the vestibular nuclei (Plate 39). These fibers carry information from receptors of the vestibular labyrinth (Plate 28), which signal the position and motion of the head in space. Vestibular projections have recently been shown to terminate in the anterior lobe as well (not shown).

*Spinocerebellar Pathways.* Two types of direct pathways carry signals from the spinal cord to the cerebellar cortex (Plate 48). Both pathways can be divided into forelimb and hindlimb components, and each is further subdivided into two functional groups.

The *dorsal spinocerebellar tract (DSCT)* and *cuneocerebellar tract (CCT)* convey analogous information from the hindlimb and the forelimb, respectively. In separate subdivisions, they appear to convey detailed information from proprioceptors (muscle and joint receptors) and exteroceptors (touch and pressure receptors) to specific regions of the cerebellar cortex.

The *proprioceptive division of the DSCT* originates from neurons in Clarke's column in the thoracic and upper lumbar parts of the spinal cord (Plate 49).

It ascends via the ipsilateral posterolateral funiculus and the inferior cerebellar peduncle to the ipsilaterally located hindlimb projection areas in the intermediate part of the anterior lobe and in the gracile lobule. The *proprioceptive division of the CCT* originates from neurons in the external cuneate nucleus and ascends via the inferior cerebellar peduncle to ipsilaterally located forelimb projection areas adjacent to the DSCT termination areas.

The information carried by the majority of proprioceptive DSCT and CCT neurons comes from muscle spindle afferents (group Ia and, to a lesser extent, group II fibers) and from Golgi tendon organ afferents (group Ib fibers), which signal muscle length and tension, respectively (Plates 34 and 35). An individual DSCT or CCT neuron receives input from only a few closely related muscles and provides detailed information about muscle activity to the cerebellum. A smaller group of DSCT and CCT neurons relays information from joint receptors. In addition, many proprioceptive DSCT and CCT neurons receive weak background excitation from high-threshold muscle afferents.

The *exteroceptive division of the DSCT* originates from neurons in Clarke's column that receive direct input from cutaneous afferent fibers. The *exteroceptive division of the CCT* originates from neurons in the rostral main cuneate nucleus, which receive cutaneous input via interneurons that are probably located in the caudal main cuneate nucleus. The axons of these neurons follow similar paths and terminate in the same regions as proprioceptive DSCT and CCT axons. The signals carried by exteroceptive DSCT and CCT neurons originate primarily from touch receptors and hair-movement receptors of the skin (Plate 13). An individual DSCT or CCT neuron receives input from a small area of skin, which means that these neurons are capable of providing detailed information about touch.

The *ventral spinocerebellar tract (VSCT)* and *rostral spinocerebellar tract (RSCT)* are a pair of pathways that inform the cerebellar cortex about the activity of interneurons within the spinal motor centers controlling the hindlimbs and forelimbs.

The *VSCT* originates from spinal border cells at the edge of the spinal anterior horn and from neurons in Rexed's laminae V, VI and VII (Plate 49). Axons of these neurons decussate, ascend in the anterolateral funiculus, and enter the cerebellum via the contralateral superior cerebellar peduncle. Within the cerebellum, VSCT axons terminate bilaterally in the spinocerebellum—most densely in the ipsilateral hindlimb region, where fibers of the DSCT also terminate.

The *RSCT* originates from neurons at the base of the posterior spinal horn. Their axons ascend in the ipsilateral posterolateral funiculus, and enter the cerebellum via both the inferior and superior cerebellar peduncles. Within the cerebellum, RSCT axons terminate widely throughout the forelimb and hindlimb portions of the spinocerebellum on both sides.

Neurons of the VSCT or RSCT receive a complex pattern of peripheral input that appears to be related to the input received by interneurons of spinal motor pathways. Many VSCT or RSCT neurons are directly excited by group I muscle afferent fibers, predominantly those originating from Golgi tendon organs. An individual neuron typically receives such excitation from a large group of leg muscles involved in a particular

pattern of movement. VSCT and RSCT neurons also receive input from multisynaptic spinal pathways that are activated by cutaneous and high-threshold muscle afferent fibers.

*Higher centers of the CNS* exert a strong influence on the activity of VSCT and RSCT neurons. The corticospinal system facilitates the excitatory or inhibitory effects produced in such neurons by cutaneous and high-threshold muscle afferent fibers, while the reticulospinal system inhibits these effects. Other descending systems, such as the rubrospinal and propriospinal pathways, produce an excitation of VSCT and RSCT neurons that is independent of afferent input at the spinal level (Plates 46 to 48).

*Reticulocerebellar pathways* act over wide areas of the cerebellum and the deep cerebellar nuclei. Reticulocerebellar fibers originate from the lateral reticular nucleus and the paramedian reticular nucleus in the medulla, from the nucleus reticularis tegmenti pontis in the pons and, to a lesser extent, from the medial (magnocellular) reticular formation. The most carefully studied pathway is that from the *lateral reticular nucleus*, although the other pathways are probably similar. This nucleus receives excitatory input from the spinal cord, cerebral cortex (principally the motor areas), red nucleus and fastigial nucleus. The spinal input originates from neurons in the anterior horn of the spinal cord, which send axons to the medulla in the anterolateral funiculus. The properties of these neurons are similar to properties of VSCT or RSCT neurons, except that they lack group I muscle input, are excited by descending vestibulospinal fibers, and typically respond to stimulation of larger areas of body surface.

*Pontocerebellar Pathways.* These pathways function as relays by which the cerebral cortex acts upon the cerebellar cortex. Pontocerebellar fibers originate from a number of discrete neuronal groups in the *pons*, each of which receives input from a restricted region of the cerebral cortex and projects via the middle cerebellar peduncles to a specific area of the contralateral cerebellar cortex. Their organization therefore consists of a point-to-point projection similar to that of the DSCT or CCT. The precise functional role of the pontocerebellar pathways is unknown, but they may be involved in relaying information about cortical motor commands.

## Climbing Fiber Pathways

All known climbing fiber pathways relay in the inferior olives, which project to the cerebellar cortex via the contralateral inferior cerebellar peduncle. An individual climbing fiber branches to innervate several Purkinje cells along a longitudinal strip of cerebellar cortex. The functional role of the uniquely strong action of climbing fibers on Purkinje cells is unclear.

The *inferior olive* receives excitatory input from the spinal cord, motor cortex, red nucleus, nucleus of Darkschewitsch, periaqueductal gray matter and accessory optic tract. The spinal input arrives via several ascending pathways that relay information from cutaneous receptors and high-threshold muscle receptors. In general, the spinal neurons projecting to one of the inferior olives are located on the side contralateral to that olive, which is therefore ipsilateral to the region of cerebellar cortex to which its climbing fibers project. □

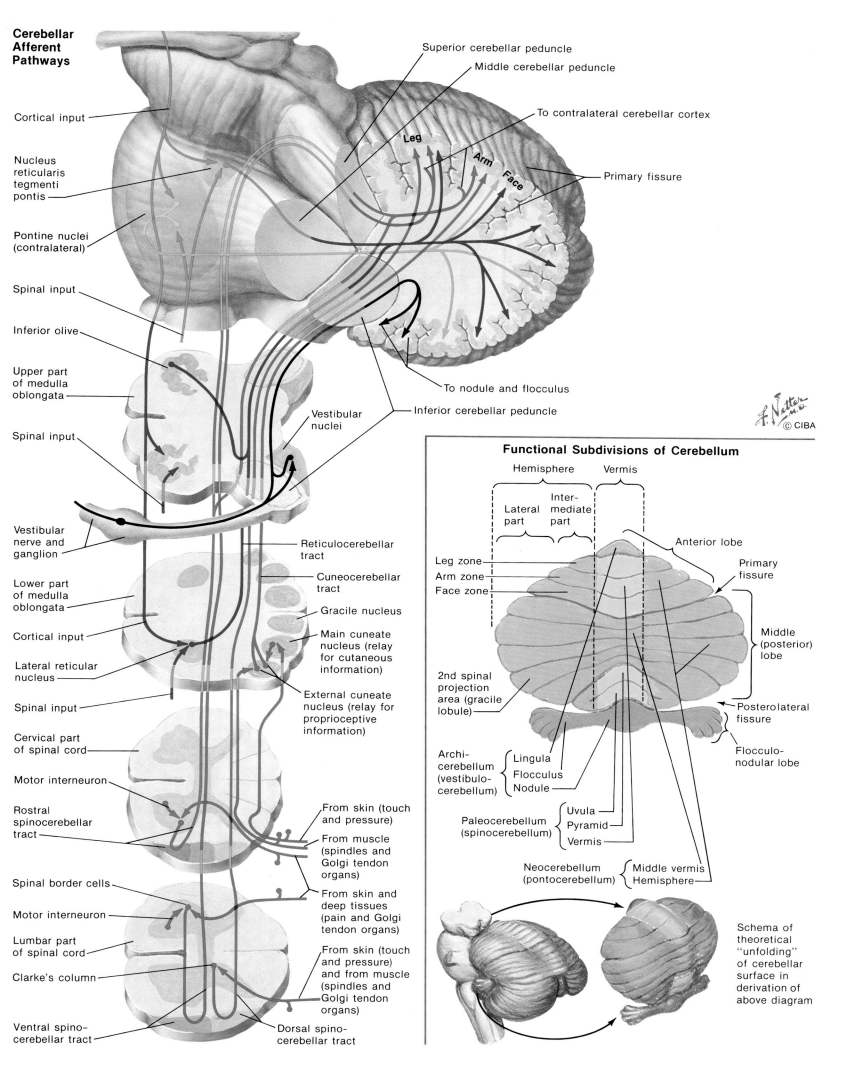

**Cerebellar Afferent Pathways**

Cortical input

Nucleus reticularis tegmenti pontis

Pontine nuclei (contralateral)

Spinal input

Inferior olive

Upper part of medulla oblongata

Spinal input

Vestibular nerve and ganglion

Lower part of medulla oblongata

Cortical input

Lateral reticular nucleus

Spinal input

Cervical part of spinal cord

Motor interneuron

Rostral spinocerebellar tract

Spinal border cells

Motor interneuron

Lumbar part of spinal cord

Clarke's column

Ventral spino-cerebellar tract

Dorsal spino-cerebellar tract

Superior cerebellar peduncle

Middle cerebellar peduncle

To contralateral cerebellar cortex

Leg

Arm

Face

Primary fissure

To nodule and flocculus

Inferior cerebellar peduncle

Vestibular nuclei

Reticulocerebellar tract

Cuneocerebellar tract

Gracile nucleus

Main cuneate nucleus (relay for cutaneous information)

External cuneate nucleus (relay for proprioceptive information)

From skin (touch and pressure)

From muscle (spindles and Golgi tendon organs)

From skin and deep tissues (pain and Golgi tendon organs)

From skin (touch and pressure) and from muscle (spindles and Golgi tendon organs)

*F. Netter M.D.*
© CIBA

**Functional Subdivisions of Cerebellum**

Hemisphere

Vermis

Lateral part

Inter-mediate part

Leg zone

Arm zone

Face zone

Anterior lobe

Primary fissure

2nd spinal projection area (gracile lobule)

Middle (posterior) lobe

Posterolateral fissure

Flocculo-nodular lobe

Archi-cerebellum (vestibulo-cerebellum) { Lingula, Flocculus, Nodule }

Paleocerebellum (spinocerebellum) { Uvula, Pyramid, Vermis }

Neocerebellum (pontocerebellum) { Middle vermis, Hemisphere }

Schema of theoretical "unfolding" of cerebellar surface in derivation of above diagram

# Cerebellar Efferent Pathways

The cerebellar efferent pathways to other parts of the CNS have a similar organization in all subdivisions of the cerebellum. *Purkinje cell* axons (Plate 36) originate from the cerebellum to terminate upon and inhibit neurons in the *deep cerebellar nuclei* and *vestibular nuclei* (Plate 39). In general, neurons inhibited by Purkinje cells are excitatory relay neurons that project to other parts of the CNS involved in *motor control*. In addition to Purkinje cell inhibition, these relay neurons also receive excitatory input from collateral fibers, which branch from cerebellar afferent fibers on their way to the cerebellar cortex. Accordingly, their activity is determined by an interaction of excitation and inhibition governed by the arrival of information in cerebellar afferent pathways, and by the processing of that information by the cerebellar cortex.

*Vermis*. The efferent pathways from the vermis involve two relay nuclei, the *dorsal part of the lateral vestibular nucleus* and the fastigial nucleus. As described on page 180, the lateral vestibular nucleus is the source of the *lateral vestibulospinal tract*. Thus, cerebellar cortical projections to this nucleus serve to regulate the activation of the descending spinal motor apparatus (Plate 48).

The *fastigial nucleus* is the most medial of the excitatory deep cerebellar nuclei. Major regions to which this nucleus projects are the *vestibular nuclei* and medial *pontomedullary reticular formation*, which are involved in the control of the spinal and extraocular motor apparatus (Plates 29 and 30) and the *lateral reticular nucleus* and *inferior olive*, which project back to the cerebellum (Plates 36 and 37). The fastigial nucleus can be further divided into an anterior part that projects to the ipsilateral side of the *brainstem* and a posterior part that projects to the contralateral side via the hook bundle of Russell. Physiological studies suggest that there may be further specialized subdivisions within each part of the nucleus. Although most fastigial efferent fibers travel in the inferior cerebellar peduncle, the nucleus also sends a few fibers rostrally via the superior peduncle. Some of these fibers may reach the *mesencephalic reticular formation*, while others may contribute to the recurrent descending projection from the superior cerebellar peduncle.

*Intermediate Zone*. The efferent pathway from the intermediate zone of the cerebellar cortex in man involves the *globose* and *emboliform nuclei*, which are analogous to the interpositus nucleus of lower mammals. These nuclei send excitatory fibers to the contralateral *red nucleus* via the superior cerebellar peduncle. At least some of these

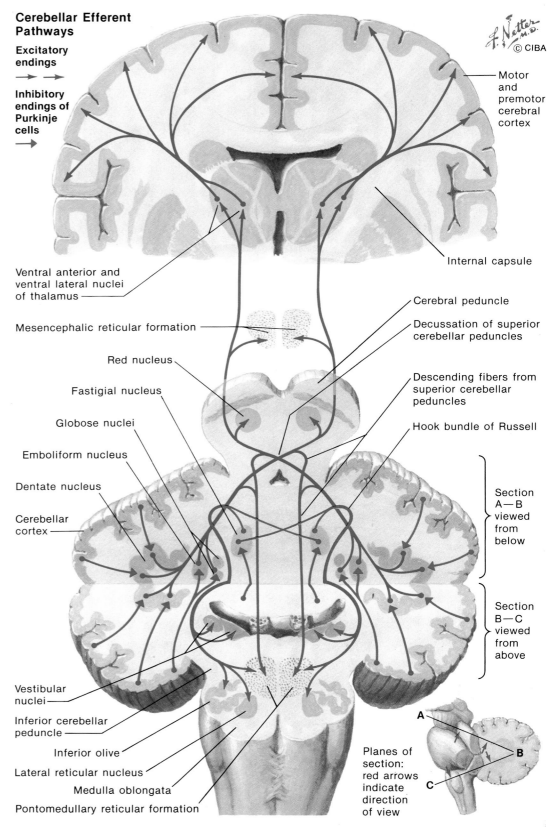

## Cerebellar Efferent Pathways

**Excitatory endings**
→  →

**Inhibitory endings of Purkinje cells**
→

Motor and premotor cerebral cortex

Internal capsule

Ventral anterior and ventral lateral nuclei of thalamus

Mesencephalic reticular formation

Red nucleus

Fastigial nucleus

Globose nuclei

Emboliform nucleus

Dentate nucleus

Cerebellar cortex

Cerebral peduncle

Decussation of superior cerebellar peduncles

Descending fibers from superior cerebellar peduncles

Hook bundle of Russell

Section A—B viewed from below

Section B—C viewed from above

Vestibular nuclei

Inferior cerebellar peduncle

Inferior olive

Lateral reticular nucleus

Medulla oblongata

Pontomedullary reticular formation

Planes of section: red arrows indicate direction of view

A   B   C

ascending excitatory fibers give off branches that continue rostrally to the ventral lateral nucleus of the thalamus. As described on page 198, the red nucleus is the source of *rubrospinal fibers* that act on the spinal motor apparatus, especially on flexor muscles of the arm and muscles of the hand.

*Hemispheres*. The efferent pathway from the cerebellar hemispheres involves the *dentate nucleus*. This nucleus is the major relay station for cerebellar action on the regions of the *cerebral cortex* involved in motor control (Plates 43 and 45). It sends excitatory fibers to the ventral lateral nucleus of the thalamus, which is the major thalamic relay nucleus to the motor cortex (the

source of the corticospinal fibers involved in motor control). It also sends fibers to the ventral anterior nucleus, which projects to frontal cortical regions, including the premotor cortex. Some dentate fibers may send branches to the red nucleus as well.

*Vestibulocerebellum*. Purkinje cells in the most ventral and lateral portions of the cerebellar cortex, which belong to the vestibulocerebellum, project directly to the *vestibular nuclei* rather than to one of the four deep cerebellar nuclei. The patterns of these projections and their role in controlling vestibular reflexes are described on page 191. ☐

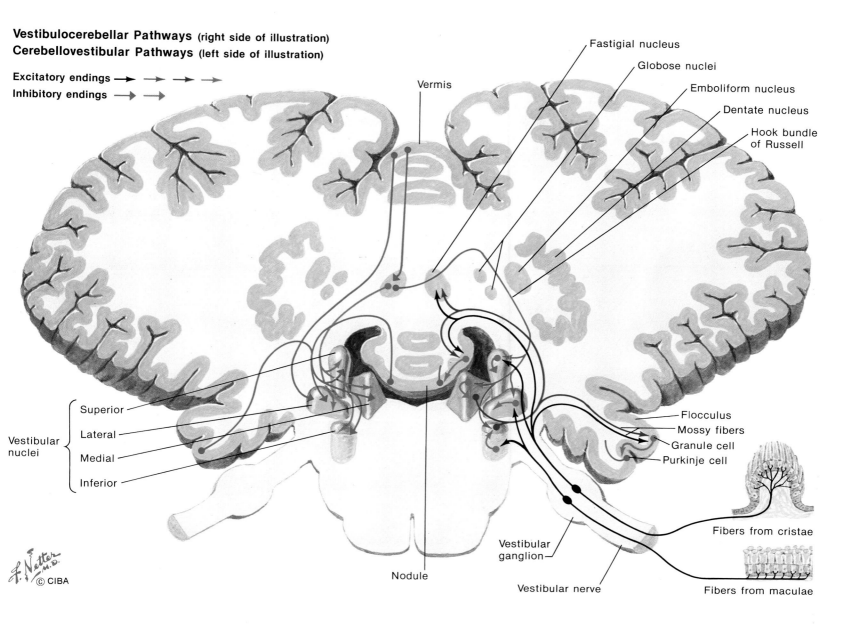

**Vestibulocerebellar Pathways** (right side of illustration)
**Cerebellovestibular Pathways** (left side of illustration)

Excitatory endings →  →  →  →
Inhibitory endings →  →

Vermis

Fastigial nucleus
Globose nuclei
Emboliform nucleus
Dentate nucleus
Hook bundle of Russell

Vestibular nuclei
Superior
Lateral
Medial
Inferior

Flocculus
Mossy fibers
Granule cell
Purkinje cell

Fibers from cristae

Nodule

Vestibular ganglion

Vestibular nerve

Fibers from maculae

*f. Netter M.D.*
© CIBA

## Vestibulocerebellar and Cerebellovestibular Pathways

The vestibular system is closely related to the phylogenetically older parts of the cerebellum, in particular to the *archicerebellum* (see page 188). As a result, this subdivision, which includes the flocculus, nodulus, lingula and parts of the uvula, is also referred to as the *vestibulocerebellum*. The vestibular system is also related to the *paleocerebellum*, which includes both the vermal region of the cortex and the most medial of the deep nuclei —the fastigial—and sends extensive projections to the vestibular nuclei.

The vestibulocerebellum receives vestibular afferent information directly from vestibular nerve fibers (mostly from fibers innervating semicircular canal receptors), and indirectly, via pathways that relay in the vestibular nuclei (Plate 29). Axons of both pathways terminate as mossy fibers upon the dendrites of cerebellar granule cells, an input that produces ordered patterns of activity within the Purkinje cells (see page 187).

Vestibulocerebellar Purkinje cells project to the *vestibular nuclei* (Plate 38), where they inhibit vestibular neurons. The most direct pathway through the vestibulocerebellum (afferent fibers from the semicircular canal to granule cells to Purkinje cells to vestibular neurons) therefore provides an inhibitory circuit that parallels semicircular canal input to the vestibular nuclei. Consequently, such pathways may adjust the amplitude of movements produced by reflexes such as the *vestibuloocular* reflex, so that they precisely compensate for head movements detected by the labyrinthine receptors. Appropriate changes in the strength of transcerebellar pathways could be induced by visual or proprioceptive signals that reach the cerebellum via climbing fibers originating in the inferior olive (Plates 22 and 37). While visual signals are known to induce corrective changes in the vestibuloocular reflex only if the vestibulocerebellum is present, the complex behavior of Purkinje cells in the flocculus of alert monkeys has raised questions as to whether the cerebellum actually modulates vestibular reflex activity or merely computes error signals that induce compensatory changes at other stages of the reflex pathway.

*Paleocerebellar projections* to the vestibular nuclei are more complex, since they involve both the vermal cortex and the fastigial nucleus. Purkinje cells in the vermal cortex project to and inhibit neurons in the *dorsal part* of the *lateral vestibular nucleus* and in the *fastigial nucleus* (Plate 38). The fastigial nucleus, in turn, sends excitatory fibers to *all four vestibular nuclei*. The projections of the rostral portion of the fastigial nucleus are ipsilateral, whereas fibers from the caudal fastigial nucleus cross in the hook bundle of Russell to excite contralateral vestibular neurons. Thus, Purkinje cells of the cerebellar vermis can depress the activity of neurons throughout the vestibular nuclei either by direct inhibition or by inhibiting the discharge of neurons in the fastigial nucleus, thereby decreasing the excitatory activity reaching vestibular neurons via fastigiovestibular pathways—an example of *disfacilitation*.

Although the paleocerebellum has a widespread action on the vestibular nuclei, it receives only a modest amount of direct *vestibular afferent input*, plus some vestibular information relayed via indirect pathways. Much more important input arrives via the *spinocerebellar tracts* (Plate 37). It therefore seems probable that the principal action of the paleocerebellum on the vestibular system is to regulate vestibular activity in response to input of information from the spinal cord. □

**Connections of Basal Ganglia**

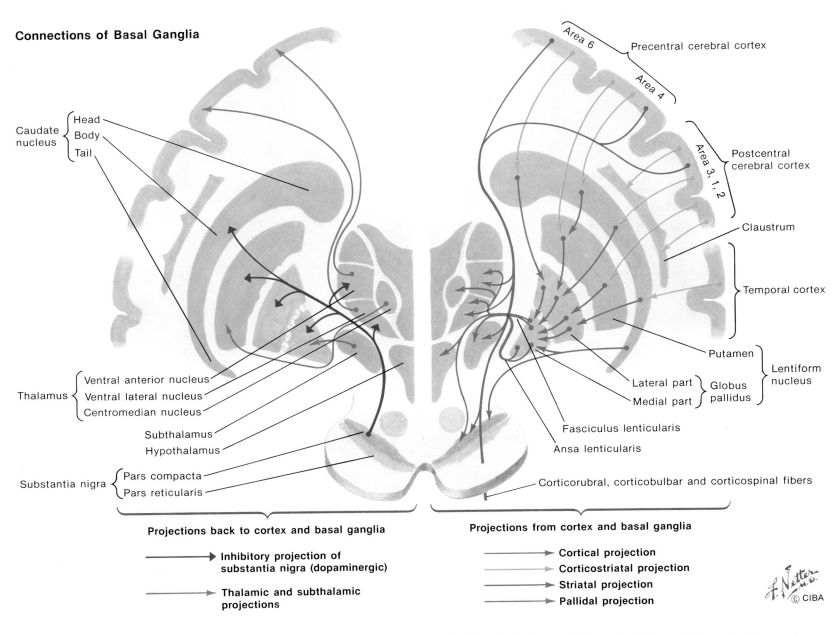

Caudate nucleus { Head, Body, Tail

Area 6
Area 4
Area 3, 1, 2
Precentral cerebral cortex
Postcentral cerebral cortex
Claustrum
Temporal cortex
Putamen
Lentiform nucleus
Lateral part } Globus pallidus
Medial part
Fasciculus lenticularis
Ansa lenticularis
Corticorubral, corticobulbar and corticospinal fibers

Thalamus { Ventral anterior nucleus, Ventral lateral nucleus, Centromedian nucleus
Subthalamus
Hypothalamus
Substantia nigra { Pars compacta, Pars reticularis

**Projections back to cortex and basal ganglia**

→ Inhibitory projection of substantia nigra (dopaminergic)

→ Thalamic and subthalamic projections

**Projections from cortex and basal ganglia**

→ Cortical projection
→ Corticostriatal projection
→ Striatal projection
→ Pallidal projection

*F. Netter M.D.* © CIBA

SECTION VIII  PLATE 40

# Basal Ganglia

The basal ganglia are the deep nuclei of the telencephalon. They form a broad, collaborative system of connections between the cerebral cortex and the thalamus, thus providing for the ease and alacrity of human movement. The principal anatomical units are the *caudate nucleus*, the *putamen* and the *globus pallidus*. The *claustrum*, which is reciprocally connected with the cerebral cortex, is usually included as a basal ganglia structure. The mesencephalic structures of the *substantia nigra* and *subthalamic nucleus* are generally included on a functional basis, while the *amygdala* (amygdaloid body), located in the temporal lobe, is functionally excluded (see Section II, Plates 4 to 6).

*Connections.* The anterior limb of the *internal capsule* carries the reciprocal fibers connecting the cerebral cortex with the basal ganglia, and separates the putamen from the head of the caudate nucleus. The head of the caudate nucleus, the anterior limb of the internal capsule and the putamen collectively form the *corpus striatum*, while

the putamen and globus pallidus form the *lenticular nucleus.*

The overall connections of the basal ganglia are not fully understood. Afferent connections are derived mainly from the cerebral cortex, thalamus and substantia nigra. *Corticostriate fibers* link each area of the cortex to a particular section of the corpus striatum, with some overlap in projection; the most profuse projections originate in the sensorimotor cortex (areas 6, 4, 3, 1 and 2), (Plates 43 and 44). The corticostriate fibers originate primarily in the small pyramidal cells in lamina V (Plate 42) and reach the corpus striatum via both the internal and external capsules; they project from the temporal cortex via sublenticular pathways. *Thalamostriate* connections are profuse and originate in the centromedian nucleus and in various other intralaminar and midline nuclei (Plate 41). *Nigrostriate fibers* arise from both the pars compacta and pars reticularis of the substantia nigra and connect with the caudate nucleus, putamen and globus pallidus, as well as with the thalamus, frontal cortex, amygdala, superior colliculi and olfactory tubercle (not shown).

*The substantia nigra* (especially the area compacta) is well developed in man and plays a significant role in basal ganglia function via the major nigrostriatal system and the nigrodiencephalic collateral fibers specified above; through its

links to the globus pallidus and thalamus, it can influence cortical activity. In turn, the substantia nigra receives multiple input from the globus pallidus, cerebral cortex, dorsal raphe nucleus, amygdaloid complex, subthalamus, septal area and stria terminalis. While the nigrostriatal pathways are dopaminergic (a fact which bears directly on the pathology and potential treatment of Parkinson's disease), input is from neurons containing serotonin and gamma-aminobutyric acid (GABA), as well as the peptide, substance P.

*Efferent Pathways.* The principal striatal efferent connections project to the *substantia nigra*, the *diencephalon* and the *cerebral cortex*. Both the caudate nucleus and the putamen project to the globus pallidus in a topically organized manner, and the caudate nucleus also projects directly to the putamen and the substantia nigra. The globus pallidus, in turn, sends fibers to the thalamus, subthalamus, hypothalamus and substantia nigra; this thick and well-myelinated *pallidofugal system* is qualitatively the most important striatal efferent pathway and consists of several distinct fiber bundles, which include the *fasciculus lenticularis* and the *ansa lenticularis*. Fibers in these bundles terminate principally in the ventral anterior, ventral lateral and centromedian nuclei of the thalamus, but some fibers synapse in the subthalamic nucleus. □

# Thalamocortical Radiations

All pathways carrying information from the periphery or the brainstem to the neocortex relay in the nuclei of the *dorsal thalamus* (see Section II, Plate 7). These nuclei can be divided into two groups on the basis of their structure, connections and function.

*Nonspecific Nuclei.* The first group includes the *midline (median)* and *intralaminar nuclei* and the medial portion of the *ventral anterior nucleus*. These nuclei receive ascending input from the mesencephalic reticular formation and from the spinal cord (paleospinothalamic tract), and descending input from the cerebral cortex. They project widely, both to other thalamic nuclei and to the cortex, especially to its frontal regions. These projections are thought to be essential in regulating the general excitability of neurons in the thalamus and cortex.

Another nucleus included in the first group is the *reticular nucleus*, which overlies the lateral surface of the thalamus. Neurons of this nucleus, which receive input from collaterals of thalamocortical fibers and project back to the thalamus, are thought to constitute a feedback pathway that regulates thalamic excitability.

*Specific Nuclei.* The second group of nuclei are referred to as "specific nuclei" because they project to restricted regions of the cortex (Plate 43). The major specific nuclei and the corresponding cortical regions to which they project are illustrated in matching colors. One set of specific nuclei are the sensory relay nuclei. The *ventral posterolateral (VPL)* and *ventral posteromedial (VPM) nuclei* receive their input from somatosensory relay neurons via the medial lemniscus, trigeminal lemnisci and the neospinothalamic tract (Plates 15 and 16). They project to the primary (Sm I) and secondary (Sm II) somatosensory cortex. The *ventral posterointermediate (VPI) nucleus* (not shown) receives input from the vestibular system and projects to the vestibular area in the parietal lobe (Plate 29). The *lateral geniculate nucleus* receives its input from the optic tract and projects to the primary visual area in the occipital lobe (Plate 22). The principal part of the *medial geniculate nucleus* receives input from auditory relay nuclei and projects to the primary auditory area in the supratemporal transverse gyrus (Plate 26).

A second set of specific nuclei is involved in the control of motor activity. The *ventral lateral (VL)* and *ventral intermediate (VI) nuclei* and the lateral portion of the *ventral anterior (VA) nucleus* receive input from the cerebellum and basal ganglia, respectively, and project to the precentral motor areas (Plates 38 and 40). These areas also receive input from the oral part of the ventral posterolateral nucleus.

The *anterior dorsal (AD)* (the least prominent of the anterior group of nuclei) and the *medial dorsal (MD) nuclei* are specifically related to the limbic system, which regulates emotional and autonomic activity (Plates 56, 63 and 64). The anterior dorsal nucleus receives input from the hippocampus

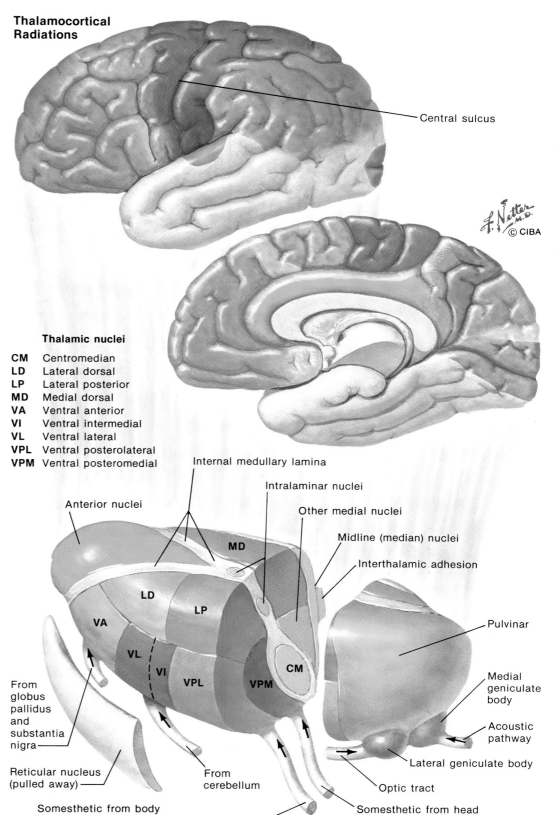

**Thalamocortical Radiations**

Central sulcus

**Thalamic nuclei**

CM  Centromedian
LD  Lateral dorsal
LP  Lateral posterior
MD  Medial dorsal
VA  Ventral anterior
VI  Ventral intermedial
VL  Ventral lateral
VPL  Ventral posterolateral
VPM  Ventral posteromedial

Internal medullary lamina
Intralaminar nuclei
Anterior nuclei
Other medial nuclei
Midline (median) nuclei
Interthalamic adhesion
MD
Pulvinar
LD
LP
VA
Medial geniculate body
VL
VI
CM
VPL  VPM
Acoustic pathway
From globus pallidus and substantia nigra
Lateral geniculate body
Reticular nucleus (pulled away)
From cerebellum
Optic tract
Somesthetic from body (spinothalamic tract and medial lemniscus)
Somesthetic from head (trigeminal nerve)

relayed via the mamillothalamic tract and projects to the cingulate gyrus. The medial dorsal nucleus receives input from the hypothalamus and amygdala and projects to the frontal lobe.

The remaining specific nuclei are related to association areas of the cortex involved in higher integrative mechanisms. They include the *lateral dorsal (LD)* and *lateral posterior (LP) nuclei* and the *pulvinar complex*. The medial, magnocellular part of the *medial geniculate nucleus*, which receives widespread convergent input from many afferent systems, should probably also be included in this category.

*Cortical Connections.* In addition to receiving the ascending input described above, all the thalamic nuclei receive descending input from the cerebral cortex, principally from the cortical regions to which they project (Plate 44). These descending projections serve as a two-way feedback system between each cortical area and its thalamic relay nucleus.

Not all the nuclei of the dorsal thalamus project to the cerebral cortex. One important nucleus without a cortical projection is the *centromedian (CM) nucleus*, which communicates only with the basal ganglia (Plate 40). □

## Types of Neurons in Cerebral Cortex

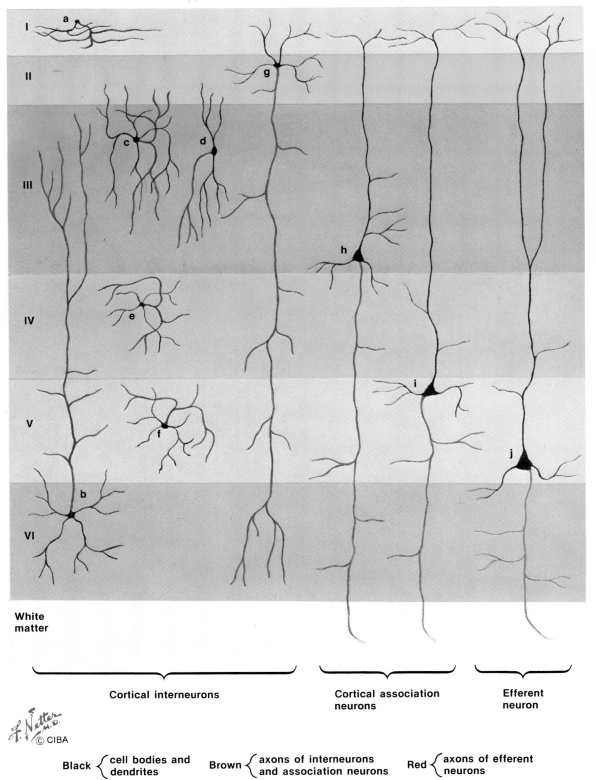

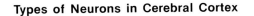

**White matter**

**Cortical interneurons**

**Cortical association neurons**

**Efferent neuron**

*f. Netter M.D.*
© CIBA

**Black** { cell bodies and dendrites

**Brown** { axons of interneurons and association neurons

**Red** { axons of efferent neurons

The six layers of the cerebral cortex contain different types of neurons, which can be broadly classified as *interneurons*, association neurons and *efferent (projection) neurons*.

*Interneurons*, which have axons that do not leave the cortex, may be of several kinds. The most common are *stellate* (star-shaped), or *granule, cells* (f), which have symmetrically branching dendritic trees and short axons that end upon nearby neurons. These cells are especially prevalent in layer IV, which is accordingly named the "granule cell layer." Other interneurons are *horizontal cells* (a), which are found in layer I; *Martinotti's cells* (b), which are located in deeper layers and send axons toward the cortical surface; and the small *pyramidal cells* of layers II and III (g), which send axons to deeper layers.

*Association neurons* (h,i) are small pyramidal cells found in the deep parts of layer III or in the superficial parts of layer V; they send axons through the white matter to other regions of the cortex.

*Efferent neurons*, which leave the cortex to innervate structures in the brainstem or spinal cord, originate from the *giant pyramidal (Betz) cells* in layer V (j) or from spindle-shaped cells in layer VI (not shown). In addition to their main axons, which leave the cortex, efferent neurons may also have collateral axons, which project to nearby cortical neurons for association.

*Afferent Fibers*. Two major classes of nerve fibers bring information to the cortex. *Specific cortical afferent fibers*, which originate in corresponding thalamic relay nuclei (Plate 41), project to layer IV to end in a highly branched terminal arborization. *Nonspecific cortical afferent fibers*, which originate in the thalamus or in other areas of the cortex and ascend through the entire depth of the cortical gray matter, giving off terminal branches in all layers. Specific afferent fibers may thus activate granule cells and efferent neurons of layers III, V and VI (via their dendrites in layer IV), while nonspecific afferents may influence all classes of cortical neurons. Neurons activated by incoming fibers relay information to other cortical neurons via intrinsic connections within the cortex.

*Cortical Organization*. An important aspect of the flow of information mediated by cortical neurons is that it occurs predominantly in a *vertical direction* across the six cortical layers. With the exception of the horizontal cells of layer I, there are very few cortical neurons that relay activity laterally over any significant distance. The vertical cell axons and dendrites are arranged within the cortex in columns of neurons that have similar properties. These columns are approximately 0.5 to 1.0 mm wide and extend across all six cortical layers. In the sensory cortex, neurons within an individual column all respond to the same stimulus; within the motor cortex, the activity of all neurons in one column is related to the activity of a single muscle or muscle group. These columns, as well as the underlying vertical neural organization, appear to represent one of the central features of information processing by the cerebral cortex. □

# Cerebral Cortex: Function and Association Pathways

In man, the cerebral cortex is highly developed, and the complexity of the interhemispheric and intrahemispheric connections parallels this degree of development. The cerebral cortex has definite areas related to specific neurological functions, either for primary sensory reception or for complex integrated activity.

*Association Pathways.* When one cortical area is activated by a stimulus, other areas also respond. This is due to the rapid activity along a large number of precisely organized, reciprocally acting association pathways. The pathways may be very short, linking neighboring areas and running only within the gray matter (Plate 42), or they may be longer (arcuate) bundles, passing through the white matter to connect gyrus to gyrus or lobe to lobe within a cerebral hemisphere — *intrahemispheric connection.* Other commissural bundles conduct *interhemispheric activity*: the most prominent are the *corpus callosum*, a large band of fibers, which lies immediately beneath the cingulum; the *anterior commissure*, which connects both temporal lobes; and the *hippocampal commissure (commissure of the fornix)*, which connects the right and left hippocampus (see Section II, Plates 5 and 6).

The reciprocal activity of the connections in the cerebral cortex ensures the coordination of sensory input and motor activity, as well as the regulation of higher function. For example, for the appreciation and integration of visual information, the primary visual sensory area of the occipital cortex is linked to the visual association areas (Plate 21). These visual centers are connected by intrahemispheric fibers to the ipsilateral parietal cortex, as well as to other areas, such as the temporal lobe, for further integrated activity. The right and left parietal and posterior temporal areas, in turn, are connected by the corpus callosum.

***The prefrontal cortex*** (which includes the three frontal gyri, the orbital gyri, most of the medial frontal gyrus and approximately half of the cingulate gyrus) is concerned with *higher mental functions*, and is involved with many behavioral aspects of man. This area receives numerous connections from the temporal and parietal lobes via pathways in the cingulum, a bundle of long association fibers lying within the cingulate gyrus (Plate 56). Bilateral lesions of the prefrontal area produce a loss of concentration, a decreased intellectual ability, and memory and judgment deficits.

***Motor and Sensory Cortices.*** The *somatosensory cortex*, which occupies contiguous parts of the frontal and parietal lobes, and the *premotor cortex* of the frontal lobe are concerned with the initiation, activation and performance of *motor activity*, and the reception of *primary sensation* of the body (Plates 44 to 48). Lesions of the somatosensory cortex result in contralateral paralysis and loss of somatosensory reception or perception.

***The parietal lobe*** is primarily concerned with the *interpretation* and *integration* of information from sensory areas: ie, the visual areas and the somatosensory cortex. Lesions in the parietal lobe

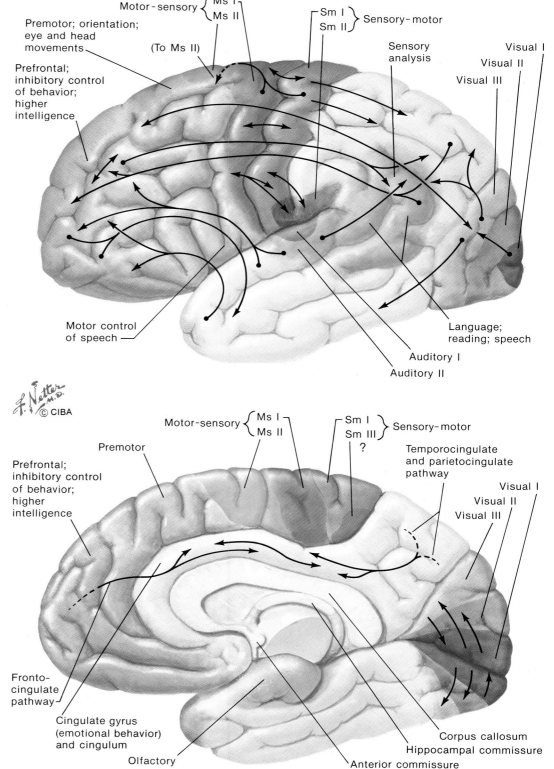

result in sensory ataxia, a loss of general awareness, defective recognition of sensory impulses, and a lack of interpretation of spatial relationships. Lesions of the striate cortex (the primary visual area) on one side result in a contralateral hemianopsia, while lesions of the secondary regions of the visual cortex cause a lack of ability to interpret visual impulses.

***Temporal Lobe.*** The *posterior part of the temporal lobe* is concerned with the reception and interpretation of *auditory information*, and with some aspects of pattern recognition and higher *visual coordination*; the interconnections of the auditory and visual segments of the occipital, temporal

and parietal lobes make this a highly integrated function (Plates 21, 26 and 27). The *anterior part of the temporal lobe* is concerned with *visceral motor activity* and certain aspects of *behavior.* Lesions here may be manifested by psychomotor seizures or, if they occur in the region of the uncus, by uncinate "fits."

***Lesions.*** In general, lesions of primary receptive areas produce identifiable deficits. A lesion in a specific area of the cerebral cortex may produce a deficit far beyond the functional identity of that particular area, since the complex interconnections beneath that cortical region may be damaged. □

# Cerebral Cortex: Efferent Pathways

The illustration gives an overall view of the projections from the cerebral cortex to the lower levels of the CNS, described in Plates 15, 16, 22, 27, 30, 41 and 45 to 48. Cortical projections to the basal ganglia are shown in Plate 40.

*Projections.* The most extensive cortical projections are those from the primary motor cortex (area 4) and sensory cortex (areas 3, 1 and 2). In man, some of the pyramidal cells of the *motor cortex* project directly to somatic muscle motor neurons located in the trigeminal motor, facial and hypoglossal nuclei in the brainstem and the anterior (ventral) horn of the spinal cord. The motor cortex also projects to the basal ganglia, thalamus, red nucleus, pontine nuclei, reticular formation, inferior olive and spinal interneurons.

The *somatosensory cortex* projects to a number of sensory relay nuclei, such as the ventral posterolateral nucleus of the thalamus, the trigeminal nuclei, the posterior column nuclei and the posterior (dorsal) horn cells of the spinal cord. These projections are believed to contribute to the control of sensory input to the CNS. The somatosensory cortex also projects to the pontine nuclei and the brainstem reticular formation.

Other sensory areas of the cerebral cortex also project to related sensory relay nuclei. The *auditory cortex* (areas 41 and 42) projects to the medial geniculate nucleus and to the inferior colliculus (Plate 27). The *visual cortex* (areas 17, 18 and 19) projects to the lateral geniculate nucleus and to the superior colliculi (Plates 22 and 30). In addition, both the auditory and visual cortices project to the pontine nuclei and the reticular formation.

*Association areas* of the parietal, temporal and frontal cortices send projections to the thalamus, pontine nuclei and reticular formation. In addition, projections from the *frontal eye fields* (areas 6 and 8) to the mesencephalon terminate in the intersitital nucleus of Cajal (Plates 30 and 31).

*CNS lesions* are seldom discrete, and diseases are rarely limited to one system. This is especially true of the intermingled descending efferent pathways, which not only regulate motor activity but also modulate sensory impulses ascending from the periphery to the brain, thus influencing reflex activity of the body, head and neck. Damage to the *posterior limb of the internal capsule* from a vascular accident will result not only in a contralateral deficit in movement, but also in some sensory loss on the side of the lesion due to damage to the pathways relaying in the thalamus (Plates 40 and 41). Visual field defects may occur if the optic radiations are affected (Plates 21 and 22). Other sensory systems affected will be efferent projections from the auditory cortex and eye field projections to the brainstem nuclei. Damage to corticobulbar efferent fibers projecting to cranial nerve nuclei results in paralysis of the muscles of facial expression, mastication and the intrinsic muscles of the tongue. Also, since the descending fibers from the brainstem reticular areas influence alpha and gamma motor neurons (Plate 35), a capsular lesion will sever cortical connections, leaving the reticular neurons without higher control. □

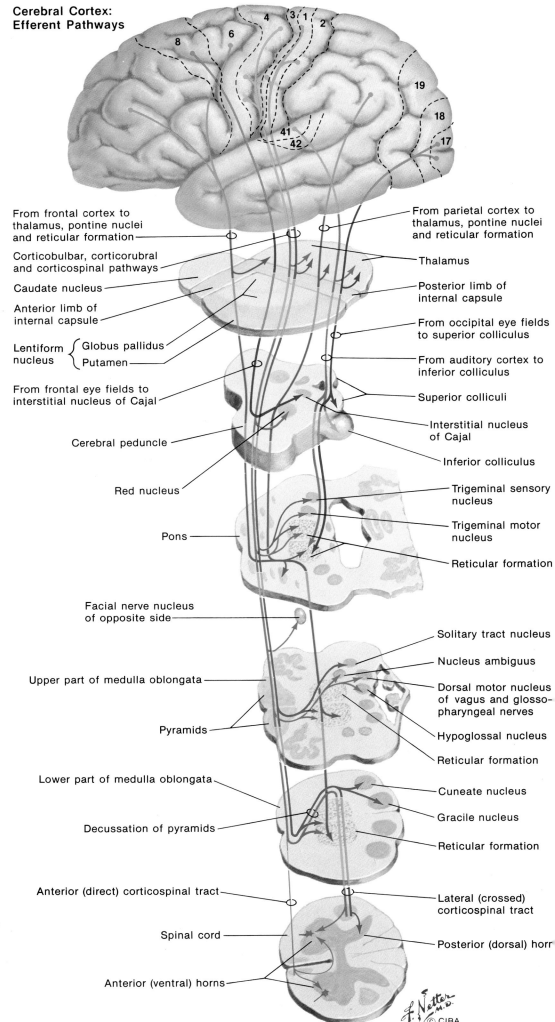

**Cerebral Cortex: Efferent Pathways**

From frontal cortex to thalamus, pontine nuclei and reticular formation

Corticobulbar, corticorubral and corticospinal pathways

Caudate nucleus

Anterior limb of internal capsule

Lentiform nucleus { Globus pallidus / Putamen

From frontal eye fields to interstitial nucleus of Cajal

Cerebral peduncle

Red nucleus

Pons

Facial nerve nucleus of opposite side

Upper part of medulla oblongata

Pyramids

Lower part of medulla oblongata

Decussation of pyramids

Anterior (direct) corticospinal tract

Spinal cord

Anterior (ventral) horns

From parietal cortex to thalamus, pontine nuclei and reticular formation

Thalamus

Posterior limb of internal capsule

From occipital eye fields to superior colliculus

From auditory cortex to inferior colliculus

Superior colliculi

Interstitial nucleus of Cajal

Inferior colliculus

Trigeminal sensory nucleus

Trigeminal motor nucleus

Reticular formation

Solitary tract nucleus

Nucleus ambiguus

Dorsal motor nucleus of vagus and glossopharyngeal nerves

Hypoglossal nucleus

Reticular formation

Cuneate nucleus

Gracile nucleus

Reticular formation

Lateral (crossed) corticospinal tract

Posterior (dorsal) horn

*F. Netter* © CIBA

**Pyramidal System**

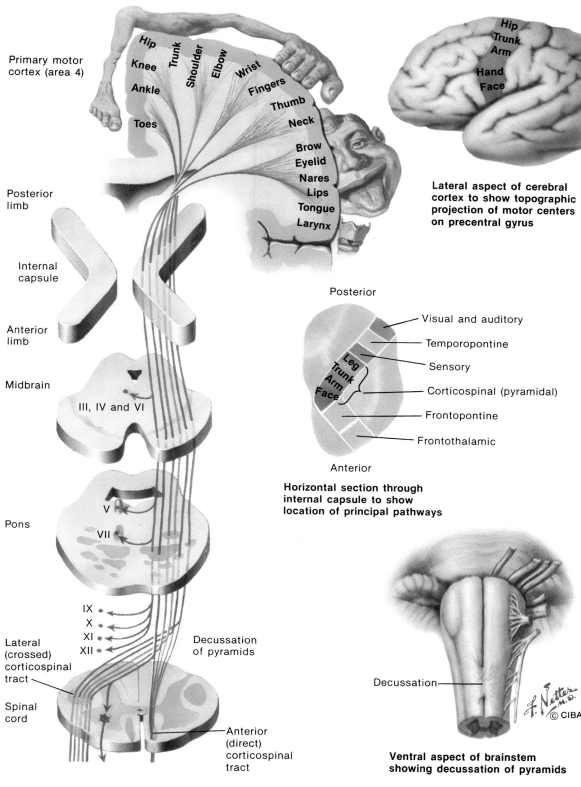

Lateral aspect of cerebral cortex to show topographic projection of motor centers on precentral gyrus

Horizontal section through internal capsule to show location of principal pathways

- Visual and auditory
- Temporopontine
- Sensory
- Corticospinal (pyramidal)
- Frontopontine
- Frontothalamic

Ventral aspect of brainstem showing decussation of pyramids

## Pyramidal System: Motor Component

The motor component of the *pyramidal tract* originates primarily in the giant pyramidal Betz cells of layer V in the primary motor cortex of the precentral gyrus (area 4), and projects to motor neurons and interneurons concerned with motor control throughout the CNS. Only the direct connections, by which cortical neurons excite motor neurons in the motor nuclei of the brainstem and spinal cord, are shown. Other illustrations show the projections of the motor cortex to the basal ganglia (Plate 40), thalamus (Plate 41), red nucleus (Plate 46), reticular formation (Plate 47) and intermediate spinal gray matter (Plate 48).

*The direct motor component* of the pyramidal tract runs from the precentral gyrus through the posterior limb of the internal capsule and into the midbrain, where it gives slips to the oculomotor, trochlear and abducens nuclei. It then enters the pons, where it gives off fibers to the trigeminal motor and facial nuclei, which control the muscles of the face. From the pons, the tract continues through the medullary pyramids, giving off fibers to the nuclei of the ninth, tenth, eleventh and twelfth cranial nerves (see Section V for details of the motor components of the cranial nerves). The major part of the tract then crosses to the opposite side of the brainstem at the *pyramidal decussation*, and the crossed fibers continue to all levels of the spinal cord as the *lateral corticospinal tract*. A smaller group of uncrossed fibers continues to the cervical spinal cord as the *anterior (direct) corticospinal tract*. The fibers end by synapsing with motor neurons in the anterior (ventral) horn of the spinal cord (Plate 49).

The pyramidal tract exhibits a *somatotopic organization* throughout its course. The homunculus at the top of the illustration indicates the orderly topographical arrangement of areas within the precentral gyrus, from which muscles in various parts of the body can be activated. The area controlling the face lies most laterally, with the areas related to the hand, arm, trunk and hip following in order toward the midline. The areas representing the leg continue downward along the medial aspect of the cortex. Within each area, distal muscles are represented posteriorly, and proximal muscles, anteriorly. The initial somatotopic organization at the cortex persists in the arrangement of fibers along the course of the tract (Plate 32).

Electrophysiological studies, using very weak electrical stimuli, have revealed that the motor cortex contains columns of neurons whose activity leads chiefly to the excitation of a single muscle.

The firing of these neurons precedes the activation of that muscle during movement, and appears to be related to both the force and the rate of increase of force produced by the muscle. Of further interest is the fact that neurons in the motor cortex receive excitation from parts of the body surface that are likely to be stimulated during the movement associated with these neurons. This positive feedback may play a role in the execution of detailed manipulatory movements involving the distal extremities.

*Lesions of the motor cortex* may produce discrete pareses, depending upon the type and size of the lesion and its somatotopic location. Irritative

lesions of the cortex can lead to abnormal movements and ultimately to Jacksonian seizures as the irritative focus spreads. Damage to the internal capsule produces contralateral paralysis, along with cranial nerve involvement (Plate 44).

Generally, pyramidal tract disturbances produce an initial flaccid paralysis and areflexia, followed by spastic paralysis and hyperactive reflexes. Brainstem lesions cause paralysis contralateral to the lesion, accompanied by ipsilateral or contralateral cranial nerve deficits, depending on the level of the lesion. Spinal cord damage to the tract is usually accompanied by alterations in the autonomic and sensory systems. □

# Rubrospinal Tract

The rubrospinal tract originates primarily from the large neurons of the caudal part of the *red nucleus* in the midbrain and extends the entire length of the spinal cord. The predominant target of its action is the motor apparatus controlling the distal muscles of the contralateral limbs, although the tract also acts to inhibit the action of cutaneous and muscle afferent fibers on spinal neurons. Within the brainstem, fibers branch from the rubrospinal tract to terminate in the facial nucleus (control of facial muscles), the lateral reticular nucleus (cerebellar afferent relay) and the gracile and cuneate nuclei (control of afferent input), (Plates 15 and 16). In addition to being the source of the rubrospinal tract, the red nucleus sends fibers to the ipsilateral inferior olive (cerebellar afferent relay) and medial reticular formation (Plate 47).

As shown in the illustration, *rubrospinal fibers decussate* almost immediately on leaving the red nucleus to descend through the lateral part of the brainstem to the spinal cord. In the cord, the tract lies in the *posterolateral funiculus*, just anterior to the lateral corticospinal tract. The distal branches of the rubrospinal fibers terminate in the intermediate regions and anterior horn (laminae V, VI and VII) of the spinal gray matter (Plate 48).

In primates, as opposed to lower mammals, many rubrospinal fibers end directly upon anterior horn motor neurons. In all species, however, the strongest rubrospinal action on these motor neurons is that which reaches them indirectly, after being relayed via both inhibitory and excitatory interneurons (Plate 35). The predominant pattern of rubrospinal action is to *excite limb flexor muscles* and *inhibit the corresponding extensor muscles*. However, a number of rubrospinal fibers have the opposite action. This allows a wide variety of movements to be executed by the selective activation of appropriate groups of rubrospinal neurons. The rubrospinal tract may thus be responsible for much of the relatively fine control of the extremities—discriminative movement that is retained when the pyramidal tract is damaged. In experimental animals, lesions involving both the pyramidal and rubrospinal tracts result in a much greater deficit in distal movement than that obtained from a lesion of either tract alone.

Rubrospinal control of *afferent input* to the spinal cord takes the form of presynaptic inhibition acting at the central posterior horn terminals of fibers from Golgi tendon organs and cutaneous receptors (Plate 34). Since these afferent fibers produce flexor responses similar to those produced by rubrospinal action, it has been suggested that inhibition of these afferent fibers gives the rubrospinal pathway exclusive control of the motor apparatus, without interference from spinal reflex pathways (Plate 33).

The two major sources of the input that controls the activity of rubrospinal neurons are the *cerebellum* and the *cerebral cortex*. As described in Plate 38, the cerebellar projection to the red nucleus consists primarily of fibers from the

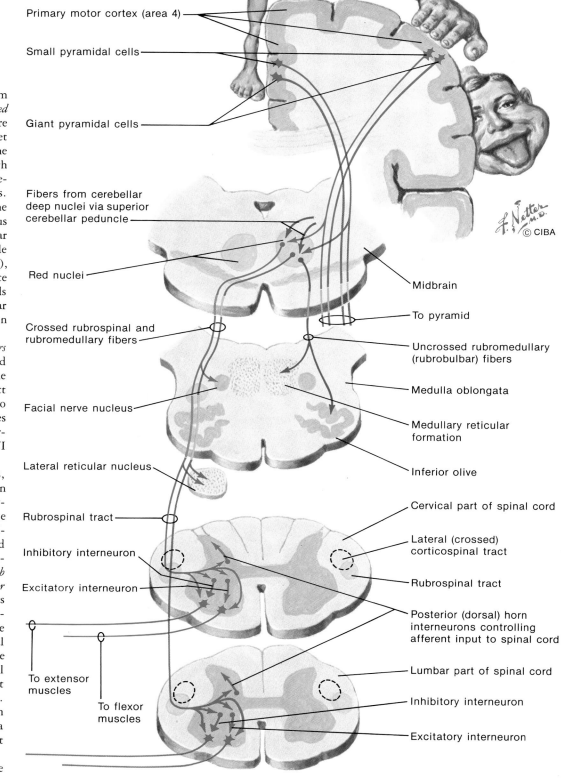

**Rubrospinal Tract**

Primary motor cortex (area 4)
Small pyramidal cells
Giant pyramidal cells
Fibers from cerebellar deep nuclei via superior cerebellar peduncle
Red nuclei
Crossed rubrospinal and rubromedullary fibers
Facial nerve nucleus
Lateral reticular nucleus
Rubrospinal tract
Inhibitory interneuron
Excitatory interneuron
To extensor muscles
To flexor muscles
Midbrain
To pyramid
Uncrossed rubromedullary (rubrobulbar) fibers
Medulla oblongata
Medullary reticular formation
Inferior olive
Cervical part of spinal cord
Lateral (crossed) corticospinal tract
Rubrospinal tract
Posterior (dorsal) horn interneurons controlling afferent input to spinal cord
Lumbar part of spinal cord
Inhibitory interneuron
Excitatory interneuron

emboliform and globose nuclei, which cross in the decussation of the superior cerebellar peduncle (brachium conjunctivum) to excite the red nucleus neurons of the opposite side. Neurons of the red nucleus are also excited by medium-conduction-velocity branches of pyramidal tract neurons from the motor cortex (Plate 45); these fibers apparently originate from small pyramidal neurons in the ipsilateral cortex. In addition, activity in fast-conduction-velocity pyramidal tract axons from giant neurons in the same cortical region exerts an opposite, inhibitory action on rubrospinal neurons, which is relayed via inhibitory interneurons. Both the input and

output of the red nucleus are *somatotopically organized*. Thus, rubrospinal fibers projecting to the lumbar part of the spinal cord originate from neurons in the lateral part of the nucleus. This same region receives input from regions of the cerebellar deep nuclei and motor cortex related to control of the lower limbs. Conversely, the medial part of the red nucleus, which contains neurons projecting to cervical levels of the spinal cord, receives input from cerebellar and cerebral regions responsible for control of the arms. This pattern of organization allows for the selective activation of individual extremities by different groups of rubrospinal neurons (Plate 32). □

# Reticulospinal and Corticoreticular Pathways

The reticulospinal pathways are important in controlling motor activity and in regulating the flow of afferent signals in the spinal cord. These pathways consist of a complex series of descending fiber connections that originate in two regions of the brainstem and project to the spinal cord via two different *reticulospinal tracts*. Both regions of origin are in the medial, magnocellular part of the brainstem reticular formation. The more rostral region is in that part of the *pontine reticular formation* which corresponds to the nucleus reticularis pontis caudalis and nucleus reticularis pontis oralis (as defined by Brodal); the more caudal region is in the nucleus gigantocellularis, in the rostromedial part of the *medullary reticular formation*. Their separate projections are described below.

*Pontine reticulospinal fibers* project to the spinal cord *via the medial reticulospinal tract only*. This tract traverses the anteromedial funiculus and extends along the entire length of the spinal cord, sending terminal branches to innervate the gray matter of the anterior horn (Plate 48). Experimental activation of the pontine reticulospinal system by electrical stimulation produces direct *excitation* of large numbers of spinal motor neurons of all types, the most pronounced excitation being that of flexor motor neurons and motor neurons controlling proximal (trunk and axial) muscles. The pontine system also has a strong, indirect influence on lumbar motor neurons, relayed by spinal interneurons (see bottom of illustration).

*The medullary reticulospinal system* has a more complex pattern of projection than that of the pontine system. Most fibers originating from the gigantocellular nucleus project to the spinal cord via the *ipsilateral lateral reticulospinal tract*, which is part of the lateral anterolateral funiculus. In addition, some medullary reticular neurons project via the *contralateral lateral reticulospinal tract*, and some join the *medial reticulospinal tract*. Within the spinal gray matter, terminations of medullary reticulospinal fibers cover an exceptionally wide area, encompassing most of the anterior horn and the basal portion of the posterior horn (Plate 48).

The physiological action of the medullary reticulospinal system on spinal motor neurons is twofold and quite complex. Stimulation of the *rostral part* of the *gigantocellular nucleus* produces *excitation* of motor neurons, whereas stimulation of its *caudal-ventral part* produces *inhibition*. Actions on axial motor neurons are mediated by direct connections, while those on limb motor neurons are relayed by spinal interneurons. Stimulation in the caudal-ventral area also produces inhibition of spinal interneurons and inhibition of afferent transmission to the spinal cord. The exact pathways mediating these various effects are unknown, but they appear to involve reticulospinal fibers descending in the dorsolateral funiculus (not shown in illustration).

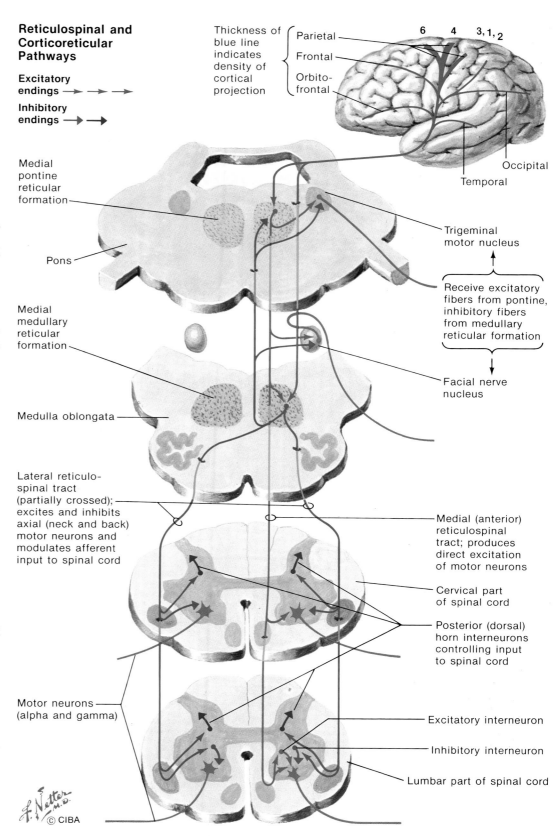

Reticulospinal and Corticoreticular Pathways

Excitatory endings → → →
Inhibitory endings → →

Thickness of blue line indicates density of cortical projection { Parietal, Frontal, Orbitofrontal

6   4   3, 1, 2

Occipital

Temporal

Medial pontine reticular formation

Pons

Trigeminal motor nucleus

Receive excitatory fibers from pontine, inhibitory fibers from medullary reticular formation

Medial medullary reticular formation

Facial nerve nucleus

Medulla oblongata

Lateral reticulospinal tract (partially crossed); excites and inhibits axial (neck and back) motor neurons and modulates afferent input to spinal cord

Medial (anterior) reticulospinal tract; produces direct excitation of motor neurons

Cervical part of spinal cord

Posterior (dorsal) horn interneurons controlling input to spinal cord

Motor neurons (alpha and gamma)

Excitatory interneuron

Inhibitory interneuron

Lumbar part of spinal cord

*Input* to the *medial brainstem reticular formation* originates from many sources. Most major sensory systems send collateral branches to one of its regions, and the most pronounced sensory input to the source of reticulospinal fibers comes from the cutaneous and high-threshold muscle receptors of the body (Plates 15 and 16). As indicated by the relative width of the particular lines in the illustration, physiological studies demonstrate that the great majority of both pontine and medullary reticulospinal neurons receive strong excitatory input from structures involved in motor control, including the motor or premotor cerebral cortex, themselves a part of an extensive corticoreticular system originating from all parts of the cortex (Plate 44), the cerebellar fastigial nucleus (Plate 38) and the superior colliculus (Plate 22). The resulting *corticoreticulospinal connections* constitute an extrapyramidal pathway by which motor regions of the cortex can act on the spinal motor apparatus. The physiological role of the projections from sensory regions of the cerebral cortex to reticulospinal neurons is less certain, but such pathways may be involved in the regulation of sensory input to the spinal cord through reticular-evoked presynaptic inhibition of spinal afferent fibers, or through postsynaptic inhibition of spinal sensory interneurons. □

# Major Descending Tracts and Ascending Pathways

In addition to their local reflex connections, spinal neurons receive input from, and send projections to, many parts of the brain (see Section II, Plate 17). The sections illustrated show the regions of the spinal gray matter within which axons of the four major descending pathways terminate, and the locations within the spinal gray matter of neurons that project to the thalamus and cerebellum (Plate 49).

*The descending pathways* shown in A, B, C and D have a variety of actions on spinal circuitry, including the modulation of somatosensory input and the production of motor output. Actions on the sensory apparatus are typically mediated by descending fibers that terminate upon neurons in the posterior (dorsal) horn (laminae I to VI) of the spinal cord. As shown in A, the specific spinal projections from the somatosensory cortex concerned with sensory control end almost entirely in the posterior horn. Some projections from the brainstem reticular formation, which also has a strong action on the sensory apparatus, also terminate in the posterior horn (C). Conversely, the vestibulospinal tracts (D), which have only a weak action on sensory processes, have relatively few terminals in the posterior horn. The rubrospinal tract (B), which has some inhibitory effect on spinal afferents, terminates in intermediate regions and in the rostral part of the anterior (ventral) horn.

By correlating the motor actions of descending pathways and the patterns of termination of those pathways within the spinal gray matter, Lawrence and Kuypers have divided the projections from the brain to the spinal cord into lateral and medial systems. The *lateral descending systems* include the lateral (crossed) corticospinal tract fibers originating in the motor cortex (A) and the rubrospinal tract (B), (Plates 45 and 46). These tracts terminate predominantly in the lateral parts of laminae V, VI, VII and IX, which are concerned with the control of the *distal musculature of the limbs*.

The *medial descending systems* include the reticulospinal tracts (C) and vestibulospinal tracts (D), (Plates 29 and 47). These tracts end most heavily in laminae VIII and IX$_M$, which are involved in controlling neck and trunk muscles. Endings are also present in the medial parts of laminae VI, VII and IX, which control the proximal muscles of the limbs. Thus, the medial systems act predominantly upon *axial* and *proximal muscles*. The functional role of the *anterior (direct) corticospinal tract* is uncertain, although its endings in lamina VIII suggest that it may be involved in the cortical control of axial muscles.

*Connections to Ascending Pathways.* Ascending projections from the spinal cord to the brain arise from many parts of the spinal gray matter. In general, however, projections to sensory structures tend to originate in the posterior horn, which is the receiving area for somatosensory input arriving via the posterior roots. The illustration shows the *ventral (anterior)* and *lateral* divisions of the *spinothalamic tract*, which are continuous with each other (Plate 15). One division originates primarily from neurons in lamina I,

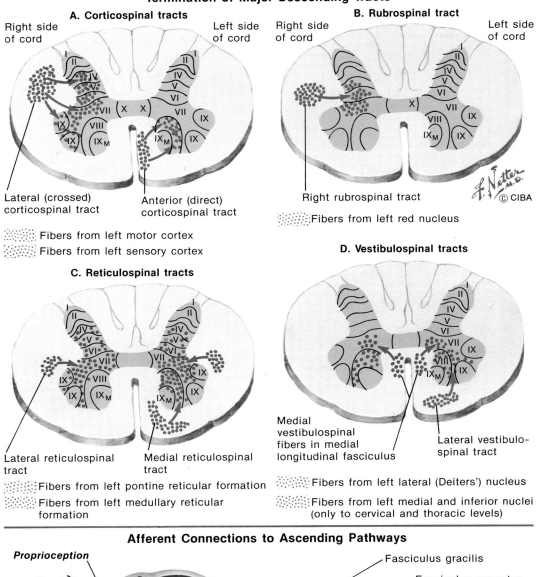

## Termination of Major Descending Tracts

### A. Corticospinal tracts

Right side of cord — Left side of cord

Lateral (crossed) corticospinal tract
Anterior (direct) corticospinal tract

:::::: Fibers from left motor cortex
:::::: Fibers from left sensory cortex

### B. Rubrospinal tract

Right side of cord — Left side of cord

Right rubrospinal tract

:::::: Fibers from left red nucleus

### C. Reticulospinal tracts

Lateral reticulospinal tract
Medial reticulospinal tract

:::::: Fibers from left pontine reticular formation
:::::: Fibers from left medullary reticular formation

### D. Vestibulospinal tracts

Medial vestibulospinal fibers in medial longitudinal fasciculus
Lateral vestibulospinal tract

:::::: Fibers from left lateral (Deiters') nucleus
:::::: Fibers from left medial and inferior nuclei (only to cervical and thoracic levels)

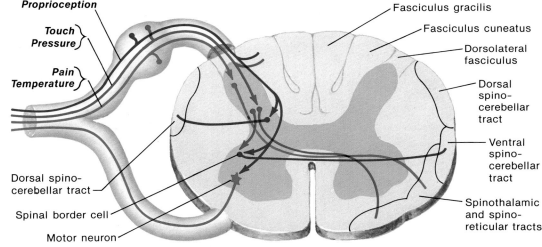

## Afferent Connections to Ascending Pathways

Proprioception
Touch Pressure
Pain Temperature

Dorsal spino-cerebellar tract
Spinal border cell
Motor neuron

Fasciculus gracilis
Fasciculus cuneatus
Dorsolateral fasciculus
Dorsal spino-cerebellar tract
Ventral spino-cerebellar tract
Spinothalamic and spino-reticular tracts

which respond chiefly to painful stimuli; the other originates from neurons located mainly in laminae IV to VI, which receive information related to a variety of somatosensory stimuli. Lamina IV also gives rise to projections to other sensory areas, such as the cuneate, gracile and lateral cervical nuclei. Laminae V to VIII give origin to the spinoreticular tract.

Ascending projections to areas involved in motor control tend to arise from laminae VI to IX, which are related to motor movements. The illustration shows two ascending pathways related to motor activity, both of which terminate in the cerebellum. The *dorsal (posterior) spinocerebellar*

*tract* originates from Clarke's column, a group of neurons located in lamina VI, and ascends in the ipsilateral posterolateral funiculus. The *ventral (anterior) spinocerebellar tract* originates from spinal border cells at the edge of lamina VII and ascends via the contralateral anterolateral funiculus. As shown, neurons projecting in both tracts receive input from muscle proprioceptors (Plate 34); some also receive indirect cutaneous input. In addition to neurons projecting to the cerebellum, the anterior horn also contains neurons projecting to other structures related to motor control, such as the inferior olive and the reticular formation. □

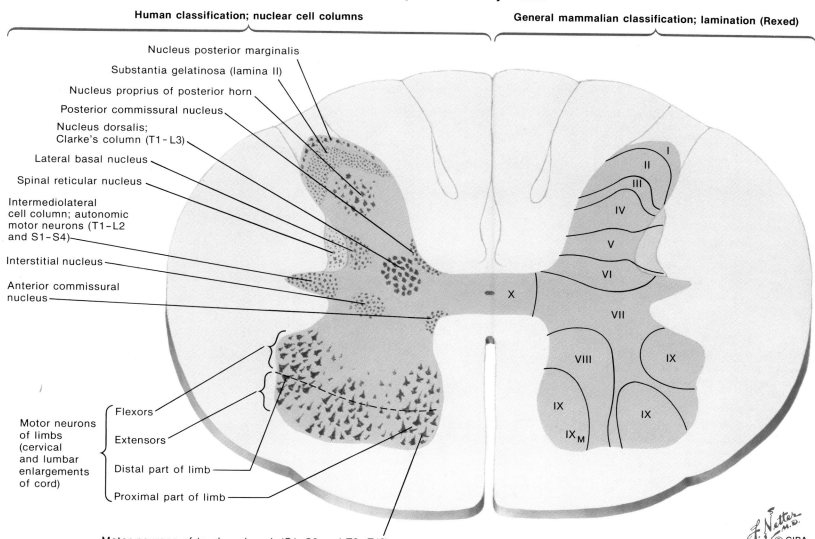

**Cytoarchitecture of Spinal Cord Gray Matter**

**Human classification; nuclear cell columns**

**General mammalian classification; lamination (Rexed)**

Nucleus posterior marginalis
Substantia gelatinosa (lamina II)
Nucleus proprius of posterior horn
Posterior commissural nucleus
Nucleus dorsalis; Clarke's column (T1–L3)
Lateral basal nucleus
Spinal reticular nucleus
Intermediolateral cell column; autonomic motor neurons (T1–L2 and S1–S4)
Interstitial nucleus
Anterior commissural nucleus
Motor neurons of limbs (cervical and lumbar enlargements of cord)
Flexors
Extensors
Distal part of limb
Proximal part of limb
Motor neurons of trunk and neck (C1–C3 and T2–T12)

I, II, III, IV, V, VI, VII, VIII, IX, IX$_M$, X

SECTION VIII    PLATE 49

# Cytoarchitecture of Spinal Cord Gray Matter

The gray matter of the spinal cord can be broadly divided into a *posterior (dorsal) horn* and an *anterior (ventral) horn*, which are further subdivided according to the size and structure of their component neuronal cell bodies. The left side of the illustration shows some of the clearly recognizable groups of neurons; the right side shows a more systematic subdivision of the spinal gray matter into 10 laminae, which were originally described by Rexed in the spinal cord of the cat, but which are useful in discussing human functional neuroanatomy.

**Posterior Horn.** Many neurons in the six laminae of the posterior horn receive direct synaptic input from spinal afferent fibers that enter the spinal cord via the posterior roots and are thus involved in sensation and in the generation of reflex responses to external or proprioceptive signals (Plate 48).

*Lamina I* of the posterior horn is a thin layer of large cells, which gives origin to the pathway relaying information about painful stimuli to the thalamus. *Laminae II and III* comprise the *substantia gelatinosa*, a tightly packed mass of tiny neurons believed to play a role in regulating afferent input to the spinal cord (Plate 17). *Lamina IV* is a collection of larger neurons (sometimes referred to as the *nucleus proprius of the posterior horn*) that projects to three sensory structures: the lateral cervical nucleus, the posterior column nuclei and the thalamus. Thus, the connections of laminae I to IV indicate their importance in sensation.

*Laminae V and VI* contain neurons of medium-to-large size, many of which receive input from afferent fibers carrying proprioceptive information, as well as other sensory information also relayed by neurons in lamina IV. These neurons probably represent an intermediate stage in the transformation of sensory input to motor output. Laminae V and VI are also the sites of origin of ascending projections to higher centers. In spinal segments T1 to L3, lamina VI contains a group of large cells known as *Clarke's column*, which projects to the cerebellum via the dorsal (posterior) spinocerebellar tract (Plate 37).

**The anterior horn** contains the cell bodies of the motor neurons supplying the somatic muscles. These cell bodies are clustered into two distinct groups, referred to by Rexed as lamina IX and IX$_M$. Lamina IX$_M$ contains the motor neurons supplying the muscles of the trunk and neck, while lamina IX contains motor neurons supplying the limbs. Lamina IX can be further divided into groups of motor neurons supplying flexor and extensor muscles in the proximal and distal parts of the limbs.

The anterior horn also contains *laminae VII and VIII*. These regions contain interneurons involved in motor control, as well as neurons that project to motor regions of the brain. The neurons of lamina VIII are particularly related to lamina IX$_M$, and thus participate in motor movements of the muscles in the trunk and neck. Conversely, neurons of lamina VII are particularly related to lamina IX, and therefore participate in motor movements of the limb muscles. Laminae VII and IX are both highly developed in the spinal enlargements that control the arms and the legs (Plate 45), whereas only laminae VIII and IX$_M$ are found in the high cervical or thoracic segments that control the neck and trunk.

In the thoracic and sacral segments, the *intermediolateral cell column*, which is not considered part of either the posterior or the anterior horn, contains the neurons of origin of preganglionic autonomic fibers. *Lamina X* contains neurons that project to the opposite side of the spinal cord, including those in the anterior and posterior commissural nuclei. □

# Interoceptors

Interoceptors are receptors that inform the CNS about the internal state of the body. They fall into three basic categories: pain receptors, chemoreceptors and stretch receptors. Typically, *pain receptors* are free nerve endings (Plate 13). They inform the CNS about intense, presumably dangerous, internal stimuli. Receptors belonging to the remaining two categories take on a variety of forms, depending upon the specific stimulus to which they must respond. The illustration shows two well-known interoceptor systems—one involving chemoreceptors, the other, stretch receptors.

*The carotid body* (glomus) contains *chemoreceptors* that are activated primarily by low oxygen levels in arterial blood and, to a lesser extent, by low blood pH or high levels of carbon dioxide in the blood. It consists of a mass of spongy tissue located at the bifurcation of the carotid artery into its internal and external carotid branches. It has its own independent arterial and venous connections. Innervation of the carotid body is via the carotid sinus nerve, which contains afferent fibers that join the glossopharyngeal (IX) nerve, and autonomic efferent fibers derived from the vagus (X) nerve (see Section V, Plates 10 and 11). Sections of the chemosensitive regions of the carotid body reveal a dense capillary plexus surrounded by two types of cells.

Because of the difficulty of determining afferent and efferent nerve fibers, two theories of the functioning of the carotid body have been advanced. The first theory, based on nerve degeneration studies, assigns the chemoreceptive function to the type II (sheath) cells and the small nerve fibers they envelop. According to this theory, the large nerve fibers and type I (glomus) cells are an efferent, or feedback, system. The second theory maintains that the type I cells and large fibers comprise the chemoreceptive system, and that the small fibers are autonomic efferents related to blood vessels; this theory is based on the finding of a cholinergic synapse in the afferent system. The connection between type I cells and large nerve fibers has the structural features of such a synapse, and it has been observed that the presynaptic vesicles within the type I cell are depleted after long periods of hypoxia, as would be expected if they contained the chemical transmitter responsible for nerve activation. Neither of these theories explains how a low oxygen level excites the receptor cells or the nerve endings. Presumably, this excitation is coupled in some way to the respiratory metabolism of the chemosensitive cells.

The afferent fibers from the carotid body play an important role in increasing respiration in response to a drop in blood oxygen levels (see CIBA COLLECTION, Volume 7, pp 22 and 290). Other chemoreceptors located in the aortic body and within the brainstem also monitor oxygen, carbon dioxide and pH levels in the blood and participate in the regulation of the respiratory and circulatory systems to maintain these levels within the proper range.

*The carotid sinus* is a thin-walled, elastic section of the internal carotid artery, the walls of which contain *stretch receptors* (C).

## Interoceptors

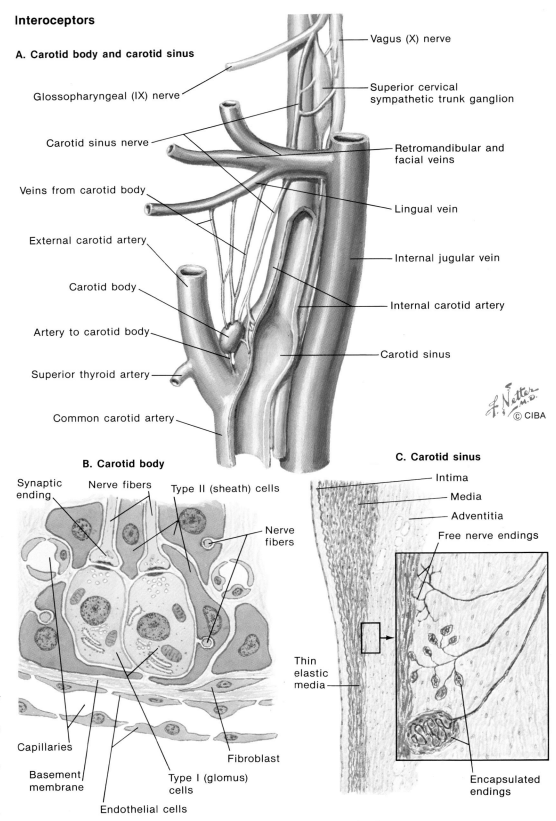

### A. Carotid body and carotid sinus

Glossopharyngeal (IX) nerve

Carotid sinus nerve

Veins from carotid body

External carotid artery

Carotid body

Artery to carotid body

Superior thyroid artery

Common carotid artery

Vagus (X) nerve

Superior cervical sympathetic trunk ganglion

Retromandibular and facial veins

Lingual vein

Internal jugular vein

Internal carotid artery

Carotid sinus

*f. Netter M.D.* © CIBA

### B. Carotid body

Synaptic ending

Nerve fibers

Type II (sheath) cells

Nerve fibers

Capillaries

Basement membrane

Type I (glomus) cells

Fibroblast

Endothelial cells

### C. Carotid sinus

Intima

Media

Adventitia

Free nerve endings

Thin elastic media

Encapsulated endings

These receptors are mechanoreceptive endings of afferent nerve fibers that reach the sinus via the glossopharyngeal (IX) and carotid sinus nerves. Section of the arterial wall shows the presence of free nerve endings and two types of encapsulated nerve endings, and it is likely that the encapsulated endings are the most sensitive stretch receptors. Presumably, the receptor transduction process in these endings resembles that in the Pacinian corpuscle (Plate 14).

Because of their location in an elastic part of the arterial wall, the carotid sinus receptors function as baroreceptors and inform the CNS about blood pressure within the artery (see CIBA COLLECTION,

Volume 5, pp 42 and 225). Strong stimulation (pressure) on these receptors results in reflex bradycardia and a marked fall in blood pressure, and may lead to loss of consciousness as well (carotid sinus syncope). Since the more sensitive baroreceptive endings are active even at normal blood pressure levels, this reflex is constantly acting to restrict the heart rate and blood pressure. Other baroreceptors are located in the aortic arch, right subclavian artery, common carotid artery, heart and pulmonary vessels. Different types of stretch receptors are found in the lungs and bladder and in the linings of the stomach and intestines. □

# General Topography of Hypothalamus

The hypothalamus, lowermost zone of the diencephalon and key neuroendocrine effector mechanism of the neuraxis, has generally well-defined boundaries. It is bordered anteriorly by the anterior commissure, lamina terminalis and optic chiasm; posteriorly, by the interpeduncular fossa; superiorly, by the hypothalamic sulcus, marking the junction with the thalamus; and inferiorly, by the bulging tuber cinereum, which tapers into the funnel-shaped infundibulum. Laterally, as seen in the subsequent frontal sections shown in Plates 52 to 54, boundaries are less distinct, due to blending of the hypothalamic gray matter with adjacent regions, such as the substantia innominata and subthalamic nucleus. In general, however, the internal capsule and its caudal continuation as the basis pedunculi provide obvious lateral limits (Plate 54).

Mostly within these boundaries, but spilling over them in places, lie more than a dozen cell clusters, the *hypothalamic nuclei*. (The number of nuclei varies in different accounts, depending on how many subsidiary clusters are recognized.) Many of these groups of cells are quite evident in some animals, and in fact the hypothalamus is remarkably similar in most vertebrates. Its commonality of effector circuitry suggests (like the uniform layout of the cranial nerves) little basic change over time. In man, however, the hypothalamic nuclei and the fine feltwork of fibers traversing them are overshadowed by more prominent nuclear regions and tracts, such as the thalamus and internal capsule. Only the supraoptic and paraventricular nuclei and the mamillary nuclear complex stand out in ordinary stained sections. The mamillary bodies, however, are more than evident in man; they are grossly prominent, a distinctive human variation on the familiar evolutionary theme.

The illustration shows the six planes of frontal (coronal) sections upon which the subsequent three diagrammatic plates are based. These planes transect each of the principal nuclear groupings of the hypothalamus: the *supraoptic* (anterior), *tuberal* (middle) and *mamillary* (posterior) *groups*.

In considering the hypothalamic nuclei, it is well to address for a moment the meaning of the neuroanatomical term *nucleus*: a cluster of nerve cell bodies in gray matter, with some evident functional role in the nervous system. This commonly used term leads to difficulty, especially in the hypothalamus, where the dendrites and the axons of the resident cells may extend for considerable distances beyond the accepted nuclear boundary. The problem is complicated by the presence, in many of these nuclei, of several histologically and neurochemically different types of

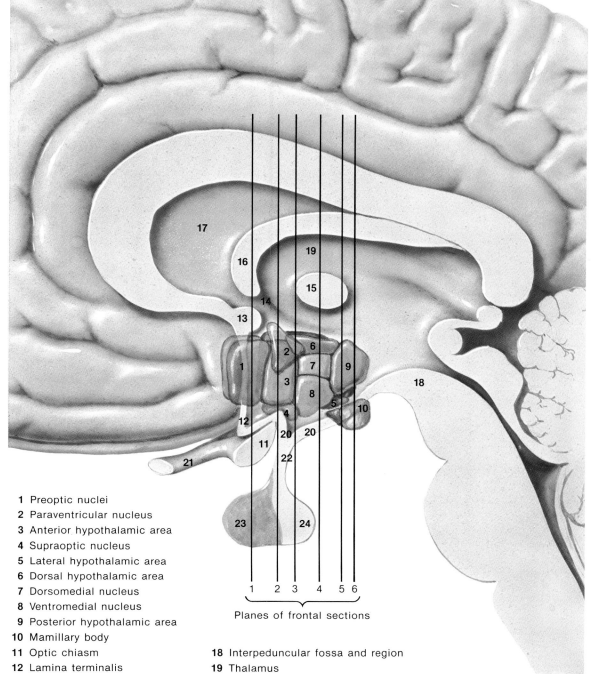

1 Preoptic nuclei
2 Paraventricular nucleus
3 Anterior hypothalamic area
4 Supraoptic nucleus
5 Lateral hypothalamic area
6 Dorsal hypothalamic area
7 Dorsomedial nucleus
8 Ventromedial nucleus
9 Posterior hypothalamic area
10 Mamillary body
11 Optic chiasm
12 Lamina terminalis
13 Anterior commissure
14 Hypothalamic sulcus
15 Interthalamic adhesion
16 Fornix
17 Septum pellucidum

18 Interpeduncular fossa and region
19 Thalamus
20 Tuber cinereum
21 Optic nerve
22 Infundibulum
23 Anterior lobe of pituitary
24 Posterior lobe of pituitary

Planes of frontal sections

neurons. Such overlapping and spreading of dendrites, extent and branching of axons and intermingling of cell types, together with much nonconformity of physiologically determined functional localization to nuclear boundaries, limit the usefulness of these anatomical subdivisions. Indeed, explicit statements of functional contributions can be made for only some of these nuclei, eg, the tuberal or supraoptic/paraventricular groups. Other efforts to define localization of function are perhaps better directed at regions, rather than specific nuclei.

Despite the limitations of nuclear boundaries, the many intrinsic and extrinsic fiber systems of

the hypothalamus (at least a dozen are evident) aid in defining the complex topography of the region. Furthermore, a knowledge of these local circuits and projections is important to the physiologist, pathologist and clinician in providing a means of descriptive communication and a framework for hypotheses. Observations based on precise localization of lesions, of points of stimulation or of the detection of electrical potentials or release of specific transmitter substances are now filling out the gaps in our knowledge of this small but complicated region, which on a weight basis (4 g versus 1,400 g) has been called by Brodal: "a trifling part of the whole brain." □

# Sections Through Hypothalamus I

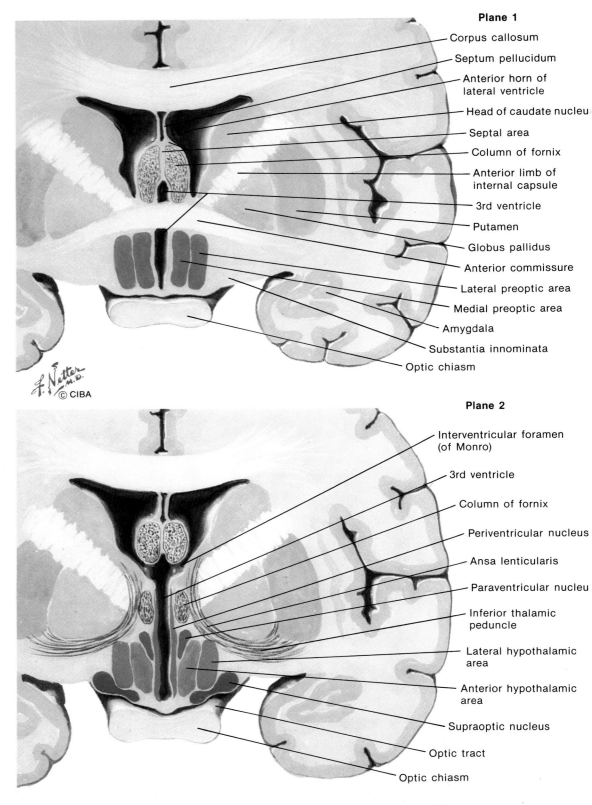

**Plane 1**

- Corpus callosum
- Septum pellucidum
- Anterior horn of lateral ventricle
- Head of caudate nucleu
- Septal area
- Column of fornix
- Anterior limb of internal capsule
- 3rd ventricle
- Putamen
- Globus pallidus
- Anterior commissure
- Lateral preoptic area
- Medial preoptic area
- Amygdala
- Substantia innominata
- Optic chiasm

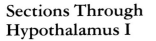

**Plane 2**

- Interventricular foramen (of Monro)
- 3rd ventricle
- Column of fornix
- Periventricular nucleus
- Ansa lenticularis
- Paraventricular nucleu
- Inferior thalamic peduncle
- Lateral hypothalamic area
- Anterior hypothalamic area
- Supraoptic nucleus
- Optic tract
- Optic chiasm

## Planes 1 and 2

The *septal* and *preoptic areas* of the telencephalon are often grouped with the diencephalic *hypothalamic nuclei*. Indeed, it is now generally considered that these three regions comprise an anatomical and functional continuum of gray matter and fiber systems, extending from the base of the septum pellucidum (Plane 1) to the interpeduncular region of the midbrain just behind the mamillary bodies (Plate 51). In particular, evidence shows that the preoptic areas participate in temperature regulation (Plate 61), as well as in regulating release of hypophyseal hormones. They are closely related to the olfactory regions laterally, and the medial forebrain bundle passes through the lateral preoptic area (Plate 55). This important olfactovisceral tract affords two-way connections between mediobasal forebrain structures, including the septal area, hypothalamus and paramedian midbrain tegmentum. Farther caudally (Plane 2), the *anterior* and *lateral hypothalamic areas* appear, the latter being infiltrated by fibers of the medial forebrain bundle. The cell population of these areas at this level is fairly uniform and consists of small, frequently isodendritic (simply branched) neurons, except for a few large neurons scattered between the conspicuous paraventricular and supraoptic nuclei.

The *paraventricular nucleus* is a slender wedge-shaped group of deeply staining neurosecretory cells, near the third ventricle and ventral to the column of the fornix. The *supraoptic nucleus* lies above the beginning of the optic tract, which separates it into two parts, a large anterolateral subnucleus and a small posteromedial one, which are united by a thin column of cells. Most of the neurons of these two nuclei are said to be *magnocellular*: large cells, with dark-staining Nissl substance (rough-surfaced endoplasmic reticulum) condensed at the periphery and a relatively clear perinuclear region. Such cells give rise to the *neuro-*

*hypophyseal tract*, which passes down the infundibular stalk into the posterior lobe of the pituitary gland (Plate 59). There, in the neurohypophysis, the axons of these neurons release two closely related hormones, *oxytocin* and *vasopressin*, into the capillaries of the pars nervosa.

The rostral part of the hypothalamus is closely related topographically to the ansa lenticularis and nearby inferior thalamic peduncle. These fiber systems afford important connections with the amygdala, substantia innominata, orbitofrontal cortex and thalamus. Connections with the septal and preoptic areas are also plentiful; these regions mediate the interactions between the

hypothalamus and the hippocampal formation in the temporal lobe (see Section II, Plates 5 and 6).

Several other smaller nuclei include the suprachiasmatic nucleus (not shown), periventricula and periventricular arcuate nuclei. The *suprachiasmatic nucleus* receives retinohypothalamic fiber from the underlying optic tracts, which, i experimental animals at least, mediate diurnal seasonal effects on pineal/hypothalamohypophyseal function. The *periventricular nuclei* contain small, lymphocytelike nerve cell bodies, some o which elaborate hypothalamohypophyseal *releasing* or *inhibiting factors*, and others serve for local integrative functions and connections. □

## Sections Through Hypothalamus II

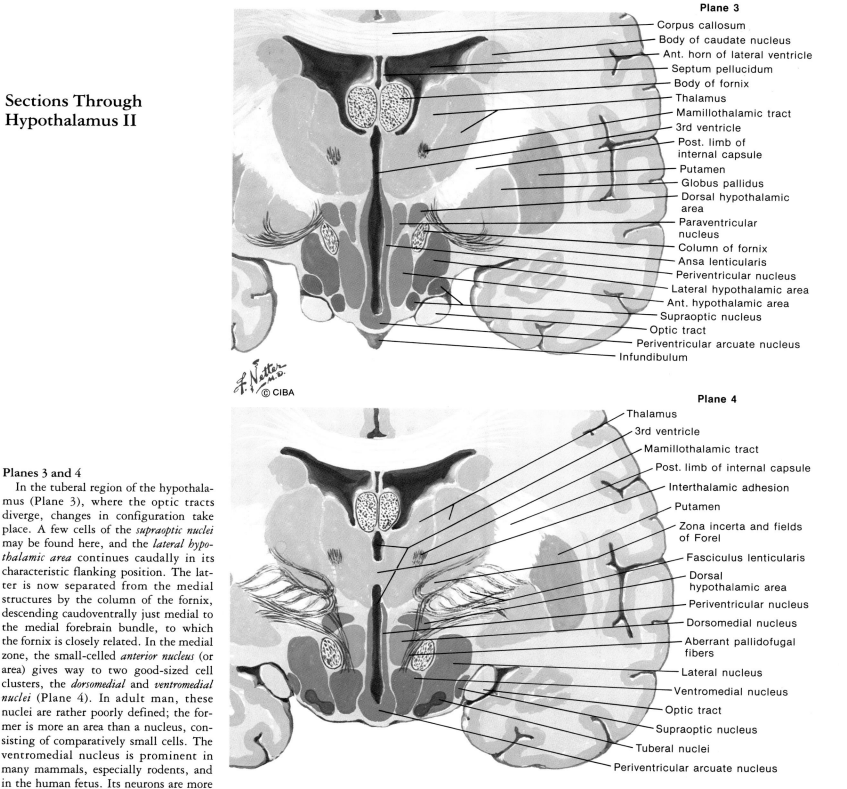

**Plane 3**
- Corpus callosum
- Body of caudate nucleus
- Ant. horn of lateral ventricle
- Septum pellucidum
- Body of fornix
- Thalamus
- Mamillothalamic tract
- 3rd ventricle
- Post. limb of internal capsule
- Putamen
- Globus pallidus
- Dorsal hypothalamic area
- Paraventricular nucleus
- Column of fornix
- Ansa lenticularis
- Periventricular nucleus
- Lateral hypothalamic area
- Ant. hypothalamic area
- Supraoptic nucleus
- Optic tract
- Periventricular arcuate nucleus
- Infundibulum

**Plane 4**
- Thalamus
- 3rd ventricle
- Mamillothalamic tract
- Post. limb of internal capsule
- Interthalamic adhesion
- Putamen
- Zona incerta and fields of Forel
- Fasciculus lenticularis
- Dorsal hypothalamic area
- Periventricular nucleus
- Dorsomedial nucleus
- Aberrant pallidofugal fibers
- Lateral nucleus
- Ventromedial nucleus
- Optic tract
- Supraoptic nucleus
- Tuberal nuclei
- Periventricular arcuate nucleus

### Planes 3 and 4

In the tuberal region of the hypothalamus (Plane 3), where the optic tracts diverge, changes in configuration take place. A few cells of the *supraoptic nuclei* may be found here, and the *lateral hypothalamic area* continues caudally in its characteristic flanking position. The latter is now separated from the medial structures by the column of the fornix, descending caudoventrally just medial to the medial forebrain bundle, to which the fornix is closely related. In the medial zone, the small-celled *anterior nucleus* (or area) gives way to two good-sized cell clusters, the *dorsomedial* and *ventromedial nuclei* (Plane 4). In adult man, these nuclei are rather poorly defined; the former is more an area than a nucleus, consisting of comparatively small cells. The ventromedial nucleus is prominent in many mammals, especially rodents, and in the human fetus. Its neurons are more densely grouped than those in the dorsomedial nucleus.

The ventromedial nucleus has important connections with the orbital cortex of the frontal lobe and amygdaloid complex (Plate 56). The medial region of the hypothalamus also has rich connections with the thalamus, in part via the ubiquitous periventricular nuclei described on page 204. These thin sheets of small, moderately dark-staining nerve cell bodies line the lower part of the third ventricle, immediately adjacent to the ependyma. Inferiorly, they expand into the *periventricular arcuate nuclei*. These neurons, among other roles that include synthesis of hormones, provide

a spiderweb of unmyelinated fibers between the thalamus and hypothalamus.

Embedded in the lateral area, some small irregular cell groupings appear, the *tuberal nuclei*. The lateral nucleus itself, hitherto uniformly composed of small cells, now contains rather dense, irregularly grouped masses of large cell bodies containing considerable Nissl substance. Such perikarya give rise to fibers that form part of the descending efferent pathways from the hypothalamus into the brainstem tegmentum. Through these nuclei pass the fibers of the medial forebrain bundle (Plate 55); many of them descend from the forebrain to the hypothalamus, others continue

down toward the reticular formation, and still others ascend from various neurochemically distinctive structures (locus ceruleus, raphe nuclei, ventral tegmental area) to hypothalamic and telencephalic targets. Thus, the lateral zone of the hypothalamus is a place of heavy impulse traffic in both directions, as well as an area of interaction of several neurotransmitter substances. The degree of this forebrain-midbrain commerce at any given moment is thought to be an important determinant of neural activity in the adjoining medial hypothalamus—important, because this medial region is the pituitary-regulating zone (Plates 58 and 59). □

# Sections Through Hypothalamus III

## Planes 5 and 6

The mamillary region contains complex and enigmatic structures. This part of the hypothalamus is bounded by the capsulopeduncular transition zone and the subthalamic nucleus, together with the "fields of Forel." These fields represent descending, hairpin-turning and then recurrent fibers from the globus pallidus ($H_2$, H and $H_1$, respectively) derived from the ansa and fasciculus lenticularis (Plates 40 and 53), bounded posteriorly by ascending fibers of the brachium conjunctivum and somesthetic systems (medial lemniscus, spinothalamic tracts, etc). The lateral hypothalamic area is considerably reduced and condensed at this level. It consists almost entirely of the large cells previously mentioned (see page 205), and the descending efferent fibers are now closely gathered, many of them poorly myelinated.

A new cell mass, the *posterior nucleus*, or *area*, appears between the third ventricle and the subthalamic nucleus. In its caudal extent, it is bounded laterally by the mamillothalamic tracts. This nucleus contains both the small cell types characteristic of the anterior nuclei and clusters of larger neurons similar to those found in the lateral nucleus. These neurons give rise to the important descending efferent pathways, which pass down through the central gray matter as the dorsal longitudinal fasciculus, or comma tract, of Schütz, and through the reticular formation of the brainstem as components of the central tegmental tract.

*The mamillary nuclear complex*, so conspicuous on the basal aspect of the forebrain, consists of a *medial nucleus* (itself divided into medial and lateral parts) and a *lateral nucleus* (quite small in man). *Satellite nuclei* include the premamillary area, nucleus intercalatus and the supramamillary area. The latter is related to the supramamillary commissure, composed largely of fibers crossing between the subthalamic nuclei.

A major input to the mamillary body comes from limbic forebrain structures, eg, the hippocampal formation and limbic lobe (cingulate and parahippocampal gyri), by way of the *fornix* (see Section II, Plate 6). This bundle descends into the lateral division of the medial mamillary nucleus, but appears to contribute fibers to all parts of the mamillary complex. In the rat, this part of the fornix comes from the subiculum, a region of the hippocampal cortical formation adjacent to the hippocampus. It is not known whether this origin is true for man. The mamillary connection is only one of the many projections of the

fornix; at least half of the fibers of this prominent cable run over the anterior commissure to ramify in the septal and preoptic areas, while half of the remaining fibers in the postcommissural column of the fornix peel away into the thalamus and other regions of the hypothalamus.

The *mamillothalamic tract* leads from the medial mamillary nucleus to the anterior thalamic nucleus, which projects in a topographically precise manner to the cingulate gyrus of the limbic lobe, in this way reciprocating the fornix input to some extent (Plates 55, 56 and 64; see also Section II, Plate 5). The *mamillotegmental tract* is comprised of collaterals of mamillothalamic

fibers; before division, the common stem of these two tracts is known as the *principal mamillary fasciculus*. This tract descends into the paramedian mesencephalon, a region frequently characterized as the "limbic midbrain area." The mamillary peduncle, inconspicuous in man, arises in this same area and terminates in the lateral mamillary nucleus, thereby reciprocating in part the mamillotegmental connection. Thus, the mamillary body is a critical part of the circuits linking the hypothalamus with the limbic forebrain and midbrain structures that lie rostral and caudal to it, respectively, and which exert powerful effects on hypothalamic activity. □

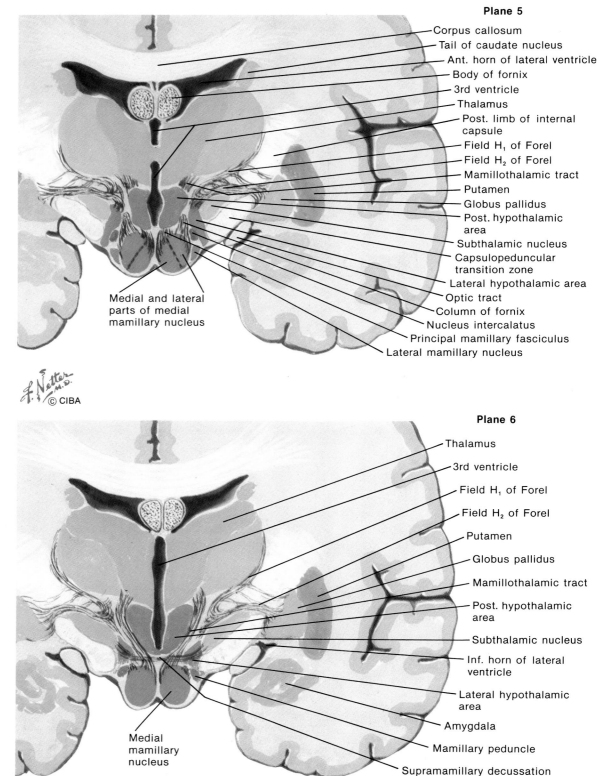

**Plane 5**
- Corpus callosum
- Tail of caudate nucleus
- Ant. horn of lateral ventricle
- Body of fornix
- 3rd ventricle
- Thalamus
- Post. limb of internal capsule
- Field $H_1$ of Forel
- Field $H_2$ of Forel
- Mamillothalamic tract
- Putamen
- Globus pallidus
- Post. hypothalamic area
- Subthalamic nucleus
- Capsulopeduncular transition zone
- Lateral hypothalamic area
- Optic tract
- Column of fornix
- Nucleus intercalatus
- Principal mamillary fasciculus
- Lateral mamillary nucleus

Medial and lateral parts of medial mamillary nucleus

**Plane 6**
- Thalamus
- 3rd ventricle
- Field $H_1$ of Forel
- Field $H_2$ of Forel
- Putamen
- Globus pallidus
- Mamillothalamic tract
- Post. hypothalamic area
- Subthalamic nucleus
- Inf. horn of lateral ventricle
- Lateral hypothalamic area
- Amygdala
- Mamillary peduncle
- Supramamillary decussation

Medial mamillary nucleus

206

# Schematic Reconstruction of Hypothalamus

This illustration of a three-dimensional reconstruction of the hypothalamic nuclei and fiber systems in sagittal aspect is highly schematic. The diffuseness of the hypothalamic cell clusters, especially in man, necessitate placement of rather arbitrary boundaries where little or no demarcation exists in the living brain. And no picture can begin to show the web of dendrites and axons—the true complexity of hypothalamic neuropil.

Overall, the hypothalamus (and the preoptic area) has three longitudinal zones—lateral, medial and periventricular. Rostrocaudally, the *lateral* and *medial preoptic nuclei* fade, respectively, into the *lateral* and *anterior hypothalamic areas*. The latter, in turn, is more or less continuous with the *dorsomedial nucleus* and overlying *dorsal hypothalamic area*. These structures are made up of fairly uniform masses of rather small neurons, interspersed with fibers of passage as well as a local feltwork (Plates 52, 53 and 54). Such small cells merge with other cell groups and infiltrate between them so as to further obscure the already indistinct nuclear boundaries. In a sense, these tiny neurons, seen in the periventricular zone and spilling outward into the medial zone, form a matrix in which the more discrete cell groupings are embedded. The posterior part of the lateral area and the *posterior nucleus* contrast with this matrix; masses of large neurons accumulate in them, which give rise to important efferent fibers of the hypothalamus. These more laterally or caudally placed nuclei receive input from regions outside the hypothalamus—such as the septal/preoptic areas, olfactory brain and ascending brainstem fiber systems—and project to structures upstream and downstream. The afferent and efferent fibers run in the *medial forebrain bundle*, which pervades this lateral zone.

The *ventromedial nucleus* is a more distinct area of small and medium-sized nerve cells reached by one fascicle of the *stria terminalis*, an amygdalofugal tract. Once considered a prime target of this bundle, it appears that few strial fibers end within the nucleus. Instead, the cell-poor zone around the nucleus is the site of largely axodendritic contacts between the stria and several nuclei in this region. These details illustrate the complex synaptology of the hypothalamus. Disturbances in the ventromedial nucleus and nearby lateral area may lead to profound behavioral disorders (Plates 62 and 63).

The neurosecretory *paraventricular* and *supraoptic nuclei* are evident, and their efferent projections (the neurohypophyseal tract; see Plates 52, 55, 59 and 60) are well established. Afferent neural connections are not clearly understood; that they exist

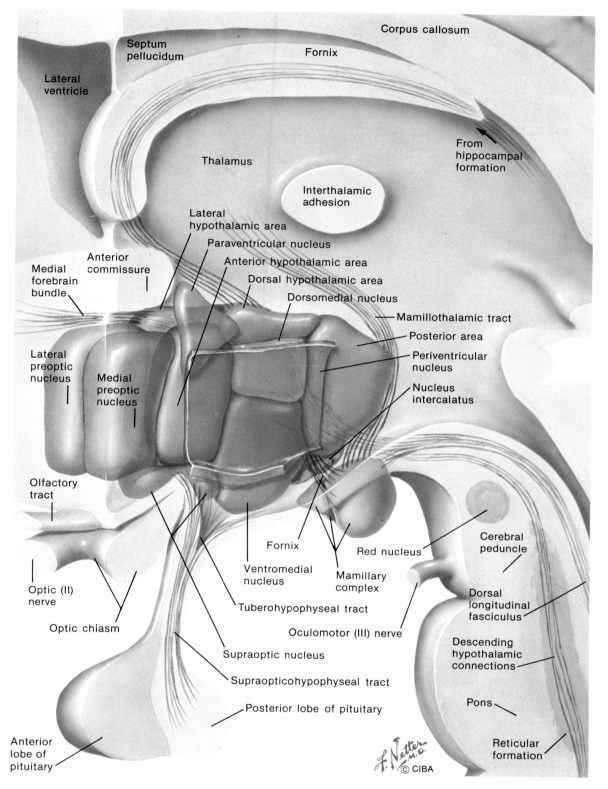

is indicated by changes in activity of this neuroendocrine system in response to noxious afferent stimuli and emotion-evoking situations. The relationship of these cells to capillaries and small blood vessels is peculiar, and this blood supply is very rich (Plate 57).

Neurosecretory fibers from the tuberal and posterior hypothalamic regions also enter the infundibular stem, and constitute the *tuberoinfundibular pathway* (Plate 58).

The *mamillary complex* is evident structurally, although knowledge of its function remains fragmentary. It has a key position in the so-called Papez circuit, a set of circularly arranged reentry

paths linking the hippocampal formation, limbic lobe and hypothalamus (Plate 54). Other connections provide reciprocal routes with the paramedian mesencephalic gray matter, a caudal continuation of hypothalamic gray matter. Its unified pattern of projection in a system of collateralizing fibers entering the *mamillothalamic* and *mamillotegmental tracts* suggests a synchronizing role for the mamillary body with regard to forebrain and midbrain activity.

The illustration shows the more obvious intrinsic and a few of the extrinsic connections of the hypothalamus. (See Plates 56 and 64 and Section II, Plate 6 for some of its other connections.) ☐

# Forebrain Regions Associated With Hypothalamus

The hypothalamus is not the only region of the CNS that provides integrative mechanisms for the performance of various autonomic and neuroendocrine activities. The cerebral cortex influences, sometimes powerfully, the "autonomic" neurovisceral outflow and the neurohumoral output of the endocrine glands—as can be demonstrated experimentally by stimulating the orbitofrontal cortex of the cingulate gyrus to produce respiratory, cardiovascular and digestive responses, as well as certain emotional reactions. The responses are less marked than those produced by stimulating the hypothalamus, but are still striking; some of them, moreover, do not depend upon the integrity of the hypothalamus, a fact that suggests mediation by corticoreticular fibers to lower "centers." In humans, subjective emotional experiences are associated with autonomic discharges (eg, tachycardia, increased blood pressure, blushing) and changes in endocrine activity (such as psychic milk letdown, stress-induced amenorrhea or anorexia nervosa).

Behavioral changes produced by cortical ablations, such as prefrontal lobotomy, are well known. Other such changes, varying from mania and hyperphagia to apathy, aphagia (Plate 62) and somnolence, result from lesions to certain parts of the hypothalamus.

Thus, hypothalamic circuitry is tied into countless other circuits—in the cerebral cortex, limbic system, brainstem reticular formation and other parts of the diencephalon. These circuits are poorly understood, but rich connections with the frontotemporal and cingulate cortex, septal/preoptic areas, amygdala, ventral mesencephalic tegmentum and numerous thalamic nuclei (midline, intralaminar, medial dorsal, anterior, etc) have been demonstrated.

Some of these connections are indicated schematically in the illustration. Connections between the *orbital cortex* of the frontal lobe and the hypothalamus have been demonstrated in certain mammals. Indirect connections with the *prefrontal areas* through the *medial dorsal thalamic nucleus* are well established. The hypothalamus is linked with the *cingulate gyrus* by way of the *anterior thalamic nuclei* and with the *hippocampal formation* via the fornix. The *amygdala* has reciprocal connections with the hypothalamus through the *ventral amygdalofugal pathway*. Additional amygdalohypothalamic connections run through the *stria terminalis*.

The hypothalamus also receives input, through *reticulohypothalamic fiber systems* departing from the main reticulothalamic stream, from the great sensory systems. Through this offshoot, the responses evolved through thalamocortical feature analysis are paralleled by responses in the visceral realm. The limbic (border) structures of the cerebral hemisphere also participate in these responses: the olfactory bulb, amygdala, frontotemporal cortex, septal nuclei, hippocampal formation and limbic lobe (see Section II, Plates 5 and 6). Stimulation of limbic structures can produce respiratory and vascular changes, and psychotropic drugs, such as mescaline, apparently exert some of their effects on the limbic system.

The stria medullaris thalami and medial forebrain bundle (not shown) deserve mention: the former bypasses the hypothalamus, the latter runs right through it (Plates 53 to 55 and 64). The *stria medullaris thalami* connects the medial olfactory area, amygdala and preoptic area with the habenular nucleus, from which fibers pass to the interpeduncular region. The *medial forebrain bundle* links the ventromedial olfactory areas with the preoptic areas, hypothalamus and mesencephalic tegmentum. A diffuse system of fine fibers, it pervades the lateral hypothalamic area and is the key fiber tract of the hypothalamus. Lastly, fibers of the *fornix* end in both medial and lateral mamillary nuclei (see page 206), as well as in the hypothalamus anterior to the mamillary region. A few fibers pass caudally into the mesencephalon. □

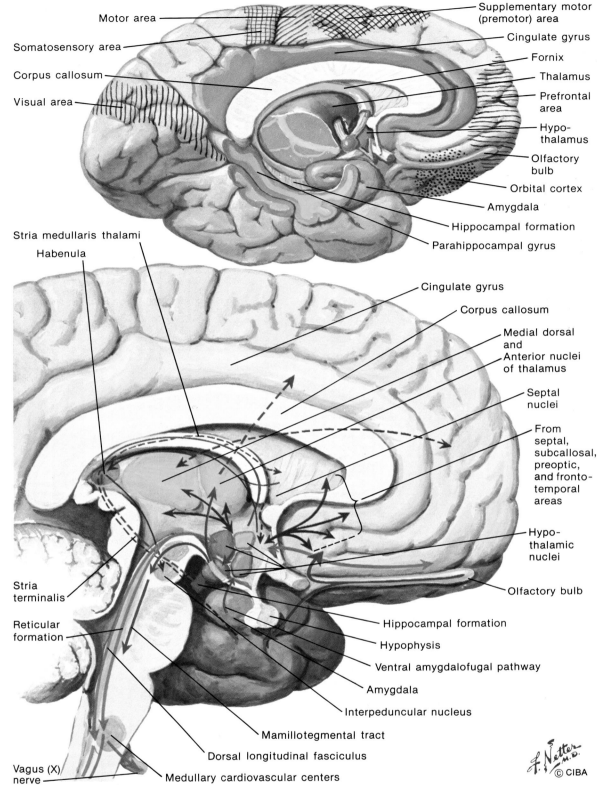

Motor area — Somatosensory area — Corpus callosum — Visual area — Supplementary motor (premotor) area — Cingulate gyrus — Fornix — Thalamus — Prefrontal area — Hypothalamus — Olfactory bulb — Orbital cortex — Amygdala — Hippocampal formation — Parahippocampal gyrus

Stria medullaris thalami — Habenula — Cingulate gyrus — Corpus callosum — Medial dorsal and Anterior nuclei of thalamus — Septal nuclei — From septal, subcallosal, preoptic, and frontotemporal areas — Hypothalamic nuclei — Olfactory bulb — Hippocampal formation — Hypophysis — Ventral amygdalofugal pathway — Amygdala — Interpeduncular nucleus — Mamillotegmental tract — Stria terminalis — Reticular formation — Dorsal longitudinal fasciculus — Vagus (X) nerve — Medullary cardiovascular centers

# Blood Supply of Hypothalamus and Pituitary Gland

*The hypothalamus* receives a rich blood supply, and certain nuclei are especially endowed in this respect. The supraoptic and paraventricular nuclei are believed to contain the most dense capillary networks in the brain, and changes in the osmolality of the blood are known to modify the activity of these neurons. Similarly, other hypothalamic neurons are strongly affected by changes in levels of electrolytes, peptides and other circulating substances.

This generous blood supply is derived from the internal carotid and basilar arteries—through small terminal branches of these vessels, which arise from the arterial circle of Willis, and from the stems of the great arteries themselves. Venous blood drains, through various tributaries, into the anterior cerebral vein rostrally, the internal cerebral vein, superiorly, and the basal vein (of Rosenthal), inferiorly (see Section II, Plates 4 and 16).

*The pituitary gland* receives blood from two groups of arteries, both of which derive from the internal carotids but are quite separate from the hypothalamic arteries. Venous drainage of the hypophysis is also different.

The branches of the *superior hypophyseal arteries*, arising either from the posterior communicating arteries or from the internal carotids themselves, wreath the upper part of the hypophyseal stalk, but do not supply blood to the anterior lobe directly. Instead, they communicate within the stalk and median eminence (the elevated part of the hypothalamus from which the stalk arises) with a *primary plexus* of looped sinusoidal capillaries). These channels lead into venules and then into small, long veins that pass down the stalk into the pars distalis of the adenohypophysis, where a *secondary plexus* of sinusoidal capillaries is formed. This tandem arrangement of capillary plexuses is called the *hypophyseal portal system.*

The portal vessels comprise an extremely complex network of whorls and loops, which spiral among the nerve fibers of the stalk and infiltrate the pars tuberalis and pars distalis. Hypothalamic releasing and inhibiting hormones (originally called factors) elaborated by the tuberal nuclei of the median eminence are transmitted to the anterior lobe by this remarkable part of the systemic circulation (Plate 58). Eventually, *venous blood* drains away through efferent lateral hypophyseal veins into the cavernous sinus, but flow may be reversed, so that hormones released in the anterior lobe can wash back into the median eminence and effect feedback modulation of their synthesis in the tuberal nuclei. And a countercurrent multiplier action, such as that seen in the kidney between the loops of Henle and their surrounding capillaries, now is postulated.

The *posterior lobe* of the pituitary gland receives blood through a similar ring of branches of the *inferior hypophyseal arteries* arising directly from the internal carotids. These vessels form arterioles and capillaries within the pars nervosa, and also contribute to some extent to the portal system described above. *Venous drainage* of the posterior lobe is also to the cavernous sinus. □

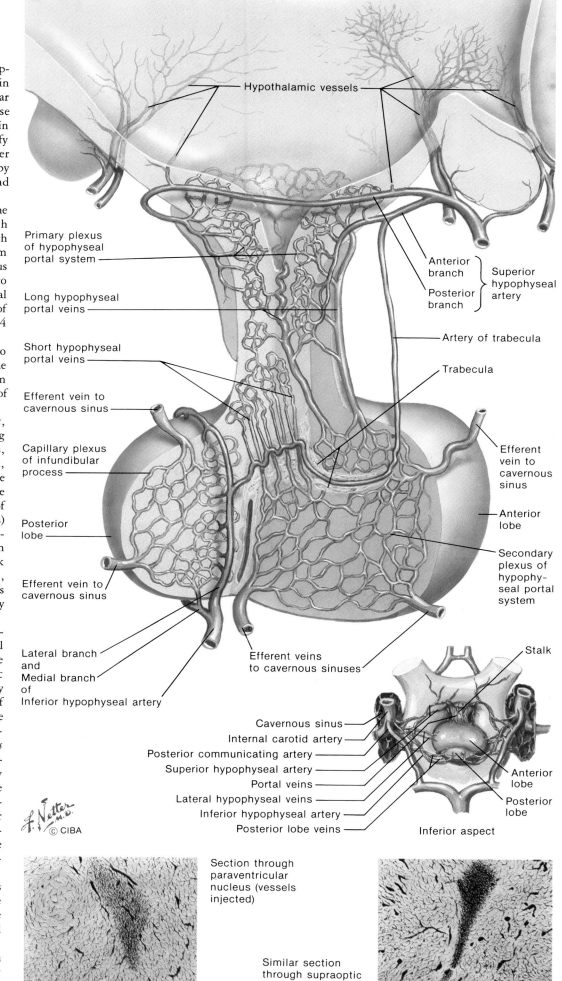

Hypothalamic vessels

Primary plexus of hypophyseal portal system

Anterior branch / Posterior branch — Superior hypophyseal artery

Long hypophyseal portal veins

Artery of trabecula

Short hypophyseal portal veins

Trabecula

Efferent vein to cavernous sinus

Efferent vein to cavernous sinus

Capillary plexus of infundibular process

Anterior lobe

Posterior lobe

Secondary plexus of hypophyseal portal system

Efferent vein to cavernous sinus

Lateral branch and Medial branch of Inferior hypophyseal artery

Efferent veins to cavernous sinuses

Stalk

Cavernous sinus
Internal carotid artery
Posterior communicating artery
Superior hypophyseal artery
Portal veins
Lateral hypophyseal veins
Inferior hypophyseal artery
Posterior lobe veins

Anterior lobe

Posterior lobe

Inferior aspect

Section through paraventricular nucleus (vessels injected)

Similar section through supraoptic nucleus

209

# Adenohypophyseal Hormones

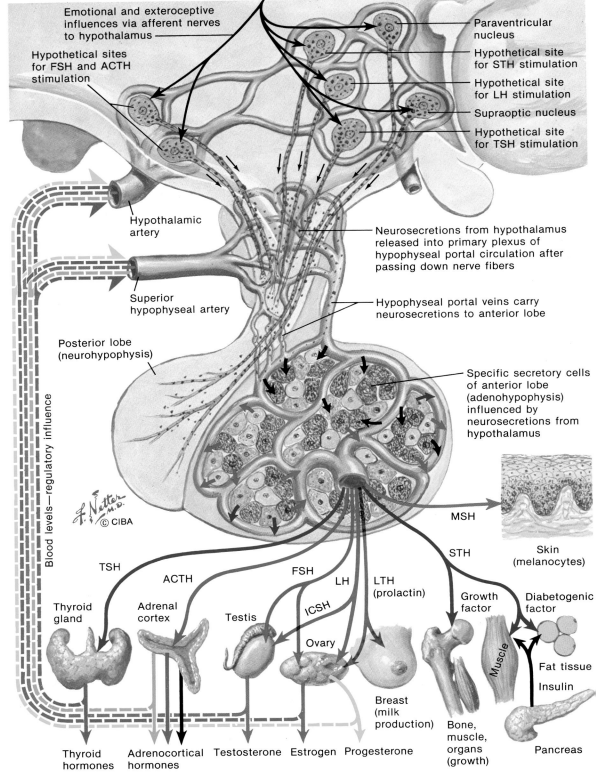

**Adenohypophyseal Hormones**

Emotional and exteroceptive influences via afferent nerves to hypothalamus

Hypothetical sites for FSH and ACTH stimulation

Paraventricular nucleus

Hypothetical site for STH stimulation

Hypothetical site for LH stimulation

Supraoptic nucleus

Hypothetical site for TSH stimulation

Hypothalamic artery

Superior hypophyseal artery

Neurosecretions from hypothalamus released into primary plexus of hypophyseal portal circulation after passing down nerve fibers

Hypophyseal portal veins carry neurosecretions to anterior lobe

Posterior lobe (neurohypophysis)

Specific secretory cells of anterior lobe (adenohypophysis) influenced by neurosecretions from hypothalamus

Blood levels—regulatory influence

MSH

STH

Skin (melanocytes)

TSH

ACTH

FSH

LH

LTH (prolactin)

Growth factor

Diabetogenic factor

Thyroid gland

Adrenal cortex

Testis

ICSH

Ovary

Muscle

Fat tissue

Insulin

Breast (milk production)

Bone, muscle, organs (growth)

Pancreas

Thyroid hormones

Adrenocortical hormones

Testosterone

Estrogen

Progesterone

F. Netter M.D. © CIBA

As emphasized on pages 204 and 209, hypothalamic neurosecretions released into the hypophyseal portal system regulate the secretory activity of anterior lobe cells. The synthesis and release of these hypothalamic-hypophyseal "releasing and inhibiting factors," or hormones, vary according to the stimuli received by the hypothalamic neurons that produce them.

These stimuli arrive through neural connections from brain regions outside the hypothalamus, through changes in the composition of the blood bathing the hypothalamus or (and probably in most cases) through a combination of both neural and vascular influences.

Thus, for example, in a nonspontaneously ovulating animal, such as the rabbit, the act of copulation stimulates hypothalamic neurons to liberate a releasing hormone that in turn promotes release of luteinizing hormone from the anterior lobe. This response depends in part upon the integrity of neural connections (in the mamillary peduncle) conveying information from the spinal cord and brainstem reticular formation into the posterior hypothalamus. On the other hand, the secretion of gonadotropic, adrenocorticotropic or thyrotropic hormones is highly dependent upon the level of gonadal, adrenocortical or thyroid hormones, respectively, circulating in the blood. In both cases, however, the hypothalamic neurons responding receive a mix of neural and vascular signals of such complexity as to warrant caution in the interpretation of cause and effect. With this caveat, the illustration is extremely helpful in elucidating hypothalamohypophyseal relationships and the general principle of blood-mediated neuroendocrine modulation of the adenohypophysis.

The cellular sources of most of the various anterior lobe hormones are now generally agreed upon. The *acidophils*, or *alpha cells*, produce prolactin, or luteotropic hormone (LTH), and

growth, or somatotropic hormone (STH). Numerous subtypes of *basophils* (beta and delta cells, with further numeric subsidiary designations) produce melanocyte-stimulating hormone (MSH), thyrotropin (TSH), adrenocorticotropin (ACTH), follicle-stimulating hormone (FSH) and luteinizing hormone (ICSH). *Chromophobes*, cells which resist staining with the varied techniques now used to study the adenohypophysis, include actively secreting, degranulated cells and primordial or resting cells.

It is evident that lesions of the hypothalamus will influence, either overtly or subtly, the output of anterior lobe hormones—by destroying, or at least interrupting the connections and impairing

the blood supply of, those diencephalic neurons which regulate anterior pituitary activities. An example of the striking effects of hypothalamic damage upon endocrine functions is the syndrome of *adiposogenital dystrophy*. This condition, which accompanies a tumor or other lesion in the hypothalamohypophyseal region or a functional imbalance that is frequently psychological in origin, involves a deficiency or delay in output of gonadotropins and sometimes other anterior lobe hormones, with consequent hypogonadism and obesity. Many other examples of damaged or disturbed hypothalamohypophyseal function are now known (see CIBA COLLECTION, Volume 4, Sections I and III). □

# Neurohypophyseal Hormones: Oxytocin and Vasopressin

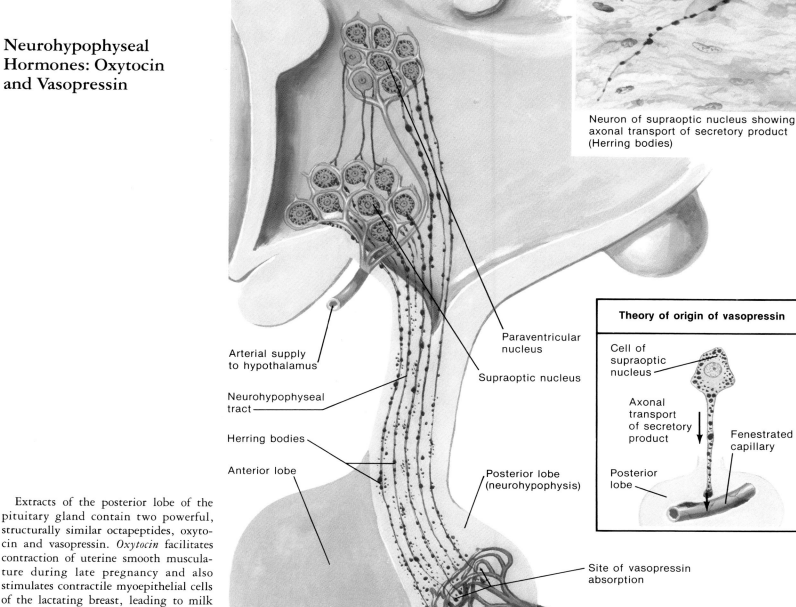

Neuron of supraoptic nucleus showing axonal transport of secretory product (Herring bodies)

Paraventricular nucleus

Arterial supply to hypothalamus

Supraoptic nucleus

Neurohypophyseal tract

Herring bodies

Anterior lobe

Posterior lobe (neurohypophysis)

**Theory of origin of vasopressin**

Cell of supraoptic nucleus

Axonal transport of secretory product

Fenestrated capillary

Posterior lobe

Site of vasopressin absorption

Venous drainage of posterior lobe

Inferior hypophyseal artery

Extracts of the posterior lobe of the pituitary gland contain two powerful, structurally similar octapeptides, oxytocin and vasopressin. *Oxytocin* facilitates contraction of uterine smooth musculature during late pregnancy and also stimulates contractile myoepithelial cells of the lactating breast, leading to milk expulsion. *Vasopressin*, also known as *antidiuretic hormone (ADH)*, promotes reabsorption of renal water by increasing the permeability of the distal convoluted and collecting tubules to water, and also exerts a pressor effect on the circulatory system by facilitating arteriolar smooth muscle contraction and thereby heightening peripheral vascular resistance (Plate 60). In the absence of vasopressin, the clinical condition of *diabetes insipidus* develops. As might be expected, the biological effects of these two related hormones overlap to some extent. (See CIBA COLLECTION, Volume 4, pages 32 to 35.)

These neurohypophyseal hormones, however, are not produced in the pituitary gland but in the overlying hypothalamus—in the paraventricular and supraoptic nuclei (Plates 52 and 55). Most accounts attribute oxytocin to the paraventricular nucleus and vasopressin, to the supraoptic, but recent immunohistochemical studies indicate that both hormones derive from both nuclei. Moreover, studies have shown that vasopressin has a

significant facilitatory effect on memory. For this and other reasons relating to their putative role as transmitters or modulators, the study of neural peptides is widening rapidly.

The neurosecretory products pass to the posterior lobe as axonally transported, stainable colloid droplets (Herring bodies) within the slender, poorly myelinated fibers of the *neurohypophyseal tract*. These droplets, which appear under the electron microscope as membrane-bound, electron-dense granules in the axon terminals of the tract, are released in the pars nervosa into the bloodstream, evidently by liberation near the walls of fenestrated capillaries.

As described on page 210, changes in the amounts of hypothalamic hormones synthesized and/or released almost certainly must reflect changes in the activity of the neurosecretory neurons responding to vascular and neural influences. The first influence consists of variations in the osmolality and other properties of the blood and tissue fluid that bathe the supraoptic and paraventricular neurons. The second influence derives from the heavy traffic of nerve impulses flowing up and down without respite through the lateral zone of the hypothalamus—the strategically located neuroendocrine effector agency of the far-flung limbic system. □

# Regulation of Water Balance

In its synthesis, transport and release of *vasopressin*, or *antidiuretic hormone (ADH)*, the supraoptic nucleus of the hypothalamus is certainly the most obvious component of the nervous system in the regulation of water balance. But functions are rarely, if ever, localized in one brain nucleus or area. On the contrary, they are carried out by many neural structures working as a team, and usually in concert with various target organs and other organ systems. The structures involved in such teamplay may appear relatively concentrated in one brain region, as is the case for neuroendocrine control mechanisms and the hypothalamus, or far-flung, as with the cerebral and spinal levels of the motor system. But in reality, most nervous regulation of body function is discharged through the specialized contributions and concerted activities of countless neurons in a widespread network—perhaps extending the length of the neuraxis. This important organizing principle of the nervous system is summed up by the words *distributed system.*

It is now known that the supraoptic nucleus is not the only source for vasopressin. As mentioned on page 210, the paraventricular nucleus is also thought to elaborate this polypeptide, and the suprachiasmatic nucleus may synthesize it as well. And while the supraoptic nucleus, in keeping with its unparalleled capillary supply, may be an ideal place for neurons that can respond to changes in the osmolality of the blood, the receptive cells may not be the same neurons that project to the posterior lobe of the pituitary. Instead, they may lie on the border of the nucleus or in its immediate vicinity, or even be distributed more widely in the anterior hypothalamus.

Moreover, osmoreception is only part of a still larger story. As well as changes in the blood, other factors—emotional states, stressful situations, painful stimuli, sleep-activity cycles and other biorhythms—may affect the activities of hypothalamic neurosecretory neurons. As pointed out on page 208, such effects are mediated through neural inputs to these cells. Afferents to the supraoptic nucleus have been described as coming from many brain regions, including the hippocampus, septal area and amygdala and especially the adjacent brainstem. While these inputs are important, it is doubtful that they can contravene the influences of osmotic changes in the blood. Nevertheless, the brainstem afferents may be monoaminergic, at least in part, and thus the action of certain drugs, such as morphine, which can change the amount of secretion of vasopressin, should be considered in the context of neurotransmitter interactions.

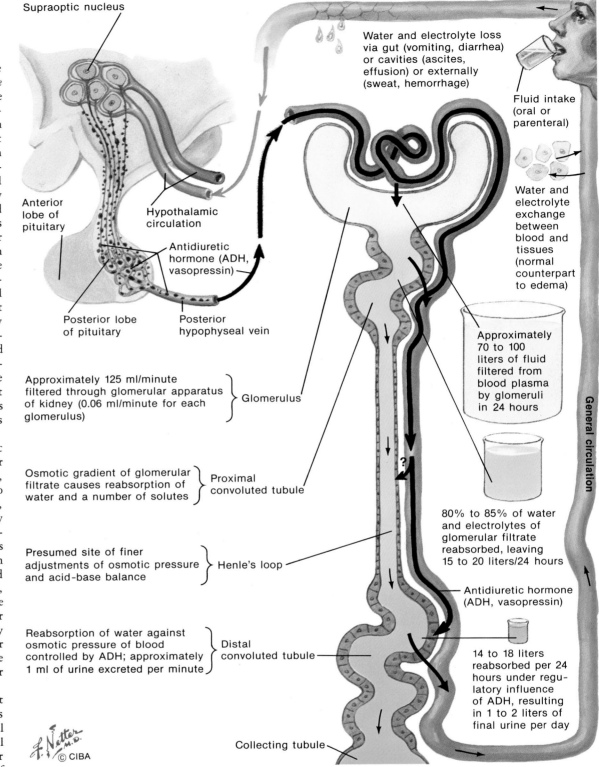

The physiology of water balance is well covered elsewhere (see CIBA COLLECTION, Volume 4, pages 33 to 35 and Volume 6, pages 51 to 59). In brief, the functioning of this mechanism is as follows. As shown in the illustration, the axons of supraoptic neurons pass down the infundibular stem (as part of the neurohypophyseal tract) and ramify extensively among the pituicytes (modified glial cells) of the posterior lobe of the pituitary. When the blood bathing the hypothalamus becomes hyperosmotic, as in dehydration, the supraoptic neurons (and other vasopressin-synthesizing cells) respond by increasing the production and/or release of ADH, and thereby raise its titer in the plasma. When ADH reaches the kidney, the hormone increases its facilitatory action upon water reabsorption in the distal convoluted and collecting tubules.

When hydration occurs, the effects are reversed. If a normal person drinks a large quantity of water or other fluid, the resulting decrease in osmolality of the blood, even though slight, inhibits the neurosecretion of ADH. As the concentration of ADH in the blood falls, the renal tubules no longer take back as much water from the urine, and water diuresis ensues until excess water is excreted and normal blood osmolality restored. □

# Temperature Regulation

Laboratory mammals with bilateral lesions of the hypothalamus can no longer maintain a stable body temperature. Clinical experience shows that man reacts in the same way, if similarly impaired. Numerous cases of postoperative hyperthermia have been noted following neurosurgical procedures for the removal of neoplasms in the immediate vicinity of the hypothalamus, such as hypophyseal tumors and suprasellar meningiomas.

While complex, hypothalamic thermoregulatory mechanisms seem to be dual: an anterior and lateral part of the region is involved in heat loss, while a posterior and lateral part regulates heat production. According to current views, only the anterolateral part of the hypothalamus contains two types of neurons sensitive to heating or cooling, respectively, of the blood, and thus act as *thermoreceptors*. Such neurons, however, are also present in the adjoining preoptic area.

Whatever the distribution of these specialized cells, they appear to serve as a major part of the hypothalamic "thermostat." When the temperature of the blood rises, one of the two types of anterior hypothalamic neurons is said to release serotonin, which activates descending pathways near the central gray matter leading to brainstem and spinal respiratory/cardiovascular mechanisms of heat loss: panting, increased peripheral blood flow and perspiration. When blood temperature falls, the other type of cell releases a catecholamine to set in motion the complex processes whereby body temperature is maintained or elevated, including increased production of body heat by shivering and heat conservation by reducing radiation through vasoconstriction.

In keeping with the principle of *distributed systems* (see page 212), other CNS regions, particularly the midbrain, take part in thermoregulation and other mechanisms are implicated in keeping body temperature within narrow limits. For example, heat production can be accelerated by a general metabolic speedup—brought about by increased hypothalamic activation (through the thyroid-stimulating hormone, or TSH) of the anterior lobe of the pituitary and its production of thyrotropic hormone (Plate 58).

Clinically, lesions of the anterior hypothalamus may result in an inability to adjust to high or low environmental temperatures. With acute trauma or unavoidable involvement of this region during surgery, the patient may fail to adapt because the

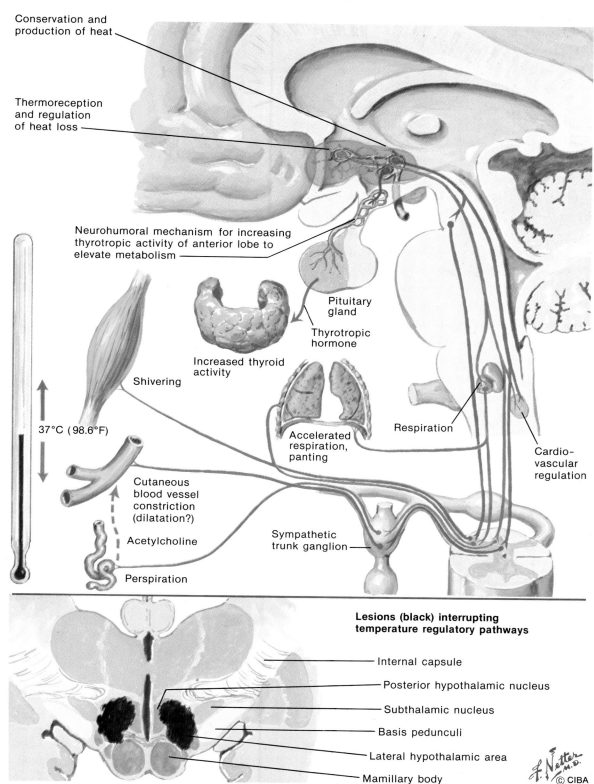

Conservation and production of heat

Thermoreception and regulation of heat loss

Neurohumoral mechanism for increasing thyrotropic activity of anterior lobe to elevate metabolism

Pituitary gland

Thyrotropic hormone

Increased thyroid activity

Shivering

37°C (98.6°F)

Accelerated respiration, panting

Respiration

Cardio-vascular regulation

Cutaneous blood vessel constriction (dilatation?)

Acetylcholine

Sympathetic trunk ganglion

Perspiration

**Lesions (black) interrupting temperature regulatory pathways**

Internal capsule

Posterior hypothalamic nucleus

Subthalamic nucleus

Basis pedunculi

Lateral hypothalamic area

Mamillary body

thermostatically unchecked temperature maintenance and heat-production mechanisms get out of control, resulting in rapidly fatal hyperthermia.

"Neurogenic" (postoperative) hyperthermia is particularly dangerous if these mechanisms are stimulated by infection or by the presence of pyrogenic substances, which appear to act selectively on the anterior hypothalamic-preoptic area. Lesions located more caudally, especially in lateral areas of the hypothalamus, depress both heat dissipation and production/conservation by interrupting the respective descending temperature regulatory pathways. In such instances, poikilothermy results.

As anticipated on page 212, precise allocation for hypothalamic functional contributions is not possible. The "thermostatic" and heat loss or conservation/production functions of the hypothalamus cannot be confined to specific nuclei. The specialized nerve cells involved in these complex and interrelated functional regulations are not segregated or grouped, but are mingled with other types of hypothalamic neurons and with one another. Such intermingling may also vary with the individual, if variations in nuclei and fiber tracts elsewhere in the CNS are any indication. Hence, the functional attributions shown only indicate regions indispensable to such functions. □

# Hypothalamic Control of Food Intake

Hunger is a basic biological drive and an important behavioral determinant. Although hunger and appetite do not necessarily go hand in hand, both are germane to the study and treatment of obesity and malnutrition. Hypothalamic damage or dysfunction may have striking effects on food intake, and the clinical concept of hypothalamic obesity, as manifested in Fröhlich's syndrome, has attracted attention for over half a century (see CIBA COLLECTION, Volume 4, page 16).

The experimental evidence is even more extensive. A vast literature has accumulated on hunger and thirst, the neural substrates of these drives and the behaviors necessary to satisfy them. These complex functions are now viewed in the context of more generalized "reward" and "punishment" mechanisms —of "pleasure" and "aversive" systems within the neuraxis, especially in the forebrain. The term "center" should be avoided, because the performance of a function is increasingly difficult to ascribe to one neural region in the face of new evidence and concepts (see pages 208 and 212).

The illustration should be interpreted in the light of the above caveats. It presents the well-known finding that localized hypothalamic lesions can have a dramatic effect on food consumption. Animals with such lesions may undergo profound behavioral changes, becoming overly withdrawn or savage, especially if they develop excessive appetite. Hyperphagic animals eat heartily, even when already amply fed. Moreover, they take hold of food and eat wolfishly, and many forego aversive behavior in their quest for food.

Since animals with hyperphagia of any cause are usually less active than normal, they easily become obese. This condition can be offset by a suitably restricted diet. Other problems, however, attend hyperphagia as a result of hypothalamic lesions: deficiencies in hypothalamohypophyseal releasing or release-inhibiting hormones and related disturbances in fat and carbohydrate metabolism.

The focal lesions shown appear to interfere with "set points" for appetite patterns—some kind of reference values that serve to keep body weight at a certain level (heavy, normal or light). A neural mechanism that includes the *ventromedial nucleus* seems important to satiety, and when this nucleus is damaged, the imbalance in the system leads to hyperphagia (and, paradoxically, to finickiness and decreased motivation for food). On the other hand, a mechanism including the *lateral hypothalamic area* appears necessary for appetite, and lesions of this region abolish the urge to eat—in

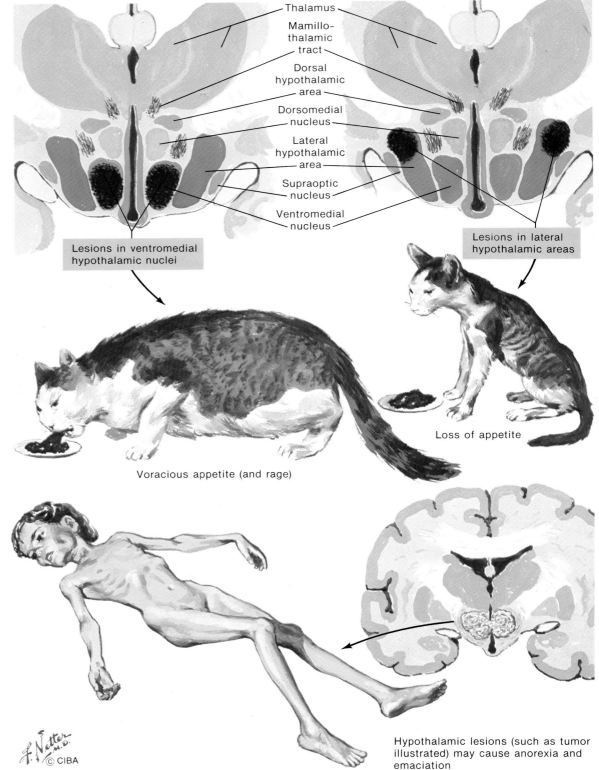

Lesions in ventromedial hypothalamic nuclei

Lesions in lateral hypothalamic areas

Thalamus
Mamillothalamic tract
Dorsal hypothalamic area
Dorsomedial nucleus
Lateral hypothalamic area
Supraoptic nucleus
Ventromedial nucleus

Voracious appetite (and rage)

Loss of appetite

Hypothalamic lesions (such as tumor illustrated) may cause anorexia and emaciation

normal animals as well as in animals hyperphagic as a result of lesions in the ventromedial nucleus.

Selective stimulation of these two hypothalamic regions produces opposite results: ie, stimulation of the ventromedial nucleus brings about suppression of feeding behavior, and stimulation of the lateral area leads to its activation.

Similar effects on other bodily functions may follow small lesions elsewhere in the hypothalamus or in the preoptic and septal nuclei. For example, changes in thirst patterns and water consumption follow destruction or stimulation of these latter regions. In such experiments, it is difficult to attribute the effects to the destruction or

stimulation of the neurons of the region destroyed or stimulated, or to the interruption or activation of fibers of passage. Recent studies with kainic acid, which sometimes destroys nerve cells without injury to extrinsic fiber systems, are interesting: injections of small amounts of this acid into the lateral hypothalamus of rats have led to aphagia and adipsia. The results indicate that the emotional changes (such as exaggerated aversiveness) that may accompany aphagia and adipsia following lesions in the lateral hypothalamus, are due to the damage to passing fiber tracts (such as the medial forebrain bundle), not to the loss of the neurons affected by the acid. □

# Hypothalamus and Emotional Behavior

In humans, the changes in emotions and in emotional expressions (the distinction is important) that follow lesions or irritative processes in the hypothalamus, include symptoms that range from apathy and depression to excitement, motor hyperactivity (including talkativeness), uncontrolled ideation and unrestrained expression—even to psychopathic and manic states.

An obvious advantage to clinical studies over animal experiments is that the investigator can question the patient to see if the observed changes in emotional expression (autonomic and somatic responses) are accompanied by changes in emotions (subjective feelings) and vice versa. A researcher cannot directly question the laboratory animal and must instead observe, measure and explain behavior in the language of stimulus, response and reward.

Thus, nobody can say for sure that the aggressive-looking cat in the illustration is really angry—that the emotion is there along with the all-too-evident emotional expression. But today it is scientifically acceptable to make this assumption, bearing in mind the degree of certainty involved.

Bilateral lesions in the ventromedial hypothalamic nuclei in previously tame cats produce, along with obesity (Plate 62), savage and vicious behavior indicative of extreme rage. This dramatic effect, also demonstrable in rats and monkeys, is irreversible; it does not respond to efforts at retaming and persists even after removal of the frontal poles or uncinate cortex of the temporal lobes. The animal tries to escape and, when cornered, growls and hisses, often attacking with fierce intensity if approached, and its overall appearance is impressive.

Removal of the cerebral cortex or high decerebration (removal of the greater parts of the basal ganglia and thalamus) in cats produces a similar effect, called "sham rage" because it was assumed that a decorticate or decerebrate animal cannot feel or direct anger. The animal arches its back, erects its fur, lashes its tail, bares its teeth and unsheathes its claws, etc, in response to the most innocuous stimuli. For the maximum picture of sham rage, the posterior hypothalamus must be left intact, although incomplete manifestations of anger still appear in high midbrain preparations. Unlike normal rage, the easily provoked sham rage ceases soon after the stimulus is removed.

Lesions in other parts of the hypothalamus cause different types of behavioral responses, such as exaggerated aversive behavior, observed after lateral hypothalamic lesions, and strong suppression of aggressive behavior and autonomic functions in general, following destruction of the

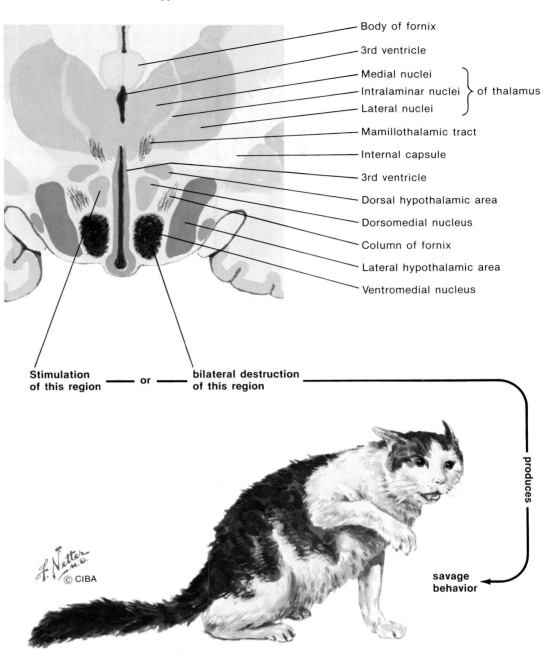

Body of fornix
3rd ventricle
Medial nuclei
Intralaminar nuclei } of thalamus
Lateral nuclei
Mamillothalamic tract
Internal capsule
3rd ventricle
Dorsal hypothalamic area
Dorsomedial nucleus
Column of fornix
Lateral hypothalamic area
Ventromedial nucleus

Stimulation of this region — or — bilateral destruction of this region — produces — savage behavior

**Note:** Paradoxically, stimulation of ventromedial nucleus is also known to produce vicious behavior. Thus, the effects of lesions and focal stimulations must be viewed as gross perturbations of complex distributed systems

mamillary region, the major source of neural output from the hypothalamus and a portal for fibers from the lower brainstem (Plates 55 and 56).

Electrical stimulation of the hypothalamus also produces a wide range of emotional responses, as well as other types of autonomic and endocrine effects. Stimulation near the fornix in the lateral and dorsal regions of the hypothalamus evokes angry behavior much like that seen in animals with ventromedial lesions: elevation in blood pressure and blood sugar, pupillary dilatation, horripilation, protrusion of claws, increased amplitude of respiration, urination, defecation, rhythmic spitting, etc. These responses, first described in complex "hanging brain" surgical preparations and later in anesthetized animals, have been elicited in unanesthetized animals, and even in awake and unrestrained ones. The classic studies of Hess, and later of Hunsperger, on the

substrates of angry behavior in the cat were based on the use of indwelling electrodes in such freely moving animals, and with increasing stimulation, the full picture of violent rage steadily unfolded until the cat sometimes attacked a stick held in front of it or the observer. These studies indicate that two indispensable substrates for the expression of anger are the perifornical region of the anterior hypothalamus and the central gray of the midbrain.

The directed nature of behaviors elicited by focal stimulation of the hypothalamus, together with the great interconnections of this region with other parts of the brain, make it clear that hypothalamic activity in the emotional realm is only part of an integrated, widely distributed system involving numerous components: the orbitofrontal cortex, uncus, amygdala, hippocampus, septal area and limbic midbrain, to name but a few. □

## Neural, Neuroendocrine and Systemic Components of Rage Reaction

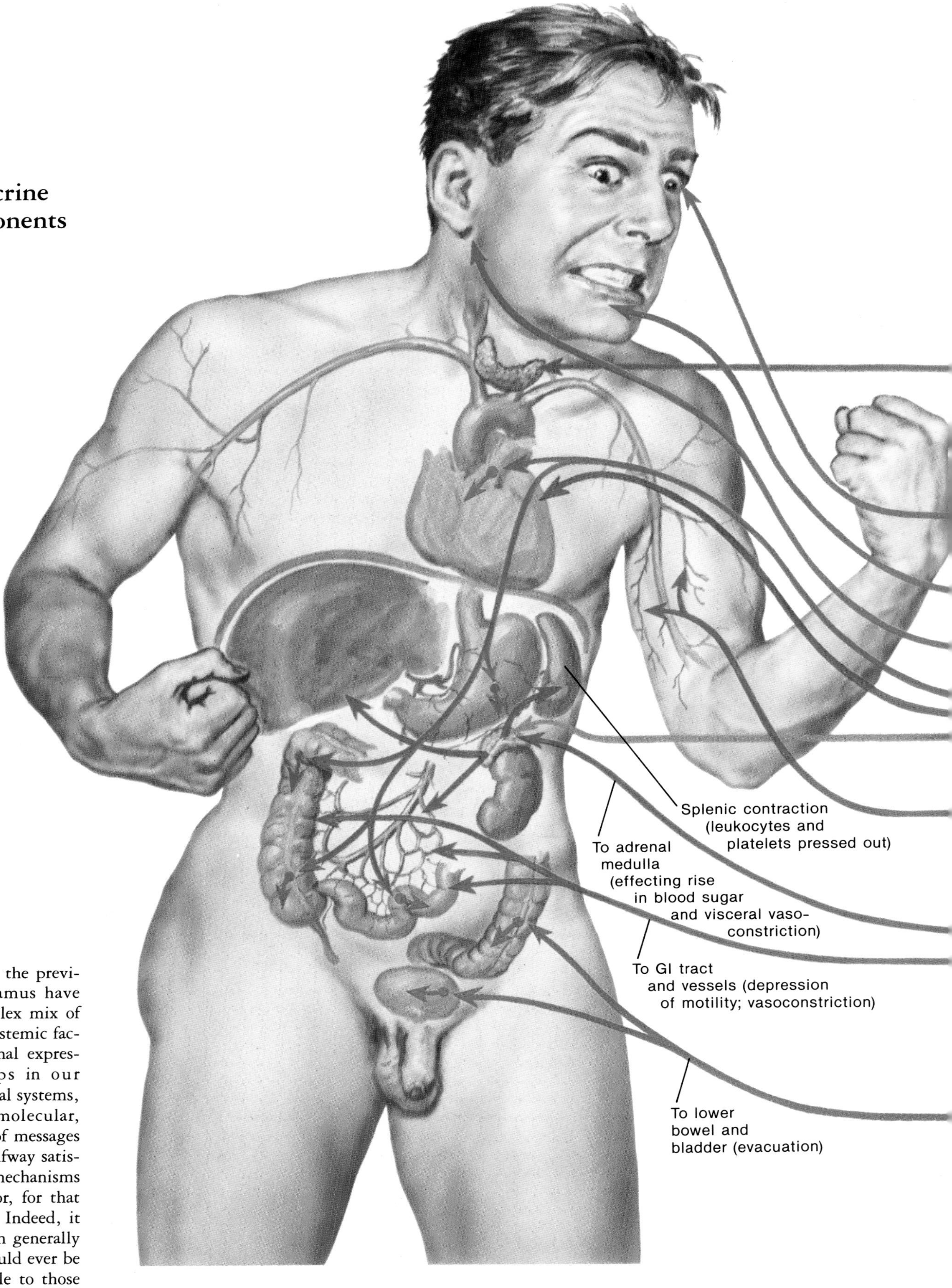

Splenic contraction
(leukocytes and
platelets pressed out)

To adrenal
medulla
(effecting rise
in blood sugar
and visceral vaso-
constriction)

To GI tract
and vessels (depression
of motility; vasoconstriction)

To lower
bowel and
bladder (evacuation)

As the texts accompanying the previous plates on the hypothalamus have attempted to show, the complex mix of neural, neuroendocrine and systemic factors in emotions and emotional expressions, and the many gaps in our knowledge of distributed neural systems, chemical transmitters and molecular, spatial and temporal coding of messages in the CNS, preclude even halfway satisfactory explanations of the mechanisms involved in angry behavior—or, for that matter, any form of behavior. Indeed, it is unlikely that an explanation generally satisfactory to neuroscience could ever be given, let alone one acceptable to those who look at human behavior from other points of view.

Still, the autonomic, glandular and general systemic concomitants of aggressive behavior are well known and familiar to everyone and, moreover, are reasonably well understood across the board. The illustration shows, in schematic form, some of the numerous neural structures, endocrine glands and target organs or organ systems that participate—in

orchestral synchrony that is nothing short of magnificent—in an outburst of rage.

The components include, but are by no means limited to, the orbitofrontal cortex and limbic system, the hypothalamus, the sympathetic and parasympathetic parts of the so-called "autonomic nervous system" (clearly a terrible misnomer), the blood vessels of the skin and the muscles and the

contractile walls of the heart and bowels. Each component participates in its own way: by excitation or inhibition, constriction or dilatation, activation or suppression of activity and so on, as indicated on the leader lines and legends.

The picture, of course, is just a picture, and a still one at that. It does not begin to show the timing and dynamic interactions of the many events

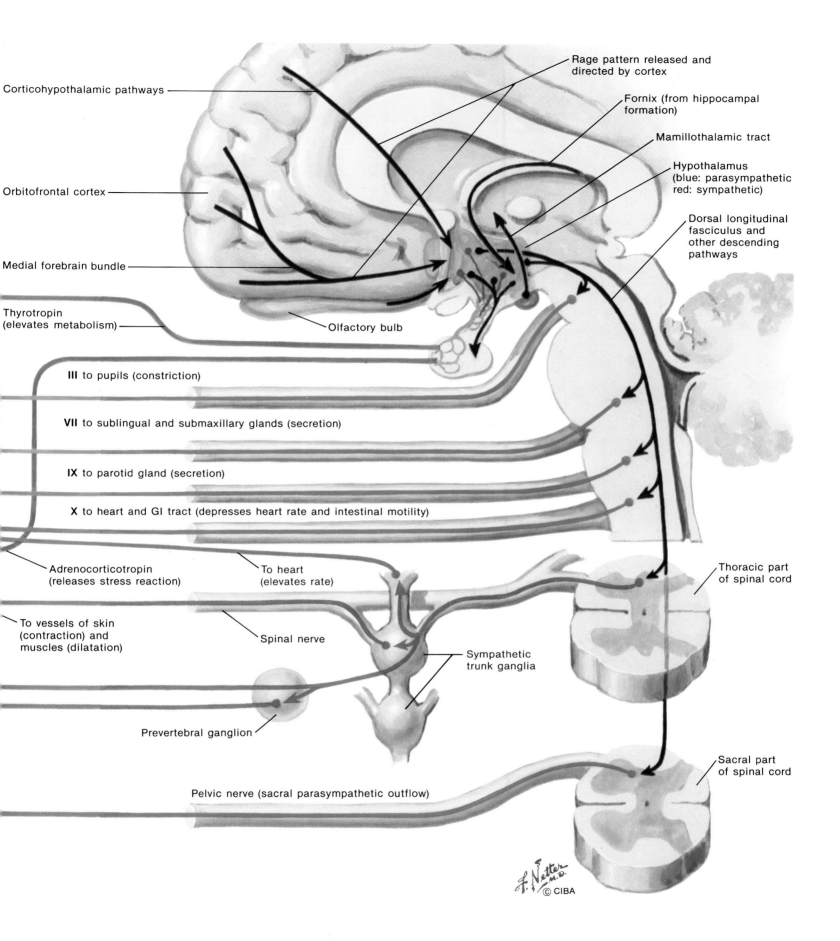

Corticohypothalamic pathways

Orbitofrontal cortex

Medial forebrain bundle

Thyrotropin
(elevates metabolism)

**III** to pupils (constriction)

**VII** to sublingual and submaxillary glands (secretion)

**IX** to parotid gland (secretion)

**X** to heart and GI tract (depresses heart rate and intestinal motility)

Adrenocorticotropin
(releases stress reaction)

To vessels of skin
(contraction) and
muscles (dilatation)

Prevertebral ganglion

Pelvic nerve (sacral parasympathetic outflow)

Rage pattern released and
directed by cortex

Fornix (from hippocampal
formation)

Mamillothalamic tract

Hypothalamus
(blue: parasympathetic
red: sympathetic)

Dorsal longitudinal
fasciculus and
other descending
pathways

Olfactory bulb

To heart
(elevates rate)

Spinal nerve

Sympathetic
trunk ganglia

Thoracic part
of spinal cord

Sacral part
of spinal cord

*f. Netter M.D.*
© CIBA

involved—those between the neuraxis and the rest of the body (including the all-reaching stream of the blood), between the various target organs themselves, and between all these effector structures and the brain itself as the loop of behavior closes back upon its source. But this remarkable illustration, which has seen wide use for over 25 years, comes as close to any picture that this writer can recall in putting across two transcendentally important organizing principles of the nervous system: unified action and all-encompassing effect, both to the end of integrated body function.

It should be noted that the actions shown for the sympathetic (red) division of the autonomic nervous system would be enhanced during the rage reaction, whereas those for the parasympa-

thetic (blue) division would be suppressed. The reverse would obtain in a hedonistic, or pleasure, reaction. In general, the two divisions of the autonomic nervous system exert antagonistic effects on their target structures, although this generalization does not adequately reflect the complexity of local autonomic interaction and balance (see Section IV). □

# Action of Drugs on Nerve Excitability

## Action of Drugs on Nerve Excitability

| Drug | Action on membrane | Changes in membrane potential and action potential | Clinical effects |
|---|---|---|---|
| Tetrodotoxin (Puffer fish toxin)<br><br>Saxitoxin (Shellfish toxin) | Blocks voltage-sensitive Na⁺ channels | Blocks action potential | Nerve block, paralysis, death |
| Tetraethylammonium (TEA) | Blocks K⁺ permeability channels | Decreases resting potential (partial depolarization); prolongs action potential | ? |
| Increased external potassium concentration | Makes K⁺ equilibrium potential ($E_{K^+}$) less negative | Decreases resting potential (partial depolarization), thereby causing accommodation that decreases action potential size and raises threshold for action potential | Nerve block, plus action on many systems causing varied clinical picture |
| Metabolic inhibitors (cyanide)<br><br>Cardiac glycosides (ouabain) | Block active transport, allowing Na⁺ to accumulate in axoplasm, K⁺ to leak out | | |
| Low external calcium concentration | Destabilizes membrane:<br><br>a. ionic permeability increased<br><br>b. increases change in Na⁺ permeability produced by depolarization | a. resting potential shifts in depolarized direction (partial depolarization)<br><br>b. threshold level shifts in hyperpolarized direction;<br><br>a. and b. may induce repetitive firing | Hyperexcitability, tetany |
| Local anesthetics (procaine) | Stabilizes membrane:<br><br>a. ionic permeability produced by depolarization<br><br>b. decreases change in Na⁺ permeability produced by depolarization | a. resting potential constant<br><br>b. threshold level shifts in depolarized direction until approaching impulse can no longer trigger action potential | Nerve block |

© CIBA

As described in Plate 4, the transmission of action potentials along nerve axons depends on two factors: the unequal distribution of sodium ions (Na⁺) and potassium ions (K⁺) across the resting axonal membrane, and the transient changes in membrane permeability to those ions during the action potential itself. The drugs listed in the left-hand column interfere with the action potential by interacting with either the metabolic machinery necessary to maintain the ionic distribution across the axonal membrane or the membrane components responsible for ionic permeability changes.

*Tetrodotoxin* and *saxitoxin* interact specifically with components of the axonal membrane that are responsible for the increase in Na⁺ permeability during the action potential. If these compounds are given in sufficient doses, the increase in Na⁺ permeability that normally occurs when the axon is depolarized is completely abolished. The axon is therefore unable to generate action potentials, and total nerve block occurs.

*Tetraethylammonium (TEA)* interacts specifically with components of the nerve membrane that are responsible for the increase in K⁺ permeability during the falling phase of the action potential. This permeability increase plays a role in the recovery (repolarization) of the axon at the end of the action potential. When this permeability increase is blocked by TEA, the depolarizing phase of the action potential is prolonged. In addition, partial depolarization of the axon occurs because TEA also decreases the resting K⁺ permeability. These changes do not result in nerve block, but they may decrease the number of action potentials the axon can transmit per second. The clinical effect of such a change is difficult to assess.

A number of different substances can alter the distribution of ions across the nerve membrane. *Metabolic inhibitors*, such as cyanide, or *cardiac glycosides*, such as ouabain, block the active transport mechanism (sodium ion pump), allowing Na⁺ to accumulate in the axoplasm and K⁺ to leak out. Direct administration of K⁺ will also decrease the ratio of internal:external concentration of K⁺. As illustrated in Plate 3, a decrease in this ratio will lead to a decrease in transmembrane

potential (depolarization). In turn, steady depolarization will activate the accommodation mechanisms that shut off Na⁺ permeability during the action potential. As accommodation builds up, the action potential size will decrease until nerve block occurs.

Lowering the *external calcium ion concentration* destabilizes the nerve membrane and causes two changes to occur. First, the ionic permeability of the membrane increases, leading to a decrease in transmembrane potential (depolarization). Secondly, the extent of the Na⁺ permeability increase caused by membrane depolarization rises, so that the threshold level for generating an action

potential becomes lower. If there is a decrease in calcium concentration, the resting membrane potential may sink to the depressed threshold level, causing repetitive firing and tetany.

*Local anesthetics*, such as procaine, act to stabilize the nerve membrane. No change in resting potential occurs, but the change in Na⁺ permeability caused by a given amount of applied transmembrane depolarization decreases. Thus, the threshold level is raised, and if this process proceeds far enough, an approaching action potential is no longer able to trigger an action potential in the next section of nerve and nerve block occurs. □

## Pharmacology of Neuromuscular Junction

| Drug | Effect on supply of acetylcholine in terminal | Effect on amount of acetylcholine released in terminal by action potential | Effect of amplitude on end plate potential | Effect of muscle response to application of acetylcholine | Direct effect on muscle membrane resting potential | Clinical effect |
|---|---|---|---|---|---|---|
| **Choline uptake inhibitors** <br><br> Hemicholinium <br> Triethylcholine | Decreased | Decreased (smaller) quanta | Decreased | — | — | Paresis |
| **Acetylcholine release blockers** <br><br> Botulinum toxin <br> Low Ca++ or high Mg++ concentration | — | Decreased (fewer quanta) | Decreased | — | — | Paralysis (low Ca++ concentration may also produce tetany by direct action on nerves) |
| **Acetylcholine (nicotinic) antagonists** <br><br> D-tubocurarine <br> Gallamine triethiodide <br> Dihydro-β-erythroidine | — | — | Decreased | Decreased | Depolarized (in high dosage) | Paralysis |
| **Cholinomimetics** <br><br> Nicotine <br> Carbamylcholine <br> Succinylcholine | — | — | Decreased (by desensitization) | Decreased (by desensitization) | Strongly depolarized | Paralysis |
| **Cholinesterase inhibitors** <br><br> Physostigmine <br> Neostigmine <br> Edrophonium | — | — | Increased; prolonged | Increased; prolonged | Depolarized slightly in high doses | Muscle power and duration of contraction increased |
| Organophosphorous compounds (nerve gases) | — | — | Increased; prolonged | Increased; prolonged | No change | Convulsions |

© CIBA

# Pharmacology of Neuromuscular Junction

Pharmacological agents can effect transmission at the neuromuscular junction (Plate 11) in three basic ways: (1) action on the motor nerve terminal to change the amount of acetylcholine released by the nerve impulse; (2) action on the muscle cell membrane to change its response to the acetylcholine released by the nerve terminal; and (3) action to block the degradation of acetylcholine by cholinesterases. Some drugs have only a single action, but many have more than one effect.

The major actions of five classes of drugs that effect neuromuscular transmission are shown. In the first class are *choline uptake inhibitors*, examples of which are hemicholinium and triethylcholine. These drugs retard the production of acetylcholine in the nerve terminal by blocking the uptake of the choline molecules that are required in its synthesis. Decreased acetylcholine synthesis results in a reduction of acetylcholine molecules in each synaptic vesicle. Thus, while each nerve impulse releases the same number of vesicles (quanta) as before, each quantum is smaller and the resulting depolarization of the muscle cell is correspondingly smaller. The net effect is a decrease in the number of muscle fibers activated per nerve impulse, and thus a decrease in the strength of muscle contraction (paresis).

In the second class of drugs are *acetylcholine release blockers*, which include botulinum toxin, and solutions containing a low concentration of calcium or a high concentration of magnesium. These agents act on the motor nerve terminal to block the process by which a nerve impulse liberates acetylcholine from synaptic vesicles into the synaptic cleft. The number of quanta released by each impulse may be decreased to the point at which the amount of acetylcholine liberated is insufficient to generate action potentials in any muscle fibers, which leads to complete paralysis.

The third class of drugs—*acetylcholine antagonists*—includes compounds such as D-tubocurarine and dihydro-β-erythroidine, which block the depolarizing action of acetylcholine on the muscle membrane. The drugs in this class are sometimes referred to as nicotinic antagonists, to differentiate them from drugs that block the action of acetylcholine at autonomic endings (nicotine mimics the action of acetylcholine at the neuromuscular junction but not at autonomic endings, see page 90). Acetylcholine antagonists are competitive inhibitors: they resemble acetylcholine and compete with it for receptor sites on the muscle membrane, thus preventing the acetylcholine from depolarizing the muscle cell. Most antagonists also have a weak depolarizing action on muscle cells, but their major effect is to block muscle activation by acetylcholine, thereby producing paralysis.

*Cholinomimetics* are drugs that mimic the action of acetylcholine. Nicotine, carbamylcholine and succinylcholine are among the cholinomimetic drugs that act at the neuromuscular junction. These drugs produce a strong, long-lasting depolarization of the muscle cells, and render these cells less sensitive to the action of the acetylcholine subsequently released by the nerve terminal (desensitization). Accommodation of the muscle cell membrane to the steady state of depolarization eventually blocks muscle action potentials completely, which leads to paralysis.

In the final class of drugs are *cholinesterase inhibitors*, which include physostigmine, edrophonium and organophosporous compounds. These drugs retard the enzymatic breakdown of acetylcholine by the cholinesterases. As a result, acetylcholine released by a nerve impulse acts for a longer time on the muscle membrane, and therefore produces a larger end plate potential. Many cholinesterase inhibitors resemble acetylcholine, and thus may themselves have a direct depolarizing action on muscle cells. □

# Selected References

## Section I

| | Plate Number |
|---|---|
| Brodie AG: *On growth pattern of human head, from third month to eighth year of life.* Am J Anat 1941, 68:209–262 | 4 |
| Ortiz MH, Brodie AG: *On growth of human head, from birth to third month of life.* Anat Rec 1949, 103:311–333 | 4 |
| Romanes GJ (ed): *Cunningham's Textbook of Anatomy,* ed 12. New York, Oxford University Press, 1981 | 1–18 |
| Scott JH: *Dento-Facial Development and Growth.* New York, Pergamon Press, 1967 | 4 |
| Williams PL, Warwick R: *Gray's Anatomy,* ed 36. Philadelphia, Lea & Febiger, 1980 | 1–18 |

## Section II

| | Plate Number |
|---|---|
| Brodal A: *Neurological Anatomy in Relation to Clinical Medicine,* ed 3. New York, Oxford University Press, 1981, pp 74–91, 185–213 | 17 |
| Carpenter MB: *Human Neuroanatomy,* ed 7. Baltimore, Williams & Wilkins, 1976, chap. 10 | 17 |
| Clark WEL: *Structure and connections of thalamus.* Brain 1932, 55:406–470 | 7 |
| Olszewski J: *Thalamus of the Macaca Mulatta.* Basel, S. Karger, 1952 | 7 |
| Walker AE: *Internal structure and afferent relations of the thalamus.* In Purpura DP, Yahr MD (eds): *The Thalamus.* New York, Columbia University Press, 1966, pp 1–12 | 7 |
| Williams PL, Warwick R: *Gray's Anatomy,* ed 36. Philadelphia, Lea & Febiger, 1980 | 1–6, 8–16 |

## Section III

| | Plate Number |
|---|---|
| Alfidi RJ, Haaga J, Weinstein M, et al: *Computed Tomography of the Human Body: Atlas of Normal Anatomy.* St. Louis, CV Mosby, 1977 | 17–18 |
| Djindjian R, et al: *Angiography of the Spinal Cord,* Kricheff, II (trans). Baltimore, University Park Press, 1970 | 19–20 |
| Doppman JL, DiChiro G, Ommaya A: *Selective Arteriography of the Spinal Cord.* St. Louis, Warren Green, 1969 | 19–20 |
| Fields WS: *Aortocranial occlusive vascular disease (Stroke).* Clin Symp 1974, 26(4):3–31 | 2–3 |
| Gordon R, Herman GT, Johnson SA: *Image reconstruction from projections.* Sci Am 1975, 223:56–57 | 17–18 |
| Goss CM (ed): *Gray's Anatomy of the Human Body,* ed 27. Philadephia, Lea & Febiger, 1959 | 1–7, 11–15, 21 |
| Greitz T, Sjogren SE: *The posterior inferior cerebellar artery.* Acta Radiol [Diagn] (Stockh) 1963, 1:284–297 | 10 |
| Hinck VC, Judkins MP, Paxton HD: *Simplified selective femorocerebral angiography.* Radiology 1967, 89:1048–1052 | 8–9 |
| Huang YP, Wolf BS: *The veins of the posterior fossa—superior or galenic draining group.* AJR 1965, 95:808–821 | 16 |

## Section III (continued)

| | Plate Number |
|---|---|
| Huang YP, Wolf BS: *Veins of the posterior fossa.* In Newton TH, Potts DG (eds): *Radiology of the Skull and Brain, II: Angiography,* book 3. St. Louis, CV Mosby, 1974, pp 2155–2219 | 16 |
| Huang YP, Wolf BS, Antin SP, et al: *The veins of the posterior fossa—anterior or petrosal draining group.* AJR 1968, 104:35–56 | 16 |
| Huang YP, Wolf BS, Okudera T: *Angiographic anatomy of the inferior vermian vein of the cerebellum.* Acta Radiol [Diagn] (Stockh) 1969, 9:327–344 | 16 |
| Mani RL, Newton TH, Glickman MG: *The superior cerebellar artery: an anatomic-roentgenographic correlation.* Radiology 1967, 91:1102–1108 | 10 |
| McCullough EC, Baker HL Jr, Houser. OW, et al: *An evaluation of the quantitative and radiation features of a scanning x-ray transverse axial tomograph: the EMI Scanner.* Radiology 1974, 111:709–715 | 17–18 |
| Naidich TP, Kricheff II, George AE, et al: *The normal anterior inferior cerebellar artery.* Radiology 1976, 119(2):355–373 | 10 |
| New PFJ, Scott WR: *Computed Tomography of the Brain and Orbit.* Baltimore, Williams & Wilkins, 1975 | 17–18 |
| Newton TH, Potts DG (eds): *Radiology of the Skull and Brain, II: Angiography,* book 1. St. Louis, CV Mosby, 1974, pp 893–1048 | 8–10 |
| Newton TH, Potts DG (eds): *Radiology of the Skull and Brain, II: Angiography,* book 2. St. Louis, CV Mosby, 1974, pp 1145–1850 | 1–7 |
| Newton TH, Potts DG (eds): *Radiology of the Skull and Brain, II: Angiography,* book 3. St. Louis, CV Mosby, 1974, pp 1851–2256 | 1–7, 11, 13 |
| Paff GH: *Anatomy of the Head and Neck.* Philadelphia, WB Saunders, 1973 | 12, 14–15 |
| Stephens RB, Stilwell DL: *Arteries and Veins of the Human Brain.* Springfield IL, Charles C Thomas, 1969 | 4–6, 12, 14–16 |
| Taveras J, Wood EH: *Diagnostic Neuroradiology, II,* ed 2. Baltimore, Williams & Wilkins, 1976 | 8–10, 14–15 |
| Turnbull IM: *Blood supply of the spinal cord.* In Vinken PJ, Bruyn GW (eds): *Handbook of Clinical Neurology, XII.* Amsterdam, North-Holland, 1972, pp 478–491 | 19–21 |
| Wallace S, Goldberg HI, Leeds NE, et al: *The cavernous branches of the internal carotid artery.* AJR 1967, 101:34–36 | 2–3, 7 |
| Wiener H: *Findings in CT.* New York, Pfizer, 1979 | 17–18 |

## Section IV

| | Plate Number |
|---|---|
| Ábráham A: *Microscopic Innervation of the Heart & Blood Vessels in Vertebrates Including Man.* New York, Pergamon Press, 1969 | 10 |
| Amassian VE: *Cortical representation of visceral afferents.* J Neurophysiol 1951, 14:433–444 | 1–2 |
| Amassian VE: *Fiber groups and spinal path-* | |

## Section IV (continued)

| | Plate Number |
|---|---|
| *ways of cortically represented visceral afferents.* J Neurophysiol 1951, 14:445–460 | 1–2 |
| Arnulf G: *La résection du plexus préaortique dans l'angine de poitrine.* J Chir (Paris) 1950, 66:97–107 | 9 |
| Auerbach L: *Fernere vorlaufige Mittheilung über den Nervenapparat des Darmes.* Virchows Arch (Pathol Anat) 1864, 30:457–460 | 14 |
| Beck LR, Boots LR: *The comparative anatomy, histology and morphology of the mammalian oviduct.* In Johnson AD, Foley CW (eds): *The Oviduct and Its Function.* New York, Academic Press, 1974 | 20–21 |
| Bernard C: *Influence du grand sympathique sur la sensibilitée et sur la calorification.* CR Soc Biol (Paris) 1851, 3:163–164 | 1–2 |
| Bernard C: *De l'influence de deux ordres des nerfs qui déterminent les variations de couleur du sang veineux dans les organes glandulaires.* CR Acad Sci (Paris) 1858, 47:245–253 | 1–2 |
| Botár J: *The Autonomic Nervous System.* Budapest, Hungarian Acad of Sciences, 1966 | 10 |
| Bourne GH (ed): *The Structure and Function of Nervous Tissue, I–VI.* New York, Academic Press, 1968–1972 | 3–4 |
| Brown-Séquard CE: *Experimental Researches Applied to Physiology and Pathology.* New York, H Baillière, 1853 | 1–2 |
| Budge J, Waller AV: *Action de la partie cervicale du nerf grand sympathique et d'une portion de la moelle épinière sur la dilatation de la pupille.* CR Acad [D] Sci (Paris) 1851, 33:370–374 | 1–2 |
| Bülbring E, et al (eds): *Smooth Muscle.* London, Edward Arnold, 1970 | 4 |
| Coupland RE: *The Natural History of the Chromaffin Cell.* London, Longmans, 1965 | 16 |
| Curtis AH, Anson BJ, Ashley FL, et al: *Anatomy of pelvic autonomic nerves in relation to gynecology.* Surg Gynecol Obstet 1942, 75:743–750 | 20–21 |
| Dale H: *Nomenclature of fibres in the autonomic system and their effects.* J Physiol (proc) 1933, 80:10–11 | 4 |
| Dale H: *Natural chemical stimulators (Sharpey Schafer memorial lecture).* Edinb Med J 1938, 45:461–480 | 4 |
| Davis L, Hart JT, Crain RC: *Pathway for visceral afferent impulses within spinal cord; experimental dilatation of biliary ducts.* Surg Gynecol Obstet 1929, 48:647–651 | 1–2 |
| Davis L, Pollock LJ, Stone TT: *Visceral pain.* Surg Gynecol Obstet 1932, 55:418–427 | 9 |
| Dixon JS, Gosling JA: *The fine structure of pacemaker cells in the pig renal calices.* Anat Rec 1973, 175:139–153 | 18–19 |
| Dogiel AS: *Die Nervenendigungen in den Nebennieren der Säugethiere.* Arch Anat Physiol Leipzig 1894, 90–104 | 16 |
| Downman CBB: *Cerebral destination of splanchnic afferent impulses.* J Physiol (Lond) 1951, 113:434–441 | 1–2 |
| Elliott TR: *The action of adrenalin.* J Physiol (Lond) 1905, 32:401–467 | 4 |
| Gaskell WH: *On the structure, distribution and function of the nerves which innervate visceral* | |

## Section IV (continued)

| | Plate Number |
|---|---|
| *and vascular systems.* J Physiol (Lond) 1886, 7:1–80 | 1–2 |
| GOSLING JA, DIXON JS: *Catecholamine-containing nerves in the submucosa of the ureter.* Experientia 1971, 27:1065–1066 | 18–19 |
| GOSLING JA, DIXON JS: *Structural evidence in support of an urinary tract pacemaker.* Br J Urol 1972, 44:550–560 | 18–19 |
| GRIGOR'EVA TA: *The Innervation of Blood Vessels.* New York, Pergamon Press, 1962 | 10 |
| HANTZ E: *Contribution à l'étude anatomique et expérimentale du plexus préaortique pour le traitement de l'angine de poitrine.* Lyon, L Pidancet, 1951 | 9 |
| HODSON N: *Nerves of the testis, epididymis and scrotum.* In JOHNSON AD, GOMES WR, VANDEMARK NL (eds): *Testis, I.* New York, Academic Press, 1970, pp 47–99 | 20–21 |
| HOLLINSHEAD WH: *Innervation of adrenal glands.* J Comp Neurol 1936, 64:449–467 | 16 |
| HOVELACQUE A: *Anatomie des Nerfs Craniens et Rachidiens et du Système Grand Sympathique Chez l'Homme.* Paris, Gaston Doin, 1927 | 18–19 |
| IRWIN DA: *Anatomy of Auerbach's plexus.* Am J Anat 1931, 49:141–166 | 14 |
| JACKSON JH: *On the anatomical and physiological localization of movements in the brain.* In TAYLOR J (ed): *Selected Writings of J. Hughlings Jackson, I.* London, Hodder and Stoughton, 1931–1932, pp 37–76 | 1–2 |
| KISS T: *Experimentell-morphologische Analyse der Nebenniereninnervation.* Acta Anat 1951, 13:81–89 | 16 |
| KUNTZ A: *The Autonomic Nervous System, ed 4.* Philadelphia, Lea & Febiger, 1953 | 14 |
| KURÉ K, WADA Y, OKINAKA S: *Spinal parasympathetic; nerve-supply of suprarenal gland.* Q J Exp Physiol 1931, 21:227–241 | 16 |
| LANGLEY JN: *The Autonomic Nervous System.* Cambridge, MA, Heffer and Sons, 1921 | 1–2 |
| LAUX G, DELMAS A, GUERRIER Y: *Innervation de la veine cave inférieure.* Quoted by Lazorthes G: *Le Système Neurovasculaire.* Paris, Masson, 1949 | 11 |
| LEVER JD: *Nerve fibres in adrenal cortex of rat.* Nature 1953, 171:882–883 | 16 |
| LOEWI O: *Über humerale Übertragbarkeit der Herznervenwirkung.* Pflugers Arch 1921, 189:239–242 | 4 |
| McCREA ED: *Abdominal distribution of vagus.* J Anat 1924, 59:18–40 | 12 |
| MEISSNER G: *Ueber die Nerven der Darmwand.* Z Rat Med 1857, 364–366 | 14 |
| MITCHELL GAG: *Innervation of distal colon.* Edinb Med J 1935, 42:11–20 | 13 |
| MITCHELL GAG: *Innervation of kidney, ureter, testicle and epididymis.* J Anat 1935, 70:10–32 | 20–21 |
| MITCHELL GAG: *Innervation of ovary, uterine tube, testis and epididymis.* J Anat 1938, 72:508–517 | 11, 20–21 |
| MITCHELL GAG: *Macroscopic study of nerve supply of stomach.* J Anat 1940, 75:50–63 | 12, 15 |
| MITCHELL GAG: *Nerve supply of kidneys.* Acta Anat 1950, 10:1–37 | 18–19 |
| MITCHELL GAG: *Intrinsic renal nerves.* Acta Anat 1951, 13:1–15 | 18–19 |
| MITCHELL GAG: *Anatomy of the Autonomic Nervous System.* Edinburgh, E & S Livingstone, 1953 | 1–21 |
| MITCHELL GAG: *Cardiovascular Innervation.* Edinburgh, E & S Livingstone, 1955 | 10 |

## Section IV (continued)

| | Plate Number |
|---|---|
| MITCHELL GAG, BROWN R, COOKSON FB: *Ventricular nerve cells in mammals.* Nature 1953, 172:812 | 9 |
| MOSELEY RL: *Preganglionic connections of intramural ganglia of urinary bladder.* Proc Soc Exp Biol Med 1936, 34:728–730 | 18–19 |
| OWMAN C, ROSENBREN E, SJÖBERG NO: *Adrenergic innervation of the human female reproductive organs: a histochemical and chemical investigation.* Obstet Gynecol 1967, 30:763–773 | 20–21 |
| PICK J: *The Autonomic Nervous System.* Philadelphia, JB Lippincott, 1970 | 1–21 |
| POPPER H, SCHAFFNER F: *Liver, Structure and Function.* New York, McGraw-Hill, 1965 | 15 |
| ROOT WS: *The urinary bladder.* In: *Macleod's Physiology in Modern Medicine.* London, H. Kimpton, 1941, pp 1127–1131 | 18–19 |
| SCHMITT FO (ed): *Neurosciences: First and Second Study Programs.* New York, Rockefeller University Press, 1967–1971 | 4 |
| SCHMITT FO (ed): *Neurosciences: Third Study Program.* Cambridge, MA, MIT Press, 1974 | 4 |
| SKAARING P, BIERRING F: *On the intrinsic innervation of normal rat liver. Histochemical and scanning electron microscopical studies.* Cell Tissue Res 1976, 171(2):141–155 | 15 |
| SUTHERLAND SD: *An evaluation of cholinesterase techniques in the study of the intrinsic innervation of the liver.* J Anat 1964, 98:321–326 | 15 |
| SUTHERLAND SD: *The intrinsic innervation of the liver.* Rev Int Hepat 1965, 15:569–578 | 15 |
| SUTHERLAND SD: *The intrinsic innervation of the gall bladder in Macaca rhesus and Cavia porcellus.* J Anat 1966, 100:261–268 | 15 |
| SWINYARD CA: *Innervation of suprarenal glands.* Anat Rec 1937, 68:417–429 | 16, 20–21 |
| TELFORD ED, STOPFORD JSB: *Autonomic nerve supply of distal colon.* Br Med J 1934, Part 1:572–574 | 13 |
| WHITE JC, GARREY WE, ATKINS JA: *Cardiac innervation: experimental and clinical studies.* Arch Surg 1933, 26:765–786 | 9 |
| WHITE JC, SMITHWICK RH, SIMEONE FA: *Autonomic Nervous System, ed 3.* London, H. Kimpton, 1952 | 1–21 |
| WHITE JC, SWEET WH: *Pain: Its Mechanisms and Neurosurgical Control.* Springfield, IL, Charles C. Thomas, 1955 | 9 |
| WILDE FR: *Perivascular neural pattern of femoral region.* Br J Surg 1951, 39:97–105 | 11 |
| YAMADA E: *Some observations on the nerve terminal on the liver parenchymal cell of the mouse as revealed by electron microscopy.* Okajimas Folia Anat Jpn 1965, 40:663–677 | 15 |

## Section V

| | Plate Number |
|---|---|
| BARNARD JW: *Hypoglossal complex of vertebrates.* J Comp Neurol 1940, 72:489–524 | 13 |
| BROUWER B: *Klinisch-anatomische Untersuchung über den Oculomotoriuskern.* Zentralbl Ges Neurol Psychiat 1918, 40:152–189 | 5–6 |
| CARTER RB, KEEN EN: *The intramandibular course of the inferior alveolar nerve.* J Anat 1971, 108:433–440 | 7 |
| CHOROBSKI J, PENFIELD W: *Cerebral vasodilator nerves and their pathway from medulla oblongata.* Arch Neurol 1932, 28:1257–1289 | 8 |

## Section V (continued)

| | Plate Number |
|---|---|
| CORBIN KB, HARRISON F: *Function of mesencephalic root of fifth cranial nerve.* J Neurophysiol 1940, 3:423–435 | 7 |
| CROSBY EC, DeJONGE BR: *Experimental and clinical studies of the central connections and central relations of the facial nerve.* Ann Otol Rhinol Laryngol 1963, 72:735–755 | 8 |
| EVANS DHL, MURRAY JG: *Histological and functional studies on fibre composition of vagus nerve of rabbit.* J Anat 1954, 88:320–337 | 11 |
| FRITSCH G: *Untersuchungen über den feinern Bau des Fischgehirns mit besonderer Berücksichtigung der Homologien bei anderen Wirbelthierklassen.* Berlin, Gutmann, 1878 | 4 |
| MARTIN H: *Surgical removal of parotid tumors.* Clin Symp 1961, 13(4):121–131 | 8 |
| McKENZIE J: *Morphology of sternomastoid and trapezius muscles.* J Anat 1955, 89:526–531 | 12 |
| MITCHELL GAG: *Autonomic nerve supply of throat, nose and ear.* J Laryngol Otol 1954, 68(8):495–516 | 8 |
| MITCHELL GAG, WARWICK R: *Dorsal vagal nucleus.* Acta Anat 1955, 25:371–395 | 11 |
| PEARSON AA: *Development and connections of mesencephalic root of trigeminal nerve in man.* J Comp Neurol 1949, 90:1–46 | 7 |
| RAMSAY-HUNT J: *The sensory system of the facial nerve and its symptomatology.* J Ophth Otolaryngol 1910, 4:89–93 | 8 |
| RAMSAY-HUNT J: *Symptomatologie sensitive et syndromes du nerf facial.* Arch Int Laryng 1910, 29:134–139 | 8 |
| RASMUSSEN GL: *Efferent fibers of the cochlear nerve and cochlear nucleus.* In RASMUSSEN GL, WINDLE WF (eds): *Neural Mechanisms of the Auditory and Vestibular Systems.* Springfield IL, Charles C Thomas, 1960 | 9 |
| RICHARDSON AP, HINSEY JC: *Functional study of nodose ganglion of vagus with degeneration methods.* Proc Soc Exp Biol Med 1933, 30:1141–1143 | 11 |
| ROSS MD: *The general visceral efferent component of the eighth cranial nerve.* J Comp Neurol 1969, 135:453–478 | 9 |
| RUSKELL GL: *The distribution of autonomic postganglionic nerve fibres to the lacrimal gland in the rat.* J Anat 1971, 109:229–242 | 5–6 |
| SPRAGUE JM: *Innervation of pharynx in rhesus monkey, and formation of pharyngeal plexus in primates.* Anat Rec 1944, 90:197–208 | 10 |
| STEWART D, WILSON SL: *Regional anaesthesia and innervation of teeth.* Lancet 1928, 2:809–811 | 7 |
| STRAUS WL JR, HOWELL AB: *Spinal accessory nerve and its musculature.* Q Rev Biol 1936, 11:387–405 | 12 |
| SZENTÁGOTHAI J: *Die innere Gliederung des Oculomotoriuskernes.* Arch Psychiatr Nervenkr 1942, 115:127–135 | 5–6 |
| SZENTÁGOTHAI J: *Functional representation in motor trigeminal nucleus.* J Comp Neurol 1949, 90:111–120 | 7 |
| TARKHAN AA, EL-MALEK SA: *On presence of sensory nerve cells on hypoglossal nerve.* J Comp Neurol 1950, 93:219–228 | 13 |
| TRUEX RC, CARPENTER MB: *Human Neuroanatomy, ed 6.* Baltimore, Williams & Wilkins, 1969 | 1–13 |
| WARWICK R: *Study of retrograde degeneration in oculomotor nucleus of rhesus monkey.* Brain 1950, 73:532–543 | 5–6 |
| WARWICK R: *Representation of extra-ocular muscles in oculomotor nuclei of monkey.* J Comp | |

## Section V (continued)

| | Plate Number |
|---|---|
| Neurol 1953, 98:449–503 | 5–6 |
| WARWICK R: *Ocular parasympathetic nerve supply and its mesencephalic sources.* J Anat 1954, 88:71–93 | 5–6 |
| WARWICK R: *So-called nucleus of convergence.* Brain 1955, 78:92–114 | 5–6 |
| WILLIAMS PL, WARWICK R: *Gray's Anatomy,* ed 36. Philadelphia, Lea & Febiger, 1980 | 1–13 |

## Section VI

| | Plate Number |
|---|---|
| CLIFFTON EE: *Unusual innervation of intrinsic muscles of the hand by median and ulnar nerve.* Surgery 1948, 23:12–31 | 5–9 |
| DAVIES F: *Note on first lumbar nerve (anterior ramus).* J Anat 1935, 70:177–178 | 10 |
| DAVIES F, LAIRD M: *Supinator muscle and deep radial (posterior interosseous) nerve.* Anat Rec 1948, 101:243–250 | 5–9 |
| EISLER P: *Der plexus lumbosacralis des Menschen.* Anat Anz 1891, 6:274 | 12 |
| HARRIS W: *The Morphology of the Brachial Plexus.* New York, Oxford University Press, 1939 | 4 |
| HOVELACQUE A: *Anatomie des Nerfs Craniens et Rachidiens et du Système Grand Sympathique.* Paris, Gaston Doin, 1927 | 5–9 |
| KEIM HA: *Low back pain.* Clin Symp 1980, 32(6):2–35 | 16 |
| KELLGREN JH, SAMUEL EP: *Sensitivity and innervation of articular capsule.* J Bone Joint Surg [Br] 1950, 32:84–92 | 12 |
| KIMMEL DL: *Innervation of spinal dura mater and dura mater of the posterior cranial fossa.* Neurology 1961, 11:800–809 | 1 |
| LAUX G, DELMAS A, GUERRIER Y: *Innervation de la veine cave inférieure.* Quoted by LAZORTHES G: *Le Système Neurovasculaire,* Paris, Masson, 1949 | 2 |
| MARINACCI AA: *The problem of unusual anomalous innervation of hand muscles.* Bull Los Angeles Neurol Soc 1964, 29:133–142 | 5–9 |
| MITCHELL GAG: *Anatomy of the Autonomic Nervous System.* Edinburgh, E & S Livingstone, 1953 | 2 |
| PAPATHANASSIOU BT: *A variant of the motor branch of the median nerve in the hand.* J Bone Joint Surg [Br] 1968, 50:156–157 | 5–9 |
| PEDERSEN HE, BLUNCK CFJ, GARDNER E: *Anatomy of lumbosacral posterior rami and meningeal branches of spinal nerves (sinuvertebral nerves), with experimental study of their functions.* J Bone Joint Surg [Am] 1956, 38:377–391 | 3 |
| PETIT-DUTAILLIS D, FLANDRIN P: *Anatomie chirurgicale des nerfs du rein.* Bull Assoc Anat (Nancy) 1923, 93(8–9):635–647 | 2 |
| ROWNTREE T: *Anomalous innervation of hand muscles.* J Bone Joint Surg [Br] 1949, 31:505–510 | 5–9 |
| SAMUEL EP: *Autonomic and somatic innervation of the articular capsule.* Anat Rec 1952, 113:53–70 | 12 |
| STOPFORD JSB: *Variation in distribution of cutaneous nerves of hand and digits.* J Anat 1918, 53:14 | 5–9 |
| SUNDERLAND S: *Nerves and Nerve Injuries.* Edinburgh, E & S Livingstone, 1968 | 4–9, 11 |
| WOODBURNE RT: *The accessory obturator nerve and the innervation of the pectineus muscle.* Anat Rec 1960, 136:367–369 | 12 |

## Section VII

| | Plate Number |
|---|---|
| AREY LB: *Developmental Anatomy,* ed 7. Philadelphia, WB Saunders, 1965 | 1–15 |
| BUNGE MB, BUNGE RP, RIS H: *Ultrastructural study of remyelination in an experimental lesion in adult cat spinal cord.* J Biophys Biochem Cytol 1961, 10:67–94 | 1–15 |
| CRELIN ES: *Anatomy of the Newborn: an Atlas.* Philadelphia, Lea & Febiger, 1969 | 1–15 |
| HAMILTON WJ, BOYD JD, MOSSMAN HW: *Human Embryology,* ed 3. Baltimore, Williams & Wilkins, 1964 | 1–15 |
| PATTEN BM: *Human Embryology,* ed 3. New York, McGraw-Hill, 1968 | 1–15 |
| WEISS L, GREEP RO: *Histology,* ed 4. New York, McGraw-Hill, 1977 | 1–15 |

## Section VIII

| | Plate Number |
|---|---|
| ANGEVINE JB JR, COTMAN CW: *Principles of Neuroanatomy.* New York, Oxford University Press, 1982 | 51–64 |
| ASANUMA H: *Recent developments in the study of the columnar arrangement of neurons within the motor cortex.* Physiol Rev 1975, 55(2):143–156 | 45 |
| BAKER R, BERTHOZ A: *Control of gaze by brain stem neurons.* In BAKER R, BERTHOZ A (eds): *Developments in Neuroscience, I.* New York, Elsevier/North-Holland, 1978 | 30 |
| BASBAUM AF, FIELDS HL: *Pain control: A new role for the medullary reticular formation.* In HOBSON JA, BRAZIER MAB (eds): *The Reticular Formation Revisited.* New York, Raven Press, 1980, pp 329–348 | 17 |
| BEIDLER LM: *The chemical senses: gustation and olfaction.* In MOUNTCASTLE VB (ed): *Medical Physiology, I,* ed 14. St. Louis, CV Mosby, 1980, pp 586–594 | 23–24 |
| BEIDLER LM: *The chemical senses: gustation and olfaction.* In MOUNTCASTLE VB (ed): *Medical Physiology, I,* ed 14. St. Louis, CV Mosby, 1980, pp 594–600 | 18 |
| BERTRAM EG, MOORE KL: *Concise Atlas of the Human Brain and Spinal Cord.* Baltimore, Williams & Wilkins, 1982 | 51–64 |
| BLOOM W, FAWCETT DW: *A Textbook of Histology,* ed 10. Philadelphia, WB Saunders, 1975 | 51–64 |
| BODIAN D: *Cytological aspects of neurosecretion in the opossom neurohypophysis.* Johns Hopkins Med J 1963, 113:57–93 | 12 |
| BRODAL A: *Neurological Anatomy, in Relation to Clinical Medicine,* ed 3. New York, Oxford University Press, 1981 | 51–64 |
| BRODAL A: *Neurological Anatomy, in Relation to Clinical Medicine,* ed 3. New York, Oxford University Press, 1981, pp 60–94, 122–141 | 15 |
| BRODAL A: *Neurological Anatomy, in Relation to Clinical Medicine,* ed 3. New York, Oxford University Press, 1981, pp 62–69 | 49 |
| BRODAL A: *Neurological Anatomy, in Relation to Clinical Medicine,* ed 3. New York, Oxford University Press, 1981, pp 84–94, 180–208 | 48 |
| BRODAL A: *Neurological Anatomy, in Relation to Clinical Medicine,* ed 3. New York, Oxford University Press, 1981, pp 94–99 | 41 |
| BRODAL A: *Neurological Anatomy, in Relation to Clinical Medicine,* ed 3. New York, Oxford University Press, 1981, pp 148–175 | 32 |

## Section VIII (continued)

| | Plate Number |
|---|---|
| BRODAL A: *Neurological Anatomy, in Relation to Clinical Medicine,* ed 3. New York, Oxford University Press, 1981, pp 180–188, 252–270 | 44 |
| BRODAL A: *Neurological Anatomy, in Relation to Clinical Medicine,* ed 3. New York, Oxford University Press, 1981, pp 194–205 | 46 |
| BRODAL A: *Neurological Anatomy, in Relation to Clinical Medicine,* ed 3. New York, Oxford University Press, 1981, pp 201–205, 470–488 | 29 |
| BRODAL A: *Neurological Anatomy, in Relation to Clinical Medicine,* ed 3. New York, Oxford University Press, 1981, pp 205–208, 394–427 | 47 |
| BRODAL A: *Neurological Anatomy, in Relation to Clinical Medicine,* ed 3. New York, Oxford University Press, 1981, pp 211–226, 260–264 | 40 |
| BRODAL A: *Neurological Anatomy, in Relation to Clinical Medicine,* ed 3. New York, Oxford University Press, 1981, pp 242–260, 273–278 | 45 |
| BRODAL A: *Neurological Anatomy, in Relation to Clinical Medicine,* ed 3. New York, Oxford University Press, 1981, pp 294–301, 308–359 | 37 |
| BRODAL A: *Neurological Anatomy, in Relation to Clinical Medicine,* ed 3. New York, Oxford University Press, 1981, pp 306–376 | 38 |
| BRODAL A: *Neurological Anatomy, in Relation to Clinical Medicine,* ed 3. New York, Oxford University Press, 1981, pp 466, 503–508 | 24 |
| BRODAL A: *Neurological Anatomy, in Relation to Clinical Medicine,* ed 3. New York, Oxford University Press, 1981, pp 470–495, 532–576 | 30 |
| BRODAL A: *Neurological Anatomy, in Relation to Clinical Medicine,* ed 3. New York, Oxford University Press, 1981, pp 488–495 | 31 |
| BRODAL A: *Neurological Anatomy, in Relation to Clinical Medicine,* ed 3. New York, Oxford University Press, 1981, pp 492–495 | 28 |
| BRODAL A: *Neurological Anatomy, in Relation to Clinical Medicine,* ed 3. New York, Oxford University Press, 1981, pp 508–532 | 16 |
| BRODAL A: *Neurological Anatomy, in Relation to Clinical Medicine,* ed 3. New York, Oxford University Press, 1981, pp 560–577 | 22 |
| BRODAL A: *Neurological Anatomy, in Relation to Clinical Medicine,* ed 3. New York, Oxford University Press, 1981, pp 578–601 | 21 |
| BRODAL A: *Neurological Anatomy, in Relation to Clinical Medicine,* ed 3. New York, Oxford University Press, 1981, pp 602–606, 636–639 | 25 |
| BRODAL A: *Neurological Anatomy, in Relation to Clinical Medicine,* ed 3. New York, Oxford University Press, 1981, pp 630–631 | 27 |
| BRODAL A: *Neurological Anatomy, in Relation to Clinical Medicine,* ed 3. New York, Oxford University Press, 1981, pp 636–639 | 26 |
| BRODAL A: *Neurological Anatomy, in Relation to Clinical Medicine,* ed 3. New York, Oxford University Press, 1981, pp 640–646 | 18 |
| BRODAL A: *Neurological Anatomy, in Relation to Clinical Medicine,* ed 3. New York, Oxford University Press, 1981, pp 640–654, 691–694 | 19 |
| BRODAL A: *Neurological Anatomy, in Relation to Clinical Medicine,* ed 3. New York, Oxford University Press, 1981, pp 797–805, 817–848 | 43 |

## Section VIII (continued)

| | Plate Number |
|---|---|
| Brodal A: *Neurological Anatomy, in Relation to Clinical Medicine,* ed 3. New York, Oxford University Press, 1981, pp 805–816 | 42 |
| Bullock TH, Orkand R, Grinnell A: *Introduction to Nervous Systems.* San Francisco, WH Freeman, 1977 | 51–64 |
| Burton H, Benjamin RM: *Central projections of the gustatory system.* In Autrum H, et al (eds): *Handbook of Sensory Physiology, IV: Chemical Sense,* part 2, *Taste;* Beidler LM (section ed). New York, Springer-Verlag, 1971 | 24 |
| Caldwell PC: *Factors governing movement and distribution of inorganic ions in nerve and muscle.* Physiol Rev 1968, 48:1–64 | 3 |
| Carpenter MB: *Human Neuroanatomy,* ed 7. Baltimore, Williams & Wilkins, 1976, pp 82–91, 551–599 | 1 |
| Carpenter MB: *Human Neuroanatomy,* ed 7. Baltimore, Williams & Wilkins, 1976, pp 115–136, 137–158, 213–237 | 2 |
| Carpenter MB: *Human Neuroanatomy,* ed 7. Baltimore, Williams & Wilkins, 1976, pp 551–599 | 43 |
| Carpenter MB, Sutin J: *Human Neuroanatomy,* ed 8. Baltimore, Williams & Wilkins, 1983 | 51–64 |
| Cooper JR, Bloom FE, Roth RH: *The Biochemical Basis of Neuropharmacology,* ed 3. New York, Oxford University Press, 1978 | 51–64 |
| Creed RS, Denny-Brown D, Eccles JC, et al: *Reflex Activity of the Spinal Cord.* New York, Oxford University Press, 1972, pp 31–38, 89 | 10 |
| Davies PW: *The action potential.* In Mountcastle VB (ed): *Medical Physiology, II,* ed 12. St. Louis, CV Mosby, 1968, p 1117 | 6 |
| Davis H: *A model for transducer action in the cochlea.* Cold Spring Harbor Symp Quant Biol 1965, 30:181–190 | 25 |
| Eccles JC: *Functional meaning of the patterns of synaptic connections in the cerebellum.* Perspect Biol Med 1965, 8:289–310 | 36 |
| Eccles JC: *The ionic mechanisms of excitatory and inhibitory synaptic action.* Ann NY Acad Sci 1966, 137:473–494 | 3, 8, 9 |
| Eccles JC: *The Physiology of Synapses.* New York, Springer-Verlag, 1973 | 7–9 |
| Eccles JC, Ito M, Szentágothai J: *The Cerebellum as a Neuronal Machine.* New York, Springer-Verlag, 1967 | 36, 38 |
| Erlanger J, Gasser HS: *The action potential in fibers of slow conduction in spinal roots and somatic nerves.* Am J Physiol 1930, 92:43–82 | 6 |
| Flock Å: *Sensory transduction in hair cells.* In Autrum H, et al (eds): *Handbook of Sensory Physiology, I: Principles of Receptor Physiology;* Loewenstein WR (section ed). New York, Springer-Verlag, 1971 pp 396–441 | 25, 28 |
| Gesteland RC: *Neural coding in olfactory receptor cells.* In Autrum H, et al (eds): *Handbook of Sensory Physiology, IV: Chemical Sense,* part 1, *Olfaction;* Beidler LM (section ed). New York, Springer-Verlag, 1971 | 18 |
| Goldstein MH Jr: *The auditory periphery.* In Mountcastle VB (ed): *Medical Physiology, I,* ed 14. St. Louis, CV Mosby, 1980, pp 428–443 | 25 |
| Granit R: *The Basis of Motor Control.* New York, Academic Press, 1970, pp 100–121 | 34–35 |

## Section VIII (continued)

| | Plate Number |
|---|---|
| Graybiel AM: *Visuo-cerebellar and cerebello-visual connections involving the ventral lateral geniculate nucleus.* Exp Brain Res 1974, 20:303–306 | 22 |
| Graziadei PPC: *The olfactory mucosa of vertebrates.* In Autrum H, et al (eds): *Handbook of Sensory Physiology, IV: Chemical Sense,* part 1, *Olfaction;* Beidler LM (section ed). New York, Springer-Verlag, 1971 | 18 |
| Grillo MA: *Electron microscopy of sympathetic tissues.* Pharmacol Rev 1966, 18:387–399 | 12 |
| Henneman E: *Organization of the motor systems —a preview.* In Mountcastle VB (ed): *Medical Physiology, II,* ed 12. St. Louis, CV Mosby, 1968, pp 1675–1680 | 2 |
| Henneman E: *Cerebellum.* In Mountcastle VB (ed): *Medical Physiology, II,* ed 12. St. Louis, CV Mosby, 1968, pp 1771–1789 | 2 |
| Henneman E: *Organization of the spinal cord.* In Mountcastle VB (ed): *Medical Physiology, II,* ed 12. St. Louis, CV Mosby, 1968, p 1720 | 6 |
| Henneman E: *Organization of the motor neuron pool: the size principle.* In Mountcastle VB (ed): *Medical Physiology, I,* ed 14. St. Louis, CV Mosby, 1980, pp 718–720 | 32 |
| Henneman E: *Organization of the spinal cord and its reflexes.* In Mountcastle VB (ed): *Medical Physiology, I,* ed 14. St. Louis, CV Mosby, 1980, pp 762–786 | 33 |
| Henneman E: *Motor functions of the cerebral cortex.* In Mountcastle VB (ed): *Medical Physiology, I,* ed 14. St. Louis, CV Mosby, 1980, pp 859–889 | 45 |
| Hille B: *Ionic channels in nerve membrane.* Prog Biophys Mol Biol 1970, 21:1–32 | 3–4 |
| Hillman DE, Lewis ER: *Morphological basis for a mechanical linkage in otolithic receptor transduction in the frog.* Science 1971, 174:416–419 | 28 |
| Hodgkin AL: *The Conduction of the Nervous Impulse.* Springfield IL, Charles C Thomas, 1964 | 4–6 |
| Hodgkin AL, Huxley AF: *Movement of sodium and potassium ions during nervous activity.* Cold Spring Harbor Symp Quant Biol 1952, 17:43–52 | 4 |
| Hogan MJ, Alvarado JA, Weddell, JE: *Histology of the Human Eye.* Philadelphia, WB Saunders, 1971, pp 393–519 | 20 |
| Hongo T, Jankowska E, Lundberg A: *The rubrospinal tract. I: Effects on alpha-motoneurones innervating hindlimb muscles in cats.* Exp Brain Res 1969, 7:344–364 | 46 |
| Houk JC: *Regulation of stiffness by skeletomotor reflexes.* Annu Rev Physiol 1979, 41:99–114 | 34–35 |
| Iggo A: *Electrophysiological and histological studies of cutaneous mechanoreceptors.* In Kenshalo DR (ed): *The Skin Senses.* Springfield IL, Charles C Thomas, 1968, pp 84–105 | 13 |
| Inch TD, Brimblecombe RW: *Antiacetylcholine drugs: chemistry, stereochemistry and pharmacology.* Int Rev Neurobiol 1974, 16(0):67–144 | 66 |
| Isaacson RL: *The Limbic System.* New York, Plenum Press, 1974 | 51–64 |
| Ito M: *Neural design of the cerebellar motor control system.* Brain Res 1972, 40:81–84 | 39 |
| Jacobson M: *Developmental Neurobiology,* ed 2. New York, Plenum Press, 1978 | 51–64 |
| Katz B: *Nerve, Muscle and Synapse.* New York, McGraw-Hill, 1966 | 3–6, 8, 11 |

## Section VIII (continued)

| | Plate Number |
|---|---|
| Klawans HL, Kramer J: *The movement disorders.* In Rosenberg RN (ed): *Diseases of the Basal Ganglia in Neurology.* New York, Grune & Stratton, 1980, pp 166–296 | 40 |
| Klinke R, Galley N: *Efferent innervation of vestibular and auditory receptors.* Physiol Rev 1974, 54:316–357 | 27 |
| Kuypers HG: *Corticobulbar connexions to the pons and lower brain-stem in man: an anatomical study.* Brain 1958, 81:364–388 | 44 |
| Lawrence DG, Kuypers HG: *The functional organization of the motor system in the monkey. I: The effects of bilateral pyramidal lesions. II: The effects of lesions of the descending brain-stem pathways.* Brain 1968, 91:1–36 | 48 |
| Lloyd DPC: *Spinal mechanisms involved in somatic activities.* In Field J (ed): *Handbook of Physiology. Section 1: Neurophysiology, II;* Magoun HW (section ed). Washington DC, Amer Physiol Soc 1960, pp 929–950 | 33 |
| Loewenstein WR, Mendelson M: *Components of receptor adaptation in a Pacinian corpuscle.* J Physiol (Lond) 1965, 177:377–397 | 14 |
| Lothman EW, Ferrendelli JA: *Disorders and diseases of the cerebellum.* In Rosenberg RN (ed): *Neurology.* New York, Grune & Stratton, 1980, pp 435–470 | 37 |
| Lothman EW, Ferrendelli JA: *Disorders and diseases of the cerebellum.* In Rosenberg RN (ed): *Neurology.* New York, Grune & Stratton, 1980, pp 450–455, 461–466 | 31 |
| Lynn B: *Somatosensory receptors and their CNS connections.* Annu Rev Physiol 1975, 37:105–127 | 15–16 |
| MacLeod P: *Structure and function of higher olfactory centers.* In Autrum H, et al (eds): *Handbook of Sensory Physiology, IV: Chemical Sense,* part 1, *Olfaction;* Beidler LM (section ed). New York, Springer-Verlag, 1971 | 19 |
| Maekawa K, Simpson JL: *Climbing fiber responses evoked in vestibulocerebellum of rabbit from visual system.* J Neurophysiol 1973, 36:649–666 | 22 |
| Massion J: *The mammalian red nucleus.* Physiol Rev 1967, 47:383–436 | 46 |
| Masterson B, Diamond IT: *Hearing: central neural mechanisms.* In Carterette EC, Friedman MP (eds): *Handbook of Perception, III: Biology of Perceptual Systems.* New York, Academic Press, 1973, pp 407–448 | 26 |
| Matthews PBC: *Mammalian Muscle Receptors and Their Central Actions.* London, Edward Arnold, 1972, pp 319–401 | 35 |
| Mendell LM, Henneman E: *Input to motor-neuron pools and its effects.* In Mountcastle VB (ed): *Medical Physiology, I,* ed 14. St. Louis, CV Mosby, 1980, pp 742–754 | 32 |
| Miles FA, Fuller JH, Braitman DJ, et al: *Long-term adaptive changes in primate vestibuloocular reflex. III: Electrophysiological observations in flocculus of normal monkeys.* J Neurophysiol 1980, 43(5):1437–1476 | 39 |
| Mosso JA, Kruger L: *Receptor categories represented in spinal trigeminal nucleus caudalis.* J Neurophysiol 1973, 36:472–488 | 16 |
| Mountcastle VB: *Neural mechanisms in somesthesis.* In Mountcastle VB (ed): *Medical Physiology, I,* ed 14. St. Louis, CV Mosby, 1980, pp 355–358 | 16 |
| Mountcastle VB: *Neural mechanisms in somesthesis.* In Mountcastle VB (ed): *Medical Physiology, I,* ed 14. St. Louis, CV Mosby, 1980, pp 365–384 | 15 |

**Section VIII** (*continued*)

Plate Number

MOUNTCASTLE VB: *Pain and temperature sensibilities.* In MOUNTCASTLE VB (ed): *Medical Physiology, I,* ed 14. St. Louis, CV Mosby, 1980, pp 418–419 — 16

MOUNTCASTLE VB: *Central nervous mechanisms in hearing.* In MOUNTCASTLE VB (ed): *Medical Physiology, I,* ed 14. St. Louis, CV Mosby, 1980, pp 457–480 — 26

MURRAY RG: *Ultrastructure of taste receptors.* In AUTRUM H, et al (eds): *Handbook of Sensory Physiology, IV: Chemical Sense,* part 2, *Taste;* BEIDLER LM (section ed). New York, Springer-Verlag, 1971 — 23

NARAHASHI T: *Drugs affecting axonal membranes.* In DIKSTEIN S (ed): *Fundamentals of Cell Pharmacology.* Springfield IL, Charles C Thomas, 1973, pp 395–424 — 65

NASTUK WI: *Neuromuscular transmission.* In MOUNTCASTLE VB (ed): *Medical Physiology, I,* ed 14. St. Louis, CV Mosby, 1980, pp 154–163 — 66

NEIL E, HOWE A: *Arterial chemoreceptors.* In AUTRUM H, et al (eds): *Handbook of Sensory Physiology, III:* part 1, *Enteroceptors;* NEIL E (section ed). New York, Springer-Verlag, 1971 — 50

NOBACK CR: *The Human Nervous System: Basic Principles of Neurobiology.* New York, McGraw-Hill, 1967 — 51–64

NOBACK CR, DEMAREST RJ: *The Nervous System: Introduction and Review,* ed 2. New York, McGraw-Hill, 1977 — 51–64

NYBERG-HANSEN R: *Functional organisation of descending supraspinal fibre systems to the spinal cord; anatomical observations and physiological correlations.* Adv Anat Embryol Cell Biol 1966, 39:3–48 — 48

OCHS S: *Elements of Neurophysiology.* New York, John Wiley, 1965, pp 287–330 — 10

OSCARSSON O: *Functional organization of spino- and cuneocerebellar tracts.* Physiol Rev 1965, 45:495–522 — 48

OSCARSSON O: *Functional organization of spino-cerebellar paths.* In AUTRUM H, et al (eds): *Handbook of Sensory Physiology, II: Somatosensory System;* IGGO A (section ed). New York, Springer-Verlag, 1973, pp 339–380 — 37

PAINTAL AS: *Cardiovascular receptors.* In AUTRUM H, et al (eds): *Handbook of Sensory Physiology, III:* part 1, *Enteroceptors;* NEIL E (section ed). New York, Springer-Verlag, 1971 — 50

PALAY SL, CHAN-PALAY V: *General morphology of neurons and neuroglia.* In BROOKHART JM, MOUNTCASTLE VB (eds): *Handbook of Physiology.* Section 1, *The Nervous System, I:* part 1,

**Section VIII** (*continued*)

Plate Number

*Cellular Biology of Neurons;* KANDEL ER (section ed). Bethesda, MD, Amer Physiol Soc, 1977 — 1

PEELE TL: *The Neuroanatomic Basis for Clinical Neurology,* ed 3. New York, McGraw-Hill, 1977 — 51–64

PETERS A, PALAY SL, WEBSTER H: *The Fine Structure of the Nervous System: The Neurons and Supporting Cells.* Philadelphia, WB Saunders, 1976 — 51–64

PETERSON BW: *Reticulospinal projections to spinal motor nuclei.* Annu Rev Physiol 1979, 41:127–140 — 47

PETRAS JM: *Cortical, tectal and tegmental fiber connections in the spinal cord of the cat.* Brain Res 1967, 6:275–324 — 47

PHILLIPS CG (ed): *Corticospinal Neurones: Their Role in Movement.* New York, Academic Press, 1977, pp 93–152, 267–320 — 45

POGGIO GF: *Central neural mechanisms in vision.* In MOUNTCASTLE VB (ed): *Medical Physiology, I,* ed 14. St. Louis, CV Mosby, 1980, pp 544–585 — 21

POGGIO GF, MOUNTCASTLE VB: *Functional organization of thalamus and cortex.* In MOUNTCASTLE VB (ed): *Medical Physiology, I,* ed 14. St. Louis, CV Mosby, 1980, pp 271–276 — 41

POGGIO GF, MOUNTCASTLE VB: *Functional organization of thalamus and cortex.* In MOUNTCASTLE VB (ed): *Medical Physiology, I,* ed 14. St. Louis, CV Mosby, 1980, pp 276–281 — 42

POGGIO GF, MOUNTCASTLE VB: *Functional organization of thalamus and cortex.* In MOUNTCASTLE VB (ed): *Medical Physiology, I,* ed 14. St. Louis, CV Mosby, 1980, pp 276–279 — 43

REXED B: *Cytoarchitectonic organization of the spinal cord in cat.* J Comp Neurol 1952, 96:415–495 — 49

REXED B: *Cytoarchitectonic atlas of spinal cord in cat.* J Comp Neurol 1954, 100:297–379 — 49

RITCHIE JM, GREENGARD P: *On the mode of action of local anesthetics.* Annu Rev Pharmacol Toxicol 1966, 6:405–430 — 65

ROBINSON DL, GOLDBERG ME: *Visual mechanisms underlying gaze: function of the superior colliculus.* In BAKER RL, BERTHOZ A (eds): *Developments in Neuroscience, I: Control of Gaze by Brain Stem Neurons,* New York, Elsevier/North-Holland, 1978, pp 445–452 — 22

SATO M: *Neural coding in taste as seen from recordings from peripheral receptors and nerves.* In AUTRUM H, et al (eds): *Handbook of Sensory Physiology, IV: Chemical Sense,* part 2, *Taste;*

**Section VIII** (*continued*)

Plate Number

BEIDLER LM (section ed). New York, Springer-Verlag, 1971, pp 116–147 — 23

SCIENTIFIC AMERICAN: *Special issue on the brain.* Sci Am 1979, 241(3) — 51–64

SCOTT BL, PEASE DC: *Electron microscopy of the salivary and lacrimal glands of the rat.* Am J Anat 1959, 104:115–161 — 12

SHEPHERD GM: *The Synaptic Organization of the Brain.* New York, Oxford University Press, 1974 — 51–64

SIDMAN RL, SIDMAN M: *Neuroanatomy: A Programmed Text, I.* Boston, Little, Brown, 1965 — 51–64

SKOGLUND S: *Anatomical and physiological studies of knee joint innervation in the cat.* Acta Physiol Scand 1956, 36(suppl 124):1–101 — 34

SZENTÁGOTHAI J: *The morphological identification of the active synaptic region: aspects of general arrangement of geometry and topology.* In ANDERSEN P, JANSEN JKS (eds): *Excitatory Synaptic Mechanisms.* Oslo, Universitetsforlaget, 1970, pp 9–26 — 7

THAEMERT JC: *Ultrastructural interrelationships of nerve processes and smooth muscle cells in three dimensions.* J Cell Biol 1966, 28:37–49 — 12

TOMITA T: *Electrical activity of vertebrate photoreceptors.* Q Rev Biophys 1970, 3:179–222 — 20

WILLIAMS PL, WARWICK R: *Functional Neuroanatomy of Man.* Philadelphia, WB Saunders, 1975 — 51–64

WILLIAMS PL, WARWICK R: *Gray's Anatomy,* ed 36. Philadelphia, Lea & Febiger, 1980, pp 1302–1304 — 23

WILLIS WD, GROSSMAN RG: *Medical Neurobiology,* ed 3. St. Louis, CV Mosby, 1981, pp 168–179 — 35

WILSON VJ: *Physiological pathways through the vestibular nuclei.* Int Rev Neurobiol 1972, 15:27–81 — 39

WILSON VJ, MELVILLE-JONES G: *Mammalian Vestibular Physiology.* New York, Plenum Press, 1979, pp 5–121 — 35

WILSON VJ, PETERSON BW: *Peripheral and central substrates of vestibulospinal reflexes.* Physiol Rev 1978, 58(1):80–105 — 29

WILSON VJ, PETERSON BW: *The role of the vestibular system in posture and movement.* In MOUNTCASTLE VB (ed): *Medical Physiology, I,* ed 14. St. Louis, CV Mosby, 1980, pp 813–836 — 28

WOLSTENCROFT JH: *The role of raphe and medial reticular neurones in control systems related to nociceptive inputs.* In HOBSON JA, BRAZIER MAB (eds): *The Reticular Formation Revisited.* New York, Raven Press, 1980, pp 349–371 — 17

# Subject Index

(Boldface page numbers refer to illustrations)

pathways in
  efferent, 196
    localization of function and association, 195
    somatosensory, 166
  postcentral and precentral, 192
  sensory, 175
  temporal, 192
Cerebrospinal fluid, 30, 32, 132
  circulation and function, 31
Cerebrum, (see also Brain)
  capsules of
    external, 26, 140
    internal, 26, 63, 137, 138, 140, 190, 192, 196, 197
  convolutions of, 132
  surfaces of, 23-25
Cervical plexus, 113
Cervical vertebrae, 12, 13
Cervix, 89
Chemical synaptic transmission, 158, 159
Chemoreceptors, 202
Chiasm, optic, 57, 58, 59, 172
Chloride ion (Cl⁻), 154, 155, 159
Choanae, 7
Choline, 162
  uptake inhibitors, 219
Cholinesterase inhibitors, 219
Cholinomimetics, 219
Chorda tympani, 69, 100, 101, 102, 103, 105, 175
Choroid, 171
Choroidal point, 52
Chromaffin cells, 84, 141, 142, 147
Chromophobes, 210
Cilia, olfactory, 169
Ciliary nerve, 69, 70, 97, 98, 99, 101, 142
Cingulate gyrus, 24, 25, 28, 132, 195, 208
Circle of Willis, 46
Cistern, subarachnoid, 31
Clarke's column, 189, 200, 201
Claustrum, 24, 26, 137, 139, 192
Climbing fibers, 187, 188
Clitoris, 89
Coccygeal plexus, 85, 122
Coccyx, 11, 19, 20
Cochlear receptors, 152, 176
Cochlea, 176, 177, 178
Colliculocentral point, 60
Colliculus, Colliculi
  facial, 32
  of midbrain, 29, 34, 35, 137, 173, 181, 196
Column, (see also Spinal column)
  of fornix, 24, 25, 28, 205, 206, 215
  gray, 136, 137
Commisural cells, 140, 141, 142, 143, 201
Commissure(s)
  anterior, 26, 138, 142, 195
  cerebral, 24-25
  of fornix (hippocampal commissure), 28, 138, 142, 195
  habenular, 142
  posterior, 142
Complex, mamillary, 207
Compounds, organophosphorous (nerve gases), 219
Computerized tomography

(CT scanning), 62-63
Concha, nasal, 5
Conduction, antidromic, 70, 71, 72
Conduction velocity, 157
Condyle, occipital, 5, 7, 8, 12, 15
Cones, 171, 172
Connection(s)
  corticoreticulospinal, 199
  intrahemispheric, 195
  thalamostriate, 192
Contraction, active, 186
Conus medullaris, 36
Convolutions, cerebral, 132
Convulsions, 219
Cords, of brachial plexus, 116, 117
Cornea, 171
Cornu, coccygeal and sacral, 19
Corpus callosum, 24, 25, 27, 30, 137, 138, 142, 195
Corpuscles, pacinian, 165, 185
Corpus striatum, 26, 132, 137, 138, 139, 192
  neurons of, 139
Cortex
  adrenal gland, 84
  cerebellar, 187, 190
    primordial, 140
  cerebral, see Cerebral cortex
  hippocampal, 138
  neopallial, 138
  prepiriform, 170
  sensory, 175
  temporal, 192
Corticoreticular pathways, 199
Cranial nerves, 91-109, 139, 144
  cells of, 153
  development of, 142, 143
  distribution of, 92-95, 93
  embryology, 134
  functions, 92-95
  nuclei of, 141
  spinal or sensory ganglion of, 145
Craniocervical ligaments, 14-15
Craniosacral outflow system, 142
Crest or Crista
  frontal, 6, 8
  galli, 8
  infratemporal, 4
  neural, 131, 133, 142, 143
    cells derived from, 141
  occipital, internal, 8
  sacral, 19
  vestibular
    fibers from, 180, 191
    section of, 179
Crus
  cerebri, 34, 35
  of fornix, 24, 25, 28
Culmen, 33, 60
Cuneocerebellar tract (CCT), 188
Cuneus, apex of, 25
Cup, optic, 131, 134
Current flow, 159
Cutaneous nerves
  of arm, 116, 117, 118, 119
  dorsal, 125, 126, 127
  femoral, 122, 123
  perforating, 122
  sural, 125, 126, 127
Cutaneous receptors, 164
Cyanide, 218
Cytoarchitecutre of spinal gray cord matter, 201
Cytoplasmic protrusion, 164

## D

Deafness, 176
Declive, 33
Decussation
  of lemnisci, 35
  pyramidal, 34, 35, 197
  of rubrospinal fibers, 198
  supramamillary, 206
Delta cell, 210
Dendrites, 140, 151, 158
  of Purkinje cell, 187
Dendritic spines (gemmules), 151
Dens of axis vertebra, 12, 15
  articular facet for, 12
Depolarization, 155, 156, 157, 159, 160, 161, 162
  of olfactory receptors, 169
  of taste cell, 174
Dermal segmentation, 128
Dermatome, 128
Descending tracts, termination of, 200
Desmosomes, 164, 174
Diabetes insipidus, 211
Diaphragma sellae, 54
Diencephalon, 29, 131, 134, 138, 192
  embryology, 137
  functions of, 135
Differentiation, cellular, 135-140
Dihydro-β-erythroidine, 219
Diocele, 131, 134
Diploë, 6
Disc(s)
  embryonic, 131
  intervertebral, 11, 16, 17, 18, 20
  lumbosacral, 17, 19
Disfacilitation, 191
Disorders
  acoustic neuroma, 177
  trigeminal, 167
Distributed system, 218
Dorsal spinocerebellar tract (DSCT), 188
Drugs, action on nerve excitability, 218
Duct
  cochlear (scala media), 176, 179
  nasolacrimal, 5
Ductus deferens, 88, 89
Duodenum, proximal, 80
Dura mater, 19, 138, 146
  cerebral, 54, 55
  meningeal arteries and, 49
  spinal, 36, 37

## E

Ear
  auditory pathways, 177, 178
  internal, 104
  middle, 178
  receptors, 176, 179
Ectoderm, 131, 133
Edrophonium, 219
Effector mechanism, spinal, 183
Efferent endings, 163
Electrical stimulation of hypothalamus, 215
Elements, costal, 17
Embryology, 139-147
  of axons, 146-147
  of brain, 131-135

cellular differentiation, 135-140
  of glial cells, 145-146
  of myelin sheath, 144-145, 146, 147
  neurohormones, 147
  of neurons, 140-142, 141, 143, 144, 145
  of satellite cells, 146
  of spinal and cranial nerves, 134, 142-144
Eminence, medial, 32
Encapsulated ending, 152, 153
Encephalitis, 173
Endings
  efferent, 163
  encapsulated, 202
  free, 185, 202
  sensory, 86
Endocrine glands, 208
Endorphin system, 168
End plate potential, 162, 219
Enkephalin, 168
Enlargements, of spinal cord, 36
Enteric plexuses, 71, 81, 82
Ependyma, of ventricle of brain, 30, 31
Ependymal cell, 132, 141
Epididymis, 88, 89
Epiglottis, 174, 175
Epinephrine (adrenaline), 72, 90, 147
Epiphysis (pineal gland), 138
Epithelium, olfactory, 169, 170
Equivalent circuit diagrams, 154, 155
Erector spinae, 20
Ergot alkaloids, 90
Esterases, 162
Estrogen, 210
Excitability, nerve, 218
Excitation, temporal and spatial summation of, 161
Excitatory postsynaptic potential (EPSP), 159, 161
Extension, contralateral, 184
Extraocular motor neurons (no x), 152
Eye, 171
  control of movement, 181
  nystagmus, 182

## F

Facets
  articular, 12, 13, 15, 16
  costal, 16
Facial (VII) nerve, 5, 7, 9, 32, 34, 52, 53, 69, 70, 92, 93, 94, 95, 102, 103, 144, 167, 175
Falx cerebelli, 54, 55
Falx cerebri, 24, 54, 55, 56, 63, 138
Fascia, thoracolumbar, 20
Fascicles, longitudinal, 15
Fasciculus
  cuneatus, 39, 166, 200
  dorsolateral (of Lissauer), 39
  gracilis, 39, 166, 200
  lenticularis, 192
  longitudinal, 39, 208, 217
  proprius, 39
  retroflexus, 27, 28
  of Schütz, 206
Feedback loop, recurrent, 152

Femoral nerve, 122, 123, 124, 125
Fiber(s), muscle, 185, 186
Fiber(s), nerve
　accessory, 108
　adrenergic, 72
　afferent (sensory), 71, 81, 82, 83, 86, 87, 88, 89, 92-95, 93, 94, 95, 99, 100, 101, 102, 103, 105, 106, 107, 109, 113, 157, 187, 188
　arcuate, 35
　of autonomic reflex pathway, 71
　of biliary tract, 83
　cerebellar, 187, 188, 189
　　climbing, 187, 188
　　mossy, 173, 187, 188, 191
　of cervical plexus, 113
　cholinergic, 72
　classification by size and conduction velocity, 157
　corticobulbar, 192, 196
　corticonuclear, 34, 35
　corticopontine, 34, 35
　corticorubral, 192
　corticospinal, 34, 35, 153, 192
　corticostriate, 192
　cranial, 94, 95, 99
　from cristae, 191
　efferent (motor), 81, 85, 94, 95, 99, 101, 102, 103, 105, 107, 108, 109, 113, 157
　excitatory, 161
　exteroceptive, 183
　facial, 102, 103, 178
　frontopontine, 34, 35
　glossopharyngeal, 105
　group Ia (Aα), 161, 183, 184, 185, 186
　group Ib (Aα), 184, 185, 186
　group II (Aβ), 184, 185
　group III (Aδ), 185
　group IV, 185
　inhibitory, 161
　intestinal, 81
　of kidneys, 86, 87
　of liver, 83
　from maculae, 191
　mixed, 94, 95
　myelinated, 153, 157, 166
　nigrostriate, 192
　nociceptive, 184
　parallel, 187
　parasympathetic, 69, 70, 71, 72, 81, 82, 83, 84, 85, 86, 87, 88, 89, 96, 98, 99, 100, 101, 102, 103, 105, 106, 107
　postganglionic, 69, 70, 71, 72, 81, 83, 84, 86, 87, 88, 89, 98
　preganglionic, 69, 70, 71, 72, 81, 83, 84, 86, 87, 88, 89, 98, 106
　properties and function, 157
　proprioceptive, 100, 101, 108, 113, 144, 183, 184, 185, 186
　of reproductive organs, 88, 89
　reticulospinal, 199
　rubromedullary, 198
　rubrospinal, 190, 198
　secretomotor, 98, 100, 101, 106, 107
　somatic, 72, 81
　sympathetic, 70, 71, 72, 81, 82, 83, 84, 85, 86, 87, 88, 89, 96, 98, 99, 100, 101, 102, 103
　temporopontine, 34, 35
　trigeminal, 100, 101
　uncrossed (rubrobulbar), 198
　unmyelinated, 157, 160
　of ureter, 86, 87
　uterine, 89
　vagus, 106, 107
　visceral, 106
Fiber systems, reticulohypothalamic, 208
Fields of Forel, 206
Filaments
　of dorsal and ventral roots, 37
　prostatic and urethral, 89
"Filtered back-projection", 62
Filum terminale, 36, 37
Fimbria of hippocampus, 24, 25, 28
Fissure(s)
　anterior median, 37
　calcarine, 172
　cerebral
　　choroid, 28, 30, 132, 136, 138
　　lateral, 47
　　longitudinal, 25
　horizontal, 33, 60
　orbital
　　inferior, 3, 4
　　superior, 3, 8, 9
　petrooccipital, 9
　petrotympanic, 7
　posterolateral, 33
　postlunate, 33, 189
　prepyramidal, 33
　primary, 33, 189
　retrotonsillar, 33
　secondary, 33
　tympanosquamous, 7
Flexion, ipsilateral, 184
Flexures, 131, 134
Flocculo-nodular lobe, 189
Flocculus, 33, 34, 189, 191
Fluid, cerebrospinal (CBF), 30, 32, 132
　circulation and function of, 31
Folds, neural, 131, 133
Folium, 33
Follicles, hair, 72, 164
Follicle-stimulating hormone (FSH), 210
Fontanelles, 6, 10
Food intake, hypothalamic control of, 214
Foramen, Foramina
　alveolar, 4
　cecum, 8, 9
　condylar, 7
　of cribriform plate, 9
　ethmoidal, 9
　incisive, 7
　infraorbital, 3
　interventricular, 27, 28, 132, 138
　　ipsilateral, 26
　　lateral, 30
　intervertebral, 11
　jugular, 5, 9, 105, 107, 108
　lacerum, 7, 9
　magnum, 5, 7, 9, 14, 15
　mastoid, 7, 9
　mental, 3, 4

ovale, 4, 7, 9
　palatine, major and minor, 7
　parietal, 6
　rotundum, 9
　sacral, pelvic, 19
　sphenopalatine, 4
　spinosum, 4, 7, 9
　stylomastoid, 7, 102, 103
　transverse, 12, 13
　vertebral, 12, 13, 16, 17
　of Vesalius, 9
　zygomatico-facial, 3, 4
Forearm, 118, 120, 121
Forebrain, 131, 134, 206
　bundle, medial, 205, 207, 208
　embryology, 138
　regions associated with hypothalamus, 208
Formation
　hippocampal, 27-28, 208
　reticular, 196, 208
　　development of, 132-133
　　medullary, 34, 35, 198, 199
　　mesencephalic, 34, 173
　　pontine, 167, 173, 181, 182
Fornix, 27, 137, 207, 208, 219
　column of, 24, 25, 28, 205, 206, 215
　commissure of, 28, 138, 142, 195
　crus, 24, 25, 28
　midline, 132
Fossa
　condylar, 7
　cranial
　　anterior, 8, 9
　　middle, 8-9
　　posterior, 8, 9, 52-53, 53, 60-61, 61
　infratemporal, 4
　jugular, 7
　lacrimal, 3
　mandibular, 7
　popliteal, 126
　pterygopalatine, 4
　temporal, 4
Fourth ventricle, 30, 31, 32, 132, 137
　ependymal roof of, 32, 139
　floor of, 32
　recesses of, 136, 139
Fovea, 171, 172
　superior, of fourth ventricle, 32
Foveola, granular, 6, 55
Free nerve endings, 152, 153, 164
Frontal bone, 3, 4
Fundus of uterus, 89
Funiculus, 143, 166, 198
Fusimotor neurons, 152

## G

Gallamine triethiodide, 219
Gallbladder, innervation of, 83
Gamma-aminobutyric acid (GABA), 72, 160, 192
Ganglion, Ganglia
　aorticorenal, 69, 81, 84, 86, 87, 88, 89
　basal, 132, 135, 139, 193
　　anatomy of, 26
　　connections of, 192
　celiac, 69, 70, 71, 72, 81, 83, 84, 87, 88, 89
　cervicothoracic (stellate), 69

ciliary, 69, 70, 97, 101, 142
　roots of, 98, 99
　of facial nerve, 92, 94, 103, 175
　of glossopharyngeal nerve, 105
　lingual, 105
　mesenteric
　　inferior, 69, 70, 72, 81, 85, 87, 88, 89
　　superior, 70, 71, 72, 81, 84, 88, 89
　otic, 69, 70, 101, 105, 142, 175
　parasympathetic, 70, 145, 152
　parasympathetic relay, 70
　pelvic, 85
　petrosal (inferior), 175
　phrenic, 83, 114
　prevertebral, 217
　pterygopalatine, 69, 70, 96, 103, 142
　renal, 84, 86, 87, 88, 89
　spinal, 36, 37, 71, 115, 143
　　dorsal root, 86, 153, 183
　spiral, 176, 177
　　of cochlea, 104
　submandibular, 69, 70, 100, 101, 102, 103, 142
　sympathetic, 38, 142, 145, 152
　sympathetic relay, 70
　sympathetic trunk, 69, 71, 72, 81, 85, 86, 89, 217
　trigeminal nerve, 92, 94, 95, 97, 101, 167
　of vagus nerve
　　nodose, 175
　　inferior and superior, 106, 107, 108
　vertebral, 69, 104
　vestibular, 179, 189, 191
Generator potentials, 165
Geniculate body, 34, 172, 177, 178, 193
Geniculostriate projections, 172
Geniculum, facial, 102
Genu
　of corpus callosum, 24, 25, 26, 27, 28
　of internal capsule, 26
Giant pyramidal (Betz) cell, 194, 197, 198
Glands
　adrenal, 72, 84
　endocrine, 208
　mammary, 115
　mucosal, 82
　olfactory (Bowman's), 169
　parotid, 100, 105
　pineal, 138, 163
　pituitary (hypophysis), 131, 135, 138, 163, 209
　salivary, 72
　submandibular, 163
　sweat, 72
Glial cells, 145-146, 152
Glial process, 151, 158
Globus pallidus, 26, 27, 140, 192, 196
Glomerulus
　cerebellar, 151, 187
　of kidney, 212
　of olfactory bulb, 170
Glossopharyngeal (IX) nerve, 7, 9, 34, 35, 52, 53, 69, 70, 72, 93, 94, 95, 102, 103, 105, 107, 144, 175, 196, 202

of medulla oblongata, 34, 35, 136,
137, 139, 142, 196
decussation, 34, 35, 197
motor component of, 197
Pyramidal cells, 141, 152, 153,
194, 196, 197, 198

## Q

3-Quinuclidinyl benzylate, 90

## R

Radial nerve, 116, 117, 118, 119
Radiations
optic, 172, 196
thalamic, 29
thalamocortical, 193
Rage reaction, 216-217
Rami, of spinal nerves, 38, 143
cervical, 114
thoracic, 115
Ramus, of lateral sulcus, 23
Ramus, of mandible, 3, 4
Ramus communicantes, 38, 70,
145
gray, 69, 71, 72, 85, 87, 115,
143
white, 69, 71, 72, 87, 115, 143
Receptors, 169
adrenergic, 90
cochlear, 176
cutaneous, 164
joint, 185
muscarinic cholinergic, 90
muscle spindle, 184, 185, 186
olfactory, 169
Pacinian corpuscle, 165
pain, 202
sensory, 151
stretch, 87
taste, 174
vestibular, 179
visual, 171
Recess(es)
infundibular, of third ventricle, 30,
136
lateral, of fourth ventricle, 32, 139
mamillary, 137
optic, 30
pineal, 136
Rectus muscle, 181, 182
Reflex(es)
arc, 71
bradycardia, 202
control of muscle tension, proprioceptive, 186
flexor withdrawal, 183, 184
hyperactive, 197
"jaw jerk," 167
muscle tension control, 186
pathways, 71
spinal, 152, 184
stretch, 183
passive, 186
reciprocal inhibition, 184
subliminal fringe of, 161
tendon organ, 184
vestibular, 180
vestibuloocular, 191
visual, 173
Region
cervicodorsal, 65
suprastriatal, 132

Renshaw cells, 153, 184
Renshaw interneuron, 153
Reproductive organs, innervation of,
88-89
Resting membrane potential
(RMP), 154, 172, 218, 219
Reticular activating system, 133
Reticular formation, 196, 208
development of, 132-133
medullary, 34, 35, 198, 199
mesencephalic, 34, 173
pontine, 167, 173, 181, 182
Reticulospinal pathway, 199
Reticulum, rough endoplasmic, 151,
153
Retina, 151, 152, 171, 172
Retinal projections, 173
Retinene, 171
Retinogeniculostriate visual path-
way, 172
Rhinencephalon, 27-28, 132
Rhinorrhea, cerebrospinal fluid, 96
Rhodopsin, 171
Rhombencephalon, 131
Rhombocele, 131, 134
Rib attachment to vertebrae, 16
Rods of retina, 171, 172
Rods of Corti, 176
Root, nerve
of accessory nerve, 106, 107, 108,
144
of ansa cervicalis, 109, 113
of brachial plexus, 116
of facial nerve, 102, 103, 104
spinal, 37, 144, 145
dorsal, 38, 84, 87, 115, 143
ventral, 38, 143
thoracic, 87, 115
trigeminal sensory, 100
Rostral spinocerebellar tract
(RSCT), 188
Rostrum, of corpus callosum, 24, 25
Rubrospinal tract, 39, 198, 200
Rudiment, axial, 131
Ruffini terminals, 164, 185

## S

Sac, yolk, 131
Saccadic movement, 181, 182
Saccule, 104, 179
Sacral plexus, 69, 85, 86, 87, 88,
89, 172
Sacrum, 11, 19
ligaments of, 20
Sarcolemma, 162
Satellite cells, 141, 144, 145, 146,
152, 153
development of, 146
Saxitoxin (shellfish toxin), 218
Scala tympani, 176
Scala vestibuli, 176
Scapular nerve, 116, 117
Schwann cell, 141, 144, 146, 152,
153, 162, 164, 169
cap, 163
Sciatic nerve, 122, 125
Sclera, 171
Scopolamine, 90
Scotomas, 172
Segmentation, dermal, 128
Seizures, Jacksonian, 197
Sella turcica, 5, 8, 9
Sensations, general, 102, 105

taste, 102
Septum
mesothelial (spinal), 37
pellucidum, 24, 132, 137, 204
Serotonin, 168, 192, 213
Sham rage, 215
Sheath(s)
arachnoid, 19
dural, 19
myelin, formation, 144-145
Sheath cells, 146, 202
Sinus(es)
carotid, 202
cavernous, 44, 97, 98, 209
intercavernous, 56
meningeal, 55
occipital, 54
petrosal, 8, 54, 56
rhomboid, 133
sagittal
inferior, 56, 138
superior, 31, 54, 55, 56, 59,
138
sigmoid, 56
sphenoidal, 5
sphenoparietal, 56
straight, 56, 59
transverse, 55, 56, 59
venous, of dura mater, 55, 56, 63
Skin, glabrous and hairy, 164
Skull
anterior aspect of, 3
base of
external aspect of, 7
internal aspect of, 8, 9
lateral aspect of, 4
midsagittal section of, 5
of newborn, 10
thickness, 6
vertex of, 6
Skullcap, 3, 5, 6, 54
dural infoldings, 54
endocranial surface of, 6
newborn, 10
Smell, sense of, 169
Smooth muscle, 163
Sodium ion (Na$^+$), 154, 162, 218
conductivity, 155
permeability, 155, 159, 162
resting membrane potential, 154
Sodium-potassium ion pump, 154,
218
Solitary tract, 92, 94, 95, 102, 103,
105, 106, 107, 175, 196
Somata, 151, 152
Somatic neuromuscular transmission, 162
Somatotropic hormone (STH), 210
Somesthetic system
body, 166
head, 167
Somite
Space
epidural, 54, 55
periaxonal, 146
subarachnoid, 19, 31, 36, 37, 54,
55
subdural, 54, 55
Spatial summation, 161
Specialized ending, 153
Sphincter ampullae, 83
Spinal border cells, 200
Spinal column, 9, 11-20, 11,
64-65, 131, 132, 134, 153

atlas and axis, 11, 12, 15
anterior view, 11
cervical vertebrae, 13
coccyx, 19, 20
curve of, 11
intervertebral disc, 11, 16, 17, 18,
20
left lateral view, 11
length of, 11
ligaments, 18, 20
craniocervical, 14, 15
lumbar vertebrae, 17
movement of, 11
posterior view, 11
sacrum, 11, 19, 20
thoracic vertebrae, 16
Spinal cord
anatomy of, 36-39, 36
membranes and nerve roots, 37
principal fiber tracts, 39
spinal nerves, 38
arteries of, 45, 64-65
central canal of, 134, 137, 140
cervical part of, 198
development of, 36
dorsolumbosacral part of, 65
embryology, 137, 140
enlargements of, 13, 36
gray matter
cytoarchitecture of, 201
distribution, 39
lesions, 166
lumbar part of, 198
middorsal region of, 64-65
myelination of, 145
in situ, 36
veins of, 66
vestibulospinal tracts to, 180
white matter distribution, 39
Spinal effector mechanisms, 183
Spinal membranes, 37
Spinal nerve, 13, 14, 36, 37, 38,
71, 87, 108, 115, 144
dermal segmentation and, 128
development of, 134, 142-144
myelinated fibers of, 153
rami of, dorsal and ventral, 38,
114, 115, 143
Spinal reflex pathway, 152, 184
Spindle, muscle, 153, 185, 186
Spines
dendritic (gemmules), 151
vertebral, 36
Spinocerebellum, 188, 189, 191
Spinocervical tract, 166
Spinoreticulothalamic pathway,
166
Spinothalamic tract, 166
Splenium, of corpus callosum, 24,
25, 26, 27, 28
Spondylolisthesis, 19, 20
Spongioblast, 141, 145
Stalk
body, 131
optic, 131, 134, 138
Stapes, 178
Stellate cells, 170, 187, 191, 194
Stomach, innervation of, 80
Stratum zonale, 29
Streak, primitive, 131, 133
Stretch receptors, 202
Stria(e)
longitudinal, of indusium griseum,
27-28, 27

# INFORMATION ON CIBA COLLECTION VOLUMES

THE CIBA COLLECTION OF MEDICAL ILLUSTRATIONS has enjoyed an enthusiastic reception from members of the medical community since the publication of its first volume. The remarkable illustrations by Frank H. Netter, M.D., and text by leading specialists make these books unprecedented in their educational, clinical, and scientific value.

**Volume 1: I**    **NERVOUS SYSTEM: Anatomy and Physiology**
"...this volume must remain a part of the library of all practitioners, scientists and educators dealing with the nervous system."
*Journal of Neurosurgery*

**Volume 1: II**    **NERVOUS SYSTEM: Neurologic and Neuromuscular Disorders**
"...Part I is a 'work of art.' Part II is even more grand and more clinical!
...This is a unique and wonderful text...rush to order this fine book."
*Journal of Neurological & Orthopaedic Medicine & Surgery*

**Volume 2**    **REPRODUCTIVE SYSTEM**
"...a desirable addition to any nursing or medical library."
*American Journal of Nursing*

**Volume 3: I**    **DIGESTIVE SYSTEM: Upper Digestive Tract**
"...a fine example of the high quality of this series."
*Pediatrics*

**Volume 3: II**    **DIGESTIVE SYSTEM: Lower Digestive Tract**
"...a unique and beautiful work, worth much more than its cost."
*Journal of the South Carolina Medical Association*

**Volume 3: III**    **DIGESTIVE SYSTEM: Liver, Biliary Tract and Pancreas**
"...a versatile, multipurpose aid to clinicians, teachers, researchers, and students..."
*Florida Medical Journal*

**Volume 4**    **ENDOCRINE SYSTEM and Selected Metabolic Diseases**
"...another in the series of superb contributions made by CIBA..."
*International Journal of Fertility*

**Volume 5**    **HEART**
"The excellence of the volume...is clearly deserving of highest praise."
*Circulation*

**Volume 6**    **KIDNEYS, URETERS, AND URINARY BLADDER**
"...a model of clarity of language and visual presentation..."
*Circulation*

**Volume 7**    **RESPIRATORY SYSTEM**
"...far more than an atlas on anatomy and physiology. Frank Netter uses his skills to present clear and often beautiful illustrations of all aspects of the system..."
*British Medical Journal*

**Volume 8: I**    **MUSCULOSKELETAL SYSTEM: Anatomy, Physiology, and Metabolic Disorders**
"...the overall value of this monumental work is nearly beyond human comprehension."
*Journal of Neurological & Orthopaedic Medicine & Surgery*

**Volume 8: II**    **MUSCULOSKELETAL SYSTEM: Developmental Disorders, Tumors, Rheumatic Diseases, and Joint Replacement**
"This book belongs in the library of every orthopaedic surgeon, medical school, and hospital."
*Journal of Bone and Joint Surgery*

Copies of all CIBA COLLECTION books may be purchased directly from CIBA-GEIGY Medical Education and Communications, 14 Henderson Drive, West Caldwell, New Jersey 07006. In countries other than the United States, please direct inquiries to the nearest CIBA-GEIGY office.